Head and Neck Cancer: Clinical Research and Challenges

Head and Neck Cancer: Clinical Research and Challenges

Edited by Katelyn Harding

hayle
medical

New York

Hayle Medical,
750 Third Avenue, 9th Floor,
New York, NY 10017, USA

Visit us on the World Wide Web at:
www.haylemedical.com

ISBN: 978-1-63241-702-2

Cataloging-in-Publication Data

Head and neck cancer : clinical research and challenges / edited by Katelyn Harding.
    p. cm.
Includes bibliographical references and index.
ISBN 978-1-63241-702-2
1. Head--Cancer. 2. Neck--Cancer. 3. Head--Cancer--Treatment.
4. Neck--Cancer--Treatment. I. Harding, Katelyn.
RC280.H4 H43 2019
616.994 91--dc23

Table of Contents

Preface

This book has been an outcome of determined endeavour from a group of educationists in the field. The primary objective was to involve a broad spectrum of professionals from diverse cultural background involved in the field for developing new researches. The book not only targets students but also scholars pursuing higher research for further enhancement of the theoretical and practical applications of the subject.

Head and neck cancer is a group of cancers that consists of oral cancer, nasopharynx cancer, tumors of the hypopharynx, laryngeal cancer, throat cancer, etc. It is classified on the basis of its histology or cell structure, and by the location in the oral cavity and neck. The stage at which the cancer is diagnosed plays a determining influence in its prognosis. Metastasis of the cancer can affect many cells and organs of the body, such as the bone marrow, the circulatory system and nervous system. Nearly 50% of all cases of head and neck cancer have advanced stage of the disease, which typically has a poor prognosis. The size of the tumor influences the probability of cure. In a significant percentage of people who have been cured of squamous cell carcinoma of the head and neck, there has been development of second primary tumors, which are a major threat to survival. Tremendous research is occurring to increase the survival rates and achieve adequate management of symptoms and complications pertaining to head and neck cancer. One such dimension explores immunotherapy with immune checkpoint inhibitors. This book contains some path-breaking studies in head and neck cancer. It covers in detail the current researches and challenges of head and neck cancer. It is a complete source of knowledge on the present status of this important type of cancer.

It was an honour to edit such a profound book and also a challenging task to compile and examine all the relevant data for accuracy and originality. I wish to acknowledge the efforts of the contributors for submitting such brilliant and diverse chapters in the field and for endlessly working for the completion of the book. Last, but not the least; I thank my family for being a constant source of support in all my research endeavours.

Editor

Swallowing interventions for the treatment of dysphagia after head and neck cancer: a systematic review of behavioural strategies used to promote patient adherence to swallowing exercises

Roganie Govender[1]*[iD], Christina H. Smith[2], Stuart A. Taylor[3], Helen Barratt[4] and Benjamin Gardner[5]

Abstract

Background: Dysphagia is a significant side-effect following treatment for head and neck cancers, yet poor adherence to swallowing exercises is frequently reported in intervention studies. Behaviour change techniques (BCTs) can be used to improve adherence, but no review to date has described the techniques or indicated which may be more associated with improved swallowing outcomes.

Methods: A systematic review was conducted to identify behavioural strategies in swallowing interventions, and to explore any relationships between these strategies and intervention effects. Randomised and quasi-randomised studies of head and neck cancer patients were included. Behavioural interventions to improve swallowing were eligible provided a valid measure of swallowing function was reported. A validated and comprehensive list of 93 discrete BCTs was used to code interventions. Analysis was conducted *via* a structured synthesis approach.

Results: Fifteen studies (8 randomised) were included, and 20 different BCTs were each identified in at least one intervention. The BCTs identified in almost all interventions were: *instruction on how to perform the behavior, setting behavioural goals* and *action planning*. The BCTs that occurred more frequently in effective interventions, were: *practical social support, behavioural practice, self-monitoring of behaviour* and *credible source* for example a skilled clinician delivering the intervention. The presence of identical BCTs in comparator groups may diminish effects.

Conclusions: Swallowing interventions feature multiple components that may potentially impact outcomes. This review maps the behavioural components of reported interventions and provides a method to consistently describe these components going forward. Future work may seek to test the most effective BCTs, to inform optimisation of swallowing interventions.

Keywords: Dysphagia, Head neck cancer, Swallowing exercises, Behavior change techniques, Adherence, Complex interventions

* Correspondence: Roganie.Govender@uclh.nhs.uk
[1]University College London, Health Behaviour Research Centre & University College London Hospital, Head & Neck Cancer Centre, Ground Floor Central, 250 Euston Road, London NW1 2PQ, UK
Full list of author information is available at the end of the article

Background

Swallowing difficulties (dysphagia), which affect 60 –75% of patients treated for head and neck cancer (HNC) [1], arise both from the presence of a tumour, and as a consequence of its treatment [2]. Dysphagia is a major patient concern after cancer treatment due to the detrimental impact on patients' quality of life (QOL) [3]. Improvement of swallowing function and earlier restoration of eating and drinking after surgery or chemoradiation treatments may be achieved with swallowing rehabilitation exercises [4, 5]. Despite this, nonadherence to swallowing exercises in this population is reported to be high [6].

The World Health Organization report defines patient adherence as "the extent to which a person's behaviour corresponds with agreed recommendations from a health care provider" [7]. This report highlights that adherence is influenced by multiple factors, and that increasing adherence to treatment could have a greater impact on health than trying to improve the efficacy of the treatment to which patients are encouraged to adhere. Adopting this perspective transforms the concept of patient adherence from a peripheral marker of study quality into a concept central to the intervention. The Medical Research Council's "complex intervention" guidelines highlight that multiple components at different levels may interact to bring about desired health outcomes [8]. Effectiveness of swallowing exercise interventions are determined not just by the exercises but also the broader 'behaviours of those delivering and receiving the intervention' (p.979). Complex interventions that take place as *pragmatic trials* under real-world conditions [9] are influenced by context factors;

how interventions are implemented (where, by whom) and how patients may respond to this (uptake/adherence) [10].

Newer paradigms in systematic reviewing such as realist reviews focus on understanding how and why interventions work in some situations and not others, rather than simply investigating whether they do or do not work [11]. Sutcliffe and colleagues [12] argue the importance of recognising and identifying the critical components of complex interventions highlighting that outcomes of complex interventions cannot be solely ascribed to the primary content, in this case swallowing exercises. Traditional systematic reviews that focus exclusively on pooling effect sizes may overlook other aspects that influence outcomes. This limits our ability to differentially examine the evidence and to gather important information that may improve future interventions.

The system in which the intervention takes place and the possible interactions that may occur can be represented as a logic model [13] (Fig. 1). Swallowing exercise interventions for patients with HNC are normally implemented by trained professionals such as speech therapists within a healthcare setting, and as part of a wider cancer care pathway. The content of the intervention tends to be focused on type, timing and intensity of different swallowing exercises. Accordingly, previous reviews have been largely concerned with these exercise parameters. Langmore and Pisegna [14] suggest that exercises such as the Shaker (head lift exercise) and Mendelsohn manoeuvre (larynx elevation exercise) have good efficacy in improving swallowing function. A general review of interventions to improve eating and drinking after HNC [15] concluded

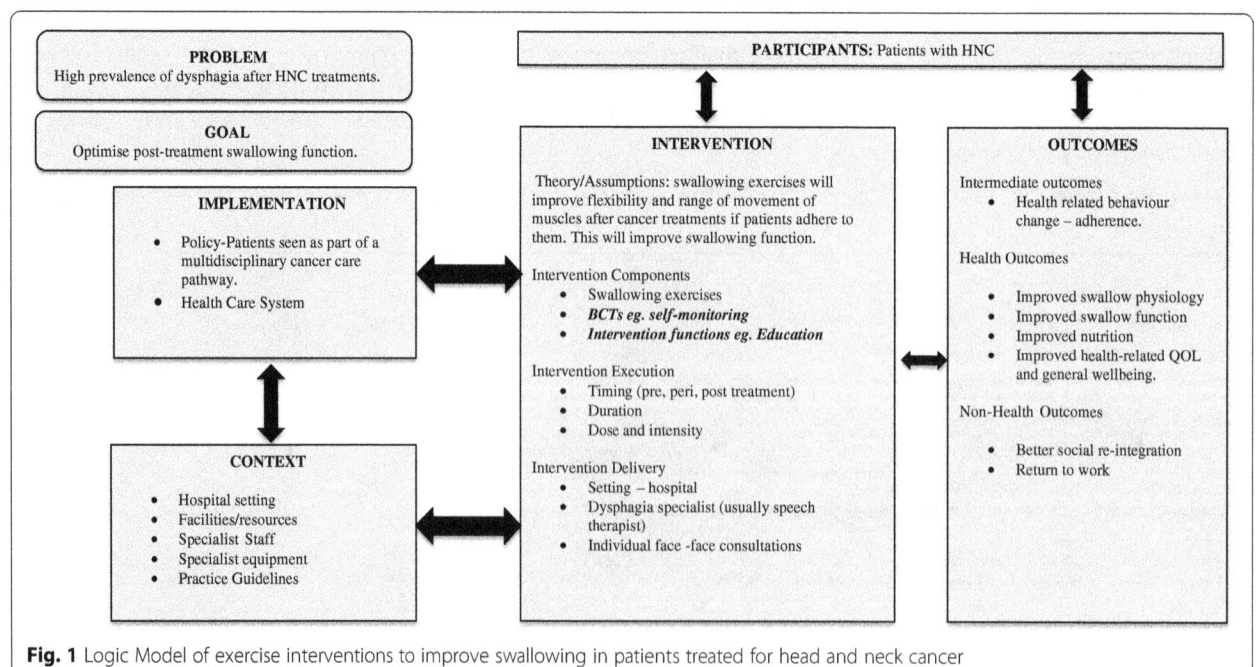

Fig. 1 Logic Model of exercise interventions to improve swallowing in patients treated for head and neck cancer

that some evidence exists to support exercises to improve swallowing function and jaw movement in patients treated for HNC but acknowledged that larger controlled studies are needed. A recent Cochrane review [16] concluded that the evidence for pre-treatment swallowing exercises in improving swallowing safety and efficiency is lacking due to insufficiently robust studies, heterogeneity of outcome measures across studies, and poor patient adherence. Whilst there is much to be learned from these reviews, the broader perspective proposed in our logic model may facilitate better understanding of the existing evidence that could improve the content and design of future studies (Fig. 1).

As highlighted in our model, behavioural strategies used to promote adherence to the exercises are an important *part of the intervention content* that may be frequently overlooked yet such strategies may have a potentially crucial influence on outcomes. This review employs established tools from Behavioural Science, in particular the Behaviour Change Technique Taxonomy (BCTTv1) [17] that defines 93 discrete behaviour change techniques (BCTs) thereby facilitating a standardised description of the techniques that can be used to change behaviour. BCTs represent the smallest observable and replicable components that may bring about a change in behaviour [17], and therefore may be potentially active ingredients in an intervention [18] The success of exercise interventions is dependent on good adherence. It is logical therefore that this aspect of the intervention be given appropriate consideration.

In this review, we aim to identify the specific behaviour change strategies reported in interventions to improve swallowing function after HNC. We also explored where possible, relationships between the presence of these components and intervention effectiveness. We propose that BCTs that occur at least twice as frequently in successful interventions may be useful to include in future interventions. We used a narrative synthesis approach [19] and as part of this we also explored the trial methods used more broadly (for example type of comparator group), providing discussion of possible associations with the study outcomes. To our knowledge this is the first attempt to apply this method of reviewing swallowing interventions within this field, and by its nature the work is exploratory.

Methods

The review is registered with PROSPERO (CRD420 15017048), and a protocol reporting full methodological detail has been published [20].

Eligibility Criteria

Studies were eligible for inclusion where they met the following PICO criteria [21]. *Participants* were adults diagnosed with head and neck cancer; treated *via* one of the key treatment modalities of surgery, radiotherapy, chemo-radiotherapy or combinations thereof. *Interventions* that were eligible included behavioural interventions to improve swallowing such as swallowing exercises or instructions to adhere to a specific diet texture, and other specific swallowing strategies. Studies that included an independent *comparator* group were eligible - these could be randomised or non-randomised studies. The comparator group could have received no treatment (non-active comparator), usual care (active or non-active) or a different treatment (active) or sham exercise (active). For inclusion, the study had to report at least one swallow-related *outcome measure* which could be for example; swallow safety, swallow efficiency, swallow related QOL, oral diet intake or a surrogate marker such as feeding tube use, and textures of food tolerated. Evaluation could be *via* an established patient reported questionnaire, clinician rated measure or instrumental assessment tool such as videofluoroscopy.

Identification of studies

Six electronic health databases were searched: Medline, CINAHL, EMBASE, AMED, PsychInfo, and the Cochrane Library including CENTRAL. Additional searches were carried out on Google Scholar, Web of Science and the meta-registries of Trials Databases (ClinicalTrials.gov and ISRCTN). Additionally, the WHO International Clinical Trials Registry Platform (ICTRP) and the Australian New Zealand Clinical Trials Register (ANZCTR) were searched. A hand-search of reference lists of directly relevant systematic reviews and included articles identified from the main screening was also undertaken.

The search strategy was developed in conjunction with a subject librarian, following an initial scoping exercise. Medical Subject Headings from key articles and other related reviews were examined to determine the final search terms. The search was limited to clinical trials and reviews published in English. No date limit was applied.

Searches were carried out by a speech and language therapist (RG) and subject librarian (DG) in December 2014, and updated in June 2015 prior to completion of the data extraction process. One study [22] found to have two additional related reports based on longer follow-up times for the same sample and intervention, was treated as one study. Figure 2 depicts the PRISMA flowchart [23] showing the study selection process (Fig. 2).

Data extraction
Study quality

For consistency with other reviews, data was extracted on study quality using an 11-item checklist [24] used previously to assess the quality of dysphagia clinical

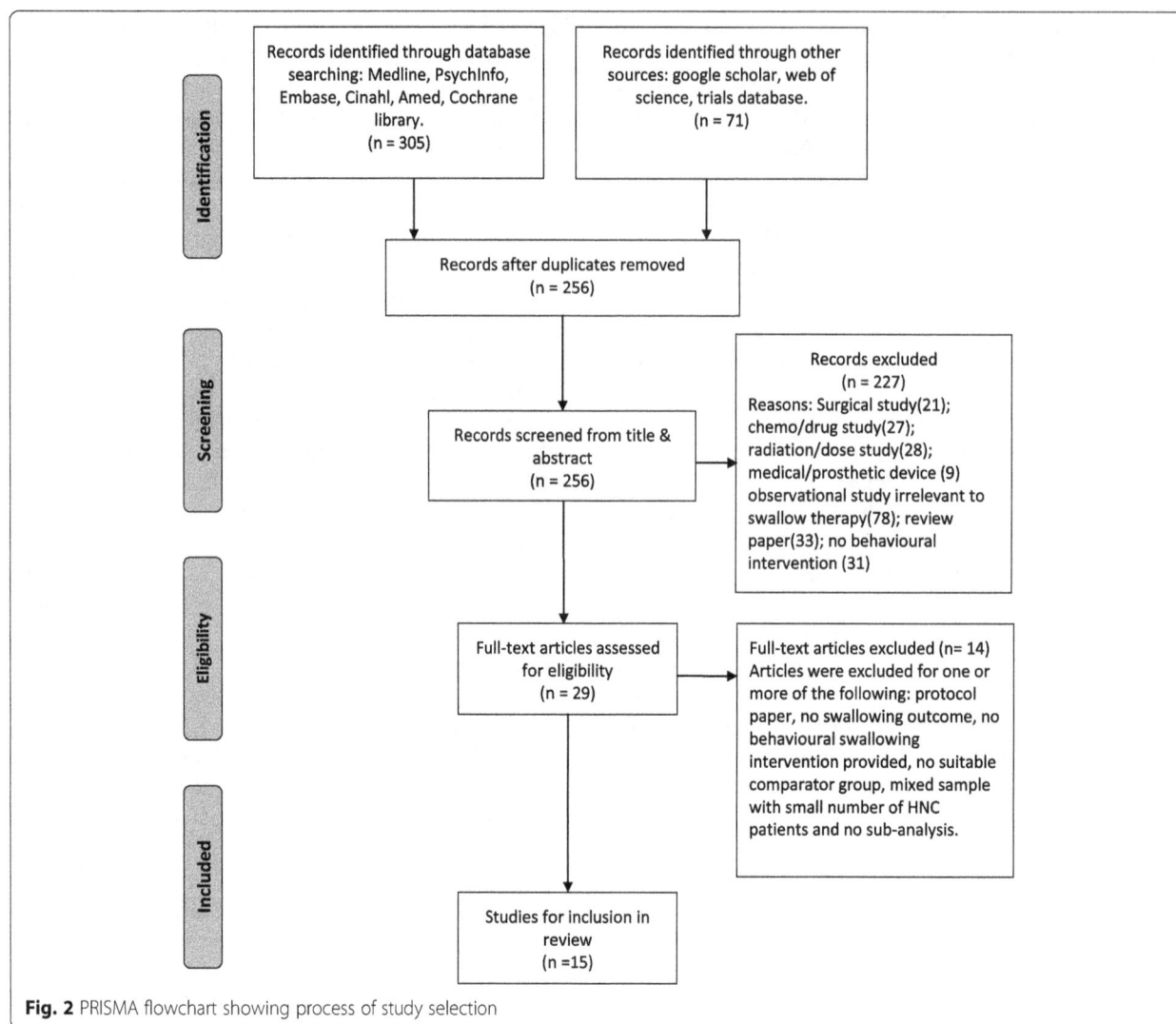

Fig. 2 PRISMA flowchart showing process of study selection

trials [25]. Each of the 11 items (Table 2) is given a score of 1 if the criterion is met, yielding a summary score of 0 (lowest) to 11 (highest quality). Van Tulder and colleagues [24] suggest that scores of ≥6 reflect studies of good quality. Studies were not excluded on the basis of quality because we aimed to ascertain any evidence, however weak, of potential links between BCTs and effects. Assessing study quality and potential risk of bias is still important when synthesizing findings even if only exploratory in nature [19].

Study characteristics
Data were extracted on study characteristics (author, year, country of origin, setting, type of study), patient characteristics (diagnostic and treatment group, sample size, age range, gender and baseline swallow function), treatment (information about the type of treatment and comparator groups), and outcome measures (length of follow-up and all swallow related outcomes). We

anticipated heterogeneity in the type and time-points of outcome measures but an attempt was made to extract data at or as close to the time intervals of 1, 3, 6 and 12 months after treatment. They included measures derived from instrumental assessments such as modified barium swallow or videofluoroscopy, clinical measurements such as weight or the water swallow test (WST) [26], functional scales such as the Functional Oral Intake Scale (FOIS) [27] and Performance Status Scale (PSS) [28], patient-reported and QOL measures such as the MD Anderson Dysphagia Inventory (MDADI) [29] and European Organisation for Research and Treatment of Cancer (EORTC QOL C-30) [30] questionnaire.

Intervention Characteristics
For this review, we were particularly interested in identifying the behaviour change strategies (Additional file 1: Table S1 and Additional file 2: Table S2) present in the interventions. We recorded the target behaviour in each

study, which was either regular performance of swallowing exercises or regular implementation of a prescribed diet modification with or without specific swallowing strategies. We intended to code for whether a named theory of behaviour or behaviour change was mentioned in the Abstract, Introduction, or Method, but no studies were found to have mentioned theory. We identified behaviour change strategies using BCTTv1. We also documented *Intervention Function* categories. Michie and colleagues [31] propose a list of nine Function categories that reflect the broad methods through which an intervention may influence behaviour: Education, Training, Enablement, Modeling, Restrictions, Environmental Restructuring, Persuasion, Incentivisation and Coercion. Both BCTs and intervention functions were only coded when they were unambiguously present in the intervention descriptions. For example if the intervention included a TheraBite device (Atos Medical, Sweden) to maintain mouth opening function – the intervention function *Education* was coded if it was clear that the intervention explicitly required that patients be informed and understand how the device and exercise works to maintain the ability to open the jaw. This may extend to information about the impact of radiotherapy on jaw movement and the consequences of doing/not doing the exercise. The function category *Training* was coded where it was clear that the patient was taught skills on how to perform the exercises using the device. The BCT *demonstration on how to perform the behaviour* was coded if the patient was presented with an observable demonstration, but not if only provided with written instructions; this was coded as *instruction on how to perform the behaviour*.

A clinician (RG) extracted data for all included studies. A speech and language therapist (CS) and health psychologist (BG) independently extracted data for four (27%) randomly selected studies. Inter-rater agreement, assessed using Cohen's kappa, was 'substantial K = 0.6' or better for selection of full-text articles assessed for inclusion (K = 0.86), study quality (K = 0.74) and BCTs (K = 0.66) [32].

Analysis

A meta-analysis was not used due to the small number of studies and the large variability. Furthermore, it would not have been as informative for the purpose of addressing our study questions. Instead we selected a qualitative method that combined the use of summary tables, and qualitative exploration of the data.

We used a synthesis approach [19] to describe and explore our findings. Results are structured and presented in line with the key steps of this approach as listed below:

1. *Developing a theory or model of how the intervention might work*: Our logic model illustrating the interaction of various components of the intervention within a health service system has been presented above.
2. *Preliminary synthesis of the findings* – We summarise the characteristics of the included studies tabulating the same features across all studies. Additionally, we present summary tables of the intervention characteristics (behavioural strategies) extracted from studies and examples of these strategies obtained from content analysis of the study reports.
3. *Exploring relationships in the data* – We present observations of relationships between studies that may explain differences in outcomes and the direction and size of intervention effects. We assumed that BCTs that featured at least twice as frequently in studies that showed a statistically significant positive effect on at least one outcome measure (p < .05) in favour of the intervention group may show some promise, or at least justify more rigorous evaluation.
4. *Assessing the robustness of the synthesis*. We reflect on the number and quality of the studies included, and the methods used in synthesizing the findings.

Results

Synthesis of study and intervention characteristics

Study selection

Of 374 articles identified from the combined searches, 254 remained after de-duplication. Twenty-nine articles were retained following title and abstract screening, of which 15 studies, each reporting one intervention, were eligible for review. No additional studies were included following the hand-search of reference lists.

Study characteristics

The 15 studies were undertaken across seven countries (USA, 7 studies; Netherlands and China, 2 studies respectively; Denmark, Sweden, Austria, Japan, 1 study respectively). All were carried out in a university hospital, medical centre or cancer centre. All studies sought to evaluate the impact of swallowing exercises, on one or more swallow related outcomes. Eight were randomised trials [22, 33–39], and seven were non-randomised controlled trials [40–46]. Six studies reported a comparator group of 'no treatment'[36–38, 42–44] and two of delayed treatment [40, 45]. In two studies, treatment as usual was described as dietary advice without exercise [33, 34]. The comparator group for the remaining studies used a different swallowing exercise protocol described as usual care for that setting.

Follow-ups took place between one and 12 months. The measure used for baseline swallowing status varied greatly, with 5 studies [40, 42–45] providing no report of swallowing function at baseline. At least 14 different outcome measures relating to swallow function were reported across the studies and at varied time intervals (Additional file 3: Table S3). The most frequently used measures (7/15) were: modified barium swallow and use of a feeding tube as a surrogate marker of swallow (dys) function. The PSS or a patient rated diet texture score, mouth opening, penetration-aspiration scale (PAS) [47], MDADI and weight measures were also used across multiple studies, although less frequently. Almost all studies reported a combination of instrumentally derived (objective), patient-reported and/or clinician rated outcomes measures. Two studies [42, 45] reported on just the MDADI, and one study [46] reported on a diet texture score alone.

Sample characteristics

A total of 995 participants were reported at the commencement of the studies (Table 1; 729 males, 257 females, nine unclear). Sample size ranged from 18 to 374. Average age across studies was 59.4 years. Both the gender and age demographics are broadly reflective of the epidemiology of HNC [48, 49].

Patients' HNC diagnosis ranged from stage II to stage IV disease. The sites included the oral cavity, oropharynx, hypopharynx, nasopharynx and larynx. The majority of studies (12/15), focused on the group of patients treated with radiotherapy or chemo-radiation. Of these 12 studies, ten focused on *pre-treatment* swallowing interventions. Three of the 15 studies [39, 42, 46] targeted patients who were treated with surgery as the main modality (Table 1).

Quality assessment

As indicated in Table 2, only one study [37] achieved a score ≥6 and met the criteria for good quality [24]. In 7/ 15 studies, there was at least one item for which information was missing or could not be deduced from the study report. Scores ranged from 0–7 out of 11. No study complied with criteria requiring that the *therapist and subject were blinded to the intervention* (15/15) (Table 2).

Intervention characteristics

Twenty individual BCTs (Table 3) were each identified in at least one intervention. The average number of BCTs per intervention was seven, with a range of four to ten. The BCT *instruction on how to perform the behaviour* was reported in all interventions (15/15), with 14/ 15 including *setting behavioural goals* (for example, perform jaw exercises 3×/day) and 13/15 including *action*

planning (for example perform exercises before mealtimes) (Additional file 1: Table S1).

A total of three Function categories were each identified in at least one intervention. *Training* was identified in all interventions (15/15), *Education* in 12/15 and *Enablement* for example providing patient with a Thera-Bite device in 5/15 (Additional file 2: Table S2).

Regular performance of the prescribed swallowing exercises was the target behaviour for all interventions. Due to the small number of studies, and the variation in exercise content we made no attempt to further group interventions according to the exercise type (Table 3).

Exploring relationships between behavioural strategies and effectiveness

Frequency of behavioral intervention components and intervention effectiveness

The three most commonly used BCTs that appeared in > 85% of interventions were *instruction on how to perform the behaviour, setting behavioural goals* and *action planning*. These BCTs may arguably form the cornerstone of exercise therapy interventions so it is unsurprising that they were identified in >85% of interventions. Four BCTs were used in at least twice as many interventions that produced positive effects relative to those with no such effects - *practical social support, behavioural practice/rehearsal, self-monitoring*, and *credible source*.

Exploring relationships between trial methods and effectiveness

Influence of comparator group on intervention effectiveness

We wished to explore any relations between active and non-active comparator groups and intervention effectiveness. Of five studies [22, 33–35, 43] reporting no evidence of a significantly positive effect of the intervention on any outcome, four had an active control group where similar behavioural strategies were used in both the intervention and comparator groups, except Ahlberg [43] who used parallel groups on different sites. The active comparator group represented either a different exercise regime (often described as usual care), or may have omitted the use of a swallowing exercise device that was included in the intervention group.

Of the ten interventions that demonstrated evidence of positive effects on at least one swallowing outcome measure (Additional file 3: Table S3), five [36–38, 42, 44] had a *non-active comparator* group. In two studies [40, 45], intervention was delayed and therefore effectively represents a non-active comparator group. Two studies had an active comparator group that received a different exercise intervention [39, 41]. One study [46] used similar exercise interventions but the intervention group included *biofeedback* by providing the patient with visual feedback of swallowing during a fibreoptic

Table 1 Study demographics and sample characteristics

Author/year Country of Origin.	Setting	Type of study	Type of intervention (I) Control (C)	Oncology Treatment, sample characteristics	Sample size T = total I = new treatment, C = control	Gender (M:F)	Sample age for (I) and (C) groups. (mean and SD/ range)	Baseline Swallowing status	Length of Follow-up
Mortensen 2015 [33] Denmark	University hospital	RCT (pre-treat)	(I) Individualised dietary advice, exercise protocol of standard exercises – 10reps/3x daily (C) = usual care, individual dietary advice. VFS and advice as needed. (active control)	Cancer of larynx, pharynx, oral cavity (T2-T4), unknown primary. Planned for radiotherapy with/ without chemo. No previous oncology treatment.	T = 39 I = 19 C = 20 NB: 5 patients excluded at start.	34:5	I = 58 (39–77) C = 59 (40–74)	(I) SPSS =1,44 (C) SPSS = 1.38	11 months
Van Den Berg 2014 [34] Netherlands	University medical centre	RCT (pre-treat)	(I) = combined diet counseling and individualized swallow therapy. (C) = weekly individual diet counseling for better nutrition. (active control)	Patients with stage II-IV HNC treated with postoperative radiation with/without chemotherapy.	T = 120 I = 60 C = 60	89:31	I = 63 (33–83) C = 60 (40–86)	(I) PSS mean =78 (SD =26) (C) PSS mean =75 (SD = 25)	30 weeks
Ohba 2014 [40] Japan	University hospital	Retro-spective case-control design (peri-treatment)	(I) = shaker exercise during CRT. (C) = Mendelsohn manoeuvre only when dysphagia developed (delayed active)	Advanced HNC, laryngeal, oropharyngeal, hypopharyngeal cancers.	T = 51 I = 21 C = 30	46:5	I = 65 (53–80) C = 63 (49–89)	Not reported	2-4 weeks
Lazarus 2014 [35] USA	Medical centre	RCT (post-treat)	(I) = isometric tongue exercises with traditional exercises. (C) = traditional exercises including ROM. (active control)	Patients with stage II-IV oral and oro-pharyngeal cancer, who previously underwent radiotherapy with/without chemo.	T = 23 I = 12 C = 11	22:1	I = 62.3 (SD, 8.06) C = 61.7 (SD, 7.27)	(I) OPSE mean = 44.63 (dysphagia if less than 39) Tongue strength =44.63 (C) OPSE =59.6 tongue strength =49.3	10 weeks
Virani 2013 [41] USA	Cancer centre	Non randomised trial – matched groups. (pre-treat)	(I) = behavioural swallow exercises (C) = repetitive swallowing tasks (active control)	Newly diagnosed HNC of the oral cavity, oropharynx, nasopharynx, larynx or unknown primary due to undergo radiotherapy with/without chemo.	T = 50 I = 26 C = 24	40:10	I = 64 (24–90) C = 60 (43–85)	(I) FOIS =6,5 (C) FOIS =6.6	3 months
Kotz 2012 [35] USA	Academic medical centre	RCT (pre-treat)	(I) = behavioural swallow exercises (5sets) (C) = no active treatment	Patients with HNC receiving CRT, excluding any surgery or previous radiation or previous history of dysphagia.	T = 26 I = 13 C = 13	20:6	I = 57 (SD,10) C = 62 (SD,11)	I) FOIS =7 PSS =100 (C) FOIS =7 PSS =100	12 months
Carnaby-Mann 2012 [37] USA	University Hospital Cancer Centre	RCT 3-arms (pre/peri)	(I) = pharyngocize and diet modification. (C) = usual care consisting of supervision for safe swallowing. Sham therapy – buccal	Newly diagnosed with oropharyngeal cancer and planned for external beam radiotherapy with/	T = 58 I = 20 C = 20 Sham =18	44:14	I =59 (SD,10.4) C =54 (SD, 11.3) sham =60 (SD, 12.2)	(I) MASA = 195.1 SD = 5.9 (C) MASA =195.5 SD =4 sham = 194.7 SD = 3.5 scores	6 months

Table 1 Study demographics and sample characteristics (Continued)

Study	Setting	Design	Intervention	Population	Sample	Gender	Age	Baseline measure	Follow-up
			extension manoeuvre – daily schedule. Active control – sham, and no treatment group	without chemo. TNM stage 1-4				>178 suggest no dysphagia.	
Zhen 2012 [42] China	University Hospital	Quasi-experiment-Parallel cluster study (post-treat)	(I) = 30 min swallow training daily for 2 weeks (C) = no active treatment	All patients were post tongue surgery. MDADI score of 60 or lower on screening.	T = 46 I = 23 C = 23	29:17	I=60.52 (SD,5.5) C = 57.5 (SD, 5.72)	Not reported	1 month
Ahlberg 2011 [43] Sweden	University Hospital	Non randomized parallel groups (pre-treat)	(I) = pre-treatment swallowing exercises. (C) = no active pretreatment intervention	Patients diagnosed with HNC due to receive curative radiotherapy	T = 374 I = 190 C = 184	253:121	I =63.6 (SD, 13.1) C = 64.1 (SD, 12)	Not reported	6 month outcomes, 2 year F/U.
Tang 2011 [38] China	University Hospital	RCT (post-treat)	(I) = exercises and jaw stretch (C) = no active exercise intervention	Previously diagnosed with nasopharyngeal cancer and received radiotherapy – long term post-treatment.	T = 46 I = 25 C = 21 3 pts excluded	32:11 (gender of patients excluded not reported)	T =49.3 (not indicated separately for groups)	(I) WST =3.6 IID =1.89 (C) = WST =3.8 IID =1.8	3 months
Van Der Molen [22] 2011 Netherlands	Cancer Centre	RCT (pre-treat)	(I) device based rehab protocol using therabite (C) standard treatment of best evidence-based exercises (active control)	Stage III-IV HNC (oral cavity, oropharynx, hypopharynx, larynx, nasopharynx) planned for curative chemo-radiation treatment.	T = 55 I = 27 C = 28	39:10 (gender of patients excluded not reported)	I = 56 (37–78) C = 57 (32–75)	Baseline function of each group not reported. Overall mean at pre-treatment: FOIS =7	*10 weeks 2 years, 6 years FU in later papers.
Logemann 2009 [39] USA	7 settings university hospitals cancer centres	RCT (post-treat)	(I) shaker exercise (C) traditional swallow therapy (active control)	Patients with prolonged oro-pharyngeal dysphagia of at least 3-month duration	T = 19 I = 8 C = 11	16:3	Not provided	All had aspiration	6 weeks
Carroll 2007 [44] USA	University hospital	2-arm Retrospective Case control Study (pre-treat)	(I) pre-treatment swallowing exercise protocol. (C) usual care -swallow rehab as problems arose post treatment. (no active pre-treat exercises)	Patients with advanced squamous cell cancer of the oropharynx, hypopharynx and larynx treated with chemo-radiation.	T = 18 I = 9 C = 9	12:6	I = 57.5 C = 60.7	Not reported	12 months
Kulbersh 2006 [45] USA	University Hospital	2-arm Prospective cohort study (pre-treat)	I) pre-treatment swallowing exercise protocol (C) exercises given at first visit after treatment. (delayed intervention)	All patients diagnosed with HNC with/without nodal disease but without metastatic disease	T = 37 I = 25 C = 12	28:9	I =55.1 (SD, 9.6) C = 66.3 (SD, 10)	Not reported	12 months
Denk 1997 [46] Austria	ENT department	Non-randomised, 2-arm parallel group study (post-treat)	(I) therapy with video-endoscopic biofeedback. (C) conventional swallow therapy. (active control)	Patients with prolonged post-operative aspiration following resection of malignant tumours of the oropharyngeal swallowing structures.	T = 33 I = 19 C = 14	25:8	I = 54 (37–68) C = 53 (37–79)	Prolonged post-op aspiration, with tube feeding	Variable, based on time to establish oral intake

Notes: (I) = intervention group; (C) = control group; T = total sample; RCT = randomised controlled trial; HNC = head and neck cancer; SPSS = swallowing performance status scale; OPSE = oro-pharyngeal swallow efficiency; FOIS = functional oral intake scale; MASA = Mann swallowing assessment; WST = water swallow test; IID = inter-incisor distance; * Later papers linked to this study include follow-up measures at 2-years, and 6 years

Table 2 Quality assessment ratings for all studies included in the review

	Mortensen	Van Den Berg	Ohba	Lazarus	Virani	Kotz	Carnaby Mann	Zhen	Ahlberg	Tang	Van Der Molen	Logemann	Caroll	Kulbersh	Denk
✓ = yes															
?=															
✗ = no															
Quality criteria															
Randomisation detailed	✓	✓	n/a	✓	n/a	?	✓	n/a	n/a	?	✓	✗	n/a	n/a	n/a
Allocation concealed	?	✗	n/a	?	n/a	✗	✓	n/a	n/a	✗	?	✗	n/a	n/a	n/a
Similar groups at baseline	✓	✓	✓	✓	✓	✓	✓	✓	✓	✓	✓	✓	✓	✗	✓
Subject blind	✗	✗	✗	✗	✗	✗	✗	✗	✗	✗	✗	✗	✗	✗	✗
Therapist blind	✗	✗	✗	✗	✗	✗	✗	✗	✗	✗	✗	✗	✗	✗	✗
Assessor blind	?	✗	✗	✓	✓	✓	✓	✗	✗	✗	✗	✓	✓	✗	✗
Co-intervention controlled	?	✗	✗	?	✗	?	✓	✗	✗	✗	?	?	?	✗	?
Acceptable compliance	✗	?	?	✗	✗	✗	✗	✓	?	✓	?	?	?	?	?
Acceptable withdrawal rate	✗	✓	✓	✗	✓	✗	✗	✓	✗	✓	✓	✗	✓	?	✓
Timing of outcome	✓	✓	✓	✓	✓	✓	✓	✗	✓	✓	✓	✓	✓	✗	✗
Intention to treat	✓	✓	✗	?	✓	✓	✓	✗	✗	✗	✓	✓	✗	✗	✗
TOTAL	4	5	3	4	5	4	7	3	2	4	5	4	4	0	2

endoscopic assessment. One study [37] had 3 groups: a treatment group receiving swallowing exercises, a group receiving sham exercises using a similar dose schedule and a usual care group who received only safe-feeding advice by the hospital team when required but not an exercise intervention. The authors found a statistically significant difference between each of the active groups (swallowing exercises and sham exercises) and the usual care group, but a smaller difference (favouring the exercise group) between the swallowing exercise group vs sham exercise group.

Again we acknowledge the small number of studies, however our findings seem to indicate that employing active comparator groups particularly when similar behavioural strategies are used, are less likely to demonstrate statistically significant positive effects. Interestingly, a positive effect was still found in one study [46] when both groups received similar exercise interventions, but different non-exercise content (intervention group received biofeedback, a named BCT).

Type and timing of outcome measures and intervention effectiveness

Outcomes that significantly improved with the exercise intervention did so mostly at 1 month post oncological treatment, with a general decline in effect at the later time-points after treatment. Four studies measured outcomes at 12 months [33, 36, 44, 45] but only one [45] showed a significant difference in favour of the intervention by this time-point. In one study [36], outcomes were measured at multiple time-points; significant differences were observed at 3 and 6 months post-treatment but not at 9 and 12 months (Additional file 3: Table S3). Another study [33] charted a rapid decline in patient adherence to swallowing exercises over the first 12 months following treatment.

Outcomes broadly classified as *objective measures* (PAS, MBS score, mouth opening, feeding tube) were more frequently improved by the intervention, when compared to patient reported and clinician rated measures.

This exploration of the data has highlighted the potential impact that BCTs and trial methods such as choice of comparator group and timing of outcome measures may have on intervention effectiveness. Implications of these findings are expanded upon in the Discussion.

Discussion

We identified 15 controlled clinical trials (8 randomised) that currently represent the best available evidence of

Table 3 Behaviour Change Techniques (BCTs) identified across included studies

Actual check ticks (✓) = BCT present	Mortensen	V.D. Berg	Ohba	Lazarus	Virani	Kotz	Carnaby	Zhen	Ahlberg	Tang	V.D. Molen	Logemann	Carroll	Kulbersh	Denk	% studies
Goals and Planning																
Goal setting (behaviour)	✓	✓	✓	✓	✓	✓	✓		✓	✓	✓	✓	✓	✓	✓	93
Problem solving	✓															7
Action planning	✓	✓	✓	✓	✓	✓	✓		✓	✓	✓	✓	✓	✓		87
Review behaviour goals							✓		✓							13
Review outcome goals															✓	7
Feedback and Monitoring																
Monitoring of behaviour by others without feedback		✓		✓										✓		20
Feedback on behaviour						✓			✓							13
Self monitoring of behaviour	✓			✓		✓	✓			✓		✓				40
Monitoring outcome of behaviour without feedback									✓							7
biofeedback															✓	7
Social Support																
Social support (unspecified)		✓		✓	✓	✓		✓	✓	✓						47
Social support (practical)	✓						✓			✓		✓			✓	33
Shaping Knowledge																
Instruction on how to perform the behaviour	✓	✓	✓	✓	✓	✓	✓	✓	✓	✓	✓	✓	✓	✓	✓	100
Comparison of behaviour																
Demonstration of the behaviour							✓									7
Associations																
Prompts and cues						✓										7
Repetition and Substitution																
Behavioural practice/rehearsal		✓	✓	✓	✓	✓	✓	✓		✓	✓	✓	✓	✓		80
Habit formation											✓		✓			13
Generalization of target behaviour	✓	✓			✓	✓				✓	✓	✓	✓			53
Comparison of outcomes																
Credible source	✓	✓				✓	✓	✓		✓		✓		✓	✓	60
Antecedents																
Adding objects to the environment				✓			✓		✓	✓	✓		✓			40
Total Number of BCTs	8	8	4	8	6	10	10	4	8	10	7	8	7	6	6	

swallowing interventions for patients with HNC, and extracted three function categories and 20 different BCTs that characterize these interventions. By specifically isolating these BCTs, we may encourage more consistent descriptions of the non-exercise content of swallowing exercise interventions in the literature increasing our ability to replicate studies more accurately. Indeed, in time it may be possible to devise interventions that test the effectiveness of specific BCTs or groups of BCTs used in swallowing exercise interventions for this patient population, and to link these to underlying theory and mechanisms of change [50]. In so doing, we may be better placed to understand why interventions work, for whom and in which contexts [11].

We also examined the data for any relationships that may elucidate the interaction of different components of this complex intervention. For example, studies that employed active comparator groups using similar BCTs to the intervention group were more likely to demonstrate non-significant results. Furthermore in a trial that employed three groups [37], (an exercise group, a sham exercise group, and a non-active control group), the authors reported that the active sham exercise group that received similar BCTs to the pharyngocize (exercise treatment) group achieved much better outcomes compared to the non-active control group. It may therefore be the constituent BCTs that were responsible for intervention effectiveness, by stimulating greater adherence to the prescribed treatment. Whilst the authors themselves did not specifically make reference to BCTs, they did question whether the 'benefits obtained from the sham group could be ascribed to the placebo effect of behavioral attention' (p.219). Equally they speculated that the sham exercise (done diligently) might have had an intrinsic benefit from the increased movement of oral musculature. Regardless, these findings raise the possibility that BCTs may be functioning as *active ingredients* influencing intervention outcomes. For most studies where both the intervention and active comparison group used similar BCTs, no statistical significance in outcomes between groups was reported. This might be because the interventions given to both groups were too similar, or because of a lack of power due to small sample sizes. However it does raise other interesting questions: What contribution do BCTs add to intervention outcomes, and how does their presence in usual care/placebo interventions impact effectiveness? Reporting of swallowing exercise interventions tends to focus mainly on the treatment group and often provides only cursory reference to the usual care group. The findings of this review highlight that the same methodological care should be taken in devising the treatment manuals for the intervention and comparator groups ensuring that behaviour change components are also specified, given

their potential to impact patient adherence and subsequent outcomes. This may prevent hasty conclusions that imply swallowing exercises have no benefit, rather than the conclusion that the "new intervention" was not shown to demonstrate any significant additional benefit over usual care.

The variability in the type and time-point of the primary outcome measures for clinical trials in this field restricts the ability to satisfactorily pool data or compute effect sizes to address the efficacy of swallowing interventions in patients with head and neck cancer. We generally observed that in studies that reported a positive outcome, this was mostly seen in the short term. One reason for this may be because patients do not continue with their exercises long term. Behavioural strategies such as *habit formation*, requires that an individual repeatedly perform the behaviour in the same context such that it becomes automatic. This automaticity may promote maintenance of exercises as it may over-ride conscious intentions [51] and could have a role to play in improving swallowing outcomes longer term. We also observed that outcomes collected after 6 months showed little difference between groups. This was especially relevant for patient-reported outcomes that arguably may also reflect patients' changing expectations and adaptation over time, and not just functional swallowing status. Furthermore, this mirrors the usual trajectory of behaviour change where short-term goals are given priority. Rothman [52] highlighted that the psychological factors that underpin initiation of a new behaviour differ from those that predict maintenance of the behaviour. By implication, different BCTs may be required for these distinct phases. It was also noted that few studies actually collected objective measures of swallowing in the longer term, making it difficult to assess changes in swallow physiology at later time-points. Standardizing outcome measures and agreement on the key evaluation time-points will greatly progress efforts to understand if swallowing exercise interventions are indeed beneficial for this group of patients and over what time period. Consideration should also be given to the expected trajectory of swallowing recovery after head and neck cancer treatment including the possible onset of late effects of treatment such as post radiation fibrosis known to impair swallow function [53, 54].

Assessing the robustness of the synthesis
According to Popay and colleagues [19], robustness of a synthesis is usually determined by 1) the methodological quality of the included studies, 2) methods used to minimise bias in the synthesis process, and 3) whether detailed information has been provided on the type of studies included/excluded. This review meets the latter two criteria by providing detailed information *via* a

published protocol. Methodological quality of the available evidence was rated as poor with only one study meeting more than 50% of the applied quality criteria. It is however acknowledged that for this type of intervention, it is usually impossible to blind the therapist and subject to the intervention. Attrition is a common feature for studies that involve a complex intervention within a multifaceted cancer care pathway, and randomised studies within this field are only beginning to emerge [16, 25]. Excluding studies that did not meet quality criteria may therefore have disadvantaged our ability to address our primary aims in this exercise. Furthermore, complex interventions may require a differing emphasis on the markers of study quality as they are frequently evaluated within the context of pragmatic clinical trials. Since developing our protocol, new methods of evaluating quality in complex interventions have begun to emerge that may be more suitable for future use [9].

Limitations and challenges

This review is limited by the fact that the accuracy of the coding scheme relies on the quality of published intervention reports, which are often not sufficiently detailed to extract all necessary components of the intervention [55]. It is possible therefore that the intervention itself may have included strategies that have not been coded in this review. Descriptions of the treatment delivered to comparator groups in particular were poor, and in some cases decisions about the presence of BCTs in the comparator group had to be based on the authors' implicit suggestions that interventions were identical apart from the specific exercise protocol used in each of the active groups.

Despite the BCT taxonomy being developed within Behavioural Science, there is ongoing debate amongst experts in behaviour change as to its merits. Critics have questioned the value of coding BCTs, suggesting it creates a level of abstraction that detracts from the detailed content analysis of interventions [56]. As a counter argument, we believe that in a clinical field that has focused mainly on exercise protocol content, drawing attention to broader more abstract process based mechanisms can only enrich our understanding of complex interventions. The taxonomy brings structure, organization and a common language to this process. For example, coding a BCT such as *self-monitoring* may not tell us how the self-monitoring was done, but it does highlight that the use of self-monitoring may be relevant to changing adherence behaviour, particularly when it is frequently observed in successful interventions.

What this review adds

This review applied a behavior change perspective to studies within head and neck cancer swallowing rehabilitation, with a specific focus on identifying the behavioral strategies that may impact patient adherence to exercises, and consequently swallowing outcomes. Such an analysis is absent in the current literature. Our aim was to instigate discussion and greater thought about the complexity of swallowing exercise interventions, their design and the reporting of such interventions. It addresses the question of *what* might bring about change by isolating the specific components within an intervention, other than the nature of the treatments to which patients are encouraged to adhere, that may influence behaviour [57]. It therefore expands on the findings from previous related reviews [15, 16, 58, 59] and goes some way to highlighting additional components that may be present and active in this complex intervention. Given the relative paucity of high quality data, the review did not attempt to definitively answer the question of which BCTs are most effective in promoting adherence, but instead aimed to highlight those that were prevalent in successful interventions. Using this as a starting point, we may begin to design future interventions incorporating specific BCTs or groups of BCTs to examine more closely whether they strengthen interventions aimed at improving swallowing function *via* swallowing exercises. Clearly BCTs are only one part of trial design and equal attention should be placed on other important aspects such as precise definition of the whole intervention package in prospective study protocols and intervention manuals.

This approach seeks to generate new discussion toward understanding the make-up of complex interventions. It also offers new perspectives in the interpretation of findings from clinical trials of swallowing exercises where it is clear that evaluating effectiveness is hampered by poor adherence.

Conclusion

The effectiveness of swallowing exercises depends in part on adherence to exercises. This review looks at BCTs – these seem to promote adherence. The review has provided preliminary information about which BCTs occur in reports of complex swallowing interventions and has highlighted that behavioural components may be *active ingredients* of change that impact intervention outcomes. It is likely that many BCTs are used in clinical practice, and there will be some bias towards the techniques that researchers tend to report. Nevertheless, introducing the taxonomy of BCTs helps equip dysphagia researchers with the tools and the language to improve consistency in how complex interventions are specified in research protocols, intervention manuals and the published literature study. In time, the approach can also be used in examining fidelity in the delivery of interventions through field testing and observational methods. Its merits and weaknesses can only be adequately evaluated as the body of work adopting this approach increases.

Additional files

Additional file 1: Table S1. BCTs, descriptions and examples from studies included in the review. NB: A complete list of BCTs in the taxonomy (BCTTv1) and a full description can be found in Michie, Atkins & West [60].

Additional file 2: Table S2. Intervention Function definitions and examples from included studies where identified. NB: Further general examples of Intervention Functions can be found in Michie, Atkins & West [60].

Addtional file 3: Table S3. Outcome measures obtained at four time points post oncology treatment.

Abbreviations
BCT: Behaviour change technique; BCTTv1: Behaviour change technique taxonomy Version 1; EORTC: European Organisation of Research and Treatment of Cancer; FOIS: Functional oral intake scale; HNC: Head and neck cancer; MBS: Modified barium swallow; MDADI: MD Anderson Dysphagia Inventory; PAS: Penetration-aspiration scale; PRISMA: Preferred Reporting of Items for Systematic reviews and Meta Analyses; PSS: Performance status scale; QOL: Quality of life; WST: Water swallow test

Acknowledgements
The authors wish to thank Daphne Grey for her assistance with the Database searches. We also thank Professors *Jane Wardle and Charles Abraham for their useful discussions and debate during the planning of this review.* Jane Wardle passed away on 20 October 2015

Funding
"This report is independent research supported by the National Institute for Health Research. (NIHR/HEE Clinical Doctoral Research Fellowship, Miss Roganie Govender, CDRF- 2013-04-020). Helen Barratt is supported by the NIHR Collaboration for Leadership in Applied Health Research and Care (CLAHRC) North Thames at Bart's Health NHS Trust. Stuart Taylor is a NIHR senior investigator supported by the UCLH Biomedical Research Centre. Department of Health Disclaimer: The views expressed are those of the author (s) and not necessarily those of the NHS, the NIHR or the Department of Health.

Authors' contributions
RG and BG conceived and designed the study. CS and ST contributed to further refinement of the protocol. RG and CS carried out screening of articles. RG extracted all data, CS and BG extracted a percentage of data and resolved discrepancies. RG analysed all data and drafted the manuscript- BG, ST, HB, CS provided critical feedback during iterative revisions. All authors approved of the final manuscript.

Competing interests
The authors declare that they have no competing interests.

Author details
¹University College London, Health Behaviour Research Centre & University College London Hospital, Head & Neck Cancer Centre, Ground Floor Central, 250 Euston Road, London NW1 2PQ, UK. ²Division of Psychology & Language Sciences University College London, London, UK. ³Centre for Medical Imaging, University College London, London, UK. ⁴Department of Applied Health Research, University College London, London, UK. ⁵Department of Psychology, Institute of Psychiatry, Psychology and Neuroscience (IoPPN), Kings College London, London, UK & UCL Department of Epidemiology & Public Health, University College London, London, UK.

References
1. Malagelada JR, Bazzoli F, Boeckxstaens G, De Looze D, Fried M, Kahrilas,P et al. World Gastroenterology Organisation Global Guidelines Dysphagia — Global Guidelines and Cascades Update. J. Clinical Gastroenterol;49:370–8
2. Manikantan K, Khode S, Sayed SI, Roe J, Nutting CM, Rhys-Evans P, et al. Dysphagia in head and neck cancer. Cancer Treat Rev. 2009;35:724–32. doi:10.1016/j.ctrv.2009.08.008.
3. Rogers SN, Heseltine N, Flexen J, Winstanley HR, Cole-Hawkins H, Kanatas A. Structured review of papers reporting specific functions in patients with cancer of the head and neck: 2006–2013. Br J Oral Maxillofac Surg 2016:1–7. doi:10.1016/j.bjoms.2016.02.012.
4. Wall LR, Ward EC, Cartmill B, Hill AJ. Physiological changes to the swallowing mechanism following (chemo) radiotherapy for head and neck cancer: a systematic review. Dysphagia. 2013;28:481–93. doi:10.1007/s00455-013-9491-8.
5. Duarte VM, Chhetri DK, Liu YF, Erman AA, Wang MB. Swallow preservation exercises during chemoradiation therapy maintains swallow function. Otolaryngol Head Neck Surg. 2013;149:878–84. doi:10.1177/0194599813502310.
6. Shinn EH, Basen-Engquist K, Baum G, Steen S, Bauman RF, Morrison W, et al. Adherence to preventive exercises and self-reported swallowing outcomes in post-radiation head and neck cancer patients. Head Neck. 2013;35:1707–12. doi:10.1002/hed.23255.
7. Sabate E. (ed) World Health Organization - Adherence to long term therapies. World Health Organization 2003. http://apps.who.int/iris/bitstream/10665/42682/1/9241545992.pdf
8. Craig P, Dieppe P, Macintyre S, Mitchie S, Nazareth I, Petticrew M. Developing and evaluating complex interventions: the new medical research council guidance. BMJ. 2008;337:979–83. doi:10.1136/bmj.a1655.
9. Barratt H, Campbell M, Moore L, Zwarenstein M, Bower P. Randomised controlled trials of complex interventions and large-scale transformation of services. In Raine R, Fitzpatrick R, barratt H, Bevan G, black N, Boaden R, et al. Challenges, solutions and future directions in the evaluation of service innovations in health care and public health. Health Serv Deliv Res. 2016; 4(16):19–36.
10. Bate P, Robert G, Fulop N, Øvretveit J, Dixon-Woods M. Perspectives on context. 2014. http://www.health.org.uk/sites/health/files/PerspectivesOnContext_fullversion.pdf.
11. Moher D, Stewart L, Shekelle P. All in the family: systematic reviews, rapid reviews, scoping reviews, realist reviews, and more. Syst Rev. 2015;4:183. doi:10.1186/s13643-015-0163-7.
12. Sutcliffe K, Thomas J, Stokes G, Hinds K, Bangpan M. Intervention component analysis (ICA): a pragmatic approach for identifying the critical features of complex interventions. Syst Rev. 2015;4:140. doi:10.1186/s13643-015-0126-z.
13. Rohwer AA, Booth A, Pfadenhauer L, Brereton L, Gerhardus A, Mozygemba K, et al. Guidance on the use of logic models in health technology assessments of complex interventions. http://www.integrate-hta.eu/wp-content/uploads/2016/02/Guidance-on-the-use-of-logic-models-inhealth-technology-assessments-of-complex-interventions.pdf. Eu/downloads/2016.
14. Langmore SE, Pisegna JM. Efficacy of exercises to rehabilitate dysphagia: A critique of the literature. Int J Speech Lang Pathol. 2015.1–8. doi:10.3109/17549507.2015.1024171
15. Cousins N, MacAulay F, Lang H, MacGillivray S, Wells M. A systematic review of interventions for eating and drinking problems following treatment for head and neck cancer suggests a need to look beyond swallowing and trismus. Oral Oncol. 2013;49:387–400. doi:10.1016/j.oraloncology.2012.12.002.
16. Perry A, Lee SH, Cotton S, Kennedy C. Therapeutic exercises for affecting post-treatment swallowing in people treated for advanced-stage head and neck cancers. Cochrane Database Syst Rev Published Online First. 2016. doi:10.1002/14651858.CD011112.

17. Michie S, Richardson M, Johnston M, Abraham C, Francis J, Hardeman W, et al. The behavior change technique taxonomy (v1) of 93 hierarchically clustered techniques: building an international consensus for the reporting of behavior change interventions. Ann Behav Med. 2013;46:81–95. doi:10.1007/s12160-013-9486-6.

18. Michie S, Abraham C, Eccles MP, Francis J, Hardeman W, Johnston M. Strengthening evaluation and implementation by specifying components of behaviour change interventions: a study protocol. Implement Sci. 2011;6:10. doi:10.1186/1748-5908-6-10.

19. Popay J, Roberts H, Sowden A, Petticrew M, Arai L, Rodgers M, et al. Guidance on the Conduct of Narrative Synthesis in Systematic Reviews: A Product from the ESRC Methods Programme. 2006:1–92. doi:10.13140/2.1. 1018.4643.

20. Govender R, Smith CH, Taylor SA, Grey D, Wardle J, Gardner B. Identification of behaviour change components in swallowing interventions for head and neck cancer patients: protocol for a systematic review. Syst Rev. 2015;4:89. doi:10.1186/s13643-015-0077-4.

21. Schardt C, Adams MB, Owens T, Keitz S, Fontelo P. Utilization of the PICO framework to improve searching PubMed for clinical questions. BMC Med Inform Decis Mak. 2007;7:16. doi:10.1186/1472-6947-7-16.

22. van der Molen L, van Rossum MA, Burkhead LM, Smeele LE, Rasch CRN, Hilgers FJM. A randomized preventive rehabilitation trial in advanced head and neck cancer patients treated with chemoradiotherapy: feasibility, compliance, and short-term effects. Dysphagia. 2011;26:155–70. doi:10.1007/s00455-010-9288-y.

23. Liberati A, Altman DG, Tetzlaff J, Mulrow C, Ioannidis JP a, Clarke M, et al. Annals of Internal Medicine Academia and Clinic The PRISMA Statement for Reporting Systematic Reviews and Meta-Analyses of Studies That Evaluate Health Care Interventions: Ann Intern Med 2009;151:W65–94. doi:10.1371/journal.pmed.1000100.

24. van Tulder M, Furlan A, Bombardier C. Updated Method Guidelines for Systematic Reviews in the Cochrane Collaboration Back Review Group 2003; 28(12):90–99.

25. Carnaby G, Madhavan A. A systematic review of randomized controlled trials in the field of dysphagia rehabilitation. Curr Phys Med Rehabil Rep. 2013;1:197–215. doi:10.1007/s40141-013-0030-1.

26. Hughes TA, Wiles CM. Clinical measurement of swallowing in health and in neurogenic dysphagia. QJM. 1996;89:109–16.

27. Crary MA, Carnaby-Mann G, Groher ME. Initial psychometric assessment of a functional oral intake scale for dysphagia in stroke patients. Arch Phys Med Rehabil. 2005;86:1516–20. doi:10.1016/j.apmr.2004.11.049.

28. List MA, Ritter-Sterr C, Lansky SB. A performance status scale for head and neck cancer patients. Cancer. 1990;66:564–9.

29. Chen AY, Frankowski R, Bishop-leone J. The Development and Validation of a Dysphagia-Specific Quality-of-Life Questionnaire for Patients With Head and Neck Cancer 2001;127:870–6.

30. Groenvold M, Klee MC, Sprangers MAG, Aaronson NK. Validation of the EORTC QLQ-C30 quality of life questionnaire through combined qualitative and quantitative assessment of patient-observer agreement. J Clin Epidemiol. 1997;50:441–50. doi:10.1016/S0895-4356(96)00428-3.

31. Michie S, van Stralen MM, West R. The behaviour change wheel: a new method for characterising and designing behaviour change interventions. Implement Sci. 2011;6:42. doi:10.1186/1748-5908-6-42.

32. Landis JR, Koch GG. The measurement of observer agreement for categorical data. Biometrics. 1977;33:159–74. doi:10.2307/2529310.

33. Mortensen HR, Jensen K, Aksglæde K, Lambertsen K, Eriksen E, Grau C. Prophylactic Swallowing Exercises in Head and Neck Cancer Radiotherapy. Dysphagia 2015:15–7. doi:10.1007/s00455-015-9600-y.

34. Van Den Berg MGA, Kalf JG, Hendriks JCM, Takes RP, Van Herpen CML, Wanten GJA et al. Normalcy of food intake in patients with head and neck cancer supported by combined dietary counseling and swallowing therapy: A randomised clinical trial. Head Neck 2015. doi:10.1002/hed.

35. Lazarus CL, Husaini H, Falciglia D, DeLacure M, Branski RC, Kraus D, et al. Effects of exercise on swallowing and tongue strength in patients with oral and oropharyngeal cancer treated with primary radiotherapy with or without chemotherapy. Int J Oral Maxillofac Surg. 2014;43:523–30. doi:10.1016/j.ijom.2013.10.023.

36. Kotz T, Federman AD, Kao J, Milman L, Packer S, Lopez-Prieto C, et al. Prophylactic swallowing exercises in patients with head and neck cancer undergoing chemoradiation: a randomized trial. Arch Otolaryngol Head Neck Surg. 2012;138:376–82. doi:10.1001/archoto.2012.187.

37. Carnaby-mann G, Crary MA, Schmalfuss I, Amdur R. Pharyngocise": randomized controlled trial of preventative exercises to maintain muscle structure and swallowing function during head-and-neck chemoradiotherapy. Radiat Oncol Biol. 2012;83:210–9. doi:10.1016/j.ijrobp.2011.06.1954.

38. Tang Y, Shen Q, Wang Y, Lu K, Peng Y. A randomized prospective study of rehabilitation therapy in the treatment of radiation-induced dysphagia and trismus. Strahlenther Onkol. 2011;187:39–44. doi:10.1007/s00066-010-2151-0.

39. Logemann JA, Rademaker A, Pauloski BR, Kelly A, Strangl-McBreen C, Antinoja J, et al. An RCT comparing the shaker exercise with traditional therapy: a preliminary study. Dysphagia. 2009;24:403–11. doi:10.1007/s00455-009-9217-0.A.

40. Ohba S, Ph JY, Kojima M, Fujimaki M, Anzai T, Komatsu H, et al. Significant Preservation of Swallowing Function in Chemoradiotherapy for Advanced Head and Neck Cancer by Prophylactic Swallowing Exercise. Neck Head 2014doi: 10.1002/hed.23913

41. Virani A, Kunduk M, Fink DS, McWhorter AJ. Effects of 2 different swallowing exercise regimens during organ-preservation therapies for head and neck cancers on swallowing function. Head Neck 2013:1–9. doi:10.1002/hed. 23570

42. Zhen Y, Wang JG, Tao D, Wang HJ, Chen WL. Efficacy survey of swallowing function and quality of life in response to therapeutic intervention following rehabilitation treatment in dysphagic tongue cancer patients. Eur J Oncol Nurs. 2012;16:54–8. doi:10.1016/j.ejon.2011.03.002.

43. Ahlberg A, Engström T, Nikolaidis P, Gunnarsson K, Johansson H, Sharp L, et al. Early self-care rehabilitation of head and neck cancer patients. Acta Otolaryngol. 2011;131:552–61. doi:10.3109/00016489.2010.532157.

44. Carroll WR, Locher JL, Canon CL, Bohannon IA, McColloch NL, Magnuson JS. Pretreatment swallowing exercises improve swallow function after chemoradiation. Laryngoscope. 2008;118:39–43. doi:10.1097/MLG. 0b013e31815659b0.

45. Kulbersh BD, Rosenthal EL, McGrew BM, Duncan RD, McColloch NL, Carroll WR, et al. Pretreatment, preoperative swallowing exercises may improve dysphagia quality of life. Laryngoscope. 2006;116:883–6. doi:10.1016/S1041-892X(07)70138-5.

46. Denk DM, Kaider A. Videoendoscopic biofeedback: a simple method to improve the efficacy of swallowing rehabilitation of patients after head and neck surgery. ORL. 1997;59:100–5.

47. Rosenbek JC, Robbins JA, Roecker EB, Coyle JL, Wood JL. A penetration-aspiration scale. Dysphagia. 1996;11:93–8. doi:10.1007/BF00417897.

48. Pytynia KB, Dahlstrom KR, Sturgis EM. Epidemiology of HPV-associated oropharyngeal cancer. Oral Oncol. 2014;50:380–6. doi:10.1016/j.oraloncology. 2013.12.019.

49. Simard EP, Torre LA, Jemal A. International trends in head and neck cancer incidence rates: differences by country, sex and anatomic site. Oral Oncol. 2014;50:387–403. doi:10.1016/j.oraloncology.2014.01.016.

50. Michie S, Carey RN, Johnston M, Rothman AJ, de Bruin M, Kelly MP, et al. From Theory-Inspired to Theory-Based Interventions: A Protocol for Developing and Testing a Methodology for Linking Behaviour Change Techniques to Theoretical Mechanisms of Action. Ann Behav Med 2016:1–12. doi:10.1007/s12160-016-9816-6.

51. Gardner B. A review and analysis of the use of "habit" in understanding, predicting and influencing health-related behaviour. Health Psychol Rev 2014;0:1–19. doi:10.1080/17437199.2013.876238.

52. Rothman AJ. Toward a theory based analysis of behavioural maintenance. Health Psychol. 2000;19:64–9.

53. Hutcheson KA, Lewin JS, Barringer DA, Lisec A, Gunn GB, Moore MWS, et al. Late dysphagia after radiotherapy-based treatment of head and neck cancer. Cancer. 2012;118:5793–9. doi:10.1002/cncr.27631.

54. King SN, Dunlap NE, Tennant PA, Pitts T. Pathophysiology of radiation-induced dysphagia in head and neck cancer. Dysphagia. 2016. doi:10.1007/s00455-016-9710-1.

55. Abraham C, Johnson BT, de Bruin M, Luszczynska A. Enhancing reporting of behavior change intervention evaluations. J Acquir Immune Defic Syndr. 2014;66 Suppl 3:S293–9.

56. Ogden J. Celebrating variability and a call to limit systematisation: the example of the Behaviour Change Technique Taxonomy and the Behaviour Change Wheel 2016;7199. doi:10.1080/17437199.2016.1190291.

57. Petticrew M, Rehfuess E, Noyes J, Higgins JPT, Mayhew A, Pantoja T, et al. Synthesizing evidence on complex interventions: How meta-analytical, qualitative, and mixed-method approaches can contribute. J Clin Epidemiol. 2013;66:1230–43. doi:10.1016/j.jclinepi.2013.06.005.

58. Speyer R, Baijens L, Heijnen M, Zwijnenberg I. Effects of therapy in oropharyngeal dysphagia by speech and language therapists: a systematic review. Dysphagia. 2010;25:40–65. doi:10.1007/s00455-009-9239-7.

59. Mccabe D, Ashford J, Wheeler-hegland K, Frymark T, Mullen R, Musson N, et al. Evidence-based systematic review: oropharyngeal dysphagia behavioral treatments. Part IV-impact of dysphagia treatment on individuals' postcancer treatments. J Rehabil Res Dev. 2009;46:205–14. doi:10.1682/JRRD. 2008.08.0092.

60. Michie S, Atkins L, West R. The Behaviour Change Wheel: A guide to designing interventions. Great Britain: Siverback Publishing; 2014.

2

EGFR copy number alterations in primary tumors, metastatic lymph nodes, and recurrent and multiple primary tumors in oral cavity squamous cell carcinoma

Shiang-Fu Huang[1,2,3]* [iD], Huei-Tzu Chien[2,4], Sou-De Cheng[5], Wen-Yu Chuang[6], Chun-Ta Liao[1,3] and Hung-Ming Wang[3,7]

Abstract

Background: The EGFR and downstream signaling pathways play an important role in tumorigenesis in oral squamous cell carcinoma (OSCC). Gene copy number alteration is one mechanism for overexpressing the EGFR protein and was also demonstrated to be related to lymph node metastasis, tumor invasiveness and perineural invasion. Therefore, we hypothesized that EGFR gene copy number alteration in the primary tumor could predict amplification in recurrent tumors, lymph node metastatic foci or secondary primary tumors.

Methods: We recruited a group of newly diagnosed OSCC patients ($n = 170$) between Mar 1997 and Jul 2004. Metastatic lymph nodes were identified from neck dissection specimens ($n = 57$). During follow-up, recurrent lesions ($n = 41$) and secondary primary tumors (SPTs, $n = 17$) were identified and biopsied. The EGFR gene amplifications were evaluated by fluorescence in situ hybridization (FISH) assay in primary tumors, metastatic lymph nodes, recurrences and SPTs.

Results: Of the 170 primary OSCCs, FISH showed low EGFR amplification/polysomy in 19 (11.4%) patients and amplification in 33 (19.8%) patients. EGFR gene amplification was related to lymph node metastasis ($\chi 2$ trend test: $p = 0.018$). Of 57 metastatic lymph nodes, nine (15.8%) had EGFR polysomy and 14 (24.6%) had EGFR gene amplification. The concordance rate of EGFR gene copy number in primary tumors and lymph node metastasis was 68.4% (McNemar test: $p = 0.389$). Of 41 recurrent tumors, five (12.2%) had EGFR polysomy and five (12.2%) had gene amplification. The concordance rate of EGFR gene copy number between primary tumors and recurring tumors was 65.9% (McNemar test: $p = 0.510$). The concordance rate between primary tumors and SPTs was 70.6%. EGFR amplification in either primary tumors, metastatic lymph nodes or recurrent tumors had no influence on patient survival.

Conclusion: We can predict two-thirds of the EGFR gene copy number alterations in lymph node metastasis or recurrent tumors from the analysis of primary tumors. For OSCC patients who are unable to provide lymph node or recurrent tumor samples for EGFR gene copy number analysis, examining primary tumors could provide EGFR clonal information in metastatic, recurrent or SPT lesions.

Keywords: Epidermal growth factor receptor (EGFR), Gene amplification, Recurrence, metastasis, Multiple primary tumors, fluorescence in situ hybridization, Oral cavity squamous cell carcinoma

* Correspondence: shiangfu.huang@gmail.com
[1]Department of Otolaryngology, Head and Neck Surgery, Chang Gung Memorial Hospital, No. 5 Fu-Shin Street, Kwei-Shan, Taoyuan, Taiwan
[2]Department of Public Health, Chang Gung University, Tao-Yuan, Taiwan
Full list of author information is available at the end of the article

Background

In Taiwan, oral cancer is the 4th most common cancer in men [1]. The consumption of areca-quid (AQ), tobacco and alcohol among Taiwanese men results in an increase in oral cancer risks about ten-fold higher than women and its incidence is rising [2]. The primary treatment for oral cavity squamous cell carcinoma (OSCC) is radical surgery with or without post-operative adjuvant radio-/chemotherapy and this treatment approach can result in good loco-regional control [3]. Some patients have recurrence and/or distant metastasis after these radical treatments. Among the poor prognostic factors for OSCC discussed by O'Brien et al., cervical lymph node metastasis is just as important as tumor stage, the extent of the tumor invasion, and perineural/lymphovascular invasion in adversely influencing tumor control [4–6]. We previously demonstrated that lymph node metastasis, tumor cell differentiation and perineural invasion and tumor stage are correlated with EGFR gene amplification [7]. Those previous findings indicate that tumor cells with EGFR amplification are invasive. These tumor cells are more likely to proliferate in recurrent tumors and metastasize to the lymph nodes. It is therefore worthwhile to investigate tumor cells with increased EGFR amplification because the number of EGFR copies plays an important role in metastasis, recurrence or development of secondary primary tumors (SPTs).

Regarding the concordance between the number of EGFR gene copies and primary tumor and metastatic lesions in non-small cell lung cancer, the discordant rate ranges from 27 to 32% [8–11]. Due to mucosal "field cancerization", OSCC patients carry a higher risk of developing SPTs in their head and neck region [12, 13]. The genetic alterations between the primary lesion and secondary primaries are more complex and reflected in markers such as TP53, microsatellite markers or the D-loop region in mitochondria [14, 15]. However, the concordance rate varies depending on the markers used. Our aim in this study was therefore to determine the clonality of EGFR from the primary tumor, metastatic lesion, recurrence and SPT lesions in OSCCs.

We hypothesized that the number of EGFR gene copy alterations in the primary tumor can predict whether tumors will reoccur or whether patients will be at risk for lymph node metastasis. Current knowledge how tumor cells with EGFR gene copy number alterations in the primary tumor are related to metastases and recurrences in OSCC is limited. More specifically, until now no investigations had been conducted in an oral cavity cancer. Therefore, in our study, the status of EGFR gene copy number was investigated in paired samples from a series of primary OSCC lesions and corresponding lymph node metastases, recurrent tumors and even multiple primary tumors. By clarifying the clonality of the EGFR gene

status in paired tumor specimens, we can determine whether EGFR amplified cells bear the invasive characters in metastasis or recurrence in oral cavity cancer.

Methods

Patients, tissue specimens and clinical diagnosis

This study was approved by the Institutional Review Board of Chang Gung Memorial Hospital. One hundred and seventy oral cancer patients treated at Chang Gung Memorial Hospital, Lin-Kuo, were recruited for participation in this study. All patients gave informed consent for participation and were interviewed uniformly before surgery by a well-trained interviewer. The questionnaire used in the interview sought detailed information on general demographic data, current and past cigarette smoking, alcohol consumption, areca-quid (AQ) chewing, and a history of family disease (Additional file 1). All patients received curative intent surgery as an initial treatment. In the surgeries, the primary tumors were excised with safety margins greater than or equal to 1 cm (for both peripheral and deep margins). The tumor margin tissue was cryosectioned to ensure that the margin was free of tumor. For each patient, clinical histological parameters were scored according to the recommendations for the reporting of specimens containing oral cavity and oropharynx neoplasms by the Association of Directors of Anatomic and Surgical Pathology (ADASP) [16].

Metastatic lymph nodes

For patients who received radical surgeries, neck dissection was performed according to the tumor stage of the patients. Two types of neck dissections were used in our patients: one was a dissection of level I-III lymph nodes (supraomohyoid neck dissection) for nodal negative patients; and the other was a dissection of level I-V lymph nodes (usually a modified radical neck dissection) for nodal positive patients. We selected pathologically proven metastatic lymph nodes from the neck dissection specimens.

Patients with advanced tumor status (T3 or T4), lymph node extracapsular spread, tumor depth ≥ 10 mm or poor differentiation, adjuvant radiotherapy or cisplatin-based concomitant chemoradiotherapy would be given after surgery.

Recurrence and secondary primary lesions

After radical surgeries with or without adjuvant chemoradiotherapy, the patients received regular follow-up visits. For tumors growing nearby the primary tumor, in the neck or distant sites, the lesions were recorded as recurrences. In the head and neck region, the mucosa carries similar risks for developing malignancies. Lesions that were located in different tumor subsites from the primary tumor or a 2 cm distance from the primary lesion in the mucosa were recorded as secondary primary lesions [17]. The secondary lesions could occur simultaneously with the primary lesion (synchronous) or be

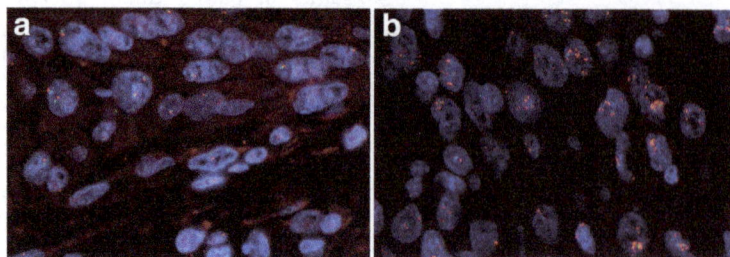

Fig. 1 *EGFR* FISH studies in tumor cells. The fields were observed using a triple band filter (630×). **a** Tumor cells with disomy (*EGFR*, SpectrumOrange, Centromere 7 SpectrumGreen). **b** Tumor with EGFR amplifications

found during regular follow-up appointments in the clinic after surgeries (metachronous).

FISH assay and analysis

EGFR gene copies were investigated with FISH using the LSI *EGFR* SpectrumOrange/CEP 7 SpectrumGreen probe (Vysis; Abbott Laboratories, Downers Grove, IL) according to the manufacturer's instructions and our previous report [7]. In brief, section slides were incubated at 56 °C overnight, deparaffinized, dehydrated, treated with 0.2 N HCl (pH 2.5) for 20 min, and treated with 1 M sodium thiocyanate (Sigma-Aldrich Corp., St. Louis, MO) in 1 M Tris (pH 8.0) at 82 °C for 20 min. Then the specimens were digested with 0.4% pepsin (Sigma-Aldrich Corp., St. Louis, MO) in 0.9% NaCl (pH 2.35) for 15 min. The samples were briefly rinsed in ddH$_2$O and 2 × SSC between steps. After fixation in 4% formaldehyde for 5 min, each slide had the probe set applied to a selected area, and the hybridization area was covered with a plastic coverslip and sealed with a glue gun before the slides were heated at 75 °C for 10 min with OmniGene (Hybaid Ltd., Middlesex, United Kingdom) to promote co-denaturation of chromosomal and probe DNAs. Hybridization was carried out in a humidified oven at 37 °C for 18 h, followed by post-washing in 0.3% Nonidet P40 (BDH, England) in 2 × SSC at 45 °C for 4 min, in 2 × SSC at 45 °C for 5 min, and finally twice in 2 × SSC at room temperature for 5 min. After being counterstained with DAPI for 5 min, the slides were mounted with Vectashield mounting medium (Vector Laboratories, Burlingame, CA) and scored under an fluorescent microscope using a Plan Neofluar 100× objective (Axiophot, Zeiss, Germany) with dual and triple pass filters (Chroma Technology Corp., Rockingham, VT). At least 100 non-overlapping nuclei per case were scored independently by two independent observers who followed strict scoring guidelines and used constant adjustment of the microscope's focus because signals were located in different focal planes. In each nucleus, the number of *EGFR* copies and chromosome 7 probes were assessed independently.

FISH patterns were classified into 3 strata based on the number of copies of the *EGFR* gene per cell as described in previous studies [7, 18, 19]. The strata were normal disomy, ≤ two copies in more than 90% of analyzed cells (Fig. 1a); and low amplification/polysomy (LA/Poly), ≥ three copies in more than 40% of analyzed cells. Gene amplification was defined as the presence of tight *EGFR* gene clusters, a ratio of gene/chromosome per cell ≥2, or ≥15 copies of *EGFR* per cell in ≥ 10% of

Table 1 Characteristics of the 170 oral cavity squamous cell carcinoma patients

Characteristic	[No. of patients (%)]
Age (yrs)	
Mean	49.55
Range	29.0–78.0
Site of primary tumor [No. of patients (%)]	
Tongue	58 (34.1)
Mouth floor	8 (4.7)
Lip	6 (3.5)
Buccal mucosa	67 (39.4)
Alveolar ridge	19 (11.2)
Hard palate	4 (2.4)
Retromolar trigone	8 (4.7)
Pathologic tumor status	
T1	30 (17.6)
T2	58 (34.1)
T3	20 (11.8)
T4	62 (36.5)
Pathologic N stage	
N0	101 (59.4)
N1	19 (11.2)
N2b	45 (26.5)
N2c	5 (2.9)
Pathologic stage	
Stage I	22 (12.9)
Stage II	32 (18.8)
Stage III	24 (14.1)
Stage IV	92 (54.1)

Table 2 EGFR gene amplification in primary cancer with recurrence, multiple primaries, and neck metastasis

EGFR gene copies	EGFR gene copies number			Discordance	P value
	Disomy [n (%)]	Polysomy [n(%)]	Amplification [n (%)]		
Recurrent tumor					
Disomy (n = 31)	24 (77.4)	4 (12.9)	3 (9.7)	14/41 (34.1%)	0.261
Polysomy (n = 5)	5 (100.0)	0 (0.0)	0 (0.0)		0.510*
Amplificaiton (n = 5)	2 (40.0)	2 (40.0)	1 (20.0)		
Second primary tumor					
Disomy (n = 12)	11 (91.7)	1 (8.3)	0 (0.0)	5/17 (29.4%)	0.264
Polysomy (n = 3)	2 (66.7)	1 (33.3)	0 (0.0)		*NA
Amplificaiton (n = 2)	1 (50.0)	1 (50.0)	0 (0.0)		
Lymph node metastasis					
Disomy (n = 34)	25 (73.5)	2 (5.9)	7 (20.6)	18/57 (31.6%)	<0.001
Polysomy (n = 9)	3 (33.3)	4 (44.4)	2 (22.2)		*0.389
Amplificaiton (n = 14)	4 (28.6)	0 (0.0)	10 (71.4)		

*McNemar test

analyzed cells (Fig. 1b). Tumors with LA/Poly or gene amplification were considered to be FISH positive.

Statistical analysis

Statistical analysis was performed using the SPSS statistical package (SPSS, Chicago, IL). Correlations between the frequency of EGFR FISH status and age, TNM stage, cigarette smoking, alcohol consumption, and AQ chewing were examined with the χ^2 test or Fisher's exact test. The concordance of EGFR gene copy alterations between primary tumors, metastatic lesions, recurrences and SPTs was analyzed with the McNemar test. Disease-free survival (DFS) was defined as the time from diagnosis to recurrence or metastasis. Overall survival (OS) was defined as the time from diagnosis to death. Survival curves were constructed using the Kaplan-Meier method, and the curves were compared using the log-rank test. A two-sided value of $p < 0.05$ was considered to be statistically significant.

Results

Patient characteristics

The clinicopathological features of the 170 OSCC male patients between Mar 1997 and Jul 2004 who took part in this study are listed in Table 1. The major primary sites were the bucca (39.4%, 67/170) and the tongue (34.1%, 58/170). Overall, 90.6% (154/170) of the patients were cigarette smokers, 68.2% (116/170) were alcohol drinkers and 91.2% (155/170) were AQ chewers. All 170 patients received surgery as their initial treatment, and 88 (51.8%) and 30 (17.6%) patients underwent additional radiation therapy and chemoradiotherapy, respectively. The median follow-up was 57.50 months.

Of 170 primary OSCCs, FISH results showed EGFR LA/polysomy in 19 (11.4%) patients and amplification in 33 (19.8%) patients. EGFR gene amplification was related to lymph node metastasis ($\chi2$ trend test: $p = 0.018$). Of 57 metastatic lymph nodes, nine (15.8%) had EGFR polysomy and 14 (24.6%) had EGFR gene amplification.

In our patients, 69 had lymph node metastasis identified in neck dissection specimens and 57 positive lymph nodes from neck dissection specimens were available for FISH assays. Fourteen patients had gene copy number amplification (24.6%, 14/57) and nine (15.8%, 9/57) patients had EGFR gene polysomy. During follow-up, 87 patients had recurrence and 41 recurrence tissues were used for analyzing the EGFR gene copy number. Five (12.2%, 5/41) had EGFR gene amplification and five (12.2%, 5/41) had increased gene copy number (LA/

Table 3 Summary for EGFR gene copy number alterations in multiple primary OSCC patients

	Case	Primary cancer site	EGFR gene copy number	Second cancer site	EGFR gene copy number	Third cancer site	EGFR gene copy number
1	OR147	Left alveolus	Polysomy	Right tongue	Trisomy with Focal amplification	Left tongue	Polysomy
2	OR218	Left alveolus	Disomy	Recurrence	Trisomy or polysomy	2nd recurrence	Polysomy
3	OR276	Left bucca	Disomy	Right hard palate	Disomy	Right alveolus	Polysomy
4	OR295	Right tongue	Disomy	Left tongue	Disomy	Hard palate (3rd primary)	Disomy
5	OR325	Right mouth floor	Disomy	Soft palatal	Disomy	Recur from 2nd primary	Disomy

Table 4 The associations between EGFR gene copies and clinicopathological parameters in recurrent tumor ($N = 41$)

	EGFR Gene Copies Number			
	Disomy [N (%)]	Polysomy [N (%)]	Amplification [N (%)]	p value
Subsites				
Local ($n = 31$)	22 (71.0)	4 (80.0)	5 (100.0)	0.643
Regional ($n = 3$)	2 (6.5)	1 (20.0)	0 (0.0)	
Distant metastasis ($n = 7$)	7 (22.5)	0 (0.0)	0 (0.0)	
Tumor status				
T null[a] ($n = 10$)	9 (29.0)	1 (20.0)	0 (0.0)	0.644
Early[b] ($n = 30$)	21 (67.7)	4 (80.0)	5 (100.0)	
Advanced[c] ($n = 1$)	1 (3.2)	0 (0.0)	0 (0.0)	
Lymph node metastasis				
Yes ($n = 12$)	10 (32.3)	2 (40.0)	0 (0.0)	0.289
No ($n = 29$)	21 (67.7)	3 (60.0)	5 (100.0)	
Radiation therapy				
Yes ($n = 29$)	22 (71.0)	4 (80.0)	3 (60.0)	0.936
No ($n = 12$)	9 (29.0)	1 (20.0)	2 (40.0)	
Chemotherapy				
Yes ($n = 7$)	7 (22.6)	0 (0.0)	0 (0.0)	0.256
No ($n = 34$)	24 (77.4)	5 (100.0)	5 (100.0)	

[a]no primary tumor recurrence, but with either lymph node or distant metastasis
[b]Early: T1/T2 lesions
[c]Advanced: T3/T4 lesions

polysomy). Twenty-six patients had secondary primary tumors. A total of 17 secondary primary lesions were suitable for FISH analysis. The results showed that two (11.8%, 2/17) had gene amplification and three (17.6%, 3/17) had an increase in gene copy number. The concordance rate of EGFR gene copy number in primary tumors and lymph node metastasis was 68.4% (McNemar test: $p = 0.389$). The concordance rate between primary tumors and recurrence tumors was 65.9% (McNemar test: $p = 0.510$), and the concordance rate between primary tumors and SPTs was 70.6% (Table 2).

In four patients with multiple primary cancers, the concordance rate of EGFR gene copy number was 100% (Table 3). In one patient (No. 2) with multiple recurrences, the EGFR copy number increased in the recurring tumor. The EGFR gene polysomy was maintained in the second recurrence.

Prognostic implications of EGFR gene copy number in metastatic lymph nodes and tumor recurrence

As shown in Table 4, *EGFR* gene amplification was significantly more prevalent in tumors at an advanced stage

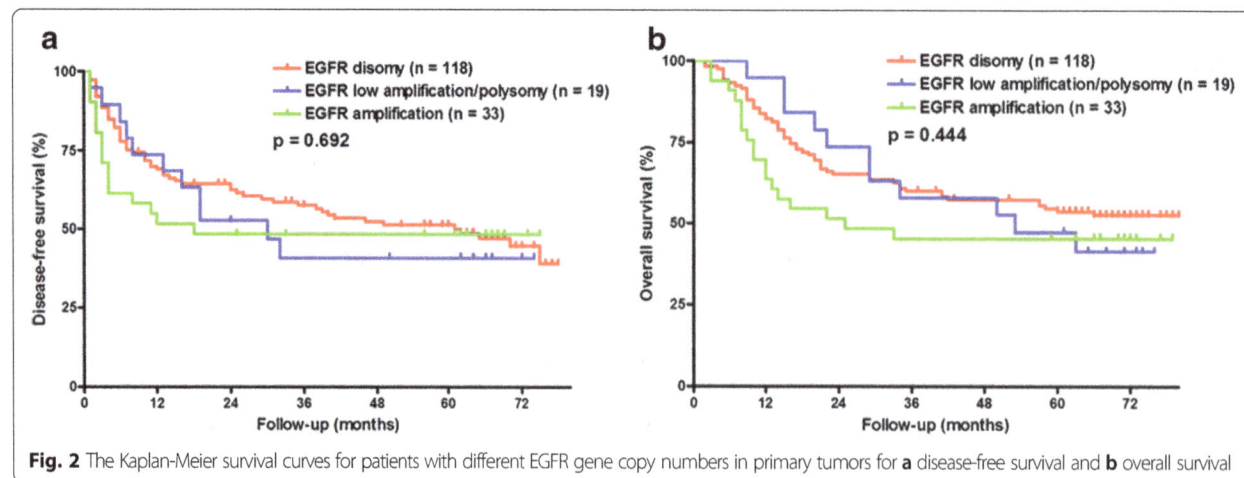

Fig. 2 The Kaplan-Meier survival curves for patients with different EGFR gene copy numbers in primary tumors for **a** disease-free survival and **b** overall survival

than tumors at early stages. Younger patients had a higher risk of EGFR gene amplification. Tumors with high levels of tumor invasion, lymph node metastasis, bone invasion and perineural invasion had a significantly higher frequency of *EGFR* gene amplification than tumors without those characteristics. However, *EGFR* gene amplification was not associated with subsites, skin invasion, AQ chewing, cigarette smoking, and alcohol consumption. We analyzed other factors that may predict EGFR gene amplification in metastatic lymph node and found no clinicopathological factors related to amplification.

The Kaplan-Meier survival curves for patients with different EGFR gene copy numbers are shown in Fig. 2. Patients showing an EGFR FISH pattern were not significantly associated with either DFS or OS (Fig. 2a, $p = 0.692$ and Fig. 2b, $p = 0.444$). The EGFR gene amplification in metastatic lymph nodes was not associated with patient survival (DFS and OS, Fig. 3a, $p = 0.872$, and Fig. 3b, $p = 0.618$, respectively). Furthermore, the EGFR FISH pattern in recurrence tumors did not predict patient survival from recurrence to death (Fig. 4, $p = 0.868$).

Discussion

For loco-regional advanced head and neck squamous cell carcinoma, concomitant radiotherapy with anti-EGFR target therapy such as Cetuximab (C225, Erbitux™) has been shown to improve locoregional control and reduce mortality [20]. A significant improvement in OS/DFS and response rate were also observed in the EX-TREME clinical trial [21]. In non-small cell lung cancer (NSCLC), several reports have also shown that EGFR-specific tyrosine kinase inhibitors, such as gefitinib and erlotinib, are capable of reducing brain and adrenal metastases [22, 23]. EGFR mutations, amplifications or gene gains have been associated with clinical responses to those inhibitors [18, 24]. A previous study demonstrated

that *EGFR* FISH analysis may be used as an alternative to gene mutation analysis as the primary laboratory test [25]. Additionally, in our previous study, the EGFR mutation rate in areca-quid-related OSCC was as low as 0.58% [26]. Gene amplification is one of the important mechanisms that influence EGFR proteins expression. We sought to better understand the clonal change of *EGFR gene* between primary tumors, metastatic lesions and recurrence tumors in OSCC.

The tumors examined in our experiments were heterogeneous and polyclonal. Park et al. demonstrated that *EGFR* mutations are not always identical in disseminated cancer cells and cells from the primary tumors in NSCLC [27]. The differences could originate from intratumoral molecular heterogeneity or the consequences of genetic instability during metastatic spread of tumor cells. In our study, we hypothesized that tumor cells with EGFR amplification were prone to recur or metastasize. Our EGFR copy number comparison analyzed primary and metastatic lesions in OSCC, and we found the concordance rate was approximately 60%. In the literature, studies on clonal changes between primary tumors and metastatic lesions in EGFR in OSCC were few and most related studies focused on lung cancer. Matsumoto et al. reported a 100% concordance for EGFR mutation status in six NSCLC patients of Asian ethnicity [28]. In a study by Kalikaki et al., the authors demonstrated significant discordance between EGFR and K-RAS mutations occurring in primary tumors and the corresponding metastases in patients with NSCLC [29]. The discordance in EGFR mutation status was 28% and the discordance for K-RAS was 24%. Similarly, two other studies of paired NSCLC tumors showed discordance rates of 32 and 27% for the EGFR gene copy number [8, 10]. The concordance rate of EGFR copy number in

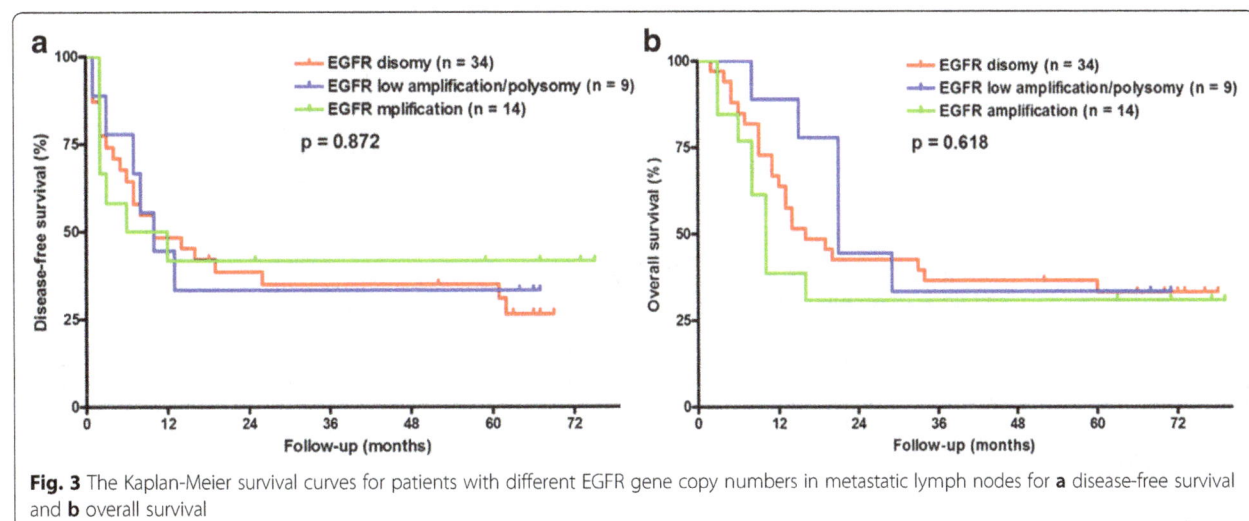

Fig. 3 The Kaplan-Meier survival curves for patients with different EGFR gene copy numbers in metastatic lymph nodes for **a** disease-free survival and **b** overall survival

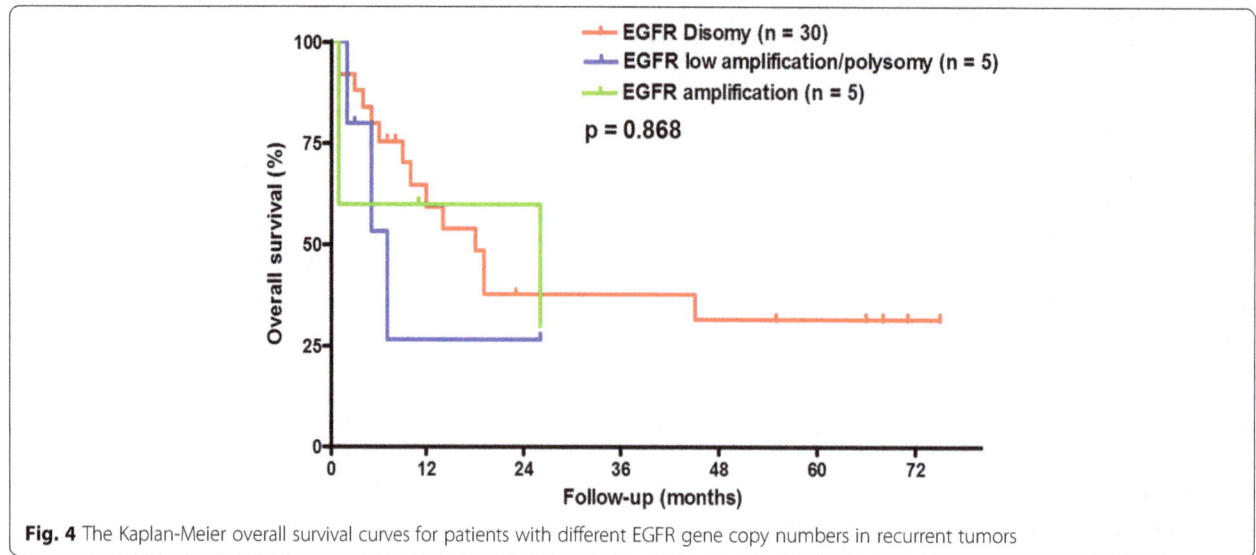

Fig. 4 The Kaplan-Meier overall survival curves for patients with different EGFR gene copy numbers in recurrent tumors

metastatic lymph nodes or recurrent OSCC from our study were within the range of concordance rates for lung cancer.

In a meta-analysis by Wang and Wang, primary NSCLC had a lower EGFR copy number rate (29.3%, 39/133) than corresponding metastases (39.8%, 53/133), but there was no significant difference [30]. In our study, the EGFR copy number in metastatic lymph node samples was higher (40.35%) than samples from primary tumors (30.59%). Although the result was statistically insignificant, tumor cells with EGFR gene amplification carried a higher propensity for lymph node metastasis. In OSCC, an increased EGFR copy number was identified in 24.39% of recurrent tumors and 29.41% of SPTs. We intended to identify the factors that would lead to a higher risk of EGFR gene amplification in patients. In Table 4, no clinical factors, such as primary tumor stage, lymph node metastasis, radiation therapy or chemotherapy, were related to increased EGFR gene copy number. To minimize the heterogeneity of our study population, none had received neo-adjuvant chemotherapy, neoadjuvant bio-chemotherapy or adjuvant bio-CCRT. Adjuvant chemo-radiotherapy for locoregional advanced OSCCs consists of cisplatin-based regimen in our patients. In the patients with tumor recurrence, 70.73% had previous radiation therapy after primary surgery and 17.07% received adjuvant chemotherapy concomitantly with radiation therapy. Interestingly, none of the recurrences had EGFR amplification if the patients had chemotherapy included in the initial treatment of OSCC. The tumor clones of increased EGFR copy number could potentially have been eliminated during the process of recurrence.

Conclusions

In OSCC, the concordance rates between primary tumors and metastatic lymph nodes, recurrence tumors or SPTs were 65.9, 68.4 and 70.6%, respectively. We could predict two-thirds of the EGFR gene copy number alterations for the lymph node metastasis group or the recurrence tumor group from analysis of the primary tumor. For OSCC patients, in whom the lymph nodes or recurrence tumors were unavailable for EGFR gene copy number analysis, studies of the primary tumor could provide part of the EGFR clonal information to predict metastatic or recurrent lesions.

Abbreviations
AQ: Areca-quid; DFS: Disease-free survival; FISH: Fluorescence in situ hybridization; LA/Poly: Low amplification/polysomy; NSCLC: Non-small cell lung cancer; OS: Overall survival; OSCC: Oral squamous cell carcinoma; SPT: Secondary primary tumor

Acknowledgements
The authors thank all the members of the Cancer Center and the Tissue Bank at Chang Gung Memorial Hospital, Linkou, for their invaluable assistance.

Funding
This study was supported by grants CMRPG3F0671, CMRPG3F2221 and CMRPB53 from Chang Gung Memorial Hospital in the writing of the manuscript and publication fee, and grants MOST 103–2314-B-182A-057-MY2 and MOST106–2314-B-182-025-MY3 from the National Science Council, Executive Yuan, Taiwan, ROC, in the design of the study, experiments, analysis and interpretation of data.

Authors' contributions
SFH and HTC conceived the idea for the manuscript, conducted a literature search, and drafted the manuscript. SFH, WYC, CTL and HMW organized the manuscript and critically revised the manuscript. SFH, SDC, WYC, CTL and HMW collected the data. HTC, SDC, WYC and SFH analyzed the data. HTC plotted the figures. SFH, HTC, SDC, WYC, CTL and HMW have given final approval of the version to be published.

Competing interest
The authors declare that they have no competing interests.

Author details

[1]Department of Otolaryngology, Head and Neck Surgery, Chang Gung Memorial Hospital, No. 5 Fu-Shin Street, Kwei-Shan, Taoyuan, Taiwan. [2]Department of Public Health, Chang Gung University, Tao-Yuan, Taiwan. [3]Taipei CGMH Head and Neck Oncology Group, Tao-Yuan, Taiwan. [4]Department of Nutrition and Health Sciences, Chang Gung University of Science and Technology, Tao-Yuan, Taiwan. [5]Department of Anatomy, Chang Gung University, Tao-Yuan, Taiwan. [6]Department of Pathology, Chang Gung Memorial Hospital, Tao-Yuan, Taiwan. [7]Division of Hematology/Oncology, Department of Internal Medicine, Chang Gung Memorial Hospital, Tao-Yuan, Taiwan.

References

1. Yarbrough WG, Shores C, Witsell DL, Weissler MC, Fidler ME, Gilmer TM. Ras mutations and expression in head and neck squamous cell carcinomas. Laryngoscope. 1994;104(11 Pt 1):1337–47.
2. Ciardiello F, Caputo R, Bianco R, Damiano V, Pomatico G, De Placido S, Bianco AR, Tortora G. Antitumor effect and potentiation of cytotoxic drugs activity in human cancer cells by ZD-1839 (Iressa), an epidermal growth factor receptor-selective tyrosine kinase inhibitor. Clin Cancer Res. 2000;6(5):2053–63.
3. Liao CT, Wang HM, Ng SH, Yen TC, Lee LY, Hsueh C, Wei FC, Chen IH, Kang CJ, Huang SF, et al. Good tumor control and survivals of squamous cell carcinoma of buccal mucosa treated with radical surgery with or without neck dissection in Taiwan. Oral Oncol. 2006;42(8):800–9.
4. O'Brien CJ, Traynor SJ, McNeil E, McMahon JD, Chaplin JM. The use of clinical criteria alone in the management of the clinically negative neck among patients with squamous cell carcinoma of the oral cavity and oropharynx. Arch Otolaryngol Head Neck Surg. 2000;126(3):360–5.
5. Woolgar JA, Scott J. Prediction of cervical lymph node metastasis in squamous cell carcinoma of the tongue/floor of mouth. Head Neck. 1995;17(6):463–72.
6. Spiro RH, Guillamondegui O Jr, Paulino AF, Huvos AG. Pattern of invasion and margin assessment in patients with oral tongue cancer. Head Neck. 1999;21(5):408–13.
7. Huang SF, Cheng SD, Chien HT, Liao CT, Chen IH, Wang HM, Chuang WY, Wang CY, Hsieh LL. Relationship between epidermal growth factor receptor gene copy number and protein expression in oral cavity squamous cell carcinoma. Oral Oncol. 2012;48(1):67–72.
8. Bozzetti C, Tiseo M, Lagrasta C, Nizzoli R, Guazzi A, Leonardi F, Gasparro D, Spiritelli E, Rusca M, Carbognani P, et al. Comparison between epidermal growth factor receptor (EGFR) gene expression in primary non-small cell lung cancer (NSCLC) and in fine-needle aspirates from distant metastatic sites. J Thorac Oncol. 2008;3(1):18–22.
9. Daniele L, Cassoni P, Bacillo E, Cappia S, Righi L, Volante M, Tondat F, Inghirami G, Sapino A, Scagliotti GV, et al. Epidermal growth factor receptor gene in primary tumor and metastatic sites from non-small cell lung cancer. J Thorac Oncol. 2009;4(6):684–8.
10. Italiano A, Vandenbos FB, Otto J, Mouroux J, Fontaine D, Marcy PY, Cardot N, Thyss A, Pedeutour F. Comparison of the epidermal growth factor receptor gene and protein in primary non-small-cell-lung cancer and metastatic sites: implications for treatment with EGFR-inhibitors. Ann Oncol. 2006;17(6):981–5.
11. Monaco SE, Nikiforova MN, Cieply K, Teot LA, Khalbuss WE, Dacic S. A comparison of EGFR and KRAS status in primary lung carcinoma and matched metastases. Hum Pathol. 2010;41(1):94–102.
12. Liao CT, Wallace CG, Lee LY, Hsueh C, Lin CY, Fan KH, Wang HM, Ng SH, Lin CH, Tsao CK, et al. Clinical evidence of field cancerization in patients with oral cavity cancer in a betel quid chewing area. Oral Oncol. 2014;50(8):721–31.
13. Slaughter DP, Southwick HW, Smejkal W. Field cancerization in oral stratified squamous epithelium; clinical implications of multicentric origin. Cancer. 1953;6(5):963–8.
14. Foschini MP, Morandi L, Marchetti C, Cocchi R, Eusebi LH, Farnedi A, Badiali G, Gissi DB, Pennesi MG, Montebugnoli L. Cancerization of cutaneous flap reconstruction for oral squamous cell carcinoma: report of three cases studied with the mtDNA D-loop sequence analysis. Histopathology. 2011;58(3):361 7.
15. Tabor MP, Brakenhoff RH, Ruijter-Schippers HJ, Kummer JA, Leemans CR, Braakhuis BJ. Genetically altered fields as origin of locally recurrent head and neck cancer: a retrospective study. Clin Cancer Res. 2004;10(11):3607–13.
16. Association of Directors of A, Surgical P. Recommendations for the reporting of specimens containing oral cavity and oropharynx neoplasms. ModPathol. 2000;13(9):1038–41.
17. Hong WK, Lippman SM, Itri LM, Karp DD, Lee JS, Byers RM, Schantz SP, Kramer AM, Lotan R, Peters LJ, et al. Prevention of second primary tumors with isotretinoin in squamous-cell carcinoma of the head and neck. N Engl J Med. 1990;323(12):795–801.
18. Hirsch FR, Varella-Garcia M, McCoy J, West H, Xavier AC, Gumerlock P, Bunn PA Jr, Franklin WA, Crowley J, Gandara DR. Increased epidermal growth factor receptor gene copy number detected by fluorescence in situ hybridization associates with increased sensitivity to gefitinib in patients with bronchioloalveolar carcinoma subtypes: a southwest oncology group study. J ClinOncol. 2005;23(28):6838–45.
19. Cappuzzo F, Hirsch FR, Rossi E, Bartolini S, Ceresoli GL, Bemis L, Haney J, Witta S, Danenberg K, Domenichini I, et al. Epidermal growth factor receptor gene and protein and gefitinib sensitivity in non-small-cell lung cancer. J NatlCancer Inst. 2005;97(9):643–55.
20. Bonner JA, Harari PM, Giralt J, Azarnia N, Shin DM, Cohen RB, Jones CU, Sur R, Raben D, Jassem J, et al. Radiotherapy plus cetuximab for squamous-cell carcinoma of the head and neck. N Engl J Med. 2006;354(6):567–78.
21. Rivera F, Garcia-Castano A, Vega N, Vega-Villegas ME, Gutierrez-Sanz L. Cetuximab in metastatic or recurrent head and neck cancer: the EXTREME trial. Expert Rev Anticancer Ther. 2009;9(10):1421–8.
22. Chiu CH, Tsai CM, Chen YM, Chiang SC, Liou JL, Perng RP. Gefitinib is active in patients with brain metastases from non-small cell lung cancer and response is related to skin toxicity. Lung Cancer. 2005;47(1):129–38.
23. Fekrazad MH, Ravindranathan M, Jones DV Jr. Response of intracranial metastases to erlotinib therapy. J Clin Oncol. 2007;25(31):5024–6.
24. Yeh KH, Yeh SH, Wan JP, Shen YC, Cheng AL. Somatic mutations in epidermal growth factor receptor underlying complete responsiveness to gefitinib in a Taiwanese female patient with metastatic adenocarcinoma of lung. Anti-Cancer Drugs. 2005;16(7):739–42.
25. Daniele L, Macri L, Schena M, Dongiovanni D, Bonello L, Armando E, Ciuffreda L, Bertetto O, Bussolati G, Sapino A. Predicting gefitinib responsiveness in lung cancer by fluorescence in situ hybridization/chromogenic in situ hybridization analysis of EGFR and HER2 in biopsy and cytology specimens. Mol Cancer Ther. 2007;6(4):1223–9.
26. Huang SF, Chuang WY, Chen IH, Liao CT, Wang HM, Hsieh LL. EGFR protein overexpression and mutation in areca quid-associated oral cavity squamous cell carcinoma in Taiwan. Head Neck. 2009;31(8):1068–77.
27. Park S, Holmes-Tisch AJ, Cho EY, Shim YM, Kim J, Kim HS, Lee J, Park YH, Ahn JS, Park K, et al. Discordance of molecular biomarkers associated with epidermal growth factor receptor pathway between primary tumors and lymph node metastasis in non-small cell lung cancer. J Thorac Oncol. 2009;4(7):809–15.
28. Matsumoto S, Takahashi K, Iwakawa R, Matsuno Y, Nakanishi Y, Kohno T, Shimizu E, Yokota J. Frequent EGFR mutations in brain metastases of lung adenocarcinoma. Int J Cancer. 2006;119(6):1491–4.
29. Kalikaki A, Koutsopoulos A, Trypaki M, Souglakos J, Stathopoulos E, Georgoulias V, Mavroudis D, Voutsina A. Comparison of EGFR and K-RAS gene status between primary tumours and corresponding metastases in NSCLC. Br J Cancer. 2008;99(6):923–9.
30. Wang S, Wang Z. Meta-analysis of epidermal growth factor receptor and KRAS gene status between primary and corresponding metastatic tumours of non-small cell lung cancer. Clin Oncol (R Coll Radiol). 2015;27(1):30–9.

3

Prognostic significance of tumor infiltrating immune cells in oral squamous cell carcinoma

Juan Fang[1†], Xiaoxu Li[1†], Da Ma[1], Xiangqi Liu[1], Yichen Chen[1], Yun Wang[1], Vivian Wai Yan Lui[2], Juan Xia[1], Bin Cheng[1*] and Zhi Wang[1*]

Abstract

Background: Prognostic factors aid in the stratification and treatment of cancer. This study evaluated prognostic importance of tumor infiltrating immune cell in patients with oral squamous cell carcinoma.

Methods: Profiles of infiltrating immune cells and clinicopathological data were available for 78 OSCC patients with a median follow-up of 48 months. The infiltrating intensity of CD8, CD4, T-bet, CD68 and CD57 positive cells were assessed by immunohistochemistry. Chi-square test was used to compare immune markers expression and clinicopathological parameters. Univariate and multivariate COX proportional hazard models were used to assess the prognostic discriminator power of immune cells. The predictive potential of immune cells for survival of OSCC patients was determined using ROC and AUC.

Results: The mean value of CD8, CD4, T-bet, CD68 and CD57 expression were 28.99, 62.06, 8.97, 21.25 and 15.75 cells per high-power field respectively. The patient cohort was separated into low and high expression groups by the mean value. Higher CD8 expression was associated with no regional lymph node metastasis ($p = 0.033$). Patients with more abundant stroma CD57$^+$ cells showed no metastasis into regional lymph node ($p = 0.005$), and early clinical stage ($p = 0.016$). The univariate COX regression analyses showed that no lymph node involvement ($p < 0.001$), early clinical stage (TNM staging I/II vs III/IV, $p = 0.007$), higher CD8 and CD57 expression ($p < 0.001$) were all positively correlated with longer overall survival. Multivariate COX regression analysis showed that no lymph node involvement ($p = 0.008$), higher CD8 ($p = 0.03$) and CD57 ($p < 0.001$) expression could be independent prognostic indicators of better survival. None of CD4, T-bet or CD68 was associated with survival in ether univariate or multivariate analysis. ROC and AUC showed that the predictive accuracy of CD8 and CD57 were all superior compared with TNM staging. CD57 (AUC = 0.868; 95% CI, 0.785–0.950) and CD8 (AUC = 0.784; 95% CI, 0.680–0.889) both provided high predictive accuracy, of which, CD57 was the best predictor.

Conclusion: Tumor stroma CD57 and CD8 expression was associated with lymphnode status and independently predicts survival of OSCC patients. Our results suggest an active immune microenvironment in OSCC that may be targetable by immune drugs.

Keywords: Tumor infiltrating immune cell, Oral squamous cell carcinoma (OSCC), Prognosis, Overall survival (OS)

---

* Correspondence: chengbin@mail.sysu.edu.cn; wangzh75@mail.sysu.edu.cn
†Equal contributors
[1]Guangdong Provincial Key Laboratory of Stomatology, Guanghua School of Stomatology, Sun Yat-Sen University, No. 56, Lingyuanwest Road, Guangzhou, Guangdong 510055, China
Full list of author information is available at the end of the article

Background

Oral squamous cell carcinoma (OSCC) is a major cause of morbidity and mortality in patients with head and neck cancer. Even with multi-modality treatment, only modest improvement of patient survival has been reported. To date, the prognosis of OSCC patients remains unsatisfactory, as indicated by the poor 5-year survival rate of less than 20% in advanced patients [1–3]. Such a poor survival in OSCC patients indicates not only the aggressiveness of this cancer, but also insufficient understanding of the disease, which hinders the development of effective treatments. Our recent understanding of the involvement of immune components in disease progression, prognostic or treatment stratification in other cancers revealed the significance of immuno-characterization of human malignancies [4, 5], which is lacking in OSCC. Our current TNM staging system for OSCC is informative for prognosis, however, it is likely that additional immuno-characterization of OSCC tumors in situ may further facilitate treatment stratification, especially for the new arrays of immune drugs for cancer [1].

Tumor infiltrating immune cells have been shown to provide prognostic values in several human malignancies [6–10]. For adaptive immune cells, CD8$^+$ cytotoxic lymphocytes (CTLs) were generally considered as the main force against cancer. Both intra- and peri-tumoral CD8 expression have been shown to predict better survival in colorectal and esophageal cancers [11–13]. CD4$^+$ cells consist of several subpopulations and its benefit was controversial [14–17]. Among these subpopulations, Th1 is considered as a critical component of tumor surveillance. T-bet is commonly used as a specific marker of Th1 cells, its expression have been shown significantly associated with survival of patients with breast or gastric cancer [18, 19]. As the important components of innate immunity, functions of macrophages and natural killer (NK) cells in tumor microenvironment draw much attention in recent decades [20–22]. CD68 has been widely used as a pan-macrophage marker, its expression was reported associated with poor prognosis in breast cancer and hepatocellular cancer [23, 24]. CD57 expression is most prominent in highly mature cytotoxic NK cells and terminally differentiated effector T-cells such as CTLs and Th cells [25]. NK cells were important effectors of both innate and adaptive immune response, their killing capacity against tumor cells enhances in absence of MHC class I molecules. Tumour CD57 expression has been reported independently predicting survival in patients with colorectal cancer, gastric cancer and prostate cancer [26–28].

Yet, the precise role of immune cells in OSCC remained poorly defined and controversial, though primary OSCC tumors are known to be heavily infiltrated with lymphocytes [29]. Thus, in this study several representative immune subsets (CD8, CD4, T-bet, CD68 and CD57) in a cohort of surgically treated OSCC patients were determined. To keep the consistency and reproducibility, the methodology recommended by an international breast cancer TILs Working Group was tested [30]. This study will provide new strategies to select the most promising immune markers for clinic trials through an integrative scope.

Methods

Study population

Our study randomly enrolled 78 OSCC patients who underwent curative operations at the Department of Oral-Maxillofacial Surgery, Stomatology Hospital Affiliated to Sun Yat-sen University, China, between 2007 and 2009. TNM staging was determined according to the Union for International Cancer Control 2002 standard (UICC2002). Pathological examination was performed by two independent pathologists according to the 2005 revised World Health Organization classification of OSCC tumors. Ethical approval was obtained from the Ethical Review Committee of Guanghua School of Stomatology, Sun Yat-sen University, China. Written informed consents had been obtained from all patients. The data were analyzed anonymously.

Immunohistochemistry

Paraffin-embedded specimens were cut into 4 μm thick sections. The slides were dewaxed by heating at 60 °C for 60 min followed by deparaffinizationin xylene and rehydration in graded alcohol. The slides were then put in Citrate Buffer solution (pH 6.0) and microwaved for 10 min at low power for antigen retrieval. Deparaffinized sections were stained with the following antibodies: CD8 1:150 (Abcam ab17147), CD4 1:250 (Abcam ab846), T-bet 1:100 (Abcam ab91109), CD68 1:100 (Dako M0814), CD57 1:150 (Abcam ab82749), Isotype Control (Abcam ab91353). The slides were then incubated in 3% H_2O_2 for 20 min for removal of endogenous peroxidase activity and subsequently incubated with secondary antibody (DAB) at 37 °C for 30 min. The tissue sections were immersed in a solution of 3, 3′-diaminobenzidine tetrahydrochloride (Dako, Hamburg, Germany) and then counterstained with hematoxylin.

Microscopic evaluation of tumor sections

By use of a standard light microscope, images were acquired with a CCD-camera using a 20× objective, transferred to a PC and semi-automatically evaluated using the image analysis software COUNT (Biomas, Erlangen, Germany). Cases were scored blindly with respect to patient history, presentation, and previous scoring by two independent observers. In case of discrepancy, a final decision was made upon further re-examination of the slides in a microscope based on consensus by both pathologists.

Immune cells were identified by their specific markers (CD8, CD4, T-bet, CD68 and CD57). For each section, 10 areas of a representative field of tumor were assessed using an ocular grid comprising a high-power field (HPF) area of 0.0314 mm^2. Tumor areas were divided into three anatomic compartments (i.e. tumor epithelial, tumor stroma and advancing tumor margin). The total number of each type of immune cells in tumor stroma, excluding cells within tumour cell nests, was counted. The average number of 10 HPFs was calculated as the final density of each section (cells per hpf).

Follow up

Phone interviews and physical examinations of each patient were carried out once every 6 months. Patients were followed till the closing date of the study or death, whichever reached first. Overall survival (OS) was determined based on the date of diagnosis until the date of death or the end of study. All patients were followed for more than two years, the median follow-up time was 48 months (ranged from 29 to 93 months).

Statistical analysis

All statistical analyses were performed using SPSS 16.0 software (SPSS, Chicago, IL, USA) and Stata/MP 14.0 software (Stata Corp, College Station, TX). Mean number of each type of immune cells was used as the cut off value separating patients into low and high infiltrated groups. Chi-square test was used to compare immune markers expression and clinicopathologic parameters. Overall survival (OS) was evaluated using the Kaplan–Meier method and the differences between survival curves were tested for statistical significance using the log-rank test. The Cox proportional hazards model was used to estimate the independent prognostic factors for OS. Receiver Operating Characteristic (ROC) and area under curve (AUC) were used to evaluate and compare the prognostic value of immune cells. All tests were two-sided and $p < 0.05$ was considered statistically significant.

Results

Patients outcome

The retrospectively registered cohort of 78 patients with OSCC who underwent a primary resection of tumor was investigated. Basic information and clinicopathological variables are summarized in Table 1. The average age of the patients was 60 years (range 24–82). The median follow up duration was 48 months (Inter-quartile range, 29–93 months). The panel consisted of about equal numbers of Stage I/II ($n = 36$, 46.15%) and Stage III/IV ($n = 42$, 53.85%) tumors. 48 (61.54%) patients were with lymphnode metastasis.

The distribution of CD8$^+$, CD4$^+$, T-bet$^+$, CD68$^+$ and CD57$^+$ cells in OSCC tissues

Positively stained immune cells demonstrated brown granules on the membrane. The majority of immune cells were located in stroma compartment around cancer

Table 1 Clinicopathological characteristics of OSCC patients

Factors		Number (range)	Percentage (%)
Age	Mean (range)	60 (24–82)	
Gender	Male	57	73.08
	Female	21	26.92
Smoking	Yes	47	60.26
	No	31	39.74
Drinking	Yes	42	53.85
	No	36	46.15
Differentiation	Well	57	73.08
	Moderate or poor	21	26.92
T stage	T1 and T2	58	74.36
	T3 and T4	20	25.64
N stage	N0	48	61.54
	N1-N3	30	38.46
Clinical stage	I and II	36	46.15
	III and IV	42	53.85

nests. Only a few were detected in the center of nests. The mean number of each cell type was shown in Table 2. CD8, CD4, T-bet, CD68 and CD57 expression in low and high infiltrated groups was shown in Fig. 1.

Relationships between clinicopathological features and density of immune cells

The relationships between clinicopathological features and density of immune cells were shown in Table 3. In the whole series, CD57 expression was associated with features of better prognosis including no lymphnode metastasis ($p = 0.005$), and early clinical stages (I/II vs III/IV, $p = 0.016$). Higher CD8 expression was significantly correlated with no lymphnode status ($p = 0.033$) and no drinking history ($p = 0.014$). T-bet was more abundant for patients older than 60 years ($p = 0.046$). CD4 and CD68 expression were not associated with any of the clinicopathological features in our OSCC cohort.

Assessment of survival by COX regression analysis
Univariate COX regression analyses and Kaplan-Meier survival curves

To determine the predictive value of immune cells infiltration, we performed the COX regression analysis. The results of the univariate COX regression analyses were summarized in Table 4.

Table 2 Mean numbers of immune cell in tumor stroma for 78 OSCC samples

	CD8	CD4	T-bet	CD68	CD57
Mean (SD) cells/hpf	28.99 (12.67)	62.06 (21.33)	8.97 (3.99)	21.25 (6.01)	15.75 (9.41)
Range	8–65	9–104	0–18	7–32	3–62

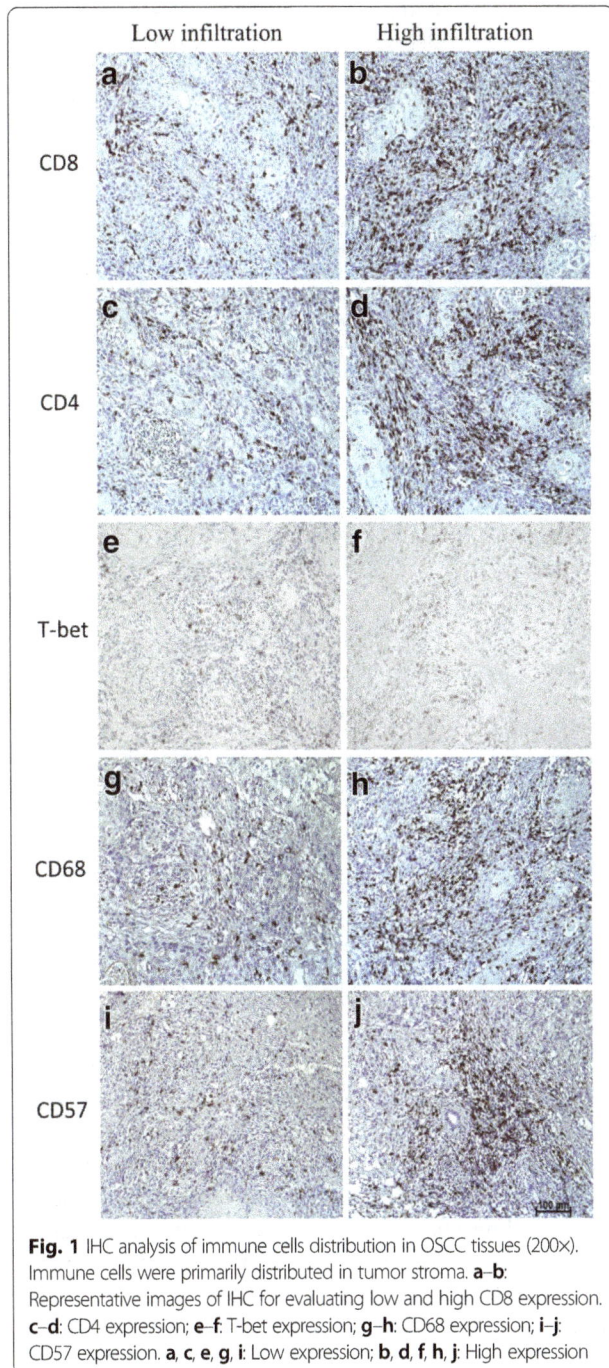

Fig. 1 IHC analysis of immune cells distribution in OSCC tissues (200×). Immune cells were primarily distributed in tumor stroma. **a–b**: Representative images of IHC for evaluating low and high CD8 expression. **c–d**: CD4 expression; **e–f**: T-bet expression; **g–h**: CD68 expression; **i–j**: CD57 expression. **a, c, e, g, i**: Low expression; **b, d, f, h, j**: High expression

Univariate analyses in all patients confirmed that both late clinical stage ($p = 0.007$) and lymph node metastasis ($p < 0.001$) were associated with a shorter survival. High CD8 and CD57 expression were significantly associated with longer survival ($p < 0.001$) in our cohort.

Figure 2a–c shows the Kaplan–Meier survival curves based on N stages and infiltration level (high and low defined by the average number) of CD8$^+$ and CD57$^+$ cells. Patients with lymphnode metastasis showed shorter survival compared with those without lymphnode involvement. The

average OS of patients with different levels of immune cells were: 21.38 months in low and 43.68 months in high CD8 expression group; 22.14 months in low and 46.2 months in high CD57 expression group. Comparison of the Kaplan–Meier curves for OS indicated that higher CD8 and CD57 expression were associated with better patient survival. CD4, T-bet and CD68 levels did not show any correlation with patient outcome.

We determined whether CD8 and CD57 could discriminate patient outcome at different N stages. Patients were stratified according to N stage (N0 and N1–3). As Fig. 2d and e showed, a strong stroma CD8 and CD57 expression correlated with favorable prognosis regardless of invasion of regional lymph nodes ($p < 0.01$).

Multivariate COX regression analysis.

The results of multivariate COX regression analysis confirmed that lymph node involvement ($p = 0.008$), CD8 expression ($p = 0.03$) and CD57 expression ($p < 0.001$) were significantly correlated with OS (Table 5). CD8 and CD57 expression can be considered as independent prognostic factors in OSCC patients. Clinical stage was not statistically significant in multivariate analysis.

Predictive accuracy for OS

To determine the predictive accuracy of immune cells on OS, we performed ROC curve analyses. As shown in Fig. 3 and Table 6, the respective predictive accuracy of CD8 and CD57 expression were all superior to TNM staging in determining patient outcome. CD57 provided the highest predictive accuracy (AUC = 0.868; 95% CI, 0.785–0.950).

Discussion

A comprehensive detection and assessment of factors influencing prognosis is important for improving patient management of OSCC. This study performed on various immune parameters in OSCC patients has shown that infiltration levels of immune cells were important predictive factors for patient outcome. Particularly, among these, stroma CD8 and CD57 expression were found to be the most powerful prognostic indicators.

We found that patients with strong CD8 expression had a significantly better clinical outcome. CD8$^+$ cell is a crucial component of cell-mediated immunity as it produces interferon-γ upon interaction with tumour targets. In agreement to our findings, strong tumour infiltration by CD8$^+$ cells has been correlated with a favorable outcome in several tumor types [31–36], including head and neck cancer [14–17, 37]. Former study on colorectal cancer with a large cohort has shown that infiltrating CD8$^+$ T cells had a prognostic value that superior to and independent of those of TNM classification [38]. In our study, CD8 expression was significantly higher in patients with

Table 3 Relationships between clinicopathological parameters of OSCC and densities of tumor infiltrating immune cells

Factors	CD8			CD4			T-bet			CD68			CD57		
	Low	High	P-Value	Low	High	P-Value	Low	High	P-Value	Low	High	P-Value	Low	High	P-Value
Age															
< 60	18	17	0.981	17	18	0.821	21	14	0.046*	21	14	0.238	23	12	0.137
≥ 60	22	21		22	21		16	27		20	23		21	22	
Gender															
Male	31	27	0.517	29	29	1	28	30	0.802	30	28	0.802	32	26	0.709
Female	9	11		10	10		9	11		11	9		12	8	
Smoking															
Yes	27	21	0.27	25	23	0.644	23	25	0.915	24	24	0.569	28	20	0.667
No	13	17		14	16		14	16		17	13		16	14	
Drinking															
Yes	27	15	0.014*	23	19	0.367	21	21	0.626	24	18	0.385	26	16	0.294
No	13	23		16	20		16	20		17	19		18	18	
Differentiation															
Well	26	31	0.101	31	26	0.205	27	30	0.984	28	29	0.319	32	25	0.937
Moderate or Poor	14	7		8	13		10	11		13	8		12	9	
T stage															
T1 and T2	29	29	0.702	29	29	1	26	32	0.435	28	30	0.199	30	28	0.158
T3 and T4	11	9		10	10		11	9		13	7		14	6	
N stage															
N0	20	28	0.033*	23	25	0.644	22	26	0.722	24	24	0.569	21	27	0.005*
N1-N3	20	10		16	14		15	15		17	13		23	7	
Clinical stage															
I and II	16	20	0.266	18	18	1	15	21	0.348	16	20	0.186	15	21	0.016*
III and IV	24	18		21	21		22	20		25	17		29	13	

P values showing statistically significance were indicated by

Table 4 Univariate COX regression analysis of overall survival

Factors	SE	P	Exp (β)	95.0% CI	
Gender	0.328	0.677	1.147	0.603	2.181
Age	0.293	0.555	0.841	0.473	1.494
Smoking	0.297	0.451	0.799	0.446	1.431
Drinking	0.299	0.277	1.384	0.771	2.485
T stage	0.319	0.301	1.391	0.744	2.600
N stage	0.313	<0.001*	3.784	2.048	6.989
Differentiation	0.315	0.307	1.379	0.744	2.557
Clinical stage	0.304	0.007*	2.264	1.248	4.109
CD8	0.329	<0.001*	3.808	1.998	7.256
CD4	0.299	0.207	0.686	0.382	1.232
T-bet	0.294	0.639	0.871	0.489	1.551
CD68	0.296	0.293	0.733	0.411	1.308
CD57	0.383	<0.001*	7.718	3.646	16.338

P values showing statistically significance were indicated by

no lymph node involvements, when stratified patients according to N stages, CD8 expression was still correlated with favorable prognosis regardless of N stages, which revealed the superior prognostic value of CD8 expression.

Detailed analysis of CD57[+] inflammatory cell activity in the host immune systems and head and neck cancer development has not been well defined. Function of tumor infiltrated CD57[+]cells remain unclear. Former studies have shown that CD57 was not an independent factor associated with survival [39, 40]. A more recent study included 57 cases of OSCC indicated that high level of CD57[+] cells correlated with longer OS in OSCC patients and CD57 expression could be considered as a powerful indicator of OS [41]. This result was accordant with our study. In the present study, high CD57 expression was significantly associated with early clinical stage and no lymph node metastasis. A strong CD57 expression was found to be an independent prognostic factor for longer survival, moreover, it represented better predictive value compared with other immune cells, including CD4 and CD8 positive cells, and TNM staging. As researchers have reported

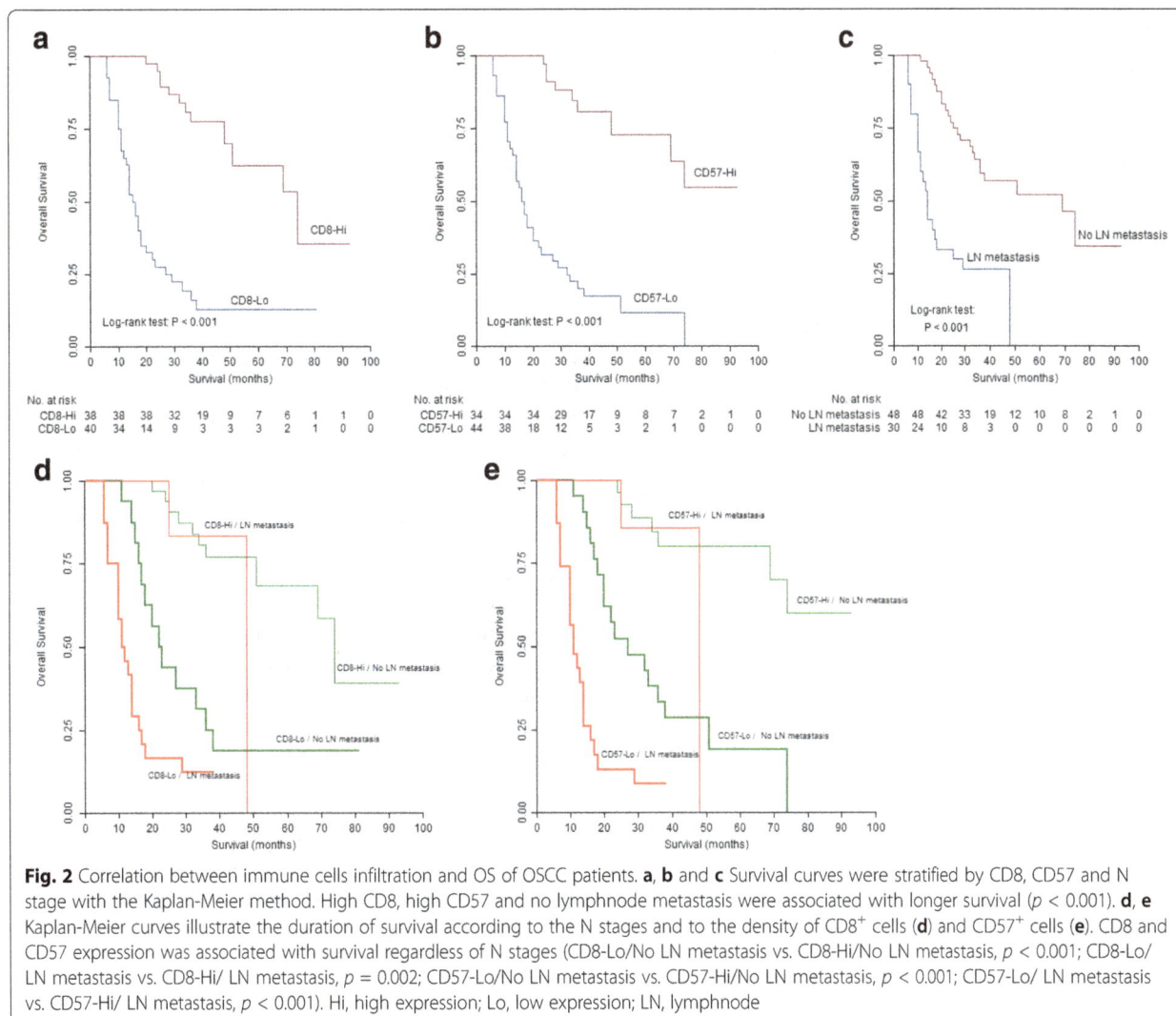

Fig. 2 Correlation between immune cells infiltration and OS of OSCC patients. **a**, **b** and **c** Survival curves were stratified by CD8, CD57 and N stage with the Kaplan-Meier method. High CD8, high CD57 and no lymphnode metastasis were associated with longer survival ($p < 0.001$). **d**, **e** Kaplan-Meier curves illustrate the duration of survival according to the N stages and to the density of $CD8^+$ cells (**d**) and $CD57^+$ cells (**e**). CD8 and CD57 expression was associated with survival regardless of N stages (CD8-Lo/No LN metastasis vs. CD8-Hi/No LN metastasis, $p < 0.001$; CD8-Lo/ LN metastasis vs. CD8-Hi/ LN metastasis, $p = 0.002$; CD57-Lo/No LN metastasis vs. CD57-Hi/No LN metastasis, $p < 0.001$; CD57-Lo/ LN metastasis vs. CD57-Hi/ LN metastasis, $p < 0.001$). Hi, high expression; Lo, low expression; LN, lymphnode

positive correlation between presence of $CD57^+$ T cells and cancer progression [25], our results indicated the potential important role of $CD57^+$ NK cells in anti-tumor immunity against OSCC, which remained to be further confirmed by co-staining for CD3.

$CD4^+$ cells serve a variety of biological functions according to their subpopulations. Th1 assist cytotoxic function of $CD8^+$ cells, while Th2, Th17 and regulatory T cells (Tregs) could negatively regulate the adaptive immunity. T-bet plays critical roles in the differentiation of Th1 and regulates the Th1/Th2 shift. In OSCC, the role of CD4 remains controversial as mixed findings have been reported. Balermpas P et al. found no correlation between CD4 expression and clinical outcome of patients with head and neck cancer [15], whereas Nguyen N et al. reported that higher CD4 levels predicted improved OS and disease-specific survival [17]. T-bet has been shown to be associated with better outcome in patients with renal cell cancer, breast cancer, gastric cancer and colorectal cancer

[19, 42–45]. We did not observe any correlation for either CD4 or T-bet expression and clinical outcome in our series. As $CD4^+$ cells consist of various subpopulations, each of them could affect tumor behavior. The clinical significance according to each phenotype remains to be established.

Another important component of innate immunity, macrophages, is functionally differentiated into pro-inflammatory "M1" and alternative anti-inflammatory "M2" phenotypes. M1 type, commonly identified by staining the CD11c antigen, was conferred a significantly better prognosis. M2 type, expressing CD163 and MRC1, promoted tumor growth, invasion, angiogenesis, and metastasis [46]. Generally speaking, CD68 is the best established marker of tumor associated macrophages (TAMs), it is expressed on both M1 and M2 phenotypes. Ni YH et al. found that $CD68^+$ TAMs infiltration in tumor stroma was correlated with high tumor grade and lymph node metastasis. More TAMs was correlated with short OS, but TAMs was not an independent predictive factor [46]. Our study showed that

Table 5 Multivariate COX regression analyses of 78 OSCC patients

Factors		SE	P	Exp (β)	95% CI	
T stage	T1/T2			Reference		
	T3/T4	0.487	0.529	1.359	0.523	3.530
N stage	N0			Reference		
	N1–N3	0.602	0.008*	4.969	1.527	16.168
Clinical stage	I and II			Reference		
	III and IV	0.667	0.282	0.488	0.132	1.804
CD8	Low	0.358	0.030*	2.174	1.078	4.384
	High			Reference		
CD4	Low	0.328	0.909	1.038	0.545	1.977
	High			Reference		
T-bet	Low	0.310	0.836	1.066	0.580	1.959
	High			Reference		
CD68	Low	0.316	0.177	1.533	0.825	2.848
	High			Reference		
CD57	Low	0.441	<0.001*	6.576	2.768	15.623
	High			Reference		

*indicated P values with statistically significance

CD68 expression was not significantly associated with OSCC patient survival in both univariate and multivariate analysis, which was consistent with a more recent study including larger cohort of 278 patients by Nguyen N et al. [17] This result indicated the counterweight of M1 and M2 in tumor microenvironment of OSCC. Further study is required to differentiate M1 and M2 to determine their respective functions in OSCC.

In this study, special attention was paid for evaluating immune infiltrates. Regarding localization of the stained markers, stroma and tumor periphery not tumor nest were evaluated, because most current studies have shown that stroma immune cells were superior and more reproducible [47, 48]. We used full section over core biopsy (such as in the settings of tissue microarrays) because up till now, there was no published evidence that Tissue Microarrays (TMAs) can mirror or reflect the potential heterogeneity of immune cells in tumor, and the number and diameter of cores in TMAs vary, which will likely affect the accuracy needed for the determination of various immune components [30]. Regarding the scoring system, a quantitative parameter of cells count per HPF was applied. Machine scoring approaches, while promising, have not been published or validated yet, which needs to be explored in future studies.

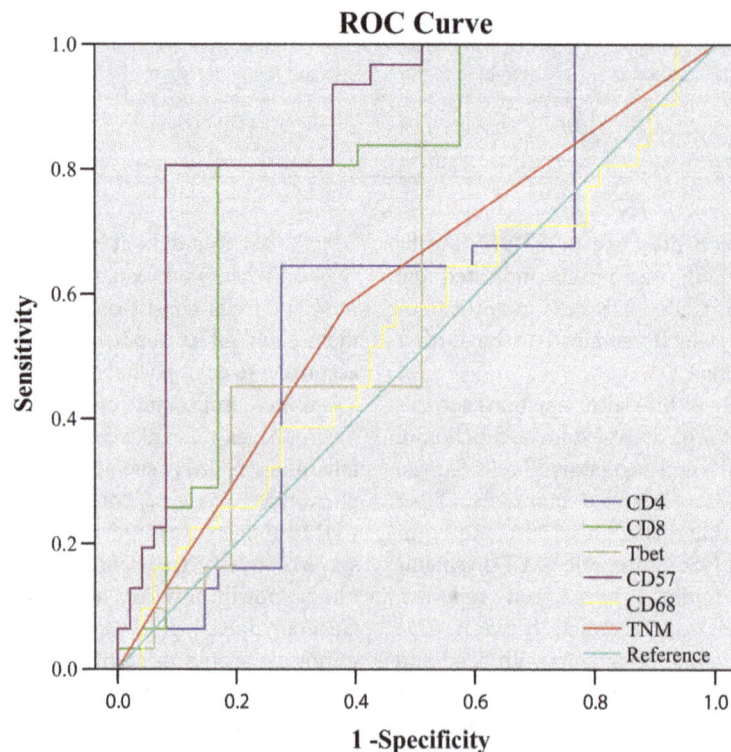

Fig. 3 ROC curves indicating predictive accuracy, sensitivity and specificity of each potential parameter. AUCs of CD8 and CD57 were 0.784 (95% CI 0.680–0.889) and 0.868 (95% CI 0.785–0.950) respectively, significantly higher than TNM staging (AUC 0.599, 95% CI 0.469–0.728)

Table 6 Summary of the OS predictive accuracy of immune cells

Predictive factors	AUC	SE	P	95% CI	
TNM	0.599	0.066	0.141	0.469	0.728
CD8	0.784	0.053	0.000	0.680	0.889
CD4	0.581	0.067	0.226	0.450	0.713
T-bet	0.651	0.063	0.024	0.528	0.774
CD68	0.533	0.068	0.624	0.399	0.667
CD57	0.868	0.042	0.000	0.785	0.950

SE standard error, *95% CI* 95% confidence interval

There were some limitations in the current study. First was the limited size of our cohort with all patients being Chinese OSCC patients. It remains unclear if Chinese ethnic background is associated with particular immunological features. Second, a critical negatively regulated factor of immune response, Tregs, has not been separately stained. As a subpopulation of CD4$^+$ cells, Tregs might contribute to the final negative results of association between CD4 and survival. Third, as CD68 expression cannot differentiate M1 and M2 subtypes of TAMs, further study should be designed including reliable markers of M1 and M2 TAMs for precise analysis. Fourth, without co-staining for CD3, the specific functions of CD57$^+$ T cell and CD57$^+$ NK cell in OSCC were not illuminated.

Conclusions

In conclusion, our study revealed that stroma CD57 and CD8 expression were independent prognostic markers for OS of OSCC patients. When compared with TNM staging, expression of CD8 and CD57 provided superior predictive function. The results from this small OSCC cohort suggest that tumor infiltrating immune cells can potentially predict patient survival, thus provide new clues to therapeutic strategies in OSCC based on utilizing host immune response.

Abbreviations

AUC: Area under the curve; CTLs: Cytotoxic lymphocytes; HPF: High-power field; NK cells: Natural killer cells; OS: Overall survival; OSCC: Oral squamous cell carcinoma; ROC: Receiver operating characteristic; TAMs: Tumor associated macrophages; TMAs: Tissue microarrays; Tregs: Regulatory T cells

Acknowledgements

Not applicable.

Funding

This project was supported by Nonprofit Industry Research Specific Fund of National Health and Family Planning Commission of China (No. 201502018), the National Natural Science Foundations of China (No. 81472524, 81,630,025, 81,500,864 and 81,602,383), Research Grant Council, Hong Kong (No.17114814, General Research Fund). The funding agency has no role in the actual experimental design, analysis, or writing of this manuscript.

Authors' contributions

JF, XXL, DM, XQL and YCC were involved in patients enrollment, collection of clinicopathological data and tissue samples; JF, XXL, YW and DM were involved in the immunohistochemistry experiments and microscopic evaluation of tumor sections; XXL, YCC, JX and YW were involved in the clinical follow-up of the patients; JF and XQL were involved in statistical analysis; JF, XXL, VL, ZW and BC were involved in the interpretation of the results. XXL, JF, VL, DM, XQL, YCC, YW, JX, ZW and BC were involved in the manuscript drafting or editing. ZW and BC were involved in the conception and design of the study. All authors have read and approved the final manuscript.

Competing interests

The authors declare that they have no competing interests.

Author details

[1]Guangdong Provincial Key Laboratory of Stomatology, Guanghua School of Stomatology, Sun Yat-Sen University, No. 56, Lingyuanwest Road, Guangzhou, Guangdong 510055, China. [2]School of Biomedical Sciences, Faculty of Medicine, The Chinese University of Hong Kong, Hong Kong, SAR, China.

References

1. Winck FV, Prado RAC, Ramos DR, et al. Insights into immune responses in oral cancer through proteomic analysis of saliva and salivary extracellular vesicles. Sci Rep. 2015;5:16305.
2. Carvalho AL, Nishimoto IN, Califano JA, Kowalski LP. Trends in incidence and prognosis for head and neck cancer in the United States: a site-specific analysis of the SEER database. Int J Cancer. 2005;114(5):806–16.
3. van der Waal I. Are we able to reduce the mortality and morbidity of oral cancer; some considerations. Med Oral Patol Oral Cir Bucal. 2013;18(1):e33–7.
4. Ujiie H, Kadota K, Nitadori JI, et al. The tumoral and stromal immune microenvironment in malignant pleural mesothelioma: a comprehensive analysis reveals prognostic immune markers. Oncoimmunology. 2015;4(6): e1009285.
5. Punt S, van Vliet ME, Spaans VM, et al. FoxP3(+) and IL-17(+) cells are correlated with improved prognosis in cervical adenocarcinoma. Cancer Immunol Immunother. 2015;64(6):745–53.
6. Lee AM, Clear AJ, Calaminici M, et al. Number of CD4+ cells and location of forkhead box protein P3-positive cells in diagnostic follicular lymphoma tissue microarrays correlates with outcome. J Clin Oncol. 2006;24(31):5052–9.
7. Englund E, Reitsma B, King BC, et al. The human complement inhibitor sushi domain-containing protein 4 (SUSD4) expression in tumor cells and infiltrating T cells is associated with better prognosis of breast cancer patients. BMC Cancer. 2015;15:737.
8. Chirica M, Le BL, Lehmann-Che J, et al. Phenotypic analysis of T cells infiltrating colon cancers: correlations with oncogenetic status. Oncoimmunology. 2015;4(8):e1016698.
9. Jia Q, Zhou J, Chen G, et al. Diversity index of mucosal resident T lymphocyte repertoire predicts clinical prognosis in gastric cancer. Oncoimmunology. 2015;4(4):e1001230.
10. Zelba H, Weide B, Martens A, Bailur JK, Garbe C, Pawelec G. The prognostic impact of specific CD4 T-cell responses is critically dependent on the target antigen in melanoma. Oncoimmunology. 2015;4(1):e955683.
11. Naito Y, Saito K, Shiiba K, et al. CD8+ T cells infiltrated within cancer cell nests as a prognostic factor in human colorectal cancer. Cancer Res. 1998; 58(16):3491–4.
12. Funada Y, Noguchi T, Kikuchi R, Takeno S, Uchida Y, Gabbert HE. Prognostic significance of CD8+ T cell and macrophage peritumoral infiltration in colorectal cancer. Oncol Rep. 2003;10(2):309–13.
13. Schumacher K, Haensch W, Roefzaad C, Schlag PM. Prognostic significance of activated CD8(+) T cell infiltrations within esophageal carcinomas. Cancer Res. 2001;61(10):3932–6.
14. Watanabe Y, Katou F, Ohtani H, Nakayama T, Yoshie O, Hashimoto K. Tumor-infiltrating lymphocytes, particularly the balance between CD8(+) T cells and CCR4(+) regulatory T cells, affect the survival of patients with oral squamous cell carcinoma. Oral Surg Oral Med Oral Pathol Oral Radiol Endod. 2010;109(5):744–52.

15. Balermpas P, Michel Y, Wagenblast J, et al. Tumour-infiltrating lymphocytes predict response to definitive chemoradiotherapy in head and neck cancer. Br J Cancer. 2014;110(2):501–9.

16. Nordfors C, Grün N, Tertipis N, et al. CD8+ and CD4+ tumour infiltrating lymphocytes in relation to human papillomavirus status and clinical outcome in tonsillar and base of tongue squamous cell carcinoma. Eur J Cancer. 2013;49(11):2522–30.

17. Nguyen N, Bellile E, Thomas D, et al. Tumor infiltrating lymphocytes and survival in patients with head and neck squamous cell carcinoma. Head Neck. 2016;38(7):1074–84.

18. Ladoire S, Arnould L, Mignot G, et al. T-bet expression in intratumoral lymphoid structures after neoadjuvant trastuzumab plus docetaxel for HER2-overexpressing breast carcinoma predicts survival. Br J Cancer. 2011;105(3):366–71.

19. Chen LJ, Zheng X, Shen YP, et al. Higher numbers of T-bet(+) intratumoral lymphoid cells correlate with better survival in gastric cancer. Cancer Immunol Immunother. 2013;62(3):553–61.

20. Lima L, Oliveira D, Tavares A, et al. The predominance of M2-polarized macrophages in the stroma of low-hypoxic bladder tumors is associated with BCG immunotherapy failure. Urol Oncol. 2014;32(4):449–57.

21. Focosi D, Petrini M. CD57 expression on lymphoma microenvironment as a new prognostic marker related to immune dysfunction. J Clin Oncol. 2007; 25(10):1289–91. author reply 1291-2

22. Greaves P, Clear A, Coutinho R, et al. Expression of FOXP3, CD68, and CD20 at diagnosis in the microenvironment of classical Hodgkin lymphoma is predictive of outcome. J Clin Oncol. 2013;31(2):256–62.

23. Medrek C, Pontén F, Jirström K, Leandersson K. The presence of tumor associated macrophages in tumor stroma as a prognostic marker for breast cancer patients. BMC Cancer. 2012;12:306.

24. Zhou J, Ding T, Pan W, Zhu LY, Li L, Zheng L. Increased intratumoral regulatory T cells are related to intratumoral macrophages and poor prognosis in hepatocellular carcinoma patients. Int J Cancer. 2009;125(7):1640–8.

25. Kared H, Martelli S, Ng TP, Pender SL, Larbi A. CD57 in human natural killer cells and T-lymphocytes. Cancer Immunol Immunother. 2016;65(4):441–52.

26. Chaput N, Svrcek M, Auperin A, et al. Tumour-infiltrating CD68+ and CD57+ cells predict patient outcome in stage II-III colorectal cancer. Br J Cancer. 2013;109(4):1013–22.

27. Ishigami S, Natsugoe S, Tokuda K, et al. Prognostic value of intratumoral natural killer cells in gastric carcinoma. Cancer. 2000;88(3):577–83.

28. Wangerin H, Kristiansen G, 0000–0003-4149-5487 AO, et al. CD57 expression in incidental, clinically manifest, and metastatic carcinoma of the prostate. Biomed Res Int. 2014. 2014: 356427.

29. Huang TY, Hsu LP, Wen YH, et al. Predictors of locoregional recurrence in early stage oral cavity cancer with free surgical margins. Oral Oncol. 2010; 46(1):49–55.

30. Salgado R, Denkert C, Demaria S, et al. The evaluation of tumor-infiltrating lymphocytes (TILs) in breast cancer: recommendations by an international TILs working group 2014. Ann Oncol. 2015;26(2):259–71.

31. Matsumoto H, Thike AA, Li H, et al. Increased CD4 and CD8-positive T cell infiltrate signifies good prognosis in a subset of triple-negative breast cancer. Breast Cancer Res Treat. 2016;156(2):237–47.

32. Liu L, Zhao G, Wu W, et al. Low intratumoral regulatory T cells and high peritumoral CD8(+) T cells relate to long-term survival in patients with pancreatic ductal adenocarcinoma after pancreatectomy. Cancer Immunol Immunother. 2016;65(1):73–82.

33. Geng Y, Shao Y, He W, et al. Prognostic role of tumor-infiltrating lymphocytes in lung cancer: a meta-analysis. Cell Physiol Biochem. 2015;37(4):1560–71.

34. Nedergaard BS, Ladekarl M, Thomsen HF, Nyengaard JR, Nielsen K. Low density of CD3+, CD4+ and CD8+ cells is associated with increased risk of relapse in squamous cell cervical cancer. Br J Cancer. 2007;97(8):1135–8.

35. Wang K, Xu J, Zhang T, Xue D. Tumor-infiltrating lymphocytes in breast cancer predict the response to chemotherapy and survival outcome: A meta-analysis. Oncotarget. 2016; DOI: 10.18632/oncotarget. 9988.

36. Mao Y, Qu Q, Chen X, Huang O, Wu J, Shen K. The prognostic value of tumor-infiltrating lymphocytes in breast cancer: a systematic Review and meta-analysis. PLoS One. 2016;11(4):e0152500.

37. Balermpas P, Rödel F, Rödel C, et al. CD8+ tumour-infiltrating lymphocytes in relation to HPV status and clinical outcome in patients with head and neck cancer after postoperative chemoradiotherapy: a multicentre study of the German cancer consortium radiation oncology group (DKTK-ROG). Int J Cancer. 2016;138(1):171–81.

38. Galon J, Costes A, Sanchez-Cabo F, et al. Type, density, and location of immune cells within human colorectal tumors predict clinical outcome. Science (80-). 2006. 313(5795): 1960–4.

39. Zancope E, Costa NL, Junqueira-Kipnis AP, et al. Differential infiltration of CD8+ and NK cells in lip and oral cavity squamous cell carcinoma. J Oral Pathol Med. 2010;39(2):162–7.

40. Fraga CA, de Oliveira MV, Domingos PL, et al. Infiltrating CD57+ inflammatory cells in head and neck squamous cell carcinoma: clinicopathological analysis and prognostic significance. Appl Immunohistochem Mol Morphol. 2012;20(3):285–90.

41. Taghavi N, Bagheri S, Akbarzadeh A. Prognostic implication of CD57, CD16, and TGF-beta expression in oral squamous cell carcinoma. J Oral Pathol Med. 2015;45(1):58–62.

42. Yu H, Yang J, Jiao S, Li Y, Zhang W, Wang J. T-box transcription factor 21 expression in breast cancer and its relationship with prognosis. Int J Clin Exp Pathol. 2014;7(10):6906–13.

43. Tosolini M, Kirilovsky A, Mlecnik B, et al. Clinical impact of different classes of infiltrating T cytotoxic and helper cells (Th1, th2, treg, th17) in patients with colorectal cancer. Cancer Res. 2011;71(4):1263–71.

44. Hennequin A, Derangère V, Boidot R, et al. Tumor infiltration by Tbet+ effector T cells and CD20+ B cells is associated with survival in gastric cancer patients. Oncoimmunology. 2016;5(2):e1054598.

45. Dielmann A, Letsch A, Nonnenmacher A, Miller K, Keilholz U, Busse A. Favorable prognostic influence of T-box transcription factor Eomesodermin in metastatic renal cell cancer patients. Cancer Immunol Immunother. 2016;65(2):181–92.

46. Ni YH, Ding L, Huang XF, Dong YC, Hu QG, Hou YY. Microlocalization of CD68 tumor-associated macrophages in tumor stroma correlated with poor clinical outcomes in oral squamous cell carcinoma patients. Tumour Biol. 2015;36(7):5291–8.

47. Kayser G, Schulte-Uentrop L, Sienel W, et al. Stromal CD4/CD25 positive T-cells are a strong and independent prognostic factor in non-small cell lung cancer patients, especially with adenocarcinomas. Lung Cancer. 2012;76(3):445–51.

48. Goc J, Germain C, Vo-Bourgais TK, et al. Dendritic cells in tumor-associated tertiary lymphoid structures signal a Th1 cytotoxic immune contexture and license the positive prognostic value of infiltrating CD8+ T cells. Cancer Res. 2014;74(3):705–15.

4

Phase I study of oral ridaforolimus in combination with paclitaxel and carboplatin in patients with solid tumor cancers

Hye Sook Chon[1], Sokbom Kang[2], Jae K. Lee[3], Sachin M. Apte[1], Mian M. Shahzad[1], Irene Williams-Elson[4] and Robert M. Wenham[1]*

Abstract

Background: Ridaforolimus is a mammalian target of rapamycin inhibitor that has activity in solid tumors. Paclitaxel and carboplatin have broad antineoplastic activity in many cancers. This phase I trial was conducted to determine the safety profile, maximal tolerated dose, and recommended phase II dose and schedule of oral ridaforolimus combined with paclitaxel and carboplatin in patients with solid tumor cancers.

Methods: Eligible patients with advanced solid tumor cancers received oral 10 to 30 mg ridaforolimus daily for 5 consecutive days per week combined with intravenous paclitaxel (175 mg/m^2) and carboplatin (area under the curve [AUC] 5–6 mg/mL/min) in 3-week cycles. A standard 3 + 3 design was used to escalate doses, with predefined changes to an alternate dosing schedule and/or changes in carboplatin AUC doses based on dose-limiting toxicity (DLT). Secondary information was collected regarding response and time to progression. Patients were continued on treatment if therapy was tolerated and if stable disease or better was demonstrated.

Results: Thirty-one patients were consented, 28 patients were screened, and 24 patients met eligibility requirements and received treatment. Two patients were replaced for events unrelated to drug-related toxicity, resulting in 22 DLT-evaluable patients. Two grade 4 DLTs due to neutropenia were observed at dose level 1. The next cohort was changed to a predefined alternate dosing schedule (days 1–5 and 8–12). DLTs were neutropenia, sepsis, mucositis, and thrombocytopenia. The most common adverse events were neutropenia, anemia, thrombocytopenia, fatigue, alopecia, nausea, pain, and leukopenia. Twenty-four patients received a median of 4 cycles (range, 1–12). Evaluable patients for response (*n* = 18) demonstrated a median tumor measurement decrease of 25%. The best response in these 18 patients included 9 patients with partial response (50%), 6 with stable disease (33%), and 3 with progressive disease (17%). Thirteen of these patients received treatment for 4 or more cycles.

Conclusions: Treatment with ridaforolimus combined with paclitaxel and carboplatin had no unanticipated toxicities and showed antineoplastic activity. The recommended phase II dose and schedule is ridaforolimus 30 mg (days 1–5 and 8–12) plus day 1 paclitaxel (175 mg/m^2) and carboplatin (AUC 5 mg/mL/min) on a 21-day cycle.

Keywords: Oral ridaforolimus, Phase 1 trial, Paclitaxel and carboplatin combination, Solid tumors

* Correspondence: Robert.Wenham@moffitt.org
[1]Department of Gynecologic Oncology, H. Lee Moffitt Cancer Center and Research Institute, 12902 Magnolia Drive, Tampa, FL 33647, USA
Full list of author information is available at the end of the article

Background

Because mammalian target of rapamycin (mTOR) inhibitors target the downstream effects of the PI3K/AKT/PTEN-related pathways, this class of drugs has broad antiproliferative activity [1]. Ridaforolimus (deforolimus; AP23573; MK 8669, AP 23573), a potent mTOR inhibitor with an IC_{50} in the nanomolar range, appears to be well tolerated in both intravenous and oral formulations as either a single agent or in combination with other chemotherapy agents [2]. In preclinical studies, ridaforolimus demonstrated antitumor activity against a broad range of human cancer cell lines in vitro and tumor xenograft models in vivo [3–6]. In phase I and II clinical trials, ridaforolimus displayed activity in various cancers, including sarcoma and hematologic malignancies [7–10]. In a phase III trial of patients with advanced sarcoma, single-agent ridaforolimus treatment (40 mg orally, once daily for 5 consecutive days every week) resulted in a statistically significant improvement in progression-free survival compared with placebo [11]. Ridaforolimus has shown additive or synergistic activity when combined with other single agents, such as paclitaxel, carboplatin, cisplatin, doxorubicin, imatinib, and trastuzumab [12, 13]. Therefore, combining chemotherapy regimens with an mTOR inhibitor with a different mechanism of action and reasonable toxicity may provide an advantageous clinical approach.

The combination of paclitaxel and carboplatin is one of the most commonly used chemotherapeutic combinations in cancer treatment, including head and neck cancer, advanced-stage non-small cell lung cancer, endometrial cancer, ovarian cancer, and others. Oral ridaforolimus has shown equivalent effectiveness comparable to the intravenous form [14]. Therefore, the potential benefit of a convenient oral dosing with paclitaxel plus carboplatin warranted investigation. In this phase I study, our aim was to determine the maximal tolerated dose (MTD) and the recommended phase 2 dose and schedule of oral ridaforolimus in combination with paclitaxel and carboplatin in patients with solid tumor cancers and to describe the safety and tolerability of this combination.

Methods

Study eligibility

Patients ≥18 years of age with solid tumor cancers not deemed curable by other therapies and who had measurable disease by Response Evaluation Criteria in Solid Tumor (RECIST) 1.1 or evaluable disease were eligible. Other eligibility criteria included Eastern Cooperative Oncology Group performance status of 0, 1, or 2; a life expectancy of at least 60 days; adequate bone marrow function, renal function, hepatic function, and neurologic function; serum cholesterol ≤350 mg/dL and triglyceride ≤400 mg/dL; and full recovery to baseline from

acute toxicities of all prior chemotherapy regimens. Patients may have had up to 3 (0–3) prior cytotoxic chemotherapeutic regimens including prior treatment with carboplatin and paclitaxel (patients who had regimens switched for toxicity rather than progression, used for radiation sensitization only, or hormonal only were not eligible). No chemotherapy, radiotherapy, biologic, hormonal, or investigational drug therapy within 28 days before start of study treatment was permitted. Patients were excluded if they had any upper gastrointestinal illness that would impair swallowing or absorption of oral medication, any intercurrent illness, were known to have human immunodeficiency virus or AIDS, had received prior therapy with an mTOR inhibitor, or had concomitant treatment with inhibitors or inducers of cytochrome P450-3A. The study protocol was approved by the University of South Florida Institutional Review Board. All patients provided written informed consent before study participation.

Study design and treatment

Patients received oral ridaforolimus daily on days 2–5, days 8–12, and days 15–19 during the first cycle of therapy and then 5 days a week (days 1–5, days 8–12, and days 15–19) throughout the remainder of therapy beginning with the second cycle of therapy. Oral ridaforolimus was administered in combination with day 1 intravenous paclitaxel (175 mg/m^2) and carboplatin (AUC = 5–6 mg/mL/min) every 3 weeks, except for the first cycle of therapy where day 1 ridaforolimus was skipped to allow for blood samples to be collected day 1 of the first 2 cycles. These were held for potential PK analyses if specific drug and temporally related toxicities were noted. All patients received steroids, antiemetics, and antihistamines before the administration of paclitaxel and carboplatin. All patients were expected to continue study treatment in the absence of disease progression, complete response, unacceptable toxicity, or voluntary choice to withdraw participation. A 3 + 3 dose escalation design was used, with ridaforolimus dose levels of 10, 20, 30, and 40 mg orally in combination with intravenous paclitaxel and carboplatin based on a predefined dose escalation scheme. Carboplatin was dosed at an AUC of 5, with a planned escalation to an AUC of 6 mg/mL/min based on dose level cohort.

The maximal tolerated dose was defined as the highest dose at which no more than 1 of 6 evaluable patients experienced a dose-limiting toxicity (DLT) due to the combination of ridaforolimus, paclitaxel, and carboplatin during the first cycle of treatment. A patient who did not complete the first cycle of treatment for reasons other than a DLT was replaced. DLT was defined as ≥ grade 3 non-hematologic toxicity (specifically, rash, mucositis, pneumonitis) with the exceptions of fatigue, hypersensitivity reaction, nausea, and vomiting; ≥ grade

3 thrombocytopenia requiring platelet transfusion; grade 4 thrombocytopenia or neutropenia >7 days duration; any grade 4 neutropenic fever requiring hospitalization; unresolved toxicity resulting in delay of retreatment >2 weeks; grade 3 or 4 non-surgical hemorrhages; and failure of administration of ridaforolimus for 5 days or more (consecutive or nonconsecutive) due to any toxicity. Growth factor support was not allowed prophylactically for cycle 1 but could be subsequently used based on investigator discretion.

A modification of the schedule that changed ridaforolimus administration to the first 2 weeks (days 1–5, days 8–12) versus all 3 weeks (days 1–5, days 8–12, days 15–18) of a cycle was predefined for 2 DLTs in a cohort that resulted from thrombocytopenia or neutropenia in the latter part of the cycle. The dose of ridaforolimus remained the same as the maximum achieved level in the prior cohort at which the DLTs were experienced. Dose escalation was to continue at each subsequent cohort until a maximum of 40 mg/day (days 1–5, days 8–12) of ridaforolimus was reached. Subsequent treatment cycles would not begin until absolute neutrophil count reached ≥ 1500 cells/mm^3 and platelet count reached $\geq 75,000$/mm^3; mucositis, nausea, and vomiting were grade 1 or less; and bilirubin was ≤ 1.5 x institutional upper limit of normal. All drugs were held during the recovery period. Therapy was delayed for a maximum of 2 weeks until these values were achieved. Patients who failed to recover adequate counts within a 2-week delay were removed from study. Adverse events were graded according to the Common Terminology Criteria for Adverse Events version 4.0.

Efficacy and safety assessments

Patients were evaluated at baseline and before each subsequent treatment cycle to assess Eastern Cooperative Oncology Group performance status, vital signs, and adverse events. Hematologic and clinical chemistry assessments, including cholesterol, triglyceride, and glucose levels, were performed at baseline and at each treatment cycle. Tumor assessment by RECIST v1.1 was performed at baseline and every 2 cycles thereafter. Patients were required to have completed a minimum of 2 cycles of therapy to be evaluable for efficacy.

Results

Patients and study treatment

Thirty-one patients were consented and 24 patients were enrolled between June 2011 and May 2014. A total of 116 cycles were initiated until January 2015. All patients who received at least one dose of study medication were included in the toxicity analyses (n = 24 patients). Two patients were replaced for DLT evaluation (see below). Patients who completed required imaging after the second

cycle were included for efficacy analyses (n = 18 patients). The mean age was 62 years (range, 30–72 years), and the median number of prior chemotherapy treatments was 2 (range, 0–3). Tumor types included ovarian/fallopian/primary peritoneal (n = 10), endometrial (n = 5), cervical (n = 3), esophageal (n = 2), and urethral, vaginal, mesothelial, and salivary (n = 1 for each). Number of cycles delivered to patients ranged from 1 to 12 (median of 5 cycles; n = 22 patients evaluable for DLT). Patient characteristics are summarized in Table 1.

Safety

The number of patients enrolled and evaluable at each dose level and the DLTs are summarized in Table 2. Two DLTs of grade 4 neutropenia were observed at dose level

Table 1 Patient Characteristics (n = 24)

Characteristics	No. of Patients (%)
Age, years	
Median	62
Range	30–72
Sex	
Male	4 (17)
Female	20 (83)
Race	
White	22 (90)
Black	0
Other	2 (10)
ECOG performance status	
ECOG 0	16 (67)
ECOG 1	7 (29)
ECOG 2	1 (4)
Tumor type	
Ovarian/fallopian/peritoneal	10 (42)
Endometrial	5 (21)
Cervical	3 (13)
Esophageal	2 (8)
Urethral	1 (4)
Vaginal	1 (4)
Mesothelial	1 (4)
Salivary	1 (4)
Prior chemotherapies[a]	
0	7 (29)
1	1 (4)
2	7 (29)
3	9 (38)

ECOG Eastern Cooperative Oncology Group
[a]Therapies that included chemotherapy for radiation sensitization only (n = 4), were discontinued due to toxicity without progression (n = 2), were radiation alone (n = 4), or were hormonal only (n = 2) were not included for eligibility

Table 2 Patients treated and DLTs by dose level

Dose Level	Ridaforolimus mg (days of cycle)	Carboplatin (AUC)	No. of Patients Enrolled	No of Patients evaluable for DLT[a]	Dose-Limiting Toxicity
1	10 (days 1–5, 8–12, 15–19)	5	4	4	Two grade 4 neutropenia
1A	10 (days 1–5, 8–12)	5	6	6	Death from sepsis
2A	20 (days 1–5, 8–12)	5	4[a]	3	None
3A	30 (days 1–5, 8–12)	5	3	3	None
4A	30 (days 1–5, 8–12)	6	7[b]	6	Grade 3 mucositis; grade 4 thrombocytopenia requiring transfusion

Slots replaced due to [a]protocol non-compliance or [b]non-treatment related issue
Paclitaxel was at 175 mg/m^2 for all cohorts

1 (ridaforolimus 10 mg from days 1–5, days 8–12, and days 15–18 combined with 175 mg/m^2 paclitaxel and carboplatin (AUC 5 mg/mL/min)). A predefined alternate dosing cohort (days 1–5, days 8–12) was opened at the same dose of ridaforolimus (dose level 1A). There was one DLT with sepsis at alternate dose level 1A (1 of 6 patients). No DLTs were observed at alternate dose levels 2A (20 mg ridaforolimus) and 3A (30 mg ridaforolimus). Dose escalations were continued to cohort 4A (30 mg ridaforolimus, 175 mg/m^2 paclitaxel, and AUC = 6 mg/mL/min carboplatin). At dose level 4A, 2 of 6 patients had DLTs (1 grade 3 mucositis and 1 grade 4 thrombocytopenia). Thus, the maximal tolerated dose was established as the 3A dose level (30 mg ridaforolimus combined with 175 mg/m^2 paclitaxel and AUC = 5 mg/mL/min carboplatin). Two patients were replaced for DLT determination during cycle 1 (1 patient from cohort 2A for noncompliance and 1 patient from cohort 4A due to *C. difficile* diarrhea and diverticulitis deemed unrelated to treatment). Allowed drug-specific dose reductions after cycle 1 were done in 9 patients after a median of 5 cycles, including for paclitaxel + carboplatin (*n* = 4), paclitaxel only (*n* = 3), and ridaforolimus (*n* = 2).

Treatment-related adverse events observed in >20% of patients are shown in Table 3. The most common adverse events were neutropenia, anemia, thrombocytopenia, fatigue, alopecia, nausea, pain, and leukopenia. The most common grade 3 and grade 4 adverse events were hematologic, including neutropenia (92% of patients: 10 with grade 3 and 12 with grade 4), anemia (42%: 10 with grade 3), thrombocytopenia (67%: 8 with grade 3 and 8 with grade 4), and leukopenia (42%: 8 with grade 3 and 2 with grade 4). Non-hematologic grade 3 and 4 adverse events were infrequent, except hypokalemia (13%; 3 with grade 3 and 1 with grade 4). Of note, two grade 3 hyperglycemia and one grade 3 mucositis were among the less frequent (<10%) high-grade non-hematologic toxicities. One patient with recurrent fallopian tube cancer died. She initiated treatment 7 days before she presented with fever, chills, and abdominal pain. An autopsy showed the cause of death due to multiorgan failure, attributed to sepsis.

With no other obvious cause, this was deemed at least possibly related to treatment. Table 4 demonstrates drug-related toxicities by dose level.

Efficacy

Eighteen of 24 patients were evaluable for antitumor response (5 were not evaluable because of DLTs and 1 patient was replaced due to discontinuation unrelated to treatment). Best response included 9 patients with partial response (50%), 6 with stable disease (33%), and 3 with progressive disease (17%). In 18 patients, 15 (83%) had stable disease or partial response at the time of first tumor assessment. Thirteen patients received 4 or more treatment cycles (range, 1–12). In the 18 patients evaluable for best response, 6 patients came off study before progression of disease was determined by RECIST. Of the remaining 12 patients with RECIST-determined progressive disease, the median duration of response was 81 days (range, 0–236 days) and median time to progression from start of therapy was 166 days (range, 42–393 days). Five patients with partial response or stable disease discontinued treatment due to patient choice; however, these patients were deemed to have no treatment-defined toxicities at the time of discontinuation. One patient remained on treatment for 4 cycles with a partial response but was replaced at cycle 1 as a DLT determination due to noncompliance with drug schedule. The 18 evaluable patients demonstrated a median RECIST 1.1 tumor size decrease of 25% as the best response in target lesion (range, −83% to 232%; Fig. 1). Notably, responses among the 3 cervical and 1 vaginal cancer patients included 1 stable disease and 3 partial responses with a total of 29 cycles (median of 8) delivered. Figure 1 demonstrates best response by RECIST. As shown in Fig. 1, the majority of patients with partial response or stable disease had received prior paclitaxel and carboplatin or carboplatin-based chemotherapy.

Discussion

This phase I study of ridaforolimus combined with paclitaxel and carboplatin demonstrated tolerability at the defined maximal tolerated dose using doses of the 3

Table 3 Number of cycles and patients with treatment-related adverse events in >20% of patients (N = 24 patients)

	Grade (number of cycles)				Patients	
	1	2	3	4	Number	%
Alkaline phosphatase increased	6				5	21%
Dysphagia	2	2	1		5	21%
Dyspnea	5	3	2		5	21%
Hypoalbuminemia	3	1	1		5	21%
Dehydration	3	5	1		7	29%
Fever	8				7	29%
Hypokalemia	11	1	4	2	7	29%
Transaminases increased	11				7	29%
Hypertriglyceridemia	7	1	1		8	33%
Peripheral sensory neuropathy	8	3			8	33%
Vomiting	7	1	4		8	33%
Anorexia	7	4			9	38%
Urinary tract infection	1	6	2		9	38%
Diarrhea	8	6	1		10	42%
Hyperglycemia	18	6	2		10	42%
Hypomagnesemia	23	6			10	42%
Mucositis oral	10	10	2		11	46%
White blood cell decreased	14	14	29	3	12	50%
Nausea	17	4	3		13	54%
Pain	7				13	54%
Alopecia	8	12			14	58%
Fatigue	14	14	1		15	63%
Anemia	21	45	15		20	83%
Platelet count decreased	32	26	14	14	20	83%
Neutrophil count decreased	8	19	26	20	21	88%

Toxicities by grade seen in >20% of patients deemed possibly, probably, or definitely related in all patients eligible for toxicity evaluation. Under grade, this is listed as: Total Number of Cycles. Under Patients, this is listed as the: Total Number of Patients for any grade. There were 24 patients who received at least 1 dose of treatment and were part of the toxicity evaluation. A patient may be counted only once for each grade of toxicity but may appear under more than one grade for each toxicity

agents considered active in patients with solid tumor cancers. Treatment with ridaforolimus showed toxicities that were expected from its known profile. Mouth sores, rash, fatigue, stomatitis, and hypertriglyceridemia have been most prevalent in phase I and II clinical trials with ridaforolimus as a single agent, with incident rates ranging from 31% to 48% [7, 9]. Previous phase I and II studies have explored combinations of ridaforolimus with capecitabine [15], weekly paclitaxel [16], bevacizumab [16, 17], dalotuzumab [18, 19], and traztuzumab [20] and have demonstrated tolerability. Doses of up to 40 mg ridaforolimus once daily as a single agent for 5 consecutive days with 2 days rest each week have been shown to be tolerable in patients with metastatic or advanced solid tumors [14, 20]. When weekly intravenous ridaforolimus was combined with weekly paclitaxel, 2 recommended doses were determined: 37.5 mg ridaforolimus +60 mg/m^2

paclitaxel and 12.5 mg ridaforolimus +80 mg/m^2 paclitaxel [16]. At these recommended doses, a DLT of mucositis was observed, with grade 3/4 neutropenia shown in 14% to 37.5% of the cohorts. In our study, hematologic adverse events were somewhat more prominent, likely because of the nature of combination with two cytotoxic chemotherapies. Non-hematologic adverse events shown in our study were similar to other trials with single-agent ridaforolimus. We had anticipated that the use of these three agents together would have greater potential for bone marrow suppression, namely neutropenia and thrombocytopenia. Therefore, we had preplanned an alternate dosing schedule that shortened the administration of ridaforolimus to 2 weeks (10 days) instead of 3 weeks (15 days). Indeed, the two DLTs of grade 4 neutropenia were observed at the starting dose level of 10 mg ridaforolimus (days 1–5, days 8–12, and days 15–18) combined with paclitaxel (175 mg/

Table 4 Drug-related toxicities by dose level for N = 24 Patients

	Level 1: RIDA 10 mg; P 175 mg/m2; C 5 (n = 4)					Level 1A: RIDA 10 mg; P 175 mg/m2; C 5 (n = 6)					Level 2A: RIDA 20 mg; P 175 mg/m2; C 5 (n = 4)					Level 3A: RIDA 30 mg; P 175 mg/m2; C 5 (n = 3)					Level 4A: RIDA 30 mg; P 175 mg/m2; C 6 (n = 7)				
	Grade				Total No. of Patients	Grade				Total No. of Patients	Grade				Total No. of Patients	Grade				Total No. of Patients	Grade				Total No. of Patients
	1	2	3	4		1	2	3	4		1	2	3	4		1	2	3	4		1	2	3	4	
Alkaline phosphatase increased	2				2	1				1						1				1	1				1
Alopecia		1			1	1	3			4		3			3	2	2			3	2	2			2
Anemia	2	2	3		4	3	4			4	3	4	2		4	1	2			2	3	4	5		6
Anorexia						1	1			2	1				1		2			2	4				4
Dehydration											1				1	1	3			3	1	2	1		3
Diarrhea		1			1	1	1			2	2	1			3						3	1	1		4
Dysphagia							1			1	1				1						1	1	1		3
Dyspnea	1				1			2		2											2	1			2
Fatigue	2	2			2	1	2			3	1	2			2	2	2			3	3	3	1		5
Fever	2				2						1				1	1				1	3				3
Hyperglycemia		1	1		1	2	2			2	2		1		2		1			1	2	2			3
Hypertriglyceridemia		1	1		1	2				2	2				2						3				3
Hypoalbuminemia	1	1			2	2		1		3															
Hypokalemia							1			1	2	1	1	1	2	1				1	2		2		3
Hypomagnesemia		1			1	2				2	2	1			2	1				1	4	2			4
Mucositis oral	1	1			2						2	2			3	2	1			2	3	3	1		4
Nausea	1				1	1				1	1	2	1		3	2	2			3	5	1			5
Neutrophil count decreased	1	1	2	2	4	4	2		4	5		1	3	1	3		2	1	2	3	2	4	4	3	6
Pain	1				1						2				2						3				3
Peripheral sensory neuropathy	1	1			1	3	1			3		1			1	1				1	2				2
Platelet count decreased	1	4			4	3		1	1	3	4	3	2	1	4	1	1	1	2	3	3	4	4	4	6
Transaminases increased											1				1	3				3	1				1
Urinary tract infection		1	1		2												1			1	1	3	1		4
Vomiting	1				1	2				2			1		1	1				1	1	1	1		3
White blood cell decreased						4	2	4		5	1	2	2	1	3				1	1	1	2	2		3

RIDA Ridaforolimus, *P* paclitaxel, *C* carboplatin

m^2) and carboplatin (AUC = 5 mg/mL/min). An alternate dosing cohort (dose level 1A; days 1–5 and days 8–12) was initiated at the same dose of ridaforolimus as the first cohort. This alternate dosing cohort (2 weeks on and 1 week off) was feasible for repeated cycles. This is similar to the results of the weekly paclitaxel study above in that patients had to switch from intravenous ridaforolimus in the latter part of the cycle (days 8 and 15) to earlier in the cycle (days 1 and 8) [16]. It appears that this earlier cycle dosing is sometimes necessary to allow sufficient marrow recovery when combined with cytotoxic chemotherapy.

Ridaforolimus has activity in cancer, particularly in disease stabilization in various tumor types. In a phase III trial of 702 patients with advanced metastatic sarcoma who had attained benefit with prior chemotherapy, administration of oral ridaforolimus as maintenance therapy resulted in a statistically significant improvement of 3.1 weeks in progression-free survival compared with placebo (hazard ratio of 0.72; 95% confidence interval, 0.61–0.85; P = 0.001) [11]. Various mTOR inhibitors, including everolimus (RA001), temsirolimus (CCI779), and ridaforolimus (AP2357), either as a single agent or combined with other chemotherapeutic or hormonal agents have been evaluated in patients with advanced or recurrent endometrial cancer with promising results [21–26]. Mutations or loss of function in PTEN (phosphatase and tensin homolog) plays a significant role in the pathogenesis of endometrial cancer. Downstream activation of the PI3K/AKT/mTOR signaling pathway triggered by the loss of function of PTEN suggests a therapeutic role of the mTOR inhibition. Paclitaxel plus carboplatin is a widely used regimen for this cancer; therefore, it would be of interest to study this combination with ridaforolimus at our recommended phase II

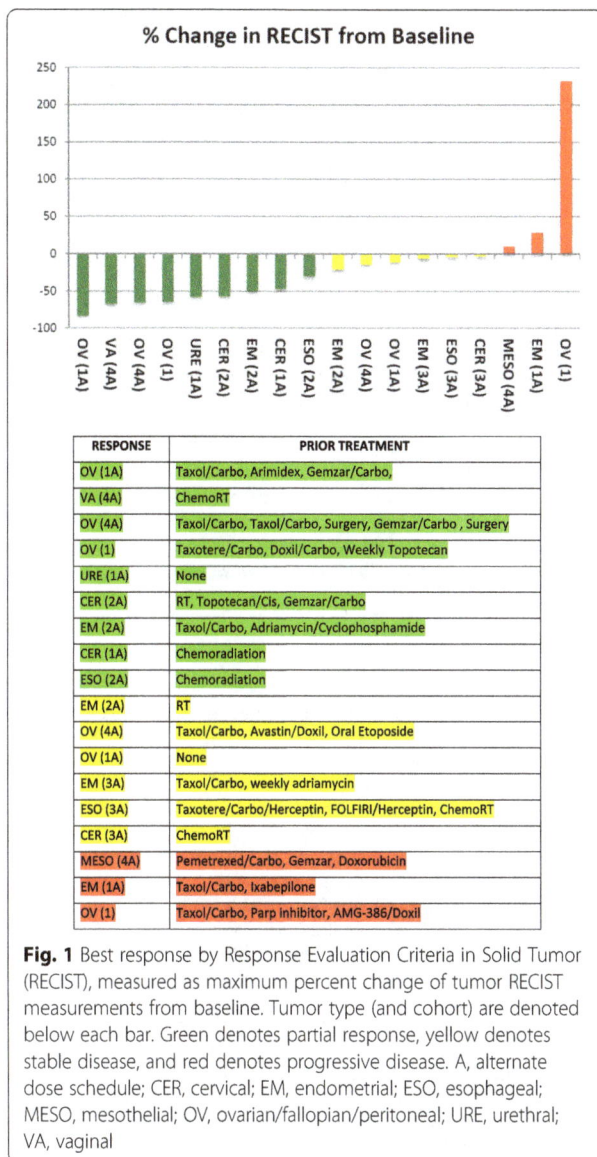

Fig. 1 Best response by Response Evaluation Criteria in Solid Tumor (RECIST), measured as maximum percent change of tumor RECIST measurements from baseline. Tumor type (and cohort) are denoted below each bar. Green denotes partial response, yellow denotes stable disease, and red denotes progressive disease. A, alternate dose schedule; CER, cervical; EM, endometrial; ESO, esophageal; MESO, mesothelial; OV, ovarian/fallopian/peritoneal; URE, urethral; VA, vaginal

33 evaluable patients, 1 patient (3.0%) had a partial response and 19 patients (57.6%) had stable disease with a duration of 6.5 months [28]. There are trials in head and neck squamous cell carcinoma with rapamycin therapy and adding everolimus to definitive chemoradiation treatment in patients with locally advanced cervical cancer. Paclitaxel combined with carboplatin is also a regimen used for the treatment of these cancers; therefore, the addition of ridaforolimus to this combination may be considered for further study, perhaps with or without bevacizumab [29]. In our study, the combination of oral ridaforolimus with intravenous paclitaxel and carboplatin had no unanticipated toxicities with antitumor activity in patients with solid tumor cancers. Given the broad activity and use of paclitaxel and carboplatin in many tumor types, there is potential to explore this triplet therapy in multiple tumors in which mTOR inhibition may be relevant.

Conclusions

Treatment with ridaforolimus in combination with paclitaxel and carboplatin had no unanticipated toxicities and showed antineoplastic activity. The recommended phase II dose and schedule is ridaforolimus 30 mg (days 1–5 and 8–12) plus day 1 paclitaxel (175 mg/m^2) and carboplatin (AUC 5 mg/mL/min) on a 21-day cycle. There is potential to explore triplet therapy with ridaforolimus combined with paclitaxel and carboplatin in multiple tumors where mTOR inhibition is relevant.

Abbreviations
AUC: Area under the curve; DLT: Dose-limiting toxicity; ECOG: Eastern Cooperative Oncology Group; mTOR: Mammalian target of rapamycin; RECIST: Response evaluation criteria in solid tumor

Acknowledgements
We thank Rasa Hamilton (Moffitt Cancer Center) for editorial assistance.

Funding
This work was supported in part by funds from the NCI comprehensive Cancer Center support grant P30-CA076292 and Moffitt Cancer Center. We thank Merck for supplying the study drug.

Authors' contributions
RMW designed and led the study. HSC and RMW were involved in manuscript writing. SK and JKL were involved in data management and trial statistician. IWE provided study management. HSC, SMA, MS and RMW recruited patients and served on the trial management group. All authors participated in reviewing and revising the manuscript, and all agreed to the final version submitted.

Competing interests
Dr. Robert M. Wenham receives trial funding from Merck. Otherwise, the authors have no competing interests.

dose and schedule in this disease. We also noted interesting activity in patients with cervical and vaginal cancer in our study. Among 3 patients with cervical cancer (1 with adenocarcinoma, 1 with squamous cell carcinoma) and 1 patient with vaginal cancer (squamous cell carcinoma), there were a total 29 cycles of treatment with 1 stable disease and 3 partial responses.

In a preclinical study, Molinolo et al. demonstrated that mTOR pathway activation was shown in most human papillomavirus-positive head and neck squamous cell carcinoma and cervical cancer squamous cell carcinoma tumor xenografts. mTOR inhibitors (rapamycin and everolimus) effectively decreased mTOR activity in vivo and caused a remarkable decrease in tumor burden ($P < 0.001$) [27]. In a phase II study of temsirolimus in patients with recurrent or metastatic cervical cancer, among

Author details

[1]Department of Gynecologic Oncology, H. Lee Moffitt Cancer Center and Research Institute, 12902 Magnolia Drive, Tampa, FL 33647, USA. [2]Division of Gynecologic Cancer Research, Center for Uterine Cancer, National Cancer Center, Ilsan-gu Madu-dong, Goyang 410-768, Korea. [3]Department of Biostatistics and Bioinformatics, H. Lee Moffitt Cancer Center and Research Institute, 12902 Magnolia Drive, Tampa, FL 33647 USA. [4]Clinical Trials Office, Phase 1 Clinical trials, H. Lee Moffitt Cancer Center and Research Institute, 12902 Magnolia Drive, Tampa, FL 33647, USA.

References

1. Schmelzle T, Hall MN. TOR, a central controller of cell growth. Cell. 2000; 103(2):253–62.
2. Dancey JE, Monzon J. Ridaforolimus: a promising drug in the treatment of soft-tissue sarcoma and other malignancies. Future Oncol. 2011;7(7):827–39.
3. Shaw RJ, Cantley LC. Ras, PI(3)K and mTOR signalling controls tumour cell growth. Nature. 2006;441(7092):424–30.
4. Fasolo A, Sessa C. mTOR inhibitors in the treatment of cancer. Expert Opin Investig Drugs. 2008;17(11):1717–34.
5. Rivera VM, Squillace RM, Miller D, Berk L, Wardwell SD, Ning Y, et al. Ridaforolimus (AP23573; MK-8669), a potent mTOR inhibitor, has broad antitumor activity and can be optimally administered using intermittent dosing regimens. Mol Cancer Ther. 2011;10(6):1059–71.
6. Squillace RM, Miller D, Cookson M, Wardwell SD, Moran L, Clapham D, et al. Antitumor activity of ridaforolimus and potential cell-cycle determinants of sensitivity in sarcoma and endometrial cancer models. Mol Cancer Ther. 2011;10(10):1959–68.
7. Chawla SP, Staddon AP, Baker LH, Schuetze SM, Tolcher AW, D'Amato GZ, et al. Phase II study of the mammalian target of rapamycin inhibitor ridaforolimus in patients with advanced bone and soft tissue sarcomas. J Clin Oncol. 2012;30(1):78–84.
8. Hartford CM, Desai AA, Janisch L, Karrison T, Rivera VM, Berk L, et al. A phase I trial to determine the safety, tolerability, and maximum tolerated dose of deforolimus in patients with advanced malignancies. Clin Cancer Res. 2009;15(4):1428–34.
9. Mita MM, Mita AC, Chu QS, Rowinsky EK, Fetterly GJ, Goldston M, et al. Phase I trial of the novel mammalian target of rapamycin inhibitor deforolimus (AP23573; MK-8669) administered intravenously daily for 5 days every 2 weeks to patients with advanced malignancies. J Clin Oncol. 2008; 26(3):361–7.
10. Rizzieri DA, Feldman E, Dipersio JF, Gabrail N, Stock W, Strair R, et al. A phase 2 clinical trial of deforolimus (AP23573, MK-8669), a novel mammalian target of rapamycin inhibitor, in patients with relapsed or refractory hematologic malignancies. Clin Cancer Res. 2008;14(9):2756–62.
11. Demetri GD, Chawla SP, Ray-Coquard I, Le Cesne A, Staddon AP, Milhem MM, et al. Results of an international randomized phase III trial of the mammalian target of rapamycin inhibitor ridaforolimus versus placebo to control metastatic sarcomas in patients after benefit from prior chemotherapy. J Clin Oncol. 2013;31(19):2485–92.
12. Mondesire WH, Jian W, Zhang H, Ensor J, Hung MC, Mills GB, et al. Targeting mammalian target of rapamycin synergistically enhances chemotherapy-induced cytotoxicity in breast cancer cells. Clin Cancer Res. 2004;10(20):7031–42.
13. Vignot S, Faivre S, Aguirre D, Raymond E. mTOR-targeted therapy of cancer with rapamycin derivatives. Ann Oncol. 2005;16(4):525–37.
14. Mita MM, Poplin E, Britten CD, Tap WD, Rubin EH, Scott BB, et al. Phase I/IIa trial of the mammalian target of rapamycin inhibitor ridaforolimus (AP23573; MK-8669) administered orally in patients with refractory or advanced malignancies and sarcoma. Ann Oncol. 2013;24(4):1104–11.
15. Perotti A, Locatelli A, Sessa C, Hess D, Vigano L, Capri G, et al. Phase IB study of the mTOR inhibitor ridaforolimus with capecitabine. J Clin Oncol. 2010; 28(30):4554–61.
16. Sessa C, Tosi D, Vigano L, Albanell J, Hess D, Maur M, et al. Phase Ib study of weekly mammalian target of rapamycin inhibitor ridaforolimus (AP23573; MK-8669) with weekly paclitaxel. Ann Oncol. 2010;21:1315–22.
17. Nemunaitis J, Hochster HS, Lustgarten S, Rhodes R, Ebbinghaus S, Turner CD, et al. A phase I trial of oral ridaforolimus (AP23573; MK-8669) in combination with bevacizumab for patients with advanced cancers. Clin Oncol (R Coll Radiol). 2013;25:336–42.
18. Di Cosimo S, Sathyanarayanan S, Bendell JC, Cervantes A, Stein MN, Brana I, et al. Combination of the mTOR Inhibitor Ridaforolimus and the Anti-IGF1R Monoclonal Antibody Dalotuzumab: Preclinical Characterization and Phase I Clinical Trial. Clin Cancer Res. 2015;21(1):49–59.
19. Seiler M, Ray-Coquard I, Melichar B, Yardley DA, Wang RX, Dodion PF, et al. Oral Ridaforolimus Plus Trastuzumab for Patients With HER2(+) Trastuzumab-Refractory Metastatic Breast Cancer. Clin Breast Cancer. 2015; 15(1):60–5.
20. Seki Y, Yamamoto N, Tamura Y, Goto Y, Shibata T, Tanioka M, et al. Phase I study for ridaforolimus, an oral mTOR inhibitor, in Japanese patients with advanced solid tumors. Cancer Chemother Pharmacol. 2012;69(4):1099–105.
21. Slomovitz BM, Lu KH, Johnston T, Coleman RL, Munsell M, Broaddus RR, et al. A phase 2 study of the oral mammalian target of rapamycin inhibitor, everolimus, in patients with recurrent endometrial carcinoma. Cancer. 2010;116(23):5415–9.
22. Oza AM, Elit L, Tsao MS, Kamel-Reid S, Biagi J, Provencher DM, et al. Phase II study of temsirolimus in women with recurrent or metastatic endometrial cancer: a trial of the NCIC Clinical Trials Group. J Clin Oncol. 2011;29(24):3278–85.
23. Colombo N, McMeekin DS, Schwartz PE, Sessa C, Gehrig PA, Holloway R, et al. Ridaforolimus as a single agent in advanced endometrial cancer: results of a single-arm, phase 2 trial. Br J Cancer. 2013;108(5):1021–6.
24. Tsoref D, Welch S, Lau S, Biagi J, Tonkin K, Martin LA, et al. Phase II study of oral ridaforolimus in women with recurrent or metastatic endometrial cancer. Gynecol Oncol. 2014;135(2):184–9.
25. Alvarez EA, Brady WE, Walker JL, Rotmensch J, Zhou XC, Kendrick JE, et al. Phase II trial of combination bevacizumab and temsirolimus in the treatment of recurrent or persistent endometrial carcinoma: a Gynecologic Oncology Group study. Gynecol Oncol. 2013;129(1):22–7.
26. Fleming GF, Filiaci VL, Marzullo B, Zaino RJ, Davidson SA, Pearl M, et al. Temsirolimus with or without megestrol acetate and tamoxifen for endometrial cancer: a gynecologic oncology group study. Gynecol Oncol. 2014;132(3):585–92.
27. Molinolo AA, Marsh C, El Dinali M, Gangane N, Jennison K, Hewitt S, et al. mTOR as a molecular target in HPV-associated oral and cervical squamous carcinomas. Clin Cancer Res. 2012;18(9):2558–68.
28. Tinker AV, Ellard S, Welch S, Moens F, Allo G, Tsao MS, et al. Phase II study of temsirolimus (CCI-779) in women with recurrent, unresectable, locally advanced or metastatic carcinoma of the cervix. A trial of the NCIC Clinical Trials Group (NCIC CTG IND 199). Gynecol Oncol. 2013;130(2):269–74.
29. Tewari KS, Sill MW, Long HJ 3rd, Penson RT, Huang H, Ramondetta LM, et al. Improved survival with bevacizumab in advanced cervical cancer. N Engl J Med. 2014;370(8):734–43.

5

Quantitation of DNA methylation in Epstein-Barr virus–associated nasopharyngeal carcinoma by bisulfite amplicon sequencing

Weilin Zhao[1,2,3], Yingxi Mo[1,3,5], Shumin Wang[1,3,6], Kaoru Midorikawa[1], Ning Ma[4], Yusuke Hiraku[1], Shinji Oikawa[1], Guangwu Huang[3], Zhe Zhang[3], Mariko Murata[1*] and Kazuhiko Takeuchi[2*]

Abstract

Background: Epigenetic changes, including DNA methylation, disrupt normal cell function, thus contributing to multiple steps of carcinogenesis. Nasopharyngeal carcinoma (NPC) is endemic in southern China and is highly associated with Epstein-Barr virus (EBV) infection. Significant changes of the host cell methylome are observed in EBV-associated NPC with cancer development. Epigenetic marks for NPC diagnosis are urgently needed. In order to explore DNA methylation marks, we investigated DNA methylation of candidate genes in EBV-associated nasopharyngeal carcinoma.

Methods: We first employed methyl-capture sequencing and cDNA microarrays to compare the genome-wide methylation profiles of seven NPC tissues and five non-cancer nasopharyngeal epithelium (NNE) tissues. We found 150 hypermethylated CpG islands spanning promoter regions and down-regulated genes. Furthermore, we quantified the methylation rates of seven candidate genes using bisulfite amplicon sequencing for nine NPC and nine NNE tissues.

Results: All seven candidate genes showed significantly higher methylation rates in NPC than in NNE tissues, and the ratios (NPC/NNE) were in descending order as follows: ITGA4 > RERG > ZNF671 > SHISA3 > ZNF549 > CR2 > RRAD. In particular, methylation levels of ITGA4, RERG, and ZNF671 could distinguish NPC patients from NNE subjects.

Conclusions: We identified the DNA methylation rates of previously unidentified NPC candidate genes. The combination of genome-wide and targeted methylation profiling by next-generation sequencers should provide useful information regarding cancer-specific aberrant methylation.

Keywords: DNA methylation, Methyl-capture sequencing, Bisulfite amplicon sequencing, Nasopharyngeal carcinoma, Epigenetic mark

* Correspondence: mmurata@doc.medic.mie-u.ac.jp;
kazuhiko@clin.medic.mie-u.ac.jp
[1]Department of Environmental and Molecular Medicine, Mie University
Graduate School of Medicine, 2-174, Edobashi, Tsu, Mie 514-8507, Japan
[2]Department of Otorhinolaryngology, Head and Neck Surgery, Mie University
Graduate School of Medicine, Tsu, Mie, Japan
Full list of author information is available at the end of the article

Background

Molecular fingerprints, including methylation changes, occur in specific human genes following exposure to environmental carcinogens [1]. Epigenetic changes play a crucial role in carcinogenesis [2]. Such epigenetic alterations include hypermethylation of CpG islands in gene promoter regions. DNA hypermethylation serves as a mechanism for inactivation of tumor suppressor genes (TSGs) in human malignancies. Nasopharyngeal carcinoma (NPC) is a rare malignancy in Western countries, but it is endemic and has become a serious health problem in Southeast Asia and southern China [3]. DNA methylation is a common event in Epstein-Barr virus (EBV)–associated NPC, and a number of tumor suppressor genes were found to be silenced or downregulated in NPC [4–6]. Aberrant DNA methylation, especially in TSG promoters, may be useful as a biomarker [7] for the early diagnosis and prognosis of NPC.

Genome-wide mapping of DNA methylation is essential to identify new disease genes and potential drug targets, as it can reveal many novel regions with epigenetic alterations in disease and provide a rich source of potential biomarkers [8]. Methyl-capture sequencing (Methyl-Cap sequencing) is a robust DNA methylation profiling approach that is based on the capture of methylated DNA using the high-affinity methyl-CpG binding domain of human MBD2 protein and subsequent next-generation sequencing analysis of enriched fragments. Methyl-Cap sequencing is theoretically able to identify methylated genomic regions located anywhere in the genome. However, certain sequential screening methods are required to establish an informative biomarker panel.

A novel method termed bisulfite amplicon sequencing (BAS), which combines the benefits of bisulfite conversion, targeted amplification, and next-generation sequencing, was developed for targeted digital quantitation of DNA methylation [9]. BAS allows for focused, accurate DNA methylation quantitation with high-throughput capabilities in both sample and target numbers. The application of BAS is useful in hypothesis-driven epigenetic studies where regions of interest have been identified [9]. Here we identify novel DNA methylation biomarker candidates for NPC using Methyl-Cap sequencing and BAS.

Methods

Clinical samples

Methyl-Cap sequencing was performed on seven tumor biopsies from untreated NPC patients (mean age ± SD, 49.4 ± 6.7 years old; four males, three females) and five non-cancer nasopharyngeal epithelium (NNE) samples from control (non-cancer) patients (47.7 ± 10.4 years old, two males, three females). BAS analysis was conducted using nine NPC samples (45.4 ± 12.1 years old, six males, three females) and nine NNE samples (39.8 ± 13.9 years old, five males, four females). All NPC samples were non-keratinizing carcinoma. The diagnoses were made by experienced pathologists according to the World Health Organization (WHO) classification. All samples were obtained from patients seen at the Department of Otolaryngology Head & Neck Surgery, First Affiliate Hospital of Guangxi Medical University, Nanning, China (with ethical review committee approval notice (2009–07-07) of the First Affiliated Hospital of Guangxi Medical University and ethical approval (no.1116) of Mie University, Japan). All patients provided written informed consent. Biopsy samples were stored in liquid nitrogen prior to DNA or RNA extraction. The tissues of all NPC patients were EBV positive and those of all NNE patients were EBV negative.

Cell culture

NPC cell line HK1_EBV and immortalized nasopharyngeal epithelial cell line NP460 were the kind gifts of Professor Sai-Wah Tsao (Hong Kong University) [10, 11]. HK1_EBV cells were maintained in RPMI 1640 medium (Gibco, 11,875–093) supplemented with 10% fetal bovine serum (Biowest, S1820), 100 U/ml penicillin, and 100 μg/ml streptomycin (Gibco, 15,070–063). NP460 cells were maintained in a 1:1 ratio of Defined Keratinocyte-SFM (Gibco, 10,744,019) supplemented with growth factors and EpiLife medium supplemented with EpiLife Defined Growth Supplement (Gibco, #S-012-5), 100 U/ml penicillin, and 100 μg/ml streptomycin. Cells were maintained at 37 °C in a 5% CO_2 incubator.

Methyl-Cap sequencing

Genomic DNA from frozen tissues and cultured cells was extracted using a QIAamp DNA Mini Kit (Qiagen, 51,304). DNA was sonicated to yield the desired size range (150 bp) using an ultra-sonicator (Covaris, Woburn, MA). After sonication, methylated DNA was selected from 12.5-μg DNA fragments using a Methyl-Miner Methylated DNA Enrichment Kit (Invitrogen, ME10025). We collected the final two fractions of highly methylated DNA, which corresponded to gradient elution buffer concentrations of 0.6 M and 2 M NaCl. The recovered DNA in the 2 M NaCl elution buffer was purified with a PureLink PCR Purification Kit (Invitrogen, K3100–02). Library construction, emulsion PCR, and sequencing were performed by Mie University Life Science Research Center using a SOLiD System (Applied Biosystems, Foster City, CA) with mapping to the human reference genome (hg 19). Partek Genomics Suite (Partek Incorporated, Saint Louis, MO) was used to map BAM files to the human CpG islands for further statistical analyses. We checked the methylation status using the Integrative Genomics Viewer (IGV) (ver1.4.05), as shown in Additional file 1: Figure S1.

Detection of gene expression using cDNA microarray analysis

Fifty nanograms of RNA from seven NPC biopsies and five NNE samples (Methyl-Cap sequencing samples) were subjected to Agilent SurePrint G3 Human GE microarray analysis (8 × 60 K, 1 color, Agilent Technologies, Santa Clara, CA) for gene expression evaluation (Hokkaido System Science).

Sodium bisulfite modification and bisulfite sequencing PCR

Genomic DNA (1 μg) from each sample was treated with sodium bisulfite using an EpiTect Bisulfite Kit (Qiagen, 59,104) and QIACube (Qiagen). Sodium bisulfite–modified DNA was subjected to PCR with bisulfite sequencing PCR primers, which were designed to amplify nucleotides in CpG islands around the transcription start sites of target genes. The primer sequences and cycling conditions for BAS are listed in Table 1. PCR products were purified using the PureLink PCR Purification Kit (Invitrogen). The purified products from individual biological samples were pooled in equimolar amounts (0.5 pmol) of 10 genes from each subject (approximately 1 μg/sample), including the seven target genes in this study.

Bisulfite amplicon sequencing (BAS)

Pooled PCR products were sheared using the Ion Shear Plus Enzyme Mix to yield appropriate insert sizes, and transformed with the Ion Xpress Plus Library kit for AB Library Builder System (Life Technologies, Carlsbad, CA) into barcoded libraries with sizes set at 200 bp.

Emulsion PCR was performed using the Ion PGM Hi-Q OT2 Kit, and sequenced using the Ion PGM Hi-Q Sequencing Kit on Ion PGM (400-bp read length) with a 318 Chip v2 BC (Life Technologies). Sequencing data were analyzed using the Bismark Bisulfite Mapper [12] with plug-in software (Life Technologies). The percent methylation in each CpG was calculated by (number of reads with methylated C/total reads) × 100. The methylation data can be viewed in the IGV using the BiSeq package in R/Bioconductor.

Bisulfite genomic sequencing (BGS)

To compare the BAS and BGS methods, sodium bisulfite–modified DNA was subjected to PCR with bisulfite sequencing primers for *ITGA4* and *ZNF549*, shown in Table 1, with an annealing time of 30 s. Subcloning and sequencing for BGS were performed as described previously [4].

Results

Selection of candidate genes with hypermethylated promoter CpG islands and reduced expression in NPC tissues

First, we targeted promoter CpG islands with overlapping regions from 1000 bp upstream to 200 bp downstream of each gene's transcription start site (about 23,000 genes). Next, we selected 150 candidate genes with hypermethylated promoter CpG islands (more than 3-fold based on Methyl-Cap sequencing data, $P < 0.05$) and down-regulated genes (relative quantity less than 0.5 based on cDNA microarray data, $P < 0.05$) in NPC compared to NNE tissues (Additional file 2: Table S1). We performed a literature search on DNA methylation in these genes, and finally chose seven genes (Table 1) for further study.

Table 1 Bisulfite sequencing PCR primers and PCR conditions for BAS samples

Gene	Sequences (5' to 3')	Product size (bp)	Annealing (°C)	Annealing Time (s)	Position from TSS	UCSC gene ID
CR2	F: GGGTGAGTTTGAGTTAAAGAGTGG R: AAAAAACCAATAAAAACAATCAAAACCAAA	514	58	50	−149 − +365	uc001hfv.3
ITGA4	F: TGTAATTTTGGGGTAGTGGT R: CCCTCCTACCTCCTTAAAAAAAAAAAA	362	58	45	+711 − +1072	uc002unu.3
RERG	F: GGAGTTTGGAGGTTTGGAAAT R: CAAAAACAAATACCAATAACCC	278	58	45	−145 − +133	uc001rct.3
RRAD	F: TTGGTGGGGGTGGATAGATA R-CCTCCCCCAACCCCCAAAT	331	61	45	−102 − +228	uc002eqo.2
SHISA3	F: GGTTGAGAGTTAAGTTTTGGGGG R: CCTCCCCACTCCTCAAAAAAA	446	58	45	−570 − −125	uc003gwp.3
ZNF549	F: TTTTAGTTTGATGGGTTTTTTTTTTTGTT R: AAACCTCAAAACCCAAATAAAAATC	502	56	45	−177 − +325	uc002qpb.2
ZNF671	F: ATTTTGTTTTTGTTAGGTTGTTTTTGG R: CTATCCTAAAACACAAAAACTACAAACACT	311	57	45	+13 − +323	uc002qpz.4

PCR cycles: 40

CR2: complement C3d receptor 2, *ITGA4*: integrin subunit alpha 4, *RERG*: RAS-like estrogen regulated growth inhibitor, *RRAD*: Ras-related glycolysis inhibitor and calcium channel regulator, *SHISA3*: shisa family member 3, *ZNF549*: zinc finger protein 549, *ZNF671*: zinc finger protein 671

Comparison of methylation rates between BAS and BGS

Using BAS, the average read depth per CpG (mean ± SD, 1274.6 ± 295.0; range 961.7–1707.1) for seven genes in 20 samples was sufficient to estimate the methylation rate. The bisulfite sequencing PCR amplicons of *ITGA4* and *ZNF549* from non-cancer cell line NP460 and NPC cell line HK1_EBV were also subjected to BGS, and at least five clones were successfully evaluated for all CpG methylation statuses (Additional file 1: Figure S2). From both sequencing results, the methylation rate in every CpG was calculated as shown in Fig. 1. Compared to NP460 cells, HK1_EBV cells were more highly methylated in the promoter CpGs of *ITGA4* (Fig. 1a) and *ZNF549* (Fig. 1b). The scatter plots show good

correlation in methylation rates between BGS and BAS (*ITGA4*, $R = 0.973$, $P = 0.000$, Fig. 1c; *ZNF549*, $R = 0.983$, $P = 0.000$, Fig. 1d).

Methylation quantification of promoter CpGs by BAS

Table 2 shows the DNA methylation rates derived by BAS analysis for NNE and NPC patients. All seven genes exhibited significant differences in DNA methylation rates between NNE and NPC patients. Among the seven genes, the ratios of the methylation rates in the two groups (NPC/NNE) were, in descending order, *ITGA4 > RERG > ZNF671 > SHISA3 > ZNF549 > CR2 > RRAD*. Fig. 2 shows the methylation rate of every CpG (average and SD, %) for the NPC and NNE subjects. High

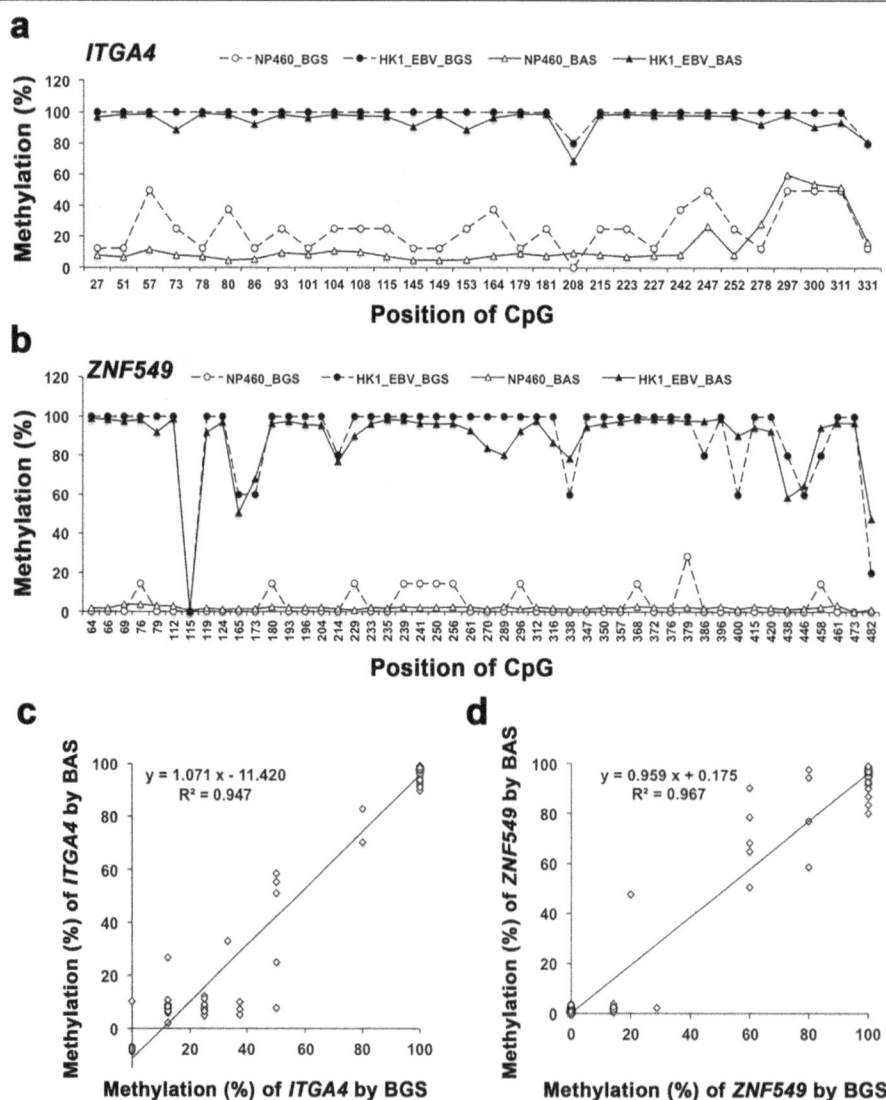

Fig. 1 Comparison of CpG methylation rates between BGS and BAS. The methylation rate of each CpG in promoter regions of *ITGA4* (**a**) and *ZNF549* (**b**) was detected by BGS (circles, dotted line) and BAS (triangles, solid line) in HK1_EBV cells (closed marker) and NP460 cells (open marker). Graphs show the correlation in methylation rates between BGS and BAS for *ITGA4* (**c**) and *ZNF549* (**d**) with Pearson's correlation coefficients

Table 2 DNA methylation rate by BAS analysis

	No. CpG	NNE (n = 9) Mean ± SD (%)	NPC (n = 9) Mean ± SD (%)	P-value by t-test	Ratio of NPC/NNE (rank[a])
CR2	47	5.3 ± 2.6	20.7 ± 11.7	0.004	3.9 (6)
ITGA4	30	3.0 ± 1.1	35.3 ± 24.6	0.004	11.8 (1)
RERG	25	3.9 ± 2.2	35.2 ± 25.0	0.006	9.1 (2)
RRAD	30	7.1 ± 2.5	15.3 ± 9.9	0.038	2.2 (7)
SHISA3	37	2.9 ± 0.7	21.1 ± 15.3	0.007	7.3 (4)
ZNF549	48	4.7 ± 2.1	19.7 ± 13.5	0.010	4.2 (5)
ZNF671	28	4.1 ± 2.0	36.4 ± 20.7	0.002	8.9 (3)

[a]: rank in descending order

methylation rates were observed in NPC patients (closed triangles) compared with NNE patients (open triangles), especially for *ITGA4*, *RERG*, and *ZNF671*.

Visualization of methylation status at a glance

BAS data were analyzed using the Bismark Bisulfite Mapper with plug-in software and the BiSeq package in R/Bioconductor, and then the resultant BED files were visualized by IGV. Fig. 3 shows the methylation status of each subject using a color scale based on methylation rate (green 0% — black 50% — red 100%), making it possible to detect differences in methylation status at a glance.

Discussion

Epigenetic changes such as DNA methylation are recognized as an important mechanism in cancer initiation and progression [13]. Inactivation of TSGs occurs as a consequence of promoter hypermethylation with gene silencing in many cancer types [14]. In NPC, a vast number of TSGs have been found to be inactivated by promoter hypermethylation [15]. Interestingly, EBV infection induces increased genome-wide gene methylation, resulting in the formation of a unique epigenotype with high CpG methylation in tumor cells [16]. Given its important functions in cancer initiation and progression, DNA methylation is being explored as a biomarker for cancer, including NPC.

Many methods are available to examine DNA methylation at single-base resolution. These are broadly classified into two categories, depending on whether they are based on microarrays or next-generation sequencing. Microarray-based technologies use a fixed number of probes with the limitation of low genome coverage and the advantage of low cost [17]. Whole-genome bisulfite sequencing can overcome this limitation but elevates the costs tremendously [17]. It is only practical to conduct whole-genome bisulfite sequencing on a limited number of samples, and coverage is usually in the range of 5–15 reads per CpG, limiting the statistical significance of results [18]. Methyl-Cap sequencing is an attractive

intermediate solution to increase the methylome coverage in large sample sets [17]. We utilized Methyl-Cap sequencing and cDNA microarray analysis to explore TSG candidates with highly methylated promoter CpG islands and gene down-regulation, resulting in 150 possibilities. Of these 150 candidate genes, several had already been reported to be epigenetic silencing of tumor suppressor genes in NPC, such as *ZFP82* [19], *ADAMTS8* [20], *INPP4B* [21], and *ATOH8* [22]. Several conventional NPC tumor suppressor genes [23], such as *RASSF1* and *CDKN2A* (*p16*), were methylated at promoter regions in NPC patients from our Methyl-Cap sequencing data, but their expression levels were not significantly down-regulated in NPC by cDNA microarray analysis. Gene *ZMYND10* (*BLU*) was significantly down-regulated in NPC, but there was no significant difference in Methyl-Cap sequencing between NNE and NPC (data not shown). Since we combined Methyl-Cap sequencing (more than 3-fold) and cDNA microarray (less than 0.5-fold) data, these TSGs were not included in our candidate gene list (Additional file 2: Table S1). Our literature review resulted in the selection of seven target genes. These genes were previously reported to exhibit DNA methylation (*CR2* [24], *ITGA4* [25], *RERG* [26], *RRAD* [4], *SHISA3* [27], *ZNF549*, and *ZNF671* [28]). Schwab and Illges found that premature B lymphocytes contained a methylated CpG island and did not express *CR2* (*CD21*) [24]. Interestingly, viral capsid protein mediated EBV binding on CR2 [29]. Gerecke et al. showed that methylation markers in the promoters of *ITGA4*, *TFPI2*, and *VIMENTIN* seemed to be suitable risk markers for inflammation-associated colon cancer [25], and Chang et al. demonstrated *ITGA4*, *SFRP2*, and *p16* promoter methylation in stool samples from patients with colorectal adenomas and carcinoma [30]. *RERG* was reported to be a tumor suppressor gene in colorectal cancer [31] and breast cancer [26]. Our previous study demonstrated that *RRAD* was frequently methylated in EBV-associated NPC, and it functioned as a tumor suppressor by inhibiting cell proliferation, colony formation, and migration in *RRAD*-overexpressing NPC cells [4].

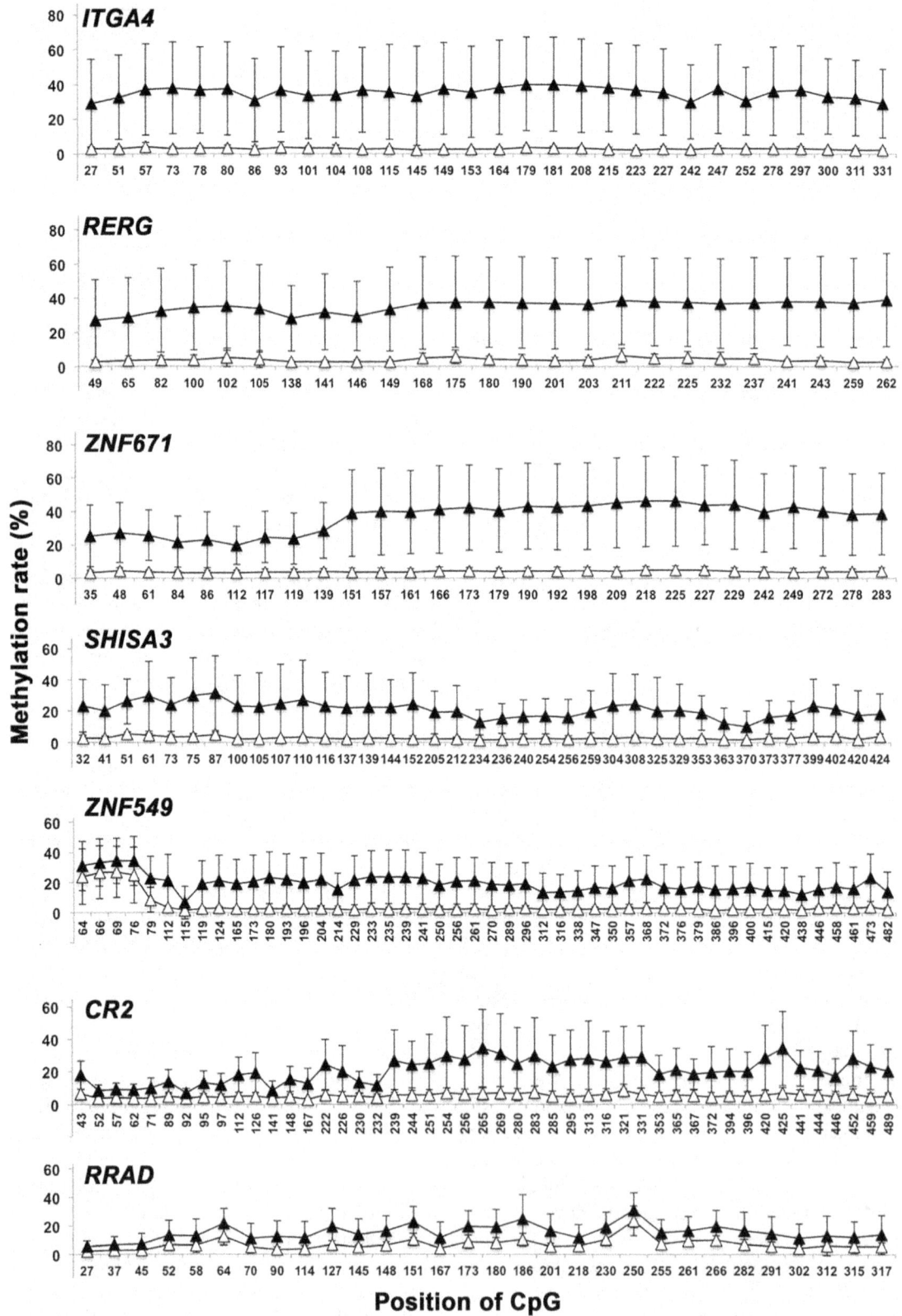

Fig. 2 CpG methylation rates in NPC and NNE tissues. Graphs show mean and SD (%) in every CpG from NPC ($n = 9$, closed triangles) and NNE ($n = 9$, open triangles)

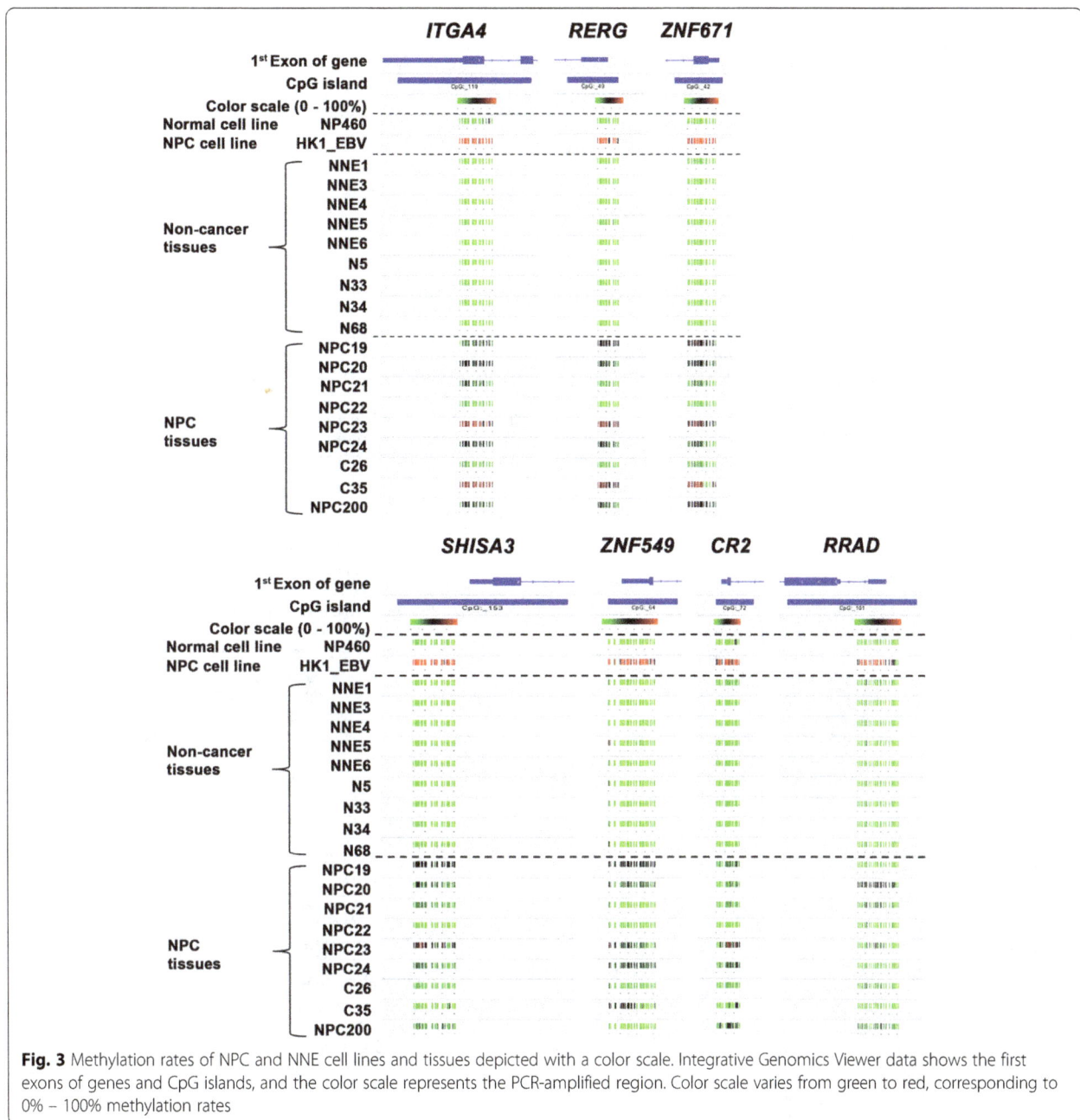

Fig. 3 Methylation rates of NPC and NNE cell lines and tissues depicted with a color scale. Integrative Genomics Viewer data shows the first exons of genes and CpG islands, and the color scale represents the PCR-amplified region. Color scale varies from green to red, corresponding to 0% – 100% methylation rates

SHISA3 was a novel tumor suppressor identified in lung cancer [32], and was found to be epigenetically inactivated in a substantial fraction of patients with colorectal cancer [27]. Yeh et al. demonstrated that *ZNF671*, an epigenetically silenced novel tumor suppressor, was a potential non-invasive biomarker for predicting urothelial carcinoma relapse [33]. Lleras et al. reported the epigenetic silencing of Kruppel-type zinc finger protein genes, including *ZNF549* and *ZNF671*, on chromosome 19q13 in oropharyngeal cancer [28]. Our results demonstrated the utility of BAS in validating findings from genome-wide methylation analysis, by showing that all

seven candidates had significantly higher average CpG methylation rates in NPC than NNE.

BAS is an efficient, cost-effective, and robust high-throughput technique for assessing DNA methylation at targeted loci of interest [18]. In our experiment, BAS coverage attained an average of over 1000 reads per CpG. BGS is another method of targeted bisulfite sequencing that includes subcloning and clone selection steps, which limits the total numbers of sequenced clones and sample sets [34]. Therefore, BGS coverage is usually in the range of around 10 clones per CpG. Due to the significantly increased throughput of next-generation sequencing, a large number of differentially methylated genes can now be identified in a single experiment, and the traditional methods of experimental validation, such as methylation-specific PCR and BGS, are no longer sufficient to keep up with increasing demand. As our results show, BAS can quantitatively and accurately measure CpG methylation levels in genomic regions of interest in a high-throughput manner, and this approach may replace traditional validation methods in the future.

Conclusions

Here we show seven candidate epigenetic marks for NPC (methylation ratios: *ITGA4 > RERG > ZNF671 > SHISA3 > ZNF549 > CR2 > RRAD*). In conclusion, the combination of genome-wide and targeted methylation profiling by next-generation sequencers provides useful information regarding cancer-specific aberrant methylation in NPC.

Additional files

Additional file 1: Figure S1. DNA methylation data visualized with IGV. This figure presents the result of methylation analysis by Methyl-Cap sequencing at promoter regions of SHISA3 in NPC and NNE sample, respectively. **Figure S2.** Methylation status of promoter regions in cell lines. Bisulfite genomic sequencing of 30 and 48 CpG sites within the promoter regions of (A) ITGA4 and (B) ZNF549, respectively, in an immortalized epithelial cell line (NP460) and an NPC cell line (HK1_EBV). At least five clones were randomly selected and sequenced for each sample. Each row represents an individual promoter allele. Open circles indicate unmethylated cytosines, and closed circles indicate methylated cytosines.

Additional file 2: Table S1. Summary of candidate genes from Methyl-Cap sequencing and cDNA microarray data.

Abbreviations

ADAMTS8: ADAM metallopeptidase with thrombospondin type 1 motif 8; *ATOH8*: Atonal bHLH transcription factor 8; BAS: Bisulfite amplicon sequencing; BGS: Bisulfite genomic sequencing; *CDKN2A (p16)*: Cyclin dependent kinase inhibitor 2A; *CR2*: Complement C3d receptor 2; IGV: Integrative Genomics Viewer; *INPP4B*: Inositol polyphosphate-4-phosphatase type II B; *ITGA4*: Integrin subunit alpha 4; Methyl-Cap sequencing: Methyl-capture sequencing; NNE: Non-cancer nasopharyngeal epithelium; NPC: Nasopharyngeal carcinoma; *RASSF1*: Ras association domain family member 1; *RERG*: Ras-like estrogen-regulated growth inhibitor; *RRAD*: Ras-related glycolysis inhibitor and calcium channel regulator; *SHISA3*: Shisa family member 3; TSG: Tumor suppressor gene; *ZFP82*: ZFP82 zinc finger protein; *ZMYND10 (BLU)*: Zinc finger MYND-type containing 10; *ZNF549*: Zinc finger protein 549; *ZNF671*: Zinc finger protein 671

Acknowledgements

We thank Mr. K. Asai and Mr. R. Ikadai (Mie University School of Medicine) for their technical support in the BGS experiments. We are deeply grateful to Professor I. Kobayashi and Dr. Y. Kobayashi (Mie University) for their valuable advice and help regarding next-generation sequencing.

Funding

This work was partly supported by JSPS KAKENHI (Grant Numbers JP25305020, JP25293149, JP16H05255, and JP16H05829), National Nature Science Foundation of China (81272983), and the Guangxi Natural Science Foundation (no. 2013GXNSFGA019002).

Authors' contributions

MM and KT conceived the project and planned the experiments. WLZ, YXM, and SMW performed experiments and analyzed the data. KM contributed to data analysis. MM, KM, and WLZ wrote the manuscript. NM, YH, SO, GWH, and ZZ critically read the manuscript and directed and supervised the experiments. All authors read and approved the final manuscript.

Competing interests

The authors declare that they have no competing interests.

Author details

[1]Department of Environmental and Molecular Medicine, Mie University Graduate School of Medicine, 2-174, Edobashi, Tsu, Mie 514-8507, Japan. [2]Department of Otorhinolaryngology, Head and Neck Surgery, Mie University Graduate School of Medicine, Tsu, Mie, Japan. [3]Department of Otolaryngology Head and Neck Surgery, First Affiliated Hospital of Guangxi Medical University, Nanning, China. [4]Graduate School of Health Science, Suzuka University of Medical Science, Suzuka, Mie, Japan. [5]Present address: Department of Research, Affiliated Tumor Hospital of Guangxi Medical University, Nanning, Guangxi, China. [6]Present address: Center for Oral Biology, University of Rochester Medical Center, Rochester, NY, USA.

References

1. Ceccaroli C, Pulliero A, Geretto M, Izzotti A. Molecular fingerprints of environmental carcinogens in human cancer. J Environ Sci Health C Environ Carcinog Ecotoxicol Rev. 2015;33(2):188–228.
2. Kasai H, Kawai K. DNA methylation at the C-5 position of cytosine by methyl radicals: a possible role for epigenetic change during carcinogenesis by environmental agents. Chem Res Toxicol. 2009;22(6):984–9.
3. Tao Q, Chan AT. Nasopharyngeal carcinoma: molecular pathogenesis and therapeutic developments. Expert Rev Mol Med. 2007;9(12):1–24.
4. Mo Y, Midorikawa K, Zhang Z, Zhou X, Ma N, Huang G, et al. Promoter hypermethylation of Ras-related GTPase gene RRAD inactivates a tumor suppressor function in nasopharyngeal carcinoma. Cancer Lett. 2012;323(2): 147–54.
5. Zhang Z, Sun D, van do N, Tang A, Hu L, Huang G. Inactivation of RASSF2A by promoter methylation correlates with lymph node metastasis in nasopharyngeal carcinoma. Int J Cancer. 2007;120(1):32–8.
6. Zhou X, Xiao X, Huang T, Du C, Wang S, Mo Y, et al. Epigenetic inactivation of follistatin-like 1 mediates tumor immune evasion in nasopharyngeal carcinoma. Oncotarget. 2016;7(13):16433–44.
7. Murata M, Thanan R, Ma N, Kawanishi S. Role of nitrative and oxidative DNA damage in inflammation-related carcinogenesis. J Biomed Biotechnol. 2012; 2012:623019.
8. Meissner A, Mikkelsen TS, Gu H, Wernig M, Hanna J, Sivachenko A, et al. Genome-scale DNA methylation maps of pluripotent and differentiated cells. Nature. 2008;454(7205):766–70.
9. Masser DR, Berg AS, Freeman WM. Focused, high accuracy 5-methylcytosine quantitation with base resolution by benchtop next-generation sequencing. Epigenetics Chromatin. 2013;6(1):33.
10. Li HM, Man C, Jin Y, Deng W, Yip YL, Feng HC, et al. Molecular and cytogenetic changes involved in the immortalization of nasopharyngeal epithelial cells by telomerase. Int J Cancer. 2006;119(7):1567–76.
11. Lo AK, Lo KW, Tsao SW, Wong HL, Hui JW, To KF, et al. Epstein-Barr virus infection alters cellular signal cascades in human nasopharyngeal epithelial cells. Neoplasia. 2006;8(3):173–80.
12. Krueger F, Andrews SR. Bismark: a flexible aligner and methylation caller for Bisulfite-Seq applications. Bioinformatics. 2011;27(11):1571–2.
13. Jones PA, Baylin SB. The fundamental role of epigenetic events in cancer. Nat Rev Genet. 2002;3(6):415–28.
14. Sharma S, Kelly TK, Jones PA. Epigenetics in cancer. Carcinogenesis. 2010; 31(1):27–36.
15. Li LL, Shu XS, Wang ZH, Cao Y, Tao Q. Epigenetic disruption of cell signaling in nasopharyngeal carcinoma. Chin J Cancer. 2011;30(4):231–9.
16. Fukayama M, Ushiku T. Epstein-Barr virus-associated gastric carcinoma. Pathol Res Pract. 2011;207(9):529–37.
17. Teh AL, Pan H, Lin X, Lim YI, Patro CP, Cheong CY, et al. Comparison of methyl-capture sequencing vs. Infinium 450K methylation array for methylome analysis in clinical samples. Epigenetics. 2016;11(1):36–48.

18. Bernstein DL, Kameswaran V, Le Lay JE, Sheaffer KL, Kaestner KH. The BisPCR(2) method for targeted bisulfite sequencing. Epigenetics Chromatin. 2015;8:27.

19. Cheng Y, Liang P, Geng H, Wang Z, Li L, Cheng SH, et al. A novel 19q13 nucleolar zinc finger protein suppresses tumor cell growth through inhibiting ribosome biogenesis and inducing apoptosis but is frequently silenced in multiple carcinomas. Mol Cancer Res. 2012;10(7): 925–36.

20. Choi GC, Li J, Wang Y, Li L, Zhong L, Ma B, et al. The metalloprotease ADAMTS8 displays antitumor properties through antagonizing EGFR-MEK-ERK signaling and is silenced in carcinomas by CpG methylation. Mol Cancer Res. 2014;12(2):228–38.

21. Yuen JW, Chung GT, Lun SW, Cheung CC, To KF, Lo KW. Epigenetic inactivation of inositol polyphosphate 4-phosphatase B (INPP4B), a regulator of PI3K/AKT signaling pathway in EBV-associated nasopharyngeal carcinoma. PLoS One. 2014;9(8):e105163.

22. Wang Z, Xie J, Yan M, Wang J, Wang X, Zhang J, et al. Downregulation of ATOH8 induced by EBV-encoded LMP1 contributes to the malignant phenotype of nasopharyngeal carcinoma. Oncotarget. 2016;7(18):26765–79.

23. Dai W, Zheng H, Cheung AK, Lung ML. Genetic and epigenetic landscape of nasopharyngeal carcinoma. Chin Clin Oncol. 2016;5(2):16.

24. Schwab J, Illges H. Regulation of CD21 expression by DNA methylation and histone deacetylation. Int Immunol. 2001;13(5):705–10.

25. Gerecke C, Scholtka B, Lowenstein Y, Fait I, Gottschalk U, Rogoll D, et al. Hypermethylation of ITGA4, TFPI2 and VIMENTIN promoters is increased in inflamed colon tissue: putative risk markers for colitis-associated cancer. J Cancer Res Clin Oncol. 2015;141(12):2097–107.

26. Hanker AB, Morita S, Repasky GA, Ross DT, Seitz RS, Der CJ. Tools to study the function of the Ras-related, estrogen-regulated growth inhibitor in breast cancer. Methods Enzymol. 2008;439:53–72.

27. Tsai MH, Chen WC, Yu SL, Chen CC, Jao TM, Huang CY, et al. DNA Hypermethylation of SHISA3 in colorectal cancer: an independent predictor of poor prognosis. Ann Surg Oncol. 2015;22(Suppl 3):S1481–9.

28. Lleras RA, Adrien LR, Smith RV, Brown B, Jivraj N, Keller C, et al. Hypermethylation of a cluster of Kruppel-type zinc finger protein genes on chromosome 19q13 in oropharyngeal squamous cell carcinoma. Am J Pathol. 2011;178(5):1965–74.

29. Barel M, Gauffre A, Lyamani F, Fiandino A, Hermann J, Frade R. Intracellular interaction of EBV/C3d receptor (CR2) with p68, a calcium-binding protein present in normal but not in transformed B lymphocytes. J Immunol. 1991; 147(4):1286–91.

30. Chang E, Park DI, Kim YJ, Kim BK, Park JH, Kim HJ, et al. Detection of colorectal neoplasm using promoter methylation of ITGA4, SFRP2, and p16 in stool samples: a preliminary report in Korean patients. Hepato-Gastroenterology. 2010;57(101):720–7.

31. Yang R, Chen B, Pfutze K, Buch S, Steinke V, Holinski-Feder E, et al. Genome-wide analysis associates familial colorectal cancer with increases in copy number variations and a rare structural variation at 12p12.3. Carcinogenesis. 2014;35(2):315–23.

32. Chen CC, Chen HY, Su KY, Hong QS, Yan BS, Chen CH, et al. Shisa3 is associated with prolonged survival through promoting beta-catenin degradation in lung cancer. Am J Respir Crit Care Med. 2014;190(4):433–44.

33. Yeh CM, Chen PC, Hsieh HY, Jou YC, Lin CT, Tsai MH, et al. Methylomics analysis identifies ZNF671 as an epigenetically repressed novel tumor suppressor and a potential non-invasive biomarker for the detection of urothelial carcinoma. Oncotarget. 2015;6(30):29555–72.

34. Huang Z, Bassil CF, Murphy SK. Bisulfite sequencing of cloned alleles. Methods Mol Biol. 2013;1049:83–94.

6

Safety and efficacy of lobaplatin combined with 5-fluorouracil as first-line induction chemotherapy followed by lobaplatin-radiotherapy in locally advanced nasopharyngeal carcinoma: preliminary results of a prospective phase II trial

Liang-Ru Ke[1,2†], Wei-Xiong Xia[1,2†], Wen-Ze Qiu[1,2], Xin-Jun Huang[1,2], Jing Yang[1,2], Ya-Hui Yu[1,2], Hu Liang[1,2], Guo-Ying Liu[1,2], Yan-Fang Ye[1,2], Yan-Qun Xiang[1,2*], Xiang Guo[1,2*] and Xing Lv[1,2*]

Abstract

Background: Due to improvements in imaging and radiological techniques as well as the use of chemotherapy, distant metastasis has become the predominant mode of treatment failure in patients with locally advanced nasopharyngeal carcinoma (LA-NPC). Platinum-based systemic chemotherapy has shown survival benefits and is now the standard strategy for systemic therapy in patients with LA-NPC. Notably, the third-generation platinum reagent lobaplatin has shown anti-tumor effects in several solid tumors with lower incidences of gastrointestinal, hepatic and renal toxicity relative to other platinum drugs. However, the safety and efficacy of lobaplatin as a first-line regimen in patients with LA-NPC are undetermined.

Methods: Patients with stage III–IVa-b NPC received lobaplatin at a dose of 30 mg/m2 on days 1 and 22 combined with a continuous 120-h intravenous injection of 5-fluorouracil at a dose of 4 g/m2 followed by lobaplatin at a dose of 50 mg/m2 on days 43 and 64 concomitant with intensity-modulated radiation therapy. Objective response rates and acute toxicity were assessed based on RECIST (1.1) and CTCAE v.3.0, respectively. Kaplan-Meier analysis was used to calculate survival rates.

Results: Fifty-nine patients were enrolled, and 44 patients (74.6%) received allocated cycles of chemotherapy. The objective response rates were 88.1% (95% confidence interval [CI], 0.77 to 0.95) and 100% after induction chemotherapy (ICT) and concurrent chemoradiotherapy (CRT), respectively. With a median follow-up period of 44 months, the 3-year estimated progression-free survival and overall survival were 86.4% (95% CI, 69.8 to 98.8) and 94.9% (95% CI, 89.5 to 100), respectively. The most common grade 3–4 toxicities were neutropenia (8.5%) and thrombocytopenia (40.7%) after ICT and CRT, respectively.

(Continued on next page)

* Correspondence: xiangyq@sysucc.org.cn; guoxiang@sysucc.org.cn; lvxing@sysucc.org.cn
†Equal contributors
[1]Department of Nasopharyngeal Carcinoma, Sun Yat-Sen University Cancer Center, 651 Dongfeng Road East, Guangzhou, Guangdong 510060, China
Full list of author information is available at the end of the article

(Continued from previous page)

Conclusion: Lobaplatin combined with 5-fluorouracil followed by lobaplatin-RT treatment showed encouraging anti-tumor effects with tolerable toxicities in patients with LA-NPC. Randomized controlled trials of lobaplatin in patients with LA-NPC are warranted.

Keywords: Lobaplatin, Nasopharyngeal carcinoma, Locally advanced, First-line, Chemotherapy

Background

Nasopharyngeal carcinoma (NPC), a malignancy derived from epithelial cells of the nasopharynx, is endemic in Southern China and Southeast Asia [1]. The development of high-resolution imaging and radiological techniques has increased the local control rate of NPC up to 95% [2], leaving distant metastasis as the major cause of treatment failure. To address this issue, a combined regimen of chemotherapy and radiotherapy has been recommended as the standard treatment strategy for locally advanced NPC (LA-NPC) [3]. However, the survival benefits of sequential chemotherapy for NPC patients are still controversial [4–8]. Induction chemotherapy (ICT) can improve both progression-free survival (PFS) and/or overall survival (OS) [8–14]. Ma J et al recently demonstrated that the introduction of cisplatin, fluorouracil, and docetaxel (TPF) induction chemotherapy to concurrent chemotherapy could significantly improve the PFS of patients with LA-NPC [15], while additional randomized controlled clinical trials to determine the role of systemic chemotherapy in NPC during the intensity modulation radiotherapy (IMRT) era are still underway.

A platinum-based regimen is recommended as the first-line chemotherapeutic strategy for NPC according to the NCCN guidelines. Cisplatin, the first anticancer reagent, has shown encouraging anti-tumor efficacy in NPC both alone and in combination with other treatments [3, 5, 16, 17]. However, cisplatin can induce severe side effects, including dose-limiting nephrotoxicity, cumulative peripheral sensory neuropathy, ototoxicity and gastrointestinal reactions, such as nausea or vomiting, which can reduce patient compliance for chemotherapy administration or even cause treatment interruptions [18]. Moreover, the requirement of a massive fluid infusion of cisplatin to avoid renal toxicity extends the inpatient period and limits the application of this treatment in patients with heart and renal dysfunction. Lobaplatin, a third-generation platinum reagent, forms DNA adducts and induces DNA damage, resulting in cell apoptosis, which is similar to the pharmacological mechanisms of other platinum reagents [19]. Lobaplatin has shown robust anti-tumor efficacy in multiple solid tumors,

such as breast cancer, hepatocellular carcinoma, non-small cell lung cancer, transitional cell carcinoma, ovarian cancer and cervical squamous carcinoma [20–23], but without the above-listed toxicities. Moreover, lobaplatin has no multidrug resistance with other platinum drugs, such as cisplatin or carboplatinum [20]. Though lobaplatin costs approximately 16-fold more than cisplatin, there is no increased economic burden to patients due to the high insurance coverage of both reagents. Major characteristics of cisplatin and lobaplatin are compared in Table 1.

A combination of lobaplatin and docetaxel has exhibited particularly effective anti-tumor activity in recurrent and metastatic NPC [24]. Herein, to further determine the anti-tumor efficacy of lobaplatin in LA-NPC, we performed a phase II clinical trial to determine the safety and efficacy of lobaplatin combined with 5-fluorouracil (5-FU) as a first-line ICT strategy followed by lobaplatin-radiotherapy (lobaplatin-RT) in LA-NPC.

Methods

Aim of study and end points

The main purpose of this trial was to test the feasibility and efficacy of delivering lobaplatin combined with 5-FU as a first-line ICT regimen followed by lobaplatin-RT in patients with LA-NPC. The primary end point was the objective response rate (ORR), and secondary end points included overall survival (OS), progression-free survival (PFS), distant metastasis-free survival (DMFS) and local recurrence-free survival (LRFS). Acute toxicities during ICT and lobaplatin-RT were also observed. The study was designed as a single arm, open-labeled phase II study.

Participant enrollment and characteristics

Regular evaluations were performed for all enrolled participants as previously described [2]. These included medical history, physical examination, pathology diagnosis, electrocardiogram, and laboratory testing, including but not limited to liver and kidney function and Epstein Barr virus (EBV) DNA copy number assessment. To ensure tumor margins were well-defined, magnetic resonance imaging (MRI) of the nasopharynx and neck were conducted in all patients, except those with contraindications (e.g., pacemaker or stent); for these cases, computed tomography (CT) was used. Regular work-ups

Table 1 Comparison of cisplatin and lobaplatin

Category	Cisplatin	Lobaplatin
Product generation	First generation	Third generation
Chemical structure		
Anti-tumor mechanism	Forms DNA-drug adducts, resulting in DNA damage and cell apoptosis	
Half-life period	Over 24 h (total platinum) [33], mainly metabolized through the kidney	131 ± 15 min (free platinum) and 6.8 ± 4.3 days (total platinum) [19], mainly metabolized through the kidney
Anti-tumor spectrum	Ovarian, testicular, bladder, colorectal, lung, head and neck cancer	Metastatic breast cancer, chronic myelogenous leukemia, and small cell lung cancer
Side effects	Nephrotoxicity, cumulative peripheral sensory neuropathy, ototoxicity, nausea and vomiting	Thrombocytopenia
Additional medication	Hydration for high dose	No
Solvent	Normal saline or glucose	Glucose
Drug resistance	Easy to produce	Rare and no cross-resistance with cisplatin
Expense per cycle for platinum drugs	¥160.0-200.0 ($23.8-29.8)	¥2800.0-3400.0 ($417.9-507.5)

including chest X-rays, abdominal sonography and bone scans, or positron emission tomography/computed tomography (PET/CT) as an optional substitution to evaluate distant metastases, were also performed based on patient preference and financial capacity. The patients were staged according to the American Joint Committee on Cancer (AJCC, 7th edition) staging system based on the above imaging results.

The following inclusion criteria were applied for enrollment: untreated patients aged 18 to 60 years; stage III or IVa-b disease; histopathologically confirmed WHO type II or III NPC; leukocytes $\geq 4.0\text{X}10\text{E}9$; neutrophils $\geq 1.5\text{X}10\text{E}9$; platelets $\geq 100\text{X}10\text{E}9$; hemoglobin ≥ 90 g/L; aminotransferase $\leq$ 2XUNL; serum creatinine $\leq$ 1.5XUNL; and no evidence of dysfunction in important organs (e.g., heart, lung, liver and kidney) or other malignancies. All participants provided informed consent. Patients who were known or suspected to be allergic to cisplatin, who had uncontrolled infection or a physical disease that could not tolerate chemotherapy/radiotherapy, or who could not coordinate contact for follow-up were excluded. Additionally, pregnant females or patients who underwent immune repressive treatment such as that following organ transplantation were also not admitted. Patients who could not tolerate the treatment toxicities or failed to receive planned treatment due to voluntary refusal or a physician's decision were withdrawn from the study.

From April 1, 2012 to Oct 31, 2012, 59 patients with confirmed undifferentiated nonkeratinizing NPC were enrolled in this study. Their demographic and clinical characteristics before treatment are listed in Table 2. The median age of the participants was 43 years. Forty-three (72.9%) males and 16 (27.1%) females were enrolled. Twenty-two participants (37.3%) had a high serum EBV DNA copy number (>4000 copies/ml) before treatment. Twenty-nine (49.2%) participants with stage III disease and 30 (50.8%) participants with stage IVa-b disease were enrolled.

Treatment

Allocated treatments including two cycles of ICT followed by two cycles of concomitant chemotherapy and radical intensity-modulated radiotherapy (IMRT) to the nasopharynx and neck were delivered to all patients. The ICT consisted of 30 mg/m^2 lobaplatin (intravenous infusion, day 1) and 4 g/m^2 5-fluorouracil (continuous 120-h intravenous injection) during each cycle. The concurrent chemotherapy consisted of 50 mg/m^2 lobaplatin (intravenous infusion, day 1) during each cycle. The interval of cycles was 3 weeks.

Radical IMRT was initiated on the same day as first concomitant chemotherapy. RT prescription doses of 68–70 Gy, 62–68 Gy and 54–60 Gy were delivered to the planning target volume (PTV) of the primary nasopharynx tumor, involved cervical lymph nodes and lymph node-negative areas, respectively. All patients received a regular fraction during RT, five fractions per week and 30–33 fractions in total.

National Cancer Institute (NCI) Common Toxicity Criteria (CTC) V.3.0 were used to determine acute adverse events. The prescription dose of chemotherapy was modified based on the toxicity induced by the previous chemotherapy cycle and was decreased to 75% of the allocated dose when a patient suffered from any of the following toxicities: granulocytopenia fever, platelet count $\leq$ 25,000/μL, or grade 3 nausea and/or vomiting. The prescription dose of

Table 2 Distribution of patient demographics and clinical characteristics before treatment

Characteristics	Patients	
	No.	%
Age, years		
Median	43	
Range	19-59	
Sex		
Male	43	72.9
Female	16	27.1
Histology, WHO type[a]		
III	59	100.0
EBV DNA copy no. (pre-treatment)		
Low (≤4000 copies/ml)	32	54.2
High (>4000 copies/ml)	22	37.3
NA	5	8.5
T stage[b]		
2	4	6.8
3	30	50.8
4	25	42.4
N stage[b]		
0	3	5.1
1	26	44.1
2	23	39.0
3	7	11.9
Clinical stage[b,c]		
III	29	49.2
IVa	23	39.0
IVb	7	11.9
ECOG score		
0	3	5.1
1	56	94.9

Abbreviation ECOG Eastern Cooperative Oncology Group; *NA* not available
[a]III, undifferentiated nonkeratinizing carcinoma
[b]According to the 7th edition AJCC staging system
[c]III, T3N0-2 M0, T1-2N2M0; IVa, T4N0-2 M0; IVb, T1-4N3M0

chemotherapy was decreased to 50% of the planned dose when a patient developed any of the following toxicities: grade 4 or greater nausea and/or vomiting or creatinine clearance around 35–49 ml/min. Prophylactic administration of hematopoietic colony-stimulating factor was performed on days 3–8 of the next chemotherapy cycle in the patients who developed grade 4 granulocytopenia. Chemotherapy was interrupted when patients developed grade 4 hematological, hepatic or kidney toxicity and was administered again if the toxicity decreased to grade 2 or less. Chemotherapy was no longer delivered to patients with a remitted time of over 2 weeks.

Of the 59 participants, 44 (74.6%) completed all cycles of planned chemotherapy, 11 (18.6%) received three cycles of chemotherapy, and four (6.8%) received only two cycles of chemotherapy (Fig. 1).

Assessment of efficacy and follow-up

Efficacy was assessed after two cycles of ICT, after concurrent chemoradiotherapy (CRT) and 3 months after CRT. Treatment response was evaluated based on Response Evaluation Criteria In Solid Tumors (RECIST 1.1). The follow-up frequency for the first 2 years and the 3rd to 5th years was 3 and 6 months, respectively. Regular examinations including physical examinations, indirect nasopharyngoscopy, fiber nasopharyngoscopy, and MRI of the nasopharynx and neck were used for efficacy evaluation and follow-up. Patients with confirmed local recurrence (LR) were diagnosed via MRI and biopsy. Diagnosis of distant metastasis (DM) was confirmed by a regular workup, including CT, MRI, bone scan or PET/CT, and needle biopsy when available. Salvage treatments including re-irradiation, surgery and/or ablation to local lesion and/or systemic chemotherapy were performed in patients with LR or DM as long as they had the indications.

Statistical analysis

SPSS 22.0 (SPSS, Chicago, IL) was used to perform all analyses in this study. A Simon Two-Stages Design was used to determine the sample size. We assumed the ORR to be 80%, and less than 60% was unacceptable. The estimated rate of loss to follow-up was 10%. We set the power to detect the effectiveness of the treatment strategy in our study as 0.9 with a two-sided significance of $P = 0.05$. Accordingly, a total of 59 evaluable patients were required. OS, PFS, LRFS and DMFS were calculated using Kaplan-Meier analysis. All time-to-event end

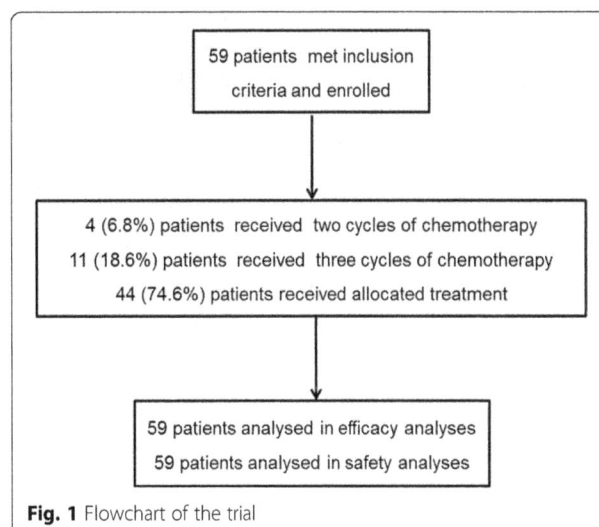

Fig. 1 Flowchart of the trial

points were calculated from the first date of treatment to the date of treatment failure or the last day of follow-up. Patients who developed either DM or LR were followed up until death or until the last scheduled day of follow-up. All efficacy analyses were performed in the intention-to-treat population. All patients who received at least one cycle of chemotherapy were included in the toxicity analysis. This trial was registered with the Chinese Clinical Trials Registry, number ChiCTR-ONC-12002060.

Results

Assessment of treatment efficacy

Fifty-two (88.1%) participants experienced an objective response (OR) after two cycles of ICT, with eight (13.6%) and 44 (74.6%) participants experiencing a complete response (CR) and a partial response (PR), respectively. After a complete course of treatment, all (100%) patients experienced an OR, with 47 (79.7%) and 12 (20.3%) participants experiencing a CR and PR, respectively. Of these 12 participants, seven and four individuals experienced residual disease in the cervical lymph nodes or nasopharynx. One patient had persistent disease in both sites after CRT. Three months after CRT, 51 (86.4%) and two (3.4%) patients experienced CR and PR, respectively, with six patients being lost to follow-up at this time (Table 3). Of the two patients who experienced PR 3 months after CRT, one had residual disease in the nasopharynx and experienced CR 6 months after CRT and the other had persistent and stable disease in the cervical lymph nodes during the close follow-up.

Failure patterns

Over a median follow-up time of 44 months (range from 1 to 47 months), eight (13.6%) patients experienced disease progression, with a range of progression time of 11 to 31 months. Of these patients, two (3.4%) developed local relapse, one in the nasopharynx and the other in the cervical lymph nodes. Moreover, six (10.2%) patients developed DM. The sites of DM were the liver ($n = 1$), the lung ($n = 3$) and

Table 3 Treatment responses in 59 patients

Treatment response	After two cycles of ICT No. (%)	After CRT No. (%)	Three months after CRT No. (%)
Complete response (CR)	8/59(13.6)	47/59(79.7)	51/59(86.4)
Partial response (PR)	44/59(74.6)	12/59(20.3)	2/59(3.4)
Stable disease (SD)	4/59(6.8)	0/59(0)	0/59(0)
Not available	3/59(5.1)	0/59(0)	6/59(10.2)
Objective response (CR + PR)	52/59(88.1)	59/59(100)	53/59(89.8)
95% CI of ORR	(0.77, 0.95)	NA	(0.82, 0.98)

Abbreviation ICT induction chemotherapy; *CRT* concurrent chemoradiotherapy; *CI* confidence interval; *ORR* objective response rate; *NA* not available

multiple organs ($n = 2$). Three (5.1%) patients with DM died of cancer progression, and the OS time ranged from 1 to 15 months.

The 3-year estimated survival rates and the 95% confidence intervals (CIs) for all time-to-event end points are listed in Table 4. Kaplan-Meier survival curves for OS or PFS and DMFS or LRFS are shown in Figs. 2 and 3. The median of all time-to-event end points had not been reached until after the paper was published.

Acute adverse events

During the ICT, the following grade 3–4 acute adverse events occurred in descending order: neutropenia ($n = 5$, 8.5%), leucopenia ($n = 4$, 6.8%), thrombocytopenia ($n = 3$, 5.1%), hepatotoxicity ($n = 2$, 3.4%) and stomatitis ($n = 1$, 1.7%). Likewise, during the CRT, the main grade 3–4 acute adverse events included thrombocytopenia ($n = 24$, 40.7%), leucopenia ($n = 20$, 33.9%), neutropenia ($n = 15$, 25.4%), anemia ($n = 10$, 16.9%), stomatitis ($n = 2$, 3.4%) and hepatotoxicity ($n = 2$, 3.4%). One (1.7%) and two (3.4%) patients developed grade 4 neutropenia during ICT and CRT, respectively. Eight (13.6%) patients developed grade 4 thrombocytopenia after the complete treatment course (Table 5). The duration time of grade 3–4 thrombocytopenia is also listed in Table 5. In addition, among the 15 patients who received only two or three cycles of chemotherapy, chemotherapy was interrupted in 12 and three patients due to persistent thrombocytopenia or leucopenia, respectively, although hematopoietic colony-stimulating factor was administered once myelosuppression occurred.

Discussion

Presently, concurrent chemotherapy with or without ICT is the standard treatment strategy for patients with LA-NPC [25]. Although the survival benefits of ICT have been inconsistent across prior studies, ICT can theoretically shrink local regional tumors and eradicate micrometastases, resulting in reduced RT volume, decreased RT dose needed for organs at risk and a slower rate of DM. Moreover, a prior study showed that changing from adjuvant cisplatin and 5-fluorouracil to induction cisplatin and capecitabine caused a favorable trend of increasing efficacy with

Table 4 Three-year estimates of time-to-event end points

End point	3-Year estimate (%)	95% Confidence interval
Progression-free survival	83.0	(69.8, 98.8)
Overall survival	94.9	(89.5, 100)
Local recurrence-free survival	96.6	(92.1, 100)
Distant metastasis-free survival	89.8	(82.4, 97.9)

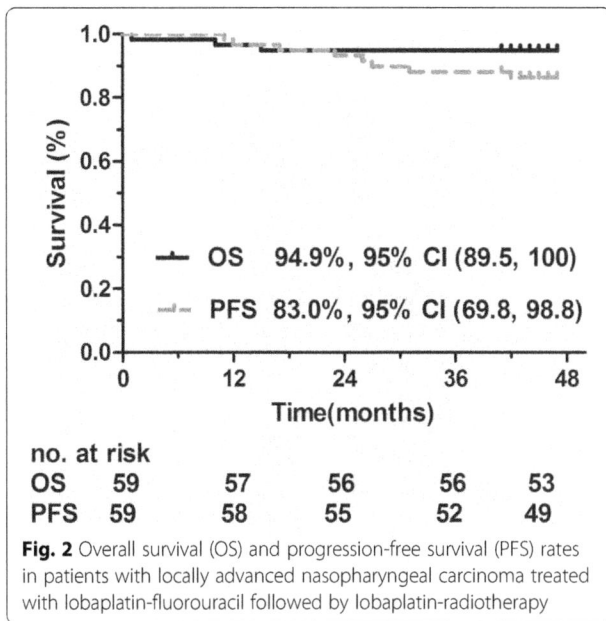

Fig. 2 Overall survival (OS) and progression-free survival (PFS) rates in patients with locally advanced nasopharyngeal carcinoma treated with lobaplatin-fluorouracil followed by lobaplatin-radiotherapy

less toxicity in LA-NPC [8]. Similarly, several phase II/III studies have shown encouraging outcomes following ICT in patients with LA-NPC [5, 8, 14, 15, 26, 27]. Platinum drugs are the most widely used agent for both ICT and CRT in patients with NPC. Lobaplatin is a third-generation platinum agent that shows less gastrointestinal, auricular, liver and renal toxicity than cisplatin or carboplatin [18]. Lobaplatin combined with or without other reagents has shown encouraging or equivalent anti-tumor efficacy but with less toxicity in squamous cell carcinoma than cisplatin [23, 28, 29]. Notably, lobaplatin combined

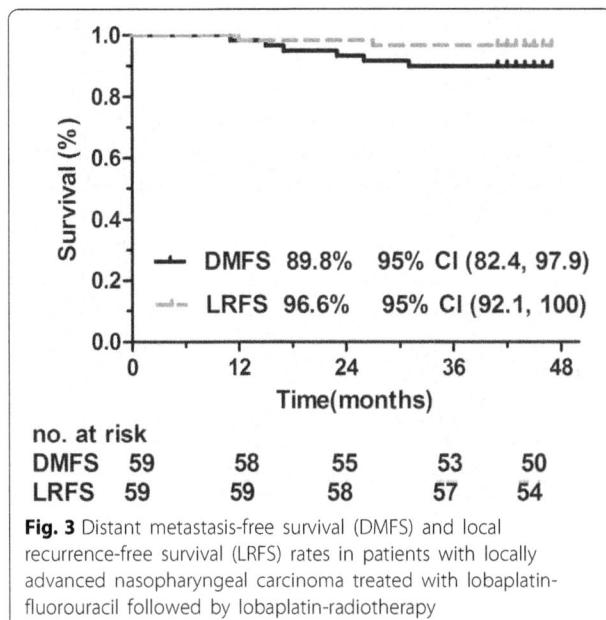

Fig. 3 Distant metastasis-free survival (DMFS) and local recurrence-free survival (LRFS) rates in patients with locally advanced nasopharyngeal carcinoma treated with lobaplatin-fluorouracil followed by lobaplatin-radiotherapy

with docetaxel also showed anti-tumor effects in recurrent or metastatic NPC [24, 30]. However, as the anti-tumor efficacy of lobaplatin as a first-line strategy in LA-NPC was not determined, we conducted the current prospective phase II clinical trial.

In previous studies, ORRs following the addition of different ICT regimens with and without CRT in LA-NPC were 79.4–90.0% and 85.3–100%, respectively, after ICT and a full course of treatment [5, 8, 17, 26]. In the present study, the ORR was encouraging after two cycles of ICT and CRT compared with a previous study in which patients with LA-NPC received cisplatin-5-fluorouracil ICT followed by cisplatin-radiotherapy (88.1% vs. 79.4%, 100% vs. 85.3%, respectively) [31]. Moreover, the 3-year OS and PFS rates of our study are also comparable with previous studies (94.9% vs. 80.0–95.0% and 86.4% vs. 54.0–89.9%) [5, 8, 17, 26, 31]. Although there is a bias in comparing our study with previous reports, we were able to estimate lobaplatin's activity as a first-line reagent in LA-NPC. However, randomized controlled studies are needed to compare the efficacy of lobaplatin and other reagents as a first-line systemic treatment for LA-NPC.

In this study, 74.6% of the patients received allocated cycles of chemotherapy, and the remaining participants received two or three cycles of chemotherapy mainly as a result of grade 3–4 thrombocytopenia, which has been reported as the major dose-limiting toxicity of lobaplatin [20]. Similarly, thrombocytopenia was also the most frequent grade 3–4 toxicity in our study. However, both thrombocytopenia and other hematological toxicities could be cured using hematopoietic colony-stimulating factor, which was acceptable. No grade 3 or 4 nausea or vomiting was observed in our study, and the rate of this complication appeared to be much lower than that following cisplatin-5-fluorouracil ICT treatment (0% vs. 23.5%) [31]. As lobaplatin has no or limited renal toxicity, a high-volume fluid infusion is not required during chemotherapy, which could shorten the inpatient period and improve patient compliance. Moreover, the lack of requirement for fluid infusion would allow patients with renal or cardiac dysfunction to receive this treatment, thus expanding the potential population with LA-NPC who could benefit from systemic chemotherapy.

A main limitation of this study is that it was not blinded. Neither the investigators nor the patients were blinded, which might have introduced observation bias from the investigators and psychological bias from the patients. Moreover, it was a single-arm trial from a single institution; therefore, the

Table 5 Acute adverse events in 59 patients

Adverse events	No. (%) of patients by toxicity grade during ICT				No. (%) of patients by toxicity grade during CRT			
	1	2	3	4	1	2	3	4
Hematological								
Anemia	28(47.5)	4(6.8)	0(0)	0(0)	22(37.3)	13(22.0)	10(16.9)	0(0)
Neutropenia	17(28.8)	17(28.8)	4(6.8)	1(1.7)	13(22.0)	22(37.3)	13(22.0)	2(3.4)
Leucopenia	20(33.9)	14(23.7)	4(6.8)	0(0)	14(23.7)	20(33.9)	20(33.9)	0(0)
Thrombocytopenia	9(15.3)	10(16.9)	3(5.1)	0(0)	4(6.8)	20(33.9)	16(27.1)	8(13.6)
Days of grade 3 or greater thrombocytopenia					≤7	8-14	≥15	
					17(28.8)	6(10.2)	1(1.7)	
Non-hematological								
Allergy	0(0)	0(0)	0(0)	0(0)	0(0)	0(0)	0(0)	0(0)
Weight loss	5(8.5)	0(0)	0(0)	0(0)	33(55.9)	5(8.5)	0(0)	0(0)
Stomatitis (mucositis)	2(3.4)	1(1.7)	1(1.7)	0(0)	49(83.1)	8(13.6)	2(3.4)	0(0)
Nausea	21(35.6)	2(3.4)	0(0)	0(0)	14(23.7)	6(10.2)	0(0)	0(0)
Vomiting	9(15.3)	2(3.4)	0(0)	0(0)	7(11.9)	6(10.2)	0(0)	0(0)
Diarrhea	1(1.7)	0(0)	0(0)	0(0)	1(1.7)	0(0)	0(0)	0(0)
Hepatotoxicity	21(35.6)	3(5.1)	2(3.4)	0(0)	23(39.0)	3(5.1)	2(3.4)	0(0)
Nephrotoxicity	10(16.9)	0(0)	0(0)	0(0)	11(18.6)	0(0)	0(0)	0(0)
Cardiotoxicity	0(0)	0(0)	0(0)	0(0)	0(0)	0(0)	0(0)	0(0)
Ototoxicity	0(0)	0(0)	0(0)	0(0)	10(16.9)	0(0)	0(0)	0(0)
Neurotoxicity	0(0)	0(0)	0(0)	0(0)	0(0)	0(0)	0(0)	0(0)
Joint and muscular ache	0(0)	0(0)	0(0)	0(0)	0(0)	0(0)	0(0)	0(0)
Alopecia	1(1.7)	0(0)	0(0)	0(0)	59(100)	0(0)	0(0)	0(0)

Abbreviation ICT induction chemotherapy; *CRT* concurrent chemoradiotherapy

superiority of lobaplatin over other platinum reagents for treatment of LA-NPC could not be defined, and the efficacy of lobaplatin in other non-endemic areas is also needed. Additionally, six patients were lost to follow-up by 3 months after treatment, leaving the lost-to-follow-up rate (about 10%) higher than in similar studies [7, 32], which might have resulted in bias when forming conclusions. Additionally, long-term follow-up is required to document the long-term efficacy and late toxicities of lobaplatin in patients with LA-NPC.

Altogether, lobaplatin showed promising anti-tumor activity with tolerable toxicity when used as a first-line treatment strategy in patients with LA-NPC; however, it might not be the best choice for patients with a low reserve of bone marrow, such as patients over 60 years old. Moreover, lobaplatin has no cross-over drug resistance with other platinum reagents [18] and therefore can be used as a substitute in patients resistant to other platinum-based agents. However, further randomized controlled trials are needed to determine the anti-tumor efficacy of lobaplatin compared with other chemotherapeutic reagents in patients with LA-NPC and to help define

the best subpopulation that will achieve maximum survival benefits with this drug.

Conclusions

We reported the short-term results produced by administering lobaplatin-5-fluorouracil ICT followed by lobaplatin-RT in patients with LA-NPC. A multi-center phase III randomized controlled trial is currently being undertaken by our group and collaborators to determine the efficacy of lobaplatin-5-fluorouracil followed by lobaplatin-RT vs. cisplatin-5-fluorouracil followed by cisplatin-RT in patients with LA-NPC. At the time of this writing, the patients in this trial were still undergoing follow-up.

Abbreviations
CI: Confidence interval; CRT: Concurrent chemoradiotherapy; DM: Distant metastasis; DMFS: Distant metastasis-free survival; ICT: Induction chemotherapy; LA-NPC: Locally advanced NPC; LR: Local recurrence; LRFS: Local recurrence-free survival; NPC: Nasopharyngeal carcinoma; ORR: Objective response rate; OS: Overall survival; PFS: Progression-free survival; RT: Radiotherapy

Acknowledgements
We thank all the participants for their participation in the study and for their cooperation during follow-up.

Funding

This trial was supported by grants from the National Nature Science Foundation of China [81572665, 81172041, 81472525], the International Cooperation Project of Science and Technology Plan of Guangdong Province [2014A050503033, 2016A050502011], the Science and Technology Plan Project of Guangdong Province [2013B021800141] and the Foundation of Science and Technology Bureau of Guangzhou City [2014Y2-00179]. The first five funders supported the design of the study and data collection. The latter two funders supported data analysis and manuscript writing.

Authors' contributions

XL, XG, and YX designed the study; WQ, XH, JY, YY, GL and HL collected the data; LK, YY and WX analyzed and interpreted the data; and LK prepared the manuscript. All authors read, revised and approved the final manuscript.

Authors' information

Detailed information for the authors can be found on the title page.

Competing interests

The authors declare that they have no competing interests.

Consent for publication

Not applicable.

Author details

[1]Department of Nasopharyngeal Carcinoma, Sun Yat-Sen University Cancer Center, 651 Dongfeng Road East, Guangzhou, Guangdong 510060, China. [2]State Key Laboratory of Oncology in Southern China, Collaborative Innovation Center for Cancer Medicine, Guangzhou, Guangdong 510060, China.

References

1. Cao SM, Simons MJ, Qian CN. The prevalence and prevention of nasopharyngeal carcinoma in China. Chin J Cancer. 2011;30:114–19.
2. Lee N, Harris J, Garden AS, Straube W, Glisson B, Xia P, Bosch W, Morrison WH, Quivey J, Thorstad W, Jones C, Ang KK. Intensity-modulated radiation therapy with or without chemotherapy for nasopharyngeal carcinoma: radiation therapy oncology group phase II trial 0225. J Clin Oncol. 2009;27: 3684–90.
3. Al-Sarraf M, LeBlanc M, Giri PG, Fu KK, Cooper J, Vuong T, Forastiere AA, Adams G, Sakr WA, Schuller DE, Ensley JF. Chemoradiotherapy versus radiotherapy in patients with advanced nasopharyngeal cancer: phase III randomized Intergroup study 0099. J CLIN ONCOL. 1998;16: 1310–17.
4. Lee AW, Ngan RK, Tung SY, Cheng A, Kwong DL, Lu TX, Chan AT, Chan LL, Yiu H, Ng WT, Wong F, Yuen KT, Yau S, Cheung FY, Chan OS, Choi H, Chappell R. Preliminary results of trial NPC-0501 evaluating the therapeutic gain by changing from concurrent-adjuvant to induction-concurrent chemoradiotherapy, changing from fluorouracil to capecitabine, and changing from conventional to accelerated radiotherapy fractionation in patients with locoregionally advanced nasopharyngeal carcinoma. Cancer Am Cancer Soc. 2015; 121:1328–38.
5. Kong L, Hu C, Niu X, Zhang Y, Guo Y, Tham IW, Lu JJ. Neoadjuvant chemotherapy followed by concurrent chemoradiation for locoregionally advanced nasopharyngeal carcinoma: interim results from 2 prospective phase 2 clinical trials. CANCER-AM CANCER SOC. 2013;119:4111–18.
6. Chen L, Hu CS, Chen XZ, Hu GQ, Cheng ZB, Sun Y, Li WX, Chen YY, Xie FY, Liang SB, Chen Y, Xu TT, Li B, Long GX, Wang SY, Zheng BM, Guo Y, Sun Y, Mao YP, Tang LL, Chen YM, Liu MZ, Ma J. Concurrent chemoradiotherapy plus adjuvant chemotherapy versus concurrent chemoradiotherapy alone in patients with locoregionally advanced nasopharyngeal carcinoma: a phase 3 multicentre randomised controlled trial. Lancet Oncol. 2012;13:163–71.
7. Fountzilas G, Ciuleanu E, Bobos M, Kalogera-Fountzila A, Eleftheraki AG, Karayannopoulou G, Zaramboukas T, Nikolaou A, Markou K, Resiga L, Dionysopoulou D, Samantas E, Athanassiou H, Misailidou D, Skarlos D, Ciuleanu T. Induction chemotherapy followed by concomitant radiotherapy and weekly cisplatin versus the same concomitant chemoradiotherapy in patients with nasopharyngeal carcinoma: a randomized phase II study conducted by the Hellenic Cooperative Oncology Group (HeCOG) with biomarker evaluation. Ann Oncol. 2012; 23:427–35.
8. Hui EP, Ma BB, Leung SF, King AD, Mo F, Kam MK, Yu BK, Chiu SK, Kwan WH, Ho R, Chan I, Ahuja AT, Zee BC, Chan AT. Randomized phase II trial of concurrent cisplatin-radiotherapy with or without neoadjuvant docetaxel and cisplatin in advanced nasopharyngeal carcinoma. J CLIN ONCOL. 2009; 27:242–49.
9. Chan AT, Teo PM, Leung TW, Leung SF, Lee WY, Yeo W, Choi PH, Johnson PJ. A prospective randomized study of chemotherapy adjunctive to definitive radiotherapy in advanced nasopharyngeal carcinoma. Int J Radiat Oncol Biol Phys. 1995;33:569–77.
10. International NCSG: Preliminary results of a randomized trial comparing neoadjuvant chemotherapy (cisplatin, epirubicin, bleomycin) plus radiotherapy vs. radiotherapy alone in stage IV (≥N2, M0) undifferentiated nasopharyngeal carcinoma: A positive effect on progression-free survival. Int J Radiat Oncol Biol Phys. 1996;35:463–9.
11. Chua DT, Sham JS, Choy D, Lorvidhaya V, Sumitsawan Y, Thongprasert S, Vootiprux V, Cheirsilpa A, Azhar T, Reksodiputro AH. Preliminary report of the Asian-Oceanian Clinical Oncology Association randomized trial comparing cisplatin and epirubicin followed by radiotherapy versus radiotherapy alone in the treatment of patients with locoregionally advanced nasopharyngeal carcinoma. Asian-Oceanian Clinical Oncology Association Nasopharynx Cancer Study Group. CANCER-AM CANCER SOC. 1998;83:2270–83.
12. Ma J, Mai HQ, Hong MH, Min HQ, Mao ZD, Cui NJ, Lu TX, Mo HY. Results of a prospective randomized trial comparing neoadjuvant chemotherapy plus radiotherapy with radiotherapy alone in patients with locoregionally advanced nasopharyngeal carcinoma. J CLIN ONCOL. 2001;19:1350–57.
13. Chua DT, Ma J, Sham JS, Mai HQ, Choy DT, Hong MH, Lu TX, Min HQ. Long-term survival after cisplatin-based induction chemotherapy and radiotherapy for nasopharyngeal carcinoma: a pooled data analysis of two phase III trials. J CLIN ONCOL. 2005;23:1118–24.
14. Hareyama M, Sakata K, Shirato H, Nishioka T, Nishio M, Suzuki K, Saitoh A, Oouchi A, Fukuda S, Himi T. A prospective, randomized trial comparing neoadjuvant chemotherapy with radiotherapy alone in patients with advanced nasopharyngeal carcinoma. CANCER-AM CANCER SOC. 2002;94: 2217–23.
15. Sun Y, Li WF, Chen NY, Zhang N, Hu GQ, Xie FY, Sun Y, Chen XZ, Li JG, Zhu XD, Hu CS, Xu XY, Chen YY, Hu WH, Guo L, Mo HY, Chen L, Mao YP, Sun R, Ai P, Liang SB, Long GX, Zheng BM, Feng XL, Gong XC, Li L, Shen CY, Xu JY, Guo Y, Chen YM, Zhang F, Lin L, Tang LL, Liu MZ, Ma J. Induction chemotherapy plus concurrent chemoradiotherapy versus concurrent chemoradiotherapy alone in locoregionally advanced nasopharyngeal carcinoma: a phase 3, multicentre, randomised controlled trial. Lancet Oncol. 2016;17:1509–20.
16. Chen Y, Sun Y, Liang SB, Zong JF, Li WF, Chen M, Chen L, Mao YP, Tang LL, Guo Y, Lin AH, Liu MZ, Ma J. Progress report of a randomized trial comparing long-term survival and late toxicity of concurrent chemoradiotherapy with adjuvant chemotherapy versus radiotherapy alone in patients with stage III to IVB nasopharyngeal carcinoma from endemic regions of China. CANCER-AM CANCER SOC. 2013;119:2230–38.
17. Gu MF, Liu LZ, He LJ, Yuan WX, Zhang R, Luo GY, Xu GL, Zhang HM, Yan CX, Li JJ. Sequential chemoradiotherapy with gemcitabine and cisplatin for locoregionally advanced nasopharyngeal carcinoma. Int J Cancer. 2013;132: 215–23.
18. Dilruba S, Kalayda GV. Platinum-based drugs: past, present and future. Cancer Chemother Pharmacol. 2016;77:1103–24.

19. Welink J, Boven E, Vermorken JB, Gall HE, van der Vijgh WJ. Pharmacokinetics and pharmacodynamics of lobaplatin (D-19466) in patients with advanced solid tumors, including patients with impaired renal of liver function. Clin Cancer Res. 1999;5:2349–58.

20. McKeage MJ. Lobaplatin: a new antitumour platinum drug. Expert Opin Investig Drugs. 2001;10:119–28.

21. Perabo FG, Muller SC. New agents for treatment of advanced transitional cell carcinoma. Ann Oncol. 2007;18:835–43.

22. Li X, Li Y. Clinical study on chemotherapy of lobaplatin combined with docetaxel in patients with relapsed ovarian cancer. Zhong Nan Da Xue Xue Bao Yi Xue Ban. 2014;39:1131–36.

23. Li WP, Liu H, Chen L, Yao YQ, Zhao EF. A clinical comparison of lobaplatin or cisplatin with mitomycine and vincristine in treating patients with cervical squamous carcinoma. Asian Pac J Cancer Prev. 2015;16:4629–31.

24. Long GX, Lin JW, Liu DB, Zhou XY, Yuan XL, Hu GY, Mei Q, Hu GQ. Single-arm, multi-centre phase II study of lobaplatin combined with docetaxel for recurrent and metastatic nasopharyngeal carcinoma patients. Oral Oncol. 2014;50:717–20.

25. Lin JC, Jan JS, Hsu CY, Liang WM, Jiang RS, Wang WY. Phase III study of concurrent chemoradiotherapy versus radiotherapy alone for advanced nasopharyngeal carcinoma: positive effect on overall and progression-free survival. J CLIN ONCOL. 2003;21:631–37.

26. Airoldi M, Gabriele AM, Garzaro M, Raimondo L, Condello C, Beatrice F, Pecorari G, Giordano C. Induction chemotherapy with cisplatin and epirubicin followed by radiotherapy and concurrent cisplatin in locally advanced nasopharyngeal carcinoma observed in a non-endemic population. Radiother Oncol. 2009;92:105–10.

27. Hong RL, Ting LL, Ko JY, Hsu MM, Sheen TS, Lou PJ, Wang CC, Chung NN, Lui LT. Induction chemotherapy with mitomycin, epirubicin, cisplatin, fluorouracil, and leucovorin followed by radiotherapy in the treatment of locoregionally advanced nasopharyngeal carcinoma. J CLIN ONCOL. 2001; 19:4305–13.

28. Wang JQ, Wang T, Shi F, Yang YY, Su J, Chai YL, Liu Z. A Randomized Controlled Trial Comparing Clinical Outcomes and Toxicity of Lobaplatin-Versus Cisplatin-Based Concurrent Chemotherapy Plus Radiotherapy and High-Dose-Rate Brachytherapy for FIGO Stage II and III Cervical Cancer. Asian Pac J Cancer Prev. 2015;16:5957–61.

29. Yang JS, Wang T, Qiu MQ, Li QL. Comparison of efficacy and toxicity profiles between paclitaxel/lobapoatin- and cisplatin/5-fluorouracil-based concurrent chemoradiotherapy of advanced inoperable oesophageal cancer. Intern Med J. 2015;45:757–61.

30. Zhang S, Chen J, Yang S, Lin S. An open-label, single-arm phase II clinical study of docetaxel plus lobaplatin for Chinese patients with pulmonary and hepatic metastasis of nasopharyngeal carcinoma. Anticancer Drugs. 2016;27: 685–88.

31. Ferrari D, Chiesa F, Codeca C, Calabrese L, Jereczek-Fossa BA, Alterio D, Fiore J, Luciani A, Floriani I, Orecchia R, Foa P. Locoregionally advanced nasopharyngeal carcinoma: induction chemotherapy with cisplatin and 5-fluorouracil followed by radiotherapy and concurrent cisplatin: a phase II study. Oncology Basel. 2008;74:158–66.

32. Songthong AP, Kannarunimit D, Chakkabat C, Lertbutsayanukul C. A randomized phase II/III study of adverse events between sequential (SEQ) versus simultaneous integrated boost (SIB) intensity modulated radiation therapy (IMRT) in nasopharyngeal carcinoma; preliminary result on acute adverse events. Radiat Oncol. 2015;10:166.

33. Himmelstein KJ, Patton TF, Belt RJ, Taylor S, Repta AJ, Sternson LA. Clinical kinetics on intact cisplatin and some related species. Clin Pharmacol Ther. 1981;29:658–64.

7

Development and external validation of nomograms to predict the risk of skeletal metastasis at the time of diagnosis and skeletal metastasis-free survival in nasopharyngeal carcinoma

Lin Yang[1,2,3†] , Liangping Xia[1,2,3†], Yan Wang[1,2,3†], Shasha He[1,2,3], Haiyang Chen[4], Shaobo Liang[5], Peijian Peng[6], Shaodong Hong[1,2,3*] and Yong Chen[1,2,3*]

Abstract

Background: The skeletal system is the most common site of distant metastasis in nasopharyngeal carcinoma (NPC); various prognostic factors have been reported for skeletal metastasis, though most studies have focused on a single factor. We aimed to establish nomograms to effectively predict skeletal metastasis at initial diagnosis (SMAD) and skeletal metastasis-free survival (SMFS) in NPC.

Methods: A total of 2685 patients with NPC who received bone scintigraphy (BS) and/or 18F–deoxyglucose positron emission tomography/computed tomography (18F–FDG PET/CT) and 2496 patients without skeletal metastasis were retrospectively assessed to develop individual nomograms for SMAD and SMFS. The models were validated externally using separate cohorts of 1329 and 1231 patients treated at two other institutions.

Results: Five independent prognostic factors were included in each nomogram. The SMAD nomogram had a significantly higher c-index than the TNM staging system (training cohort, $P = 0.005$; validation cohort, $P < 0.001$). The SMFS nomogram had significantly higher c-index values in the training and validation sets than the TNM staging system ($P < 0.001$ and $P = 0.005$, respectively). Three proposed risk stratification groups were created using the nomograms, and enabled significant discrimination of SMFS for each risk group.

Conclusion: The prognostic nomograms established in this study enable accurate stratification of distinct risk groups for skeletal metastasis, which may improve counseling and facilitate individualized management of patients with NPC.

Keywords: Nasopharyngeal carcinoma, Skeletal metastasis at the time of diagnosis (SMAD), Skeletal metastasis free survival (SMFS), Prognosis, Nomograms

* Correspondence: hongshd@sysucc.org.cn; chenyong@sysucc.org.cn
†Equal contributors
[1]Sun Yat sen University Cancer Center, 651 East Dong Feng Road, Guangzhou 510060, China
Full list of author information is available at the end of the article

Background

Nasopharyngeal carcinoma (NPC) is a malignant head and neck cancer with a distinct ethnic and geographic pattern of distribution; the highest incidences of NPC (30–80 cases per 10,000/year) are observed in southern China and South East Asia [1]. Developments in advanced imaging modalities and instrumentation have enabled more precise tumor staging. Currently, approximately 5–8% of cases of NPC have distant metastasis (M1) at first diagnosis; the skeleton is the most common distant metastasis site, representing 70% to 80% cases of M1 disease [2–4]. Distant metastasis at diagnosis is associated with poorer survival outcomes and reduced quality of life. Moreover, research on M1 disease is sparse due to the poor survival outcomes of patients with skeletal metastases. However, increasing evidence indicates long-term survival and even a complete response can be achieved among a small proportion of patients with skeletal metastases, especially those who receive aggressive treatment [5]. This indicates different treatment methods could significantly improve the prognosis of selected high-risk M1 cases. However, solely relying on the TNM classification to predict the outcomes of patients with skeletal metastasis may result in inaccurate assessment, leading to unnecessary treatment and financial burdens or – even worse – the patient receiving a suboptimal treatment strategy. Moreover, individualized follow-up and treatment strategies may be required for specific subgroups of patients with different risks of skeletal metastasis.

Bone scintigraphy (BS) remains is the leading diagnostic method for bone metastasis during initial work-up as it is widely available and low cost. However, BS is not routinely conducted during follow-up as it has a low diagnostic sensitivity, especially for early bone metastatic lesions; metastases mainly located in the bone marrow are frequently not detected by BS [6]. Although 18F–FDG PET/CT has a higher sensitivity than BS for detecting bone metastases in primary NPC, 18F–FDG PET/CT technique is expensive [7]. However, differentiation of malignant and benign lesions on BS and 18F–FDG PET remains problematic, even for experienced nuclear physicians.

As far as we are aware, research on the frequency of bone metastases at initial diagnosis (SMAD) and skeletal metastasis-free survival (SMFS) in NPC is rare and narrowly-focused [8–11]. The lack of such data hampers accurate patient staging and risk stratification and delays the design of more reliable treatment protocols, as the M1 category is a "catch-all" classification that includes patients whose treatment response could be potentially curable or incurable. Identifying subgroups of patients with different risks of bone metastasis could help determine the appropriate imaging techniques and follow-up timing in a more personalized manner. Furthermore, more accurate prediction of the risk of skeletal metastasis could provide valuable decision-making information for clinicians and patients.

Nomograms incorporate a variety of important factors and have been demonstrated to be reliable prediction tools for quantifying individual risk in cancer. Nomograms can provide more precise prognoses than the traditional TNM staging system in several tumor types. To date, there has been no attempt to establish nomograms to predict SMAD and SMFS in NPC. We hypothesized nomograms combining T category, N category and other objective laboratory indexes could generate more accurate predictive models for SMAD and SMFS. Therefore, we assessed the prognostic risk factors for SMAD and SMFS in a large cohort of patients with NPC and validated the resulting nomograms using an external cohort treated at two other institutions.

Methods

Training cohort

The training cohort was derived from patients treated at Sun Yat-sen University Cancer Center between and December, 2012. The inclusion criteria were: (i) pathologically confirmed NPC; (ii) complete pretreatment clinical information and laboratory data; (iii) BS and/or 18F–FDG PET/CT at diagnosis of NPC; and (iv) complete follow-up data. Exclusion criteria were incomplete follow-up data, death due to non-NPC-associated accident, or previous/synchronous malignant tumors. Ethical approval was obtained from the institutional review boards. The requirement for informed consent was waived as this was a retrospective study. The study protocol complied with the Declaration of Helsinki and was approved by the Ethics Committee of Sun Yat-sen University Cancer Center.

A standardized form was designed to retrieve all relevant data, including sociodemographic data (age, gender, smoking history, alcohol exposure, family history of malignant tumors, family history of NPC); baseline laboratory data including plasma Epstein-Barr virus (EBV) DNA copy number, serum calcium, serum magnesium, serum phosphorus, serum albumin(ALB), serum globulin (GLB), serum aspartate transaminase (AST), serum alanine transaminase (ALT), serum alkaline phosphatase (ALP), serum lactate dehydrogenase (LDH), serum C-reactive protein (CRP); T category [primary tumor location, size, extension], N category [number/location of lymph node metastases); and treatment data (radiotherapy technique, fractions, dosage; chemotherapy). Clinical stage was assessed using the seventh edition of the AJCC/UICC TNM staging system.

Treatment

All patients were treated using definitive radiotherapy (RT). The dose ranges for the nasopharynx, node-positive region and node-negative regions were 60–80, 60–70, and 50–60 Gy, respectively. Patients with stage I or II NPC did not receive chemotherapy; patients with stage III or IV

NPC received induction, concurrent or adjuvant chemotherapy (or a combination of these strategies) as recommended by the institutional guidelines. Induction or adjuvant chemotherapy were cisplatin with 5-fluorouracil; cisplatin with taxoids; or cisplatin, 5-fluorouracil and taxoids (every 3 weeks; two to three cycles). Concurrent chemotherapy was cisplatin in weeks 1, 4 and 7 of radiotherapy or cisplatin weekly.

Validation cohort

To examine the general applicability of the model, an independent external validation cohort of 1329 consecutive patients with NPC who received definitive radiotherapy at the Fifth affiliated hospital of Sun-Yat Sen University and the First hospital of the Foshan between January, 2006 and December, 2012 were included. Inclusion and exclusion were the same as the training cohort. Sufficient data was available for all patients to score all variables in the nomograms established in this study.

Statistical analysis

SMAD was defined as the presence of skeletal metastasis on BS or 18F–FDG PET/CT at initial diagnosis (before receiving any treatment). SMFS was measured as time from diagnosis to detection of skeletal metastasis or censorship at last follow-up. In the training set, continuous variables were expressed as mean (± standard deviation), medians and ranges were transformed into dichotomous variables using the median value. Categorical variables were compared using the chi-square test or Fisher's exact test; categorical/continuous variables, univariate logistic regression. Variables achieving significance at the level of $P < 0.05$ were entered into multivariate logistic regression analyses via stepwise procedures. In the training set, survival curves for different variables were plotted using the Kaplan-Meier method and compared using the log-rank test. Significant variables ($P < 0.05$) were entered into the Cox proportional hazards multivariate analyses to identify independent prognostic factors via forward stepwise procedures ($P < 0.05$). Statistical data analyses were performed using SPSS 22.0 (SPSS, Chicago, IL, USA).

Based on multivariate analyses, nomograms were generated to provide visualized risk prediction using the survival and rms packages of R 2.14.1 (http://www.r-project.org). Nomograms were subjected to bootstrap resampling ($n = 1000$) for interval and external validation to correct the concordance index (c-index) and explain variance with respect to over-optimism. The ability of the nomograms and TNM staging system to predict survival were compared using the c-index, a variable equivalent to the area under curve (AUC) of receiver operating characteristic curves for censored data. The maximum c-index value is 1.0, which indicates perfect prediction, while 0.5 indicates the probability of correctly predicting the outcomes by

random chance. The nomogram and TNM staging system were compared using rcorrp.cens in the Hmisc module of R. The nomogram for 1-, 3-, and 5-year SMFS was calibrated by comparing predicted and actual observed survival rates. During external validation, the nomogram point scores were calculated for individual patients, then Cox regression analysis was performed using total point scores as a predictor in the validation cohort.

In addition to numerically comparing discriminative ability by c-index, we also attempted to confirm the superior independent discriminative ability of the nomograms over the standard TNM staging system. The training cohort were evenly grouped into three risk groups by nomogram score, then we investigated the predictive ability of the risk stratification cut-off points and different subgroups (TNM stage) using Kaplan-Meier survival curve analysis. A two-sided P value <0.05 was deemed significant. Details of the R code used to generate the nomograms can be assessed in the additional information online (Additional file 1). This trial was registered with Clinical Trials.Gov (NCT00705627); all data has been deposited at Sun Yat-sen University Cancer Center for future reference (number RDD RDDA2017000293).

Results
Patient characteristics and survival

A total of 2685 and 1329 patients in the training and external validation cohorts were eligible for the SMAD analyses (Additional file 2: Figure S1). Median age was 45-years-old (range, 23 to 78-years-old) for the training cohort and 45-years-old (range, 19 to 70-years-old) for the validation cohort. After excluding patients with distant metastasis at diagnosis, 2469 and 1231 patients were included in the analyses for SMFS. Median follow-up for SMFS in the training cohort was 65.0 months and 61.8 months in the validation cohort. Five-year SMFS was 86% in the training cohort and 85.4.0% in the validation cohort. In both cohorts, a total of 391 patients (9.7%) developed skeletal metastases after initial diagnosis, and 287 patients (7.7%) were confirmed to have skeletal metastases at initial diagnosis. The characteristics of the cohorts are summarized in Table 1 and Additional file 3: Table S1.

Univariate and multivariate analyses

The factors associated with significantly poorer SMAD included in the univariate logistic regression model were sex (male); elevated LDH, CRP, ALP, platelets, monocytes, neutrophils and plasma EBV DNA; decreased hemoglobin (HGB) and ALB; and advanced clinical N category. All significant variables were entered into multivariate logistic regression; ALP, LDH, HGB, plasma EBV DNA and N category retained independent prognostic significance for SMAD.

Table 1 Associations between the clinical and laboratory characteristics of the patients and SMAD as indicated by the chi-square test or Fisher's exact test

Characteristic	Number (%)	Training cohort SMAD		P-value	Validation cohort Number (%)
		Absent	Present		
Age, years				0.379	
< 45	1404 (52.3%)	1311 (93.4%)	93 (6.6%)		679 (51.1%)
≥ 45	1281 (47.7%)	1185 (92.5%)	96 (7.5%)		650 (48.9%)
Sex				0.025	
Male	2131 (79.4%)	1969 (92.4%)	162 (7.6%)		986 (74.2%)
Female	554 (20.6%)	527 (95.1%)	27 (4.9%)		343 (25.8%)
Smoking Status				0.055	
Absent	1708 (63.3%)	1600 (93.7%)	108 (6.3%)		795 (59.8%)
Present	977 (36.4%)	896 (91.7%)	81 (8.3%)		534 (40.2%)
Drinking Status				0.873	
Absent	2382 (88.7%)	2215 (93.0%)	167 (7.0%)		1117 (84.0%)
Present	303 (11.3%)	281 (92.7%)	22 (7.3%)		212 (16.0%)
Family history				0.566	
Absent	1926 (71.7%)	1787 (92.8%)	139 (7.2%)		967 (72.8%)
Present	759 (28.3%)	709 (93.4%)	50 (6.6%)		362 (27.2%)
Calcium, mmol/L				0.932	
< 2.4	1370 (51.0%)	1273 (92.9%)	97 (7.1%)		501 (37.7%)
≥ 2.4	1315 (49.0%)	1223 (93.0%)	92 (7.0%)		828 (62.3%)
Phosphorus, mmol/L				0.587	
< 1.15	1398 (52.1%)	1296 (92.7%)	102 (7.3%)		676 (50.9%)
≥ 1.15	1287 (47.9%)	1200 (93.2%)	87 (6.8%)		653 (49.1%)
Magnesium, mmol/L				0.308	
< 0.93	1410 (52.2%)	1304 (92.5%)	106 (7.5%)		919 (69.1%)
≥ 0.93	1275 (47.5%)	1192 (93.5%)	83 (6.5%)		410 (30.9%)
CRP, mg/L				< 0.001	
< 1.91	1345 (50.1%)	1283 (95.4%)	62 (4.6%)		722 (54.3%)
≥ 1.91	1340 (49.9%)	1213 (90.5%)	127 (9.5%)		607 (45.7%)
WBCs, ×10^9				0.137	
< 6.9	1376 (51.2%)	1289 (93.7%)	87 (6.3%)		677 (50.9%)
≥ 6.9	1309 (48.8%)	1207 (92.2%)	102 (7.8%)		652 (49.1%)
Neutrophils, ×10^9				0.001	
< 4.2	1356 (50.5%)	1283 (94.6%)	73 (5.4%)		691 (52.0%)
≥ 4.2	1329 (49.5%)	1213 (91.3%)	116 (8.7%)		638 (48.0%)
HGB, g/L				0.007	
< 145	1379 (51.4%)	1264 (91.7%)	115 (8.3%)		758 (57.0%)
≥ 145	1306 (48.6%)	1232 (94.3%)	74 (5.7%)		571 (43.0%)
Platelets, ×10^9				0.013	
< 229	1343 (50.0%)	1265 (94.2%)	78 (5.8%)		638 (48.0%)
≥ 229	1342 (50.0%)	1231 (91.7%)	111 (8.3%)		691 (52.0%)
ALT, U/L				0.392	
< 22.2	1345 (50.1%)	1256 (93.4%)	89 (6.6%)		725 (54.6%)

Table 1 Associations between the clinical and laboratory characteristics of the patients and SMAD as indicated by the chi-square test or Fisher's exact test *(Continued)*

≥ 22.2	1340 (49.9%)	1240 (92.5%)	100 (7.5%)		604 (45.4%)
AST, U/L				0.092	
< 21	1366 (50.9)	1281 (93.8%)	85 (6.2%)		675 (50.8%)
≥ 21	1319 (49.1)	1215 (92.1%)	104 (7.9%)		654 (49.2%)
ALP, U/L				< 0.001	
< 70	1357 (50.5%)	1304 (96.1%)	53 (3.9%)		744 (56.0%)
≥ 70	1328 (49.5%)	1192 (89.8%)	136 (10.2%)		585 (44.0%)
LDH, U/L				< 0.001	
< 172.2	1344 (50.1%)	1287 (95.8%)	57 (4.2%)		706 (53.1%)
≥ 172.2	1341 (49.9%)	1209 (90.2%)	132 (9.8%)		623 (46.9%)
ALB, g/L				0.003	
< 44.9	1351 (50.3%)	1236 (91.5%)	115 (8.5%)		576 (43.3%)
≥ 44.9	1334 (49.7%)	1260 (94.5%)	74 (5.5%)		753 (56.7%)
GLB, g/L				0.507	
< 30.5	1341 (49.9%)	1251 (93.3%)	90 (6.7%)		793 (59.7%)
≥ 30.5	1344 (50.1%)	1245 (92.6%)	99 (7.4%)		536 (40.3%)
Cholesterol, mmol/L				0.054	
< 5.12	1353 (50.4%)	1245 (92.0%)	108 (8.0%)		576 (43.3%)
≥ 5.2	1332 (49.6%)	1251 (93.9%)	81 (6.1%)		753 (56.7%)
T lymphocytes, ×10^9				0.289	
< 1.8	1392 (51.8%)	1287 (92.5%)	105 (7.5%)		622 (46.8%)
≥ 1.8	1293 (48.2%)	1209 (93.5%)	84 (6.5%)		707 (53.2%)
Monocytes, ×10^9				0.005	
< 0.4	1385 (51.6%)	1306 (94.3%)	79 (5.7%)		462 (34.8%)
≥ 0.4	1300 (48.4%)	1190 (91.5%)	110 (8.5%)		867 (65.2%)
Pathology				0.852	
Undifferentiated	2592 (96.5%)	2410 (93.0%)	182 (7.0%)		1300 (97.8%)
Differentiated	93 (3.5%)	86 (92.5%)	7 (7.5%)		29 (2.2%)
Cranial nerve injury				0.730	
Absent	2498 (93.0%)	2321 (92.9%)	177 (7.1%)		1234 (92.9%)
Present	187 (7.0%)	175 (93.6%)	12 (6.4%)		95 (7.1%)
EBV-DNA, copies/ml				< 0.001	
< 1000	1130 (42.1%)	1092 (96.6%)	38 (3.4%)		526 (39.6%)
1000–9999	585 (21.8%)	555 (94.9%)	30 (5.1%)		265 (19.9%)
10,000–99,999	599 (22.3%)	555 (92.7%)	44 (23.3%)		325 (24.5%)
100,000–999,999	290 (10.8%)	245 (84.5%)	45 (15.5%)		156 (11.7%)
≥ 1,000,000	81 (3.0%)	49 (60.5%)	32 (39.5%)		57 (4.3%)
T category				0.804	
1	167 (6.2%)	158 (94.6%)	37 (5.4%)		81 (6.1%)
2	525 (19.6%)	488 (93.0%)	37 (7.0%)		328 (24.7%)
3	1374 (51.2%)	1278 (93.0%)	96 (7.0%)		630 (47.4%)
4	619 (23.1%)	572 (92.4%)	47 (7.6%)		290 (21.8%)
N category				< 0.001	
0	319 (11.9%)	312 (97.8%)	7 (2.2%)		250 (18.8%)

Table 1 Associations between the clinical and laboratory characteristics of the patients and SMAD as indicated by the chi-square test or Fisher's exact test *(Continued)*

1	921 (34.3%)	887 (96.3%)	34 (3.7%)		449 (33.8%)
2	775 (28.9%)	697 (89.9%)	78 (10.1%)		370 (27.8%)
3	549 (20.4%)	494 (90.0%)	55 (10.0%)		243 (18.3%)
4	121 (4.5%)	106 (87.6%)	15 (12.4%)		17 (1.3%)
Radiotherapy technique				0.451	
IMRT +3DCRT	1341(49.9%)	1252 (93.4%)	89 (6.6%)		705(65.9%)
CRT	1344(51.1%)	1244 (92.6%)	100 (7.4%)		624(34.1%)
Treatment method				$P < 0.001$	
Radiotherapy	505(18.8%)	481 (95.2%)	24 (4.8%)		318 (24.1%)
CCRT	1136 (42.3%)	1086 (95.6%)	50(4.4%)		425 (32.2%)
Neo + radiotherapy	483 (18.0%)	419 (86.7%)	64 (13.3%)		265 (20.1%)
Neo + CCRT	561(20.9%)	510 (90.9%)	51(9.1%)		311 (23.5%)
SMAD					
Absent	2496 (93.0%)				1231 (92.6%)
Present	189 (7%)				98 (7.4%)

Abbreviations: SMAD skeletal metastasis at time of diagnosis, *WBCs* white blood cells, *HGB* hemoglobin, *GLB* globulin, *ALB* albumin, *ALT* alanine transaminase, *AST* aspartate transaminase, *ALP* alkaline phosphatase, *LDH* lactate dehydrogenase, *CRP* C-reactive protein, *GGT* gamma glutamyl transpeptidase, *EBV-DNA* Epstein-Barr virus DNA, *Undifferentiated* undifferentiated non-keratinizing carcinoma, *Differentiated* differentiated carcinoma, *CRT* conventional radiotherapy, *IMRT* intensity modulated radiation therapy, *3D–CRT* three dimensional conformal radiation therapy, *RT* radiotherapy, *CCRT* concurrent radiotherapy, *Neo* neoadjuvant chemotherapy

The factors associated with significantly poorer SMFS in the univariate Cox regression models were advanced age; elevated LDH, CRP, ALP, monocytes and plasma EBV-DNA; decreased globulin (GLB) and ALB; and advanced clinical N category. ALP, LDH, CRP, plasma EBV DNA and N category retained independent prognostic value in multivariate logistic regression. Detailed summaries of the multivariate analyses are shown in Tables 2 and 3.

Nomograms for predicting SMAD and SMFS

The independent prognostic factors for SMAD and SMFS were used to construct nomograms (Fig. 1). Each variable was assigned a score. By determining the total score for all variables on the total point scale, the probabilities of specific outcomes could be determined by drawing a vertical line from the total score. Plasma EBV DNA copy number was the most important factor for prediction of both SMAD and SMFS.

In the training cohort, the SMAD nomogram had a bootstrap-corrected c-index of 0.83 (95% CI, 0.78–0.87), significantly higher than the TNM classification (0.73; 95% CI, 0.70–0.77; $P = 0.005$). The c-index of the nomogram for SMFS (0.70; 95% CI, 0.67–0.74) was also significantly higher than the TNM classification (0.59; 95% CI, 0.56–0.63; $P < 0.001$). In the external validation cohort, the c-index value of the nomogram for SMAD was 0.76 (95% CI, 0.71–0.79) and 0.61 (95% CI, 0.55–0.66) for SMFS; both of which were significantly better

than the c-index values for the TNM classification with respect to SMAD (0.64; 95% CI, 0.60–0.67; $P < 0.001$) and SMFS (0.58; 95% CI, 0.54–0.63; $P = 0.005$), respectively (Table 4).

The calibration plots demonstrated good agreement between the nomogram predictions and actual 1-, 3-, and 5-year SMFS rates observed in both the training and the validation cohorts (Fig. 2).

Nomograms for risk stratification

We determined the cut-off values for the nomogram-generated scores by which the patients in the training cohort could be stratified into three risk groups. Each group had a distinct prognosis (Additional file 3: Table S2). This stratification could effectively predict SMFS for the three proposed risk groups in both the training and validation cohorts (Fig. 3). The risk stratification even provided significant distinction between the Kaplan-Meier SMFS curves for each of the three risk groups within each TNM stage (Fig. 3).

Discussion

This is the first study to retrospectively assess a very large number of patients with NPC to evaluate the prognostic value of a wide range of clinical and laboratory parameters in order to establish effective prognostic tools for skeletal metastasis. The nomograms established in this analysis demonstrated superior discriminative ability compared to the TMM classification of the

Table 2 Associations between the clinical and laboratory characteristics of the patients and SMAD in univariate and multivariate logistic regression analysis

Characteristic	Univariate			Multivariate		
	HR	95% CI	P-value	HR	95% CI	P-value
Age (≥ 45 vs. < 45 years)	1.142	0.850–1.535	0.379			
Gender (Male vs. Female)	0.623	0.410–0.946	0.027			
Smoking Status (Present vs. Absent)	1.139	0.993–1.807	0.056			
Drinking Status (Present vs. Absent)	1.038	0.655–1.647	0.873			
Family history (Present vs. Absent)	0.907	0.649–1.267	0.566			
Calcium, mmol/L (≥ 2.4 vs. < 2.4)	0.987	0.734–1.327	0.932			
Phosphorus, mmol/L (≥ 1.15 vs. < 1.15)	0.921	0.685–1.239	0.587			
Magnesium, mmol/L (≥ 0.93 vs. < 0.93)	0.857	0.636–1.154	0.308			
CRP, mg/L (≥ 1.91 vs. < 1.91)	2.167	1.583–2.965	< 0.001			
WBCs, ×10^9 (≥ 6.9 vs. < 6.9)	1.252	0.931–1.684	0.137			
Neutrophils, ×10^9 (≥ 4.2 vs. < 4.2)	1.681	1.241–2.276	0.001			
HGB, g/L (≥ 145 vs. < 145)	0.660	0.488–0.893	0.007	0.672	0.477–0.948	0.023
Platelets, ×10^9 (≥ 229 vs. < 229)	1.462	1.083–1.974	0.013			
ALT, U/L (≥ 22.2 vs. < 22.2)	1.138	0.846–1.530	0.392			
AST, U/L (≥ 21 vs. < 21)	1.290	0.958–1.736	0.093			
ALP, U/L (≥ 70 vs. < 70)	2.807	2.024–3.893	< 0.001	2.148	1.509–3.056	< 0.001
LDH, U/L (≥ 172.2 vs. < 172.2)	2.465	1.789–3.396	< 0.001	1.512	1.069–2.139	0.019
ALB, g/L (≥ 44.9 vs. < 44.9)	0.631	0.466–0.854	0.003			
GLB, g/L (≥ 30.5 vs. < 30.5)	1.105	0.822–1.486	0.507			
Cholesterol, mmol/L (≥ 5.12 vs. < 5.12)	0.746	0.554–1.006	0.055			
T lymphocytes, ×10^9 (≥ 1.8 vs. < 1.8)	0.852	0.632–1.147	0.290			
Monocytes, ×10^9 (≥ 0.4 vs. < 0.4)	1.528	1.133–2.062	0.006			
Pathology (Differentiated vs. Undifferentiated	1.078	0.492–2.363	0.852			
Cranial nerve injury (Absent vs. Present)	0.899	0.491–1.646	0.899			
EBV-DNA, copies/ml			< 0.001			< 0.001
< 1000	1.000	1.000		1.000	1.000	
1000–9999	1.553	0.952–2.534	0.078	1.293	0.784–2.131	0.314
10,000–99,999	2.278	1.459–3.558	< 0.001	1.588	0.998–2.530	0.051
100,000–999,999	5.278	3.354–8.307	< 0.001	3.234	1.982–5.279	< 0.001
≥ 1,000,000	18.767	10.822–32.544	< 0.001	10.703	5.876–19.498	< 0.001
T category			0.805			
1	1.000	1.000				
2	1.331	0.629–2.818	0.455			
3	1.319	0.653–2.663	0.440			
4	1.443	0.692–3.007	0.328			
N category			< 0.001			0.002
0	1.000	1.000		1.000	1.000	
1	1.708	0.750–3.893	0.202	1.292	0.559–2.984	0.549
2	4.988	2.276–10.933	< 0.001	2.924	1.304–6.557	0.009
3	4.962	2.232–11.035	< 0.001	2.299	0.996–5.306	0.051
4	6.307	2.504–15.887	< 0.001	2.606	0.983–6.905	0.054

Abbreviations: SMAD skeletal metastasis at the time of diagnosis, *WBCs* white blood cells, *HGB* hemoglobin, *GLB* globulin, *ALB* albumin, *ALT* alanine transaminase, *AST* aspartate transaminase, *ALP* alkaline phosphatase, *LDH* lactate dehydrogenase, *CRP* C-reactive protein, *GGT* gamma glutamyl transpeptidase, *EBV-DNA* Epstein-Barr virus DNA, *Undifferentiated* undifferentiated non-keratinizing carcinoma, *Differentiated* differentiated carcinoma

Table 3 Associations between the clinical and laboratory characteristics of the patients and SMFS in univariate and multivariate logistic regression analysis

Characteristic	Univariate			Multivariate		
	HR	95% CI	P-value	HR	95% CI	P-value
Age (≥ 45 vs. < 45 years)	1.288	1.008–1.647	0.043			
Gender (Male vs. Female)	0.867	0.635–1.184	0.371			
Smoking Status (Present vs. Absent)	1.120	0.871–1.440	0.376			
Drinking Status (Present vs. Absent)	0.911	0.615–1.349	0.642			
Family history (Present vs. Absent)	0.831	0.627–1.010	0.198			
Calcium, mmol/L (≥ 2.4 vs. < 2.4)	0.927	0.725–1.186	0.548			
Phosphorus, mmol/L (≥ 1.15 vs. < 1.15)	0.927	0.725–1.185	0.545			
Magnesium, mmol/L (≥ 0.93 vs. < 0.93)	0.804	0.552–1.172	0.257			
CRP, mg/L (≥ 1.91 vs. < 1.91)	2.092	1.618–2.706	< 0.001	1.450	1.108–1.897	0.007
WBCs, ×10^9 (≥ 6.9 vs. < 6.9)	1.050	0.822–1.342	0.694			
Neutrophils, ×10^9 (≥ 4.2 vs. < 4.2)	1.177	0.921–1.504	0.193			
HGB, g/L (≥ 145 vs. < 145)	0.835	0.653–1.068	0.150			0.023
Platelets, ×10^9 (≥ 229 vs. < 229)	1.134	0.887–1.449	0.315			
ALT, U/L (≥ 22.2 vs. < 22.2)	0.971	0.760–1.241	0.814			
AST, U/L (≥ 21 vs. < 21)	1.283	1.003–1.641	0.047			
ALP, U/L (≥ 70 vs. < 70)	2.023	1.570–2.606	< 0.001	1.654	1.275–2.145	< 0.001
LDH, U/L (≥ 172.2 vs. < 172.2)	1.951	1.514–2.514	< 0.001	1.424	1.098–1.847	< 0.001
ALB, g/L (≥ 44.9 vs. < 44.9)	0.694	0.542–0.889	0.004			
GLB, g/L (≥ 30.5 vs. < 30.5)	1.594	1.242–2.047	< 0.001			
Cholesterol, mmol/L (≥ 5.12 vs. < 5.12)	0.955	0.747–1.220	0.710			
T lymphocytes, ×10^9 (≥ 1.8 vs. < 1.8)	0.913	0.714–1.167	0.468			
Monocytes, ×10^9 (≥ 0.4 vs. < 0.4)	1.431	1.118–1.832	0.004			
Pathology (Differentiated vs. Undifferentiated	0.410	0.153–1.101	0.077			
Cranial nerve injury (Absent vs. Present)	1.075	0.666–1.736	0.767			
EBV-DNA, copies/ml			< 0.001			< 0.001
< 1000	1.000	1.000		1.000	1.000	
1000–9999	1.955	1.349–2.832	< 0.001	1.521	1.045–2.215	0.029
10,000–99,999	2.757	1.959–3.881	< 0.001	1.822	1.277–2.601	0.001
100,000–999,999	4.569	3.147–6.631	< 0.001	2.706	1.829–4.004	< 0.001
≥ 1,000,000	7.451	4.221–13.151	< 0.001	4.764	1.829–8.533	< 0.001
Treatment method				0.040		
Radiotherapy	1.000	1.000				
CCRT	1.064	0.639–1.773	0.811			
Neo + Radiotherapy	0.188	0.834–2.521	0.188			
Neo + CCRT	0.752	0.426–1.325	< 0.001			
Radiotherapy technology (IMRT + 3DCRT vs. CRT)	0.745	0.378–1.471	0.397			
T category			0.021			
1	1.000	1.000				
2	3.190	1.269–8.020	0.014			
3	3.752	1.538–9.157	0.004			
4	3.966	1.596–9.856	0.003			

Table 3 Associations between the clinical and laboratory characteristics of the patients and SMFS in univariate and multivariate logistic regression analysis *(Continued)*

N category			< 0.001			< 0.001
0	1.000	1.000		1.000	1.000	
1	1.731	0.928–3.230	0.085	1.432	0.765–2.681	0.262
2	3.017	1.638–5.558	< 0.001	2.149	1.156–3.995	0.016
3	5.987	3.281–10.925	< 0.001	3.613	1.947–6.704	< 0.001
4	6.310	3.079–12.933	< 0.001	3.629	1.742–7.559	0.001

Abbreviations: SMFS skeletal metastasis-free survival, *WBCs* white blood cells, *HGB* hemoglobin, *GLB* globulin, *ALB* albumin, *ALT* alanine transaminase, *AST* aspartate transaminase, *ALP* alkaline phosphatase, *LDH* lactate dehydrogenase, *CRP* C-reactive protein, *GGT* gamma glutamyl transpeptidase, *EBV-DNA* Epstein-Barr virus DNA, *Undifferentiated* undifferentiated non-keratinizing carcinoma, *Differentiated*, differentiated carcinoma

seventh edition of the UICC/AJCC staging system and enabled risk scoring for individual patients. The independent prognostic factors for skeletal metastasis (SMAD, SMFS) included N category, circulating EBV-DNA, LDH, ALP, HGB and CRP; each of these factors has been previously reported to play a vital role in tumor progression or metastasis.

Advanced N category was significantly associated with skeletal metastasis in this study, which reflects the assumption that the tumor cells responsible for distant

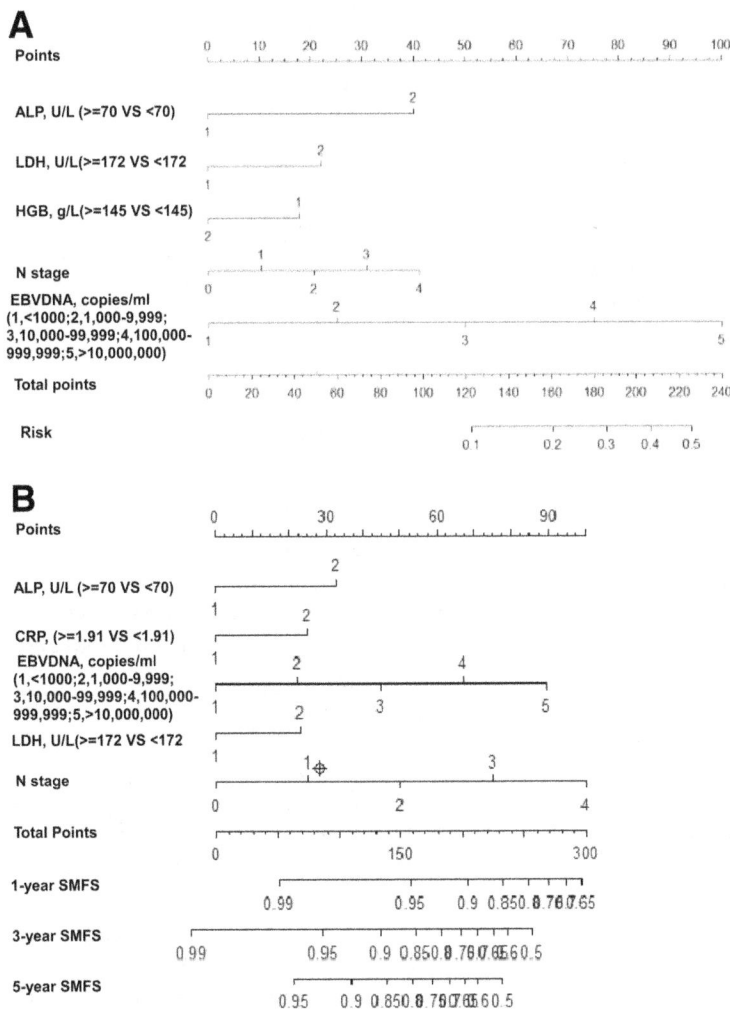

Fig. 1 Nomograms for predicting SMAD (**a**) and SMFS (**b**) in NPC. Points refers to the value of each factor included in the nomogram; total points, total points for all factors; 1/3/5-year survival, survival probability based on total points; ALP, alkaline phosphatase; HGB, hemoglobin; LDH, lactate dehydrogenase; CRP, C-reactive protein; EBV, Epstein-Barr virus; SMAD, skeletal metastasis at diagnosis; SMFS, skeletal-metastasis free survival

Table 4 The c-index values for performance of the multivariate model and the TNM classification for prediction of SMAD and SMFS in the training set and validation set

Model	Training set			Validation set		
	C-index	95% CI	P-value	C-index	95% CI	P-value
Nomograms (SMAD)	0.83	0.78–0.87	0.005	0.76	0.71–0.79	< 0.001
TNM classification (SMAD)	0.73	0.70–0.77		0.64	0.60–0.67	
Nomograms (SMFS)	0.70	0.67–0.74	< 0.001	0.61	0.55–0.0.66	0.005
TNM classification (SMFS)	0.59	0.56–0.63		0.58	0.54–0.63	

Abbreviations: SMAD skeletal metastasis at the time of diagnosis, SMFS skeletal metastasis-free survival

metastasis disseminate from the lymph nodes, rather than the primary tumor. In agreement with our findings, high serum ALP has also previously been reported to be a negative prognostic factor for skeletal metastasis and is used in the clinic to predict the presence of bone metastases in a range of cancers, including lung cancer and prostate cancer [12, 13]. The hydrolase ALP dephosphorylates a variety of molecules. Serum ALP is usually low in healthy individuals, but increases during pregnancy and in patients with bile duct obstruction, kidney disease, hepatocellular carcinoma or bone metastasis [14–18]. Yang et al. reported a high serum LDH level was an independent, unfavorable

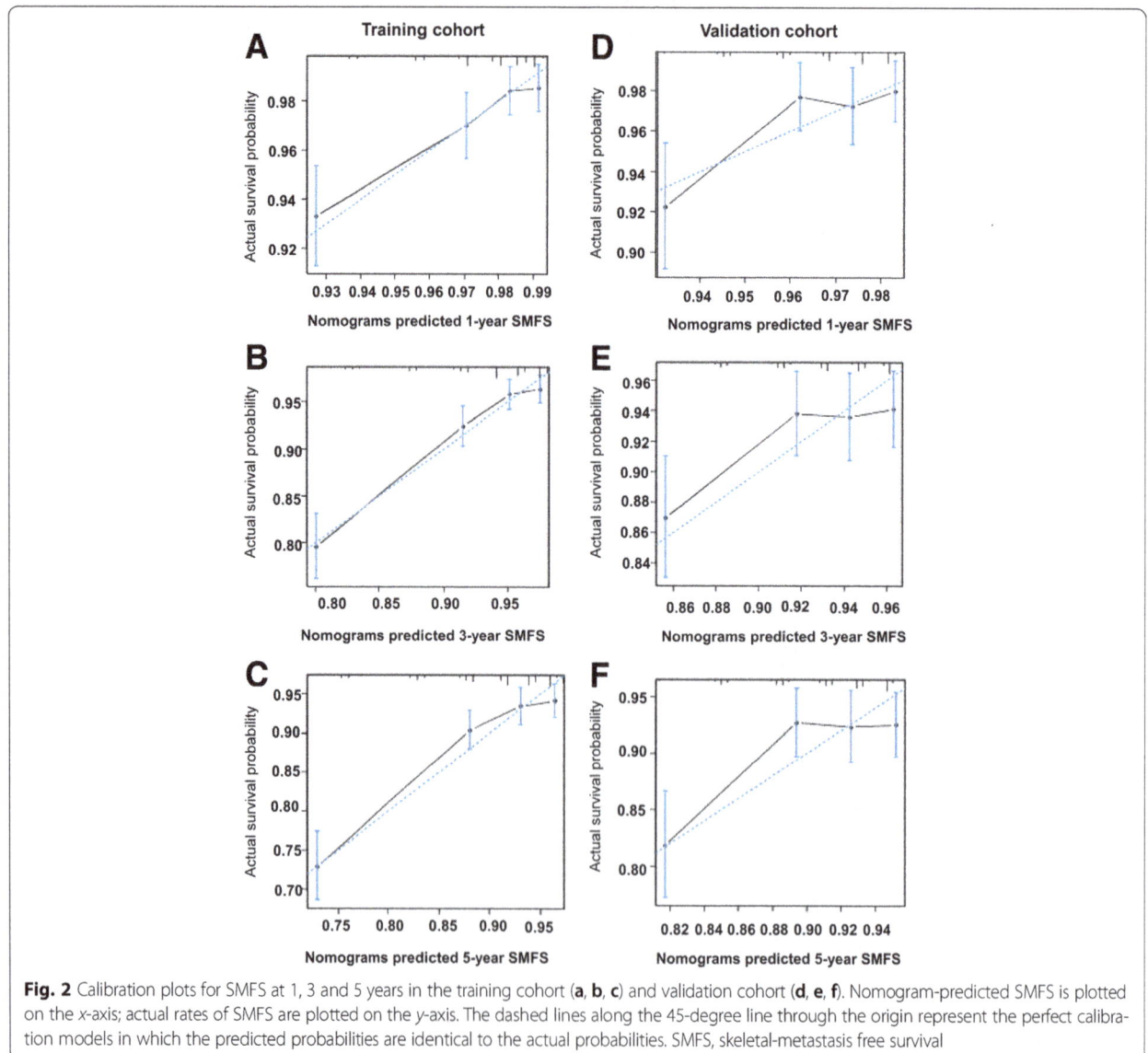

Fig. 2 Calibration plots for SMFS at 1, 3 and 5 years in the training cohort (**a**, **b**, **c**) and validation cohort (**d**, **e**, **f**). Nomogram-predicted SMFS is plotted on the *x*-axis; actual rates of SMFS are plotted on the *y*-axis. The dashed lines along the 45-degree line through the origin represent the perfect calibration models in which the predicted probabilities are identical to the actual probabilities. SMFS, skeletal-metastasis free survival

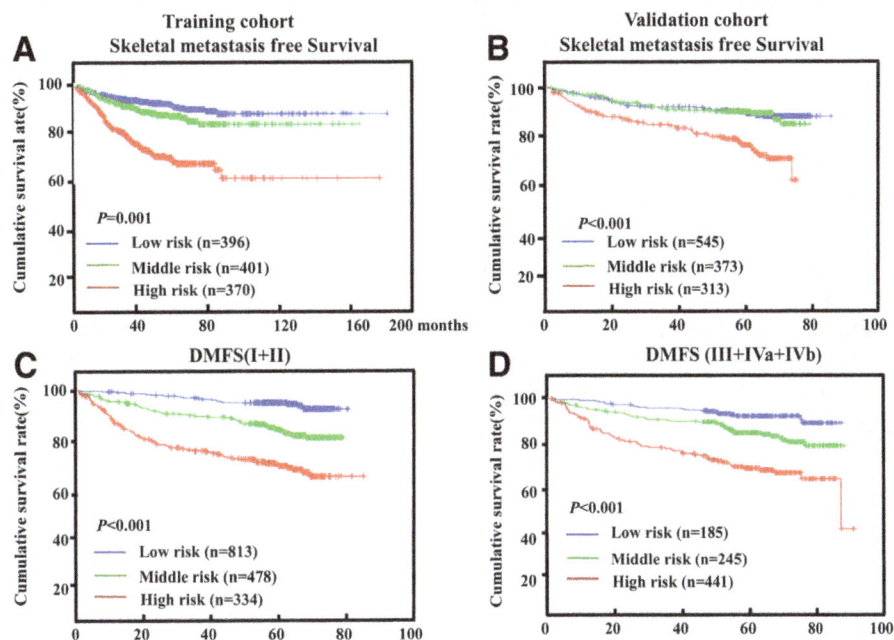

Fig. 3 Kaplan–Meier curves of SMFS for the three risk group stratifications. Nomogram risk group stratifications for the 33 and 66 percentiles are shown for the training cohort (**a**, **c**) and validation cohort (**b**, **d**). SMFS, skeletal-metastasis free survival

risk factor for overall survival (OS) and distant-metastasis free survival (DMFS) in non-metastatic NPC [19]. This study provides the first evidence that high serum LDH is an independent prognostic factor for skeletal metastasis in NPC. Rapid tumor cell proliferation initiates anaerobic glycolysis to produce energy, which requires the transformation of pyruvate to lactate by LDH, a key enzyme of glycolysis [20]. In addition, increased LDH levels lead to a low extracellular pH and activate the hypoxia-inducible factor (HIF) pathway, which is well-recognized to promote tumor growth, aggressiveness and distant metastasis [21–25].

In the regions where NPC is endemic, EBV infection is associated with an increased risk of NPC, and plasma EBV DNA is a useful prognostic marker in both early and advanced NPC [26, 27]. The present study indicates that circulating EBV DNA is also an independent prognostic factor for skeletal metastasis in NPC. Leung et al. reported that the EBV DNA cutoff value of 4000 copies/mL could categorize patients with early-stage NPC into a high-risk subgroup (with similar survival outcomes to patients with stage III disease) and a low-risk subgroup (with similar survival outcomes to stage I disease) [28]. A previously-established nomogram for disease-free survival (DFS) revealed incorporation of plasma EBV DNA increased the C-index compared to the model that did not include EBV DNA [29]. In further confirmation of its prognostic value, plasma EBV DNA was incorporated as a significant factor into the prognostic models for SMAD and SMFS in this study,

and resulted in more accurate risk discrimination for individual patients.

Reduced HGB was also an independent prognostic factor for poor SMAD, consistent with the report by Ong et al. [30]. Anemia is more common in patients with advanced stage disease and/or a poor performance status, both of which are associated with a higher probability of skeletal metastasis in NPC. Elevated CRP has been associated with advanced tumor classification, bone invasion and lymph node metastasis in NPC [31]. Similarly, CRP moderately enhanced the predictive ability of the SMFS nomogram in this study. The link between inflammation and cancer is well-recognized; prolonged exposure to proinflammatory cytokines may eventually result in the induction of CRP synthesis and is considered to be a prognostic factor in NPC [32, 33]. In the future, improving nutrition status, inflammatory status and immune function could potentially further improve the clinical outcome of patients with NPC.

The present study has several limitations. First, the time span of data collection was nearly 7 years for the data set. Therefore, the question of whether the nomograms can be applied to patients currently receiving treatment should be asked. However, at our institution, the pathologic examination has not changed during this period of time. Second, patient comorbidities were not assessed. Liu et al. previously reported that comorbidity could affect OS to some extent in NPC [34]. However, the diversity of comorbidities makes it difficult to establish categorized variables and quantify risk. Therefore, the prognostic significance of comorbidities should be assessed in future nomogram studies. Finally, whether this nomogram can be applied to younger patients (aged <18-years-old) or patients in areas with a low occurrence of NPC remains to be determined.

In summary, we have developed and externally-validated nomograms to predict SMAD and SMFS based on analyses of a relatively large number of patients with NPC. The nomograms provide significantly better discrimination than the current seventh TNM classification of the AJCC staging system and also enable individualized prognostication of skeletal metastasis. Moreover, the accuracy of the nomograms was validated using large datasets for patients treated at other two institutions. In conclusion, these nomograms represent useful tools for predicting skeletal metastasis, facilitating patient counseling, and providing timely surveillance and clinical assessments.

Conclusion

This is the first large cohort study to establish a prediction nomogram for skeletal metastasis in non-metastatic NPC; the predictive accuracy of the model was validated in an external cohort.

Abbreviations
18-FDG PET/CT: 18F–deoxyglucose positron emission tomography/computed tomography; ALB: Albumin; ALP: Alkaline phosphatase; ALT: Alanine transaminase; AST: Aspartate transaminase; AUC: Area under curve; BS: Bone scintigraphy; CRP: C-reactive protein; DMFS: Distant-metastasis free survival; EBV: Epstein-Barr virus; GLB: Globulin; HGB: Hemoglobin; HIF: Hypoxia-inducible factor; LDH: Lactate dehydrogenase; NPC: Nasopharyngeal carcinoma; OS: overall survival; RT: radiotherapy; SMAD: Skeletal metastasis at initial diagnosis; SMFS: Skeletal metastasis-free survival

Acknowledgements
Not applicable

Funding
There was no funding for this research.

Authors' contributions
YL, XLP and CY made substantial contributions to study conception and design; YL, WY, HSS, HSD, LSB, CHY and PPJ collected the data; YL, WY, and XLP analyzed the data and drafted the manuscript; LSB, CHY and PPJ analyzed the data; YL gave final approval of the version to be published; HSD and CY revised it critically for important intellectual content; CY agreed to be accountable for all aspects of the work and ensuring questions related to the accuracy or integrity of this work are appropriately investigated and resolved. All authors (YL, XLP, WY, CHY, HSS, CHY, LSB, PPJ, HSD and CY) have read and approved the final manuscript.

Competing interests
The authors declare that they have no competing interests.

Author details
[1]Sun Yat-sen University Cancer Center, 651 East Dong Feng Road, Guangzhou 510060, China. [2]State Key Laboratory of Oncology in Southern China, Guangzhou, China. [3]Collaborative Innovation Center for Cancer Medicine, Guangzhou, China. [4]The Six Affiliated Hospital of Sun Yat-sen University, Guangzhou, China. [5]The First Hospital of Foshan, Foshan, China. [6]The Fifth Affiliated Hospital of Sun Yat-sen University, Zhuhai, China.

References
1. Cao SM, Simons MJ, Qian CN. The prevalence and prevention of nasopharyngeal carcinoma in China. Chinese J Cancer. 2011;30(2):114–9.
2. Fong KW, Chua EJ, Chua ET, Khoo-Tan HS, Lee KM, Lee KS, Sethi VK, Tan BC, Tan TW, Wee J, et al. Patient profile and survival in 270 computer tomography-staged patients with nasopharyngeal cancer treated at the Singapore General Hospital. Ann Acad Med Singap. 1996;25(3):341–6.
3. Heng DM, Wee J, Fong KW, Lian LG, Sethi VK, Chua ET, Yang TL, Khoo Tan HS, Lee KS, Lee KM, et al. Prognostic factors in 677 patients in Singapore with nondisseminated nasopharyngeal carcinoma. Cancer. 1999;86(10):1912–20.
4. Tan EH, Khoo KS, Wee J, Fong KW, Lee KS, Lee KM, Chua ET, Tan T, Khoo-Tan HS, Yang TL, et al. Phase II trial of a paclitaxel and carboplatin combination in Asian patients with metastatic nasopharyngeal carcinoma. Ann Oncol. 1999; 10(2):235–7.
5. Fandi A, Bachouchi M, Azli N, Taamma A, Boussen H, Wibault P, Eschwege F, Armand JP, Simon J, Cvitkovic E. Long-term disease-free survivors in metastatic undifferentiated carcinoma of nasopharyngeal type. J Clin Oncol. 2000;18(6):1324–30.
6. Algra PR, Bloem JL, Tissing H, Falke TH, Arndt JW, Verboom LJ. Detection of vertebral metastases: comparison between MR imaging and bone scintigraphy. Radiographics. 1991;11(2):219–32.
7. Liu FY, Chang JT, Wang HM, Liao CT, Kang CJ, Ng SH, Chan SC, Yen TC. [18F]fluorodeoxyglucose positron emission tomography is more sensitive than skeletal scintigraphy for detecting bone metastasis in endemic nasopharyngeal carcinoma at initial staging. J Clin Oncol. 2006;24(4):599–604.
8. Tsuya A, Kurata T, Tamura K, Fukuoka M. Skeletal metastases in non-small cell lung cancer: a retrospective study. Lung cancer. 2007;57(2):229–32.
9. Sun JM, Ahn JS, Lee S, Kim JA, Lee J, Park YH, Park HC, Ahn MJ, Ahn YC, Park K. Predictors of skeletal-related events in non-small cell lung cancer patients with bone metastases. Lung cancer. 2011;71(1):89–93.
10. Sekine I, Nokihara H, Yamamoto N, Kunitoh H, Ohe Y, Tamura T. Risk factors for skeletal-related events in patients with non-small cell lung cancer treated by chemotherapy. Lung cancer. 2009;65(2):219–22.
11. Delea T, Langer C, McKiernan J, Liss M, Edelsberg J, Brandman J, Sung J, Raut M, Oster G. The cost of treatment of skeletal-related events in patients with bone metastases from lung cancer. Oncology. 2004;67(5–6):390–6.
12. Min JW, Um SW, Yim JJ, Yoo CG, Han SK, Shim YS, Kim YW. The role of whole-body FDG PET/CT, Tc 99m MDP bone scintigraphy, and serum alkaline phosphatase in detecting bone metastasis in patients with newly diagnosed lung cancer. J Korean Med Sci. 2009;24(2):275–80.
13. Schindler F, Lajolo PP, Pinczowski H, Fonseca FL, Barbieri A, Massonetto LH, Katto FT, Del Giglio A. Bone and total alkaline phosphatase for screening skeletal metastasis in patients with solid tumours. European J Cancer Care. 2008;17(2):152–6.
14. Bashiri A, Katz O, Maor E, Sheiner E, Pack I, Mazor M. Positive placental staining for alkaline phosphatase corresponding with extreme elevation of serum alkaline phosphatase during pregnancy. Arch Gynecol Obstet. 2007;275(3):211–4.
15. Al Mamari S, Djordjevic J, Halliday JS, Chapman RW. Improvement of serum alkaline phosphatase to <1.5 upper limit of normal predicts better outcome and reduced risk of cholangiocarcinoma in primary sclerosing cholangitis. J Hepatol. 2013;58(2):329–34.
16. Damera S, Raphael KL, Baird BC, Cheung AK, Greene T, Beddhu S. Serum alkaline phosphatase levels associate with elevated serum C-reactive protein in chronic kidney disease. Kidney Int. 2011;79(2):228–33.
17. Lu Y, Lu Q, Chen HL. Diagnosis of primary liver cancer using lectin affinity chromatography of serum alkaline phosphatase. J Exp Clin Cancer Res. 1997;16(1):75–80.
18. Sonpavde G, Pond GR, Berry WR, de Wit R, Armstrong AJ, Eisenberger MA, Tannock IF. Serum alkaline phosphatase changes predict survival independent of PSA changes in men with castration-resistant prostate cancer and bone metastasis receiving chemotherapy. Urol Oncol. 2012; 30(5):607–13.

19. Yang L, Hong S, Wang Y, He Z, Liang S, Chen H, He S, Wu S, Song L, Chen Y. A novel prognostic score model incorporating CDGSH iron sulfur Domain2 (CISD2) predicts risk of disease progression in laryngeal squamous cell carcinoma. Oncotarget. 2016;7(16):22720–32

20. Warburg O. On the origin of cancer cells. Science. 1956;123(3191):309–14.

21. Axelson H, Fredlund E, Ovenberger M, Landberg G, Pahlman S. Hypoxia-induced dedifferentiation of tumor cells–a mechanism behind heterogeneity and aggressiveness of solid tumors. Semin Cell Dev Biol. 2005;16(4–5):554–63.

22. Colgan SM, Mukherjee S, Major P. Hypoxia-induced lactate dehydrogenase expression and tumor angiogenesis. Clin Colorectal Cancer. 2007;6(6):442–6.

23. Maxwell PH. The HIF pathway in cancer. Semin Cell Dev Biol. 2005;16(4–5): 523–30.

24. Rofstad EK. Microenvironment-induced cancer metastasis. Int J Radiat Biol. 2000;76(5):589–605.

25. Stubbs M, McSheehy PM, Griffiths JR, Bashford CL. Causes and consequences of tumour acidity and implications for treatment. Mol Med Today. 2000;6(1): 15–9.

26. McDermott AL, Dutt SN, Watkinson JC. The aetiology of nasopharyngeal carcinoma. Clinical otolaryngology and allied sciences. 2001;26(2):82–92.

27. Lo YM, Chan AT, Chan LY, Leung SF, Lam CW, Huang DP, Johnson PJ. Molecular prognostication of nasopharyngeal carcinoma by quantitative analysis of circulating Epstein-Barr virus DNA. Cancer Res. 2000;60(24):6878–81.

28. Leung SF, Zee B, Ma BB, Hui EP, Mo F, Lai M, Chan KC, Chan LY, Kwan WH, Lo YM, et al. Plasma Epstein-Barr viral deoxyribonucleic acid quantitation complements tumor-node-metastasis staging prognostication in nasopharyngeal carcinoma. J Clin Oncol. 2006;24(34):5414–8.

29. Tang LQ, Li CF, Li J, Chen WH, Chen QY, Yuan LX, Lai XP, He Y, Xu YX, Hu DP, et al. Establishment and Validation of Prognostic Nomograms for Endemic Nasopharyngeal Carcinoma. J Natl Cancer Inst. 2016;108(1).

30. Ong YK, Heng DM, Chung B, Leong SS, Wee J, Fong KW, Tan T, Tan EH. Design of a prognostic index score for metastatic nasopharyngeal carcinoma. Eur J Cancer. 2003;39(11):1535–41.

31. Chen HH, Chen IH, Liao CT, Wei FC, Lee LY, Huang SF. Preoperative circulating C-reactive protein levels predict pathological aggressiveness in oral squamous cell carcinoma: a retrospective clinical study. Clin Otolaryngol. 2011;36(2):147–53.

32. Balkwill F, Mantovani A. Cancer and inflammation: implications for pharmacology and therapeutics. Clin Pharmacol Ther. 2010;87(4):401–6.

33. Allin KH, Nordestgaard BG. Elevated C-reactive protein in the diagnosis, prognosis, and cause of cancer. Crit Rev Clin Lab Sci. 2011;48(4):155–70.

34. Liu H, Chen QY, Guo L, Tang LQ, Mo HY, Zhong ZL, Huang PY, Luo DH, Sun R, Guo X, et al. Feasibility and efficacy of chemoradiotherapy for elderly patients with locoregionally advanced nasopharyngeal carcinoma: results from a matched cohort analysis. Radiat Oncol. 2013;8:70.

8

Clinical outcomes of transoral videolaryngoscopic surgery for hypopharyngeal and supraglottic cancer

Yorihisa Imanishi[1,2*], Hiroyuki Ozawa[1], Koji Sakamoto[3], Ryoichi Fujii[4], Seiji Shigetomi[5], Noboru Habu[6], Kuninori Otsuka[7], Yoichiro Sato[2], Yoshihiro Watanabe[1], Mariko Sekimizu[1], Fumihiro Ito[1], Toshiki Tomita[1] and Kaoru Ogawa[1]

Abstract

Background: Transoral videolaryngoscopic surgery (TOVS) was developed as a new distinct surgical procedure for hypopharyngeal cancer (HPC) and supraglottic cancer (SGC) staged at up to T3. However, long-term treatment outcomes of TOVS remain to be validated.

Methods: Under a straight broad intraluminal view provided by combined use of a distending laryngoscope and a videolaryngoscope, we performed en bloc tumor resection via direct bimanual handling of the ready-made straight-form surgical instruments and devices. We retrospectively analyzed functional and oncologic outcomes of 72 patients with HPC ($n = 58$) or SGC ($n = 14$) whose minimum follow-up was 24 months or until death.

Results: The cohort comprised nine patients of Tis, 23 of T1, 33 of T2, and 7 of T3. Among 36 patients (50%) who underwent neck dissection simultaneously, all but one were pathologically node-positive. Twelve patients underwent postoperative concurrent chemoradiation (CCRT) as adjuvant treatment, and another four patients underwent radiation or CCRT for second or later primary cancer. The endotracheal tube was removed in an operation room in all but two patients who underwent temporary tracheostomy. Pharyngeal fistula was formed transiently in two patients. The median time until patients resumed oral intake and could take a soft meal was 2 and 5 days, respectively. Eventually, 69 patients (96%) took normal meals. The 5-year cause-specific survival (CSS), overall survival (OS), larynx-preserved CSS, and loco-regional controlled CSS were 87.3%, 77.9%, 86.0%, and 88.0%, respectively. Multivariate analysis revealed N2-3 as an independent prognostic factor in both CSS (hazard ratio [HR] = 25.51, $P = 0.008$) and OS (HR = 4.90, $P = 0.022$), which indirectly reflected higher risk of delayed distant metastasis.

Conclusions: Considering its sound functional and oncological outcomes with various practical advantages, TOVS can be a dependable, less invasive, and cost-effective surgical option of an organ-function preservation strategy for HPC and SGC.

Keywords: Transoral videolaryngoscopic surgery (TOVS), Hypopharyngeal cancer, Supraglottic cancer, Organ-function preservation, Long-term treatment outcomes, Survival, Prognostic factor

* Correspondence: yorihisa@ja2.so-net.ne.jp
[1]Department of Otorhinolaryngology–Head and Neck Surgery, Keio University School of Medicine, 35 Shinanomachi, Shinjuku, Tokyo 160-8582, Japan
[2]Department of Otorhinolaryngology, Kawasaki Municipal Kawasaki Hospital, Kawasaki, Kanagawa 210-0013, Japan
Full list of author information is available at the end of the article

Background

Hypopharyngeal cancer (HPC) affects 0.8–1.3 per 100,000 persons per year in the US, accounting for approximately 6.5% of all head and neck squamous cell carcinomas (SCC) [1]. Unfortunately, prognosis of the patients with HPC reportedly remains the worst among all head and neck subsites, largely because the vast majority of the patients present at a locally advanced stage [2]. Since radical resection for HPC inevitably impairs laryngopharyngeal function, such as vocalization, swallowing, and breathing through the natural airway, organ-function preservation strategies have been increasingly developed, even for treatment of HPC, since the 1990s [3, 4].

Practically, there are three major options that meet the concept of organ-function preservation in the laryngopharyngeal region: radiation (RT) or chemoradiation (CRT), open partial pharyngolaryngectomy (PPL), and transoral surgery. RT or CRT has long been representative of non-surgical treatments, and concurrent CRT (CCRT), in particular, has been recognized as one of the standard therapies for advanced-staged HPC and supraglottic cancer (SGC) [5–7]. However, intensified CCRT with a high-dose regimen results in severe long-term adverse effects including subsequent loss of function in preserved organs [8–12]. Open PPL has also been established as a surgical organ-function preserving procedure for selected cases of early T-staged HPC and SGC [13–15]. Although both oncological and functional outcomes of open PPL have shown to be eventually satisfactory, the surgical invasiveness associated with external incision, reconstruction procedure, and tracheostomy necessitate cautious postoperative managements and relatively long rehabilitation periods, which may make this procedure less popular.

Transoral surgery has emerged as another therapeutic option for laryngopharyngeal lesions. Because of its less invasiveness compared to CCRT regarding treatment-induced long-term toxicity and to open PPL regarding direct histological damage to the surrounding normal tissues, transoral surgery is expected to be an ideal alternative for the treatment of HPC patients. Traditionally, application of transoral surgery had been confined to early tumors in oral, oropharyngeal (except for tongue base), and glottic regions, because of the anatomically limited visualization and manipulation due to a lack of suitable optical instruments. Technological advancements in microscopic/endoscopic monitoring and surgical supporting devices have enabled development of various transoral surgical methods that can approach the hypopharyngeal and supraglottic regions, such as transoral laser microsurgery (TLM) using a microscope since the late 1990s [16–22], and more recently, transoral robotic surgery (TORS) using a surgical robot since the late 2000s [23–30].

Besides the above-mentioned procedures, Shiotani et al. have developed a distinct, unique, non-robotic surgical method custom-built for transoral partial pharyngolaryngectomy since the 2000s; this was subsequently renamed "transoral videolaryngoscopic surgery (TOVS)" [31–33]. In this system, combined use of a distending laryngoscope with a rigid endoscope (videolaryngoscope) can provide a broad intraluminal field of view and a wide working space throughout the upper aero-digestive tract, which facilitates en bloc tumor resection via direct bimanual handling and application of the ready-made straight-form surgical instruments and devices. Favorable oncological outcomes and good functional results have been achieved so far by employing TOVS for T1, T2, and selected T3 cancers of the hypopharynx, supraglottis, and oropharynx [32, 33]. However, because it has not been long since this promising method was introduced, the long-term treatment outcome of TOVS remains to be validated.

The aim of this paper was to retrospectively evaluate clinical outcomes of TOVS for a cohort of patients with HPC and SGC in a tertiary referral center.

Methods

Indication for TOVS

All patients were staged according to the UICC TNM classification and staging system [34]. TOVS was applied to patients with HPC and/or SGC staged at Tis, T1, T2, and T3 (classified mainly by size criteria) for the curative resection of a primary lesion. Patients with neck lymph node metastasis were also included unless nodal lesions were considered unresectable.

The exclusion criteria were as follows: (1) medical contraindication to general anesthesia; (2) involvement of the thyroid cartilage, cricoid cartilage, or hyoid bone (i.e., T4 tumor); (3) invasion of bilateral arytenoid cartilages; or (4) extension to more than a semi-circumference of the esophageal entrance. Those patients underwent other treatments including RT, CRT, open PPL, total laryngectomy, or total pharyngolaryngectomy.

Pre-surgical evaluation

In the pre-therapeutic evaluation, transnasal endoscopic observation is performed routinely with Valsalva maneuver and head torsion to gain a maximally expanded intraluminal view of the hypopharynx [35–37]. This method enables accurate visualization of tumor extension on the mucosal surface and detailed inspection of the hypopharynx for any other possible lesion down to the esophageal entrance (Fig. 1a and b). Simultaneously, morphological changes in intramucosal microvascular structure (so-called "intra-epithelial papillary capillary loop (IPCL)") are observed using the narrow band imaging (NBI) mode, an image-enhancing technique equipped in the flexible endoscope ENF-VT2/VQ/VH (Olympus, Japan), to screen for intraepithelial cancer (carcinoma in situ [CIS]) in which loss of typical IPCL can be visualized as a "brownish area"

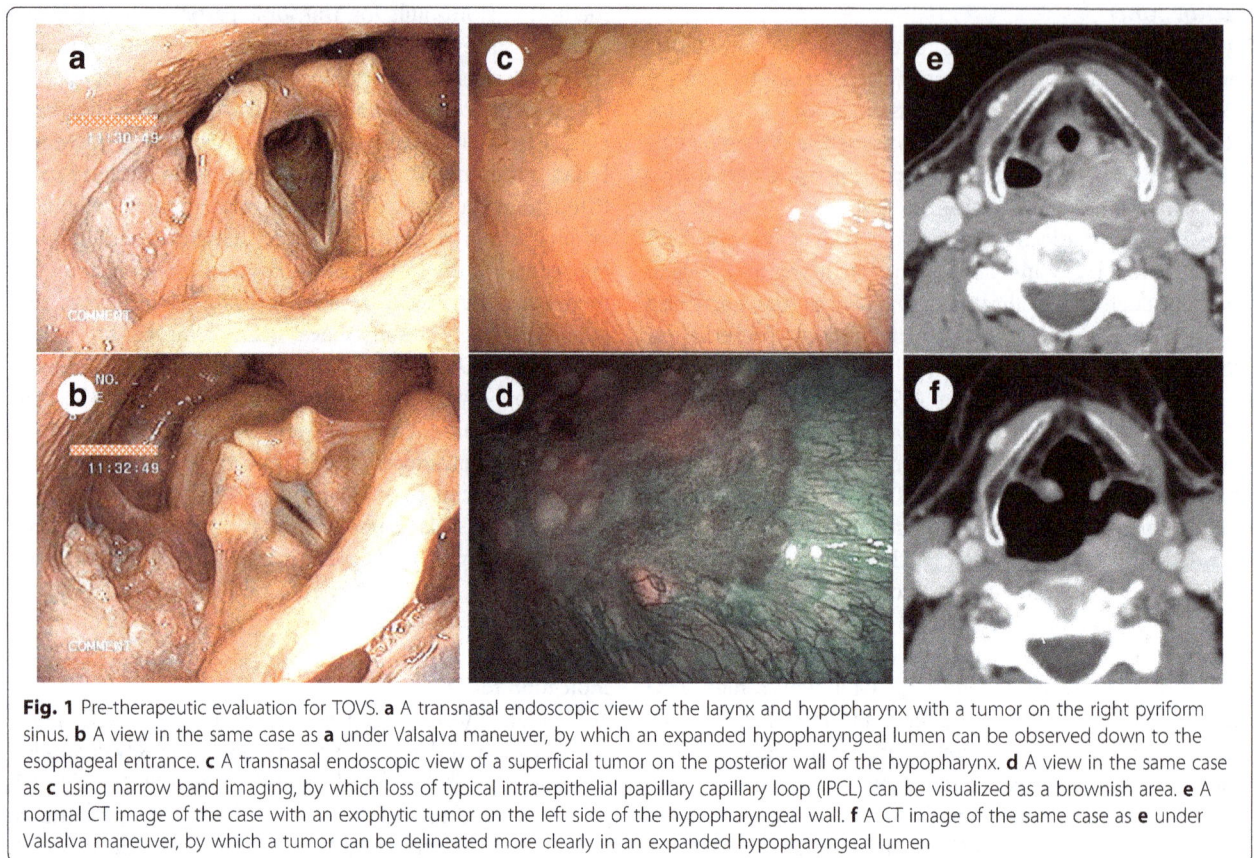

Fig. 1 Pre-therapeutic evaluation for TOVS. **a** A transnasal endoscopic view of the larynx and hypopharynx with a tumor on the right pyriform sinus. **b** A view in the same case as **a** under Valsalva maneuver, by which an expanded hypopharyngeal lumen can be observed down to the esophageal entrance. **c** A transnasal endoscopic view of a superficial tumor on the posterior wall of the hypopharynx. **d** A view in the same case as **c** using narrow band imaging, by which loss of typical intra-epithelial papillary capillary loop (IPCL) can be visualized as a brownish area. **e** A normal CT image of the case with an exophytic tumor on the left side of the hypopharyngeal wall. **f** A CT image of the same case as **e** under Valsalva maneuver, by which a tumor can be delineated more clearly in an expanded hypopharyngeal lumen

[38–41] (Fig. 1c and d). The Valsalva maneuver is also incorporated in pre-therapeutic CT scanning, by which the usually collapsed hypopharyngeal lumen can expand maximally, especially in the anteroposterior direction, leading to clearer delineation and size measurement of depth and width of a tumor, especially in an exophytic shape [35, 42] (Fig. 1e, f). These assessments are considered indispensable in decision-making regarding applicability of TOVS.

Under general anesthesia, thorough inspection is first performed routinely using the aforementioned flexible endoscope with NBI mode and mucosal staining with 1.5% iodine solution that allow visualization of the CIS as an unstained area. For this purpose, laryngeal elevation using a curved rigid pharyngolaryngeal blade (Fig. 2a) (Nagashima Medical Instruments, Japan) is helpful in keeping the hypopharynx expanded, thus providing a favorable view of the entire pharyngolaryngeal lumen, although its benefit is limited to a flexible endoscope [43]. In this step, the exact resection line can be determined based on both the mucosal extent visualized by iodine staining and submucosal extent estimated by evaluating tumor mobility through direct palpation using forceps.

Surgical procedures

To provide a straight surgical view with broad working space for TOVS, the pharyngolaryngeal lumen is kept expanded using a Weerda distending laryngoscope (Fig. 2b) (8858BV, 17 cm in length of the upper spatula, Karl Storz, Germany), distending diverticuloscope (Fig. 2c) (12067 V, 24 cm in length of the upper spatula, Karl Storz), or FK-WO retractor system (Fig. 2d) (Olympus), of which the appropriate position is determined depending on the tumor location and size. A rigid endoscope (videolaryngoscope) 4 mm in diameter (8575AV, 17 cm in length, 15 degree; or 12067VA, 24 cm in length, 0 degree; Karl Storz) connected to an HD camera (OTV-S7ProH-HD-L08E, OTV-S7ProH-HD-12E, or CH-S190-XZ-E; Olympus) is inserted, either by being attached to the distending scope or manually by a surgical assistant, to display an optimal surgical field on a monitor (Fig. 2e, f).

After a tumor's boundary is confirmed by iodine staining, marking dots on the mucosa are made on the circumference of the lesion with a safety margin ≥5 mm, using a fine needle electrode with tip diameter of 0.45 mm (Fig. 3a) (No.20191-084, Erbe, Germany), tip diameter of 0.15 mm (Fig. 3b) (No.20191-083, Erbe), or tip-shaft diameter of 0.8 mm (Fig. 3c) (No.21191-020 or 21191-070, Erbe) attached to a slim-line hand switch system (Fig. 3d) (No.20190-095, Erbe), in the Soft Coag mode of an electrosurgical generator VIO300D (Fig. 3e) (Erbe). A mixed solution consisting of sodium hyaluronate (MucoUp; Johnson & Johnson K.K., Japan), epinephrine,

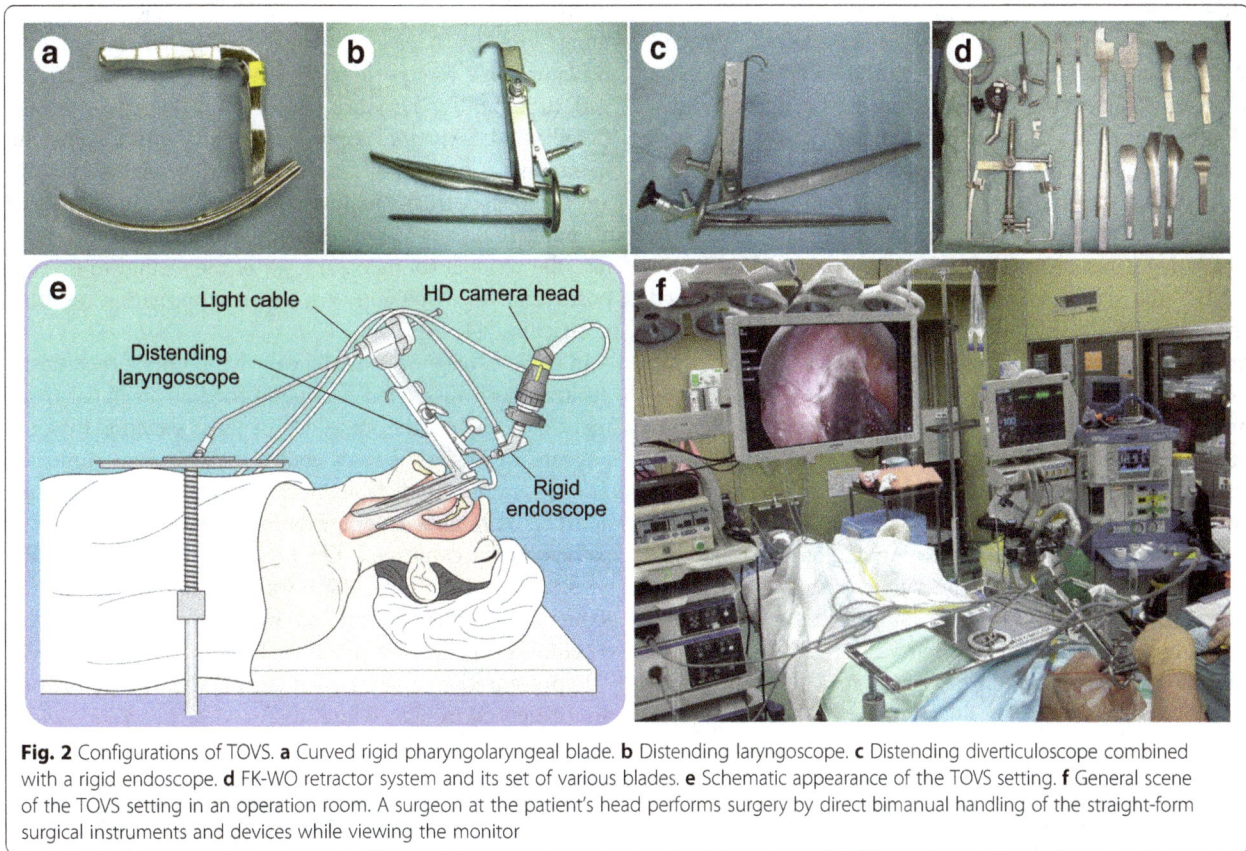

Fig. 2 Configurations of TOVS. **a** Curved rigid pharyngolaryngeal blade. **b** Distending laryngoscope. **c** Distending diverticuloscope combined with a rigid endoscope. **d** FK-WO retractor system and its set of various blades. **e** Schematic appearance of the TOVS setting. **f** General scene of the TOVS setting in an operation room. A surgeon at the patient's head performs surgery by direct bimanual handling of the straight-form surgical instruments and devices while viewing the monitor

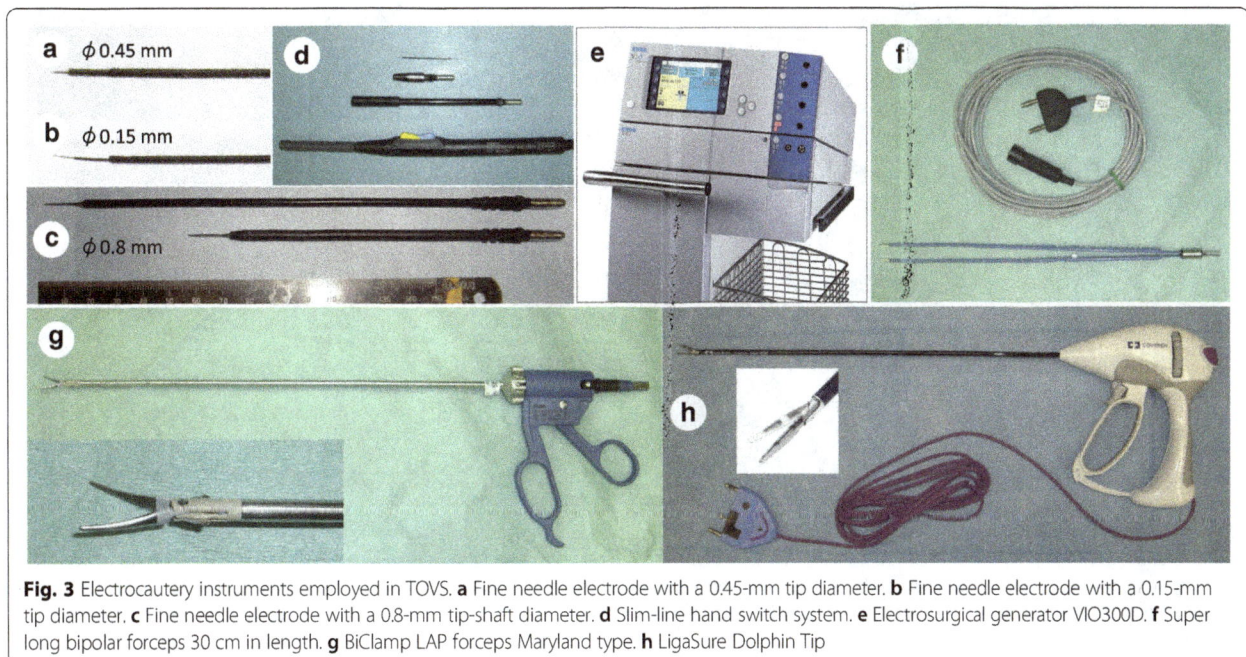

Fig. 3 Electrocautery instruments employed in TOVS. **a** Fine needle electrode with a 0.45-mm tip diameter. **b** Fine needle electrode with a 0.15-mm tip diameter. **c** Fine needle electrode with a 0.8-mm tip-shaft diameter. **d** Slim-line hand switch system. **e** Electrosurgical generator VIO300D. **f** Super long bipolar forceps 30 cm in length. **g** BiClamp LAP forceps Maryland type. **h** LigaSure Dolphin Tip

physiological saline, and indigocarmine is injected through the 25G (gauge) laryngeal fine needle (length, 28 cm) (Nagashima) into the layer beneath the lesion to expand a safety cushion vertically by lifting up the lesion. Before use of electrocautery, a Nelaton soft catheter (12-14 Fr in size) with several additional small holes bored at its tip is inserted transnasally, and the tip is placed just ahead of a the endoscope tip, so that the catheter can evacuate vapor efficiently, which maintains a clear endoscopic view during surgery.

After the mucosa around the marking dots is incised circumferentially with a fine needle electrode in Dry Cut mode, the entire lesion is dissected step-by-step using the same electrode in Dry Cut, Auto Cut, or Swift Coag mode until en bloc resection is accomplished. During the procedure, a surgeon bimanually handles a variety of ready-made straight-form surgical instruments and devices, which enables adequate counter-traction by grasping a margin of the lesion using forceps with one hand, while the other hand manipulates another instrument such as a needle electrode, suction tube, or hemostatic device.

Bleeding points and/or exposed vessels are efficiently co-agulated using a super long bipolar forceps 30 cm in length (Fig. 3f) (No.20195-109, Erbe). In case hemorrhage is uncontrollable with the aforementioned method or a bulky tumor can be hauled up from the constrictor muscle, BiClamp LAP forceps Maryland type (Fig. 3g) (No.20195-146, Erbe) and/or LigaSure Dolphin Tip (Fig. 3h) (LS1500, Covidien, USA) are applied to exert more powerful hemostasis. After tumor resection and thorough hemostasis are completed, triamcinolone acetonide solution (Kenacort; 40 mg/mL; Bristol-Meyers Squibb, Japan) is injected evenly into the residual submucosal layer of the wound to prevent postoperative edema and excessive scar formation resulting in stricture [44, 45].

In patients diagnosed as clinically lymph node metastasis-positive, neck dissection was performed as an initial treatment basically on the same day in most patients. In some patients, in whom the resectability of the primary tumor by TOVS was not predictable, neck dissection was performed at a later date after a completeness of tumor resection was pathologically confirmed. On the other hand, in case the resectability of the neck lesion was unpredictable, neck dissection was performed first and was followed by TOVS after a pathological curability of the neck lesion was ascertained.

Representative cases in which TOVS was performed are presented in Figs. 4 and 5.

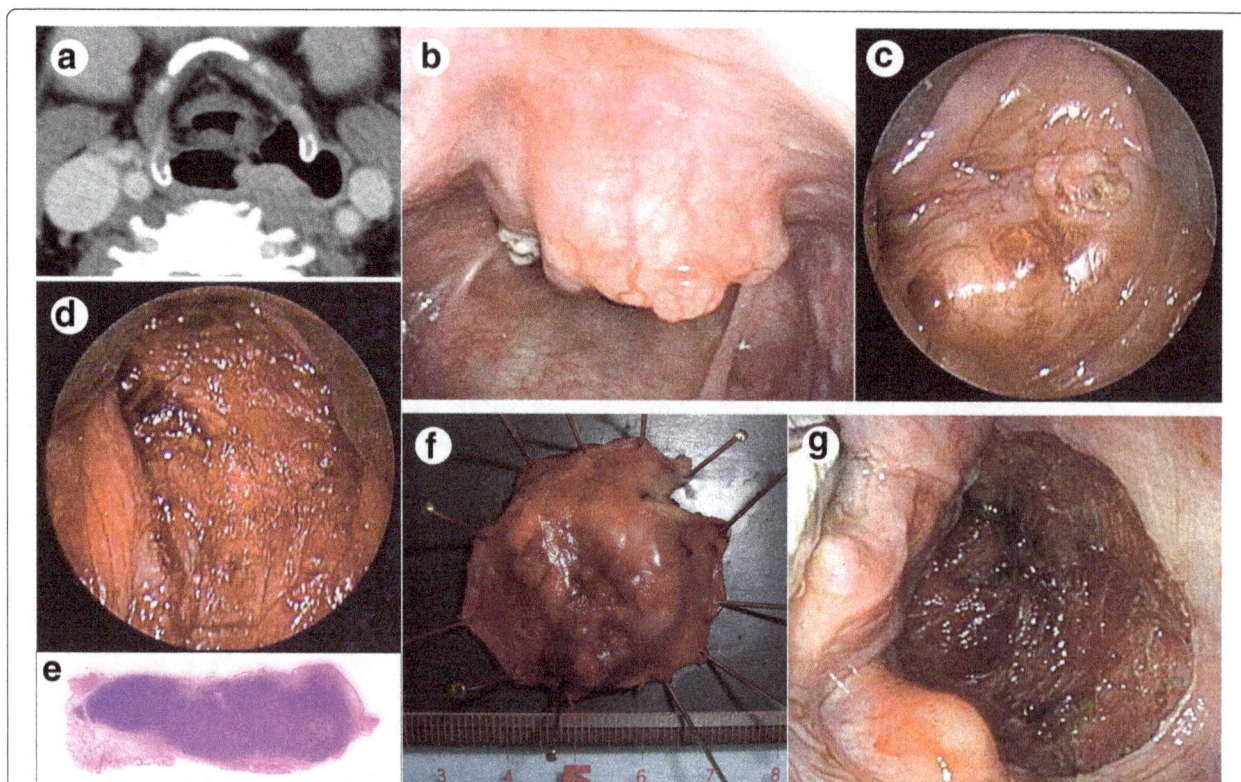

Fig. 4 A case in which TOVS was performed for a tumor on the posterior wall. **a** CT image under Valsalva maneuver showing a T2 tumor on the posterior wall of the hypopharynx. **b** Transnasal endoscopic view of the tumor under Valsalva maneuver. **c** Endoscopic view of the tumor just before resection. **d** Endoscopic view of the wound just after resection. **e** Section of the tumor specimen stained with hematoxylin and eosin. **f** Macroscopic view of the tumor specimen resected. **g** Transnasal endoscopic view of the wound just after thorough hemostasis. Inferior pharyngeal constrictor muscle was widely exposed

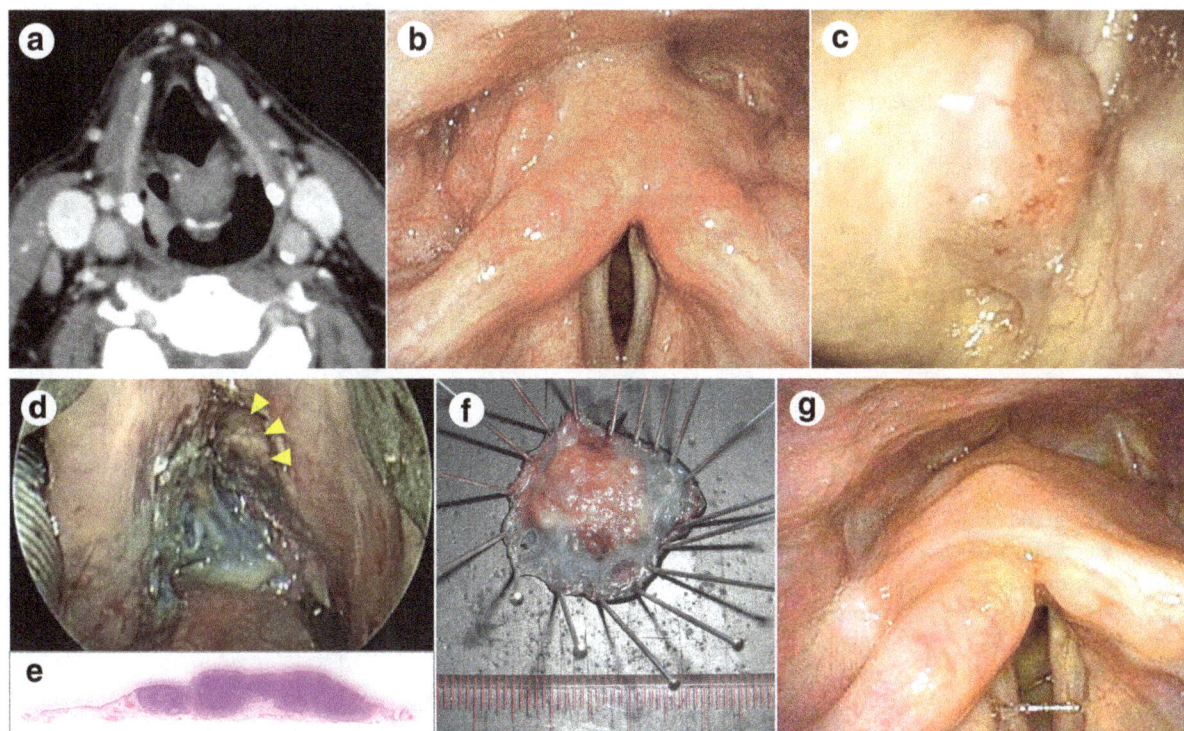

Fig. 5 A case in which TOVS was performed for a tumor on the pyriform sinus. **a** CT image under Valsalva maneuver showing a T1 tumor on the right pyriform sinus of the hypopharynx. **b** Transnasal endoscopic view of the tumor under Valsalva maneuver. **c** Endoscopic view of the tumor just before resection. **d** Endoscopic view of the wound just after resection. Thyroid cartilage was partially exposed (arrow heads). **e** Section of the tumor specimen stained with hematoxylin and eosin. **f** Macroscopic view of the tumor specimen resected. **g** Transnasal endoscopic view of the hypopharynx 3 months after resection

Adjuvant treatments

Regarding the surgical margin in the final histopathology, if the horizontal margin was undoubtedly positive, reoperation of TOVS was considered. If the vertical margin was obviously positive despite a curative intent, the patients underwent open PPL and were excluded from the study.

Concerning pathologically positive lymph node metastasis, if pathological N (pN)-stage was pN0, pN1, or pN2a, we held to a strict observation policy. In patients with pN2b or more, if the number of positive nodes was more than three, positive nodes were distributed in more than one level, or extracapsular spread was revealed, adjuvant cis-platinum (CDDP)-based CCRT was administered. Otherwise, we retained strict observation.

Patient population

From April 2007 to March 2014, 85 patients with HPC or SGC who met the aforementioned criteria underwent TOVS with or without neck dissection at the Department of Otorhinolaryngology–Head and Neck Surgery, Keio University Hospital (Tokyo, Japan). Among them, patients who subsequently underwent open PPL due to

positive vertical margin ($n = 4$), those whose tumor was residual or recurrent after an initial treatment elsewhere ($n = 3$), those treated without a curative intent ($n = 2$), those with simultaneous distant metastasis ($n = 2$), and those with non-SCC malignancy ($n = 2$) were excluded from the study. The remaining 72 patients, who had a minimum follow-up period of 24 months or until the patient's death, were considered eligible for inclusion in this cohort.

Detailed clinical data of the patients were retrieved from the database. Treatment outcomes were analyzed to evaluate the clinical validity of TOVS as a surgical organ preservation strategy.

Outcome measures and statistical analysis

All survival probabilities were estimated by using the Kaplan-Meier method. Cause-specific survival (CSS, events: death due to the disease [any of TNM]), overall survival (OS, events: all death), larynx-preserved CSS (LP-CSS, events: total laryngectomy, total pharyngolaryngectomy, or TNM-related death), and loco-regional controlled CSS (LRC-CSS, events: local or regional relapse, or TNM-related death) were analyzed as oncological endpoints.

The generalized Wilcoxon test and the univariate Cox proportional hazards model were used to examine the significance of differences in survival outcomes associated with patient/disease characteristics, including age, sex, tumor site, T stage, N stage, existence of multiple cancers, and history of radiation on the neck. The estimated hazard ratio (HR) and 95% confidence interval (CI) were calculated. The multivariate Cox proportional hazards model further assessed independent significance of the aforementioned variables without sequential and/or stepwise variable selection. P values <0.05 were considered statistically significant. All statistical analyses were performed using EXCEL Multivariate Analyses for MAC Ver. 3.0 (Esumi Co., Ltd., Tokyo).

Results

Patient characteristics

Demographic and disease characteristics of the 72 patients, including age, sex, primary tumor site, T stage, N stage, and disease stage, are summarized in Table 1. Notably, while 37 patients belonged to N0 (51.4%), the remaining 35 patients (48.6%) had lymph node metastasis. Regarding disease stage distribution, one-third of the patients ($n = 24$, 33.3%) were stage IV. Furthermore, 54 patients (75.0%) had multiple cancers in the head and neck region, other regions, or both; as well as synchronously, metachronously, or both, by the time of the last follow-up. Among them, 12 patients (16.7%) had a history of radiation on the neck for other previous cancers.

Surgical results and additional treatments

As summarized in Table 2, we achieved en bloc tumor resection by TOVS in 66 patients. On the other hand, blockwise resection was necessary in the remaining six patients due to relatively wider and/or deeper lesions, including three patients with a T3 invasive tumor that spread over the arytenoid, pyriform sinus, and postcricoid; two with a T2 tumor that extended to the cervical esophagus; and one with a T2 superficial tumor that spread across a semi-circumference of the hypopharynx just above the esophageal entrance. However, such blockwise resections in all these patients were performed in the first 3 years when the surgeons had relatively less experience, but they were not performed afterward.

Regarding the surgical margin status, obviously positive horizontal margin was not found in the final histopathology of any patient who underwent TOVS with a curative intent. This is thought to be a result of appropriate confirmation of the tumor's boundary on the mucosal surface, sufficient additional resection in case the margin was suspected to be positive, and in part with the help of abovementioned blockwise resection in case en bloc resection was impossible. On the other hand,

positive vertical margin was observed in seven of the 13 patients who underwent TOVS but were excluded from the study, which included four patients who subsequently underwent open PPL, two patients treated without a curative intent, and one patient with pharyngeal synovial sarcoma who also subsequently underwent open PPL. All cases of incomplete resection due to the positive vertical margin occurred in the first 2 years when the surgeons' expertise was likely insufficient.

Table 1 Patient characteristics ($n = 72$)

Characteristics		No.	%
Age, y			
	Median (range)	68 (46-88)	
	Mean ± SD	66 ± 9	
Sex			
	Men	67	93.1
	Women	5	6.9
Tumor site			
	Hypopharynx	58	80.6
	Supraglottis	14	19.4
T stage			
	Tis	9	12.5
	T1	23	31.9
	T2	33	45.8
	T3	7	9.7
N stage			
	N0	37	51.4
	N1	11	15.3
	N2a	1	1.4
	N2b	18	25.0
	N2c	4	5.6
	N3	1	1.4
Stage			
	0	9	12.5
	I	14	19.4
	II	13	18.1
	III	12	16.7
	IVA	23	31.9
	IVB	1	1.4
Multiple cancer			
	No	18	25.0
	Yes	54	75.0
Previous RT on the neck			
	No	60	83.3
	Yes	12	16.7

SD Standard deviation, *RT* Radiotherapy

Table 2 Surgical results and additional treatments (*n* = 72)

Outcomes		No.	%
Primary resection			
	En bloc	66	91.7
	Blockwise	6	8.3
Neck dissection			
	No	36	50.0
	Unilateral	32	44.4
	Bilateral	4	5.6
Additional RT			
	No	56	77.8
	Adjuvant	12	16.7
	Secondary	4	5.6

Table 3 Complication and dysfunction (*n* = 72)

Category	No.	%
Complication		
Respiration-related		
Temporary tracheostomy	2	2.8
Prolonged mechanical ventilation	0	0.0
Surgical site-related		
Pharyngeal fistula	2	2.8
Subcutaneous emphysema	4	5.6
Dysfunction		
Swallowing-related		
Nasogastric tube placement	16	22.2
Preventive balloon dilation	3	4.2
Gastrostomy tube placement	0	0.0
Aspiration pneumonia	2	2.8
Persistent dysphasia	3	4.2
Phonation-related		
Permanent vocal dysfunction	0	0.0

Neck dissections were performed as an initial treatment in 36 patients (50.0%), in which 32 patients were unilateral and four were bilateral, for therapeutic purposes based on clinical N stage. Regarding the timing of neck dissection, it was done on the same day as TOVS in 26 patients, at a later date within 2 weeks after TOVS in seven patients, and within 3 weeks before TOVS in three patients. All but one patient (i.e., *n* = 35, 48.6%) were pathologically positive in the lymph node. Among them, two patients additionally underwent neck dissection on the contralateral side due to delayed neck metastasis that developed in the untreated side.

Postoperative CDDP-based CCRT (50-66 Gy) was administered to 12 patients as adjuvant therapy, including nine patients with N2b, two with N2c, and one with N3. The reasons for adjuvant CCRT were extracapsular spread (*n* = 2), more than three positive lymph nodes (*n* = 2), or both (*n* = 5); or were very close to or had an equivocal surgical margin at the primary site (*n* = 3). Furthermore, another four patients who belonged to N2a (*n* = 1) or N2b (*n* = 3) and repeatedly developed multiple second primary cancers in the pharyngolaryngeal region ultimately underwent CCRT (*n* = 1), RT plus weekly cetuximab (*n* = 1), or RT alone (*n* = 2). Thus, in total, RT was administered to 16 patients (22.2%). Since other 12 patients had a history of radiation on the neck, the remaining 44 patients (61.1%) were spared from RT during the follow-up period.

Regarding 17 patients who underwent additional surgery for second or later primary tumor in the pharyngolaryngeal region, TOVS was repeated in 12 patients with relatively smaller tumors, open PPL was applied to three patients with relatively larger tumors, and the other two patients who had a history of previous RT on the neck ultimately underwent total laryngectomy as salvage therapy.

Surgical complications
Complications related to TOVS are summarized in Table 3. The endotracheal tube was removed in an operation room

after the surgery regardless of additional neck dissection in most patients (*n* = 70). In only two patients who developed laryngopharyngeal edema following a blockwise resection of T3 tumor associated with a unilateral neck dissection, a transient tracheostomy was placed before extubation and closed within a week. No patient required prolonged mechanical ventilation or an intensive care unit stay postoperatively.

A pharyngeal fistula formed in two patients who underwent resection of tumor on the pyriform sinus followed by an ipsilateral neck dissection. In the first case, a fistula was noticed just after extubation because of continuous leakage of expiratory air into the drainage tube placed under the neck skin, so it was located immediately in reoperation and closed by suturing mucosal layers with the sternohyoid muscle. In the second case, a fistula was found during an extended neck dissection for N3. Although the fistula was closed cautiously during surgery and drainage tubes were extracted uneventfully, a small subcutaneous abscess formed in the same position shortly afterward and required local treatments and interruption of oral intake for a week until ultimate closure. No other patients experienced surgical site infections.

Although four patients who did not undergo neck dissection developed cervical subcutaneous emphysema supposedly owing to pharyngeal fissure opened to the surrounding soft tissues, all were absorbed spontaneously. Other minor surgical complications included postoperative minor hemorrhage, partial tooth damage, and injuries of the upper lip.

Functional results

Postoperative dysfunctions are summarized in Table 3. Fifty-six patients (78%), including all who had Tis or T1 tumors, resumed oral intake on the first or second post-operative day without obvious dysphasia.

In the other 16 patients (22%), all of whom had a T2 or T3 tumor resected, nasogastric feeding tubes were placed for a median of 4 (range: 1–12) days. The indication depended on the extent of estimated risk of postoperative dysphasia owing to various factors, including structural changes in the supraglottis leading to aspiration, narrowed esophageal entrance associated with transient mucosal edema, hypersecretion of mucus discharge, history of previous RT on the neck, and wound pain. Among them, two patients, who had T3N2b SGC and underwent adjuvant CCRT, developed aspiration pneumonia during or after CCRT, although they recovered after conservative treatment in association with swallowing rehabilitation. Other three patients, whose T2 HPC required a resection beyond the esophageal entrance, underwent balloon dilation periodically or irregularly to prevent a progressive stricture for 4 to 12 weeks. No patient underwent gastrostomy tube placement.

Overall, the median time until patients resumed oral intake was 2 days (range 1–8 days) and that until patients could take a soft meal was 5 days (range 1–21 days). Eventually, 69 patients (96%) were able to take normal meals. The remaining three patients, comprised of one patient who developed aspiration pneumonia and needed prolonged swallowing rehabilitation, one patient whose progressive stricture of the esophageal entrance could not be avoided, and another patient with Tis HPC who had a history of RT on the neck for previous oropharyngeal cancer, retained persistent dysphasia, although they did not require additional intervention. No patients complained of vocal dysfunction 1 month after the surgery.

Oncological outcomes and survival analyses

The median follow-up period of all patients (n = 72) and that of the patients alive at the time of the analysis (n = 56) were 45 (range, 7–105) and 52 (range, 24–105) months, respectively (Table 4). During follow-up, eight patients (11.1%) died of the index cancer (seven of distant metastasis and one of locoregional recurrence), and eight patients (11.1%) died of other causes. At the last follow-up, 54 patients (75.0%) were alive without the disease (including 12 patients who underwent either salvage surgery or CCRT/RT or both, and remained recurrence-free), and two patients (2.8%) were alive with the disease (both with distant metastasis).

The 3-year CSS and OS rates were 89.4% (95% CI, 82.0–96.9%) and 81.9% (95% CI, 72.6–91.2%), respectively (Fig. 6a). The 3-year LP-CSS and LRC-CSS rates

Table 4 Follow-up information (n = 72)

Median follow-up period		Months (range)	
of all patients		45 (7-105)	
of survivors (n = 56)		52 (24-105)	
Last status		No.	%
NED		54	75.0
AWD		2	2.8
DOD		8	11.1
DOC		8	11.1

NED No evidence of the disease, *AWD* Alive with the disease, *DOD* Died of the disease, *DOC* Died of other causes

were 86.0% (95% CI, 77.4–94.6%) and 88.0% (95% CI, 80.2–95.9%), respectively (Fig. 6b). Furthermore, 5-year CSS and OS rates were 87.3% (95% CI, 78.8–95.7%) and 77.9% (95% CI, 67.5–88.3%), respectively, whereas the 5-year LP-CSS and LRC-CSS rates remained the same as those of the 3-year rates, respectively. Because the cohort included nine patients with Tis lesions who inevitably raise the survival rates, each endpoint was also evaluated for the remaining 63 patients; 5-year CSS, OS, LP-CSS, and LRC-CSS rates were 81.4%, 76.6%, 80.5%, and 81.2%, respectively. However, these results were not significantly worse than those described above.

The results of the Cox proportional hazards model analysis are summarized in Table 5. In univariate analysis, patients with N2-3 showed significantly worse CSS (P = 0.010) and OS (P = 0.032) than those with N0-1, whereas no other factor was significantly associated with CSS or OS. Kaplan-Meier survival curves according to N stage with generalized Wilcoxon tests are shown in Fig. 6c and d. The 5-year CSS rates were 96.4% (95% CI: 89.6–100.0) for N0-1 and 69.2% (95% CI: 50.0–88.4) for N2-3 (P = 0.0003, Fig. 6c), whereas the 5-year OS rates were 87.3% (95% CI: 76.8–97.9) for N0-1 and 59.9% (95% CI: 39.3–80.4) for N2-3 (P = 0.005, Fig. 6d). Multivariate analysis using the Cox proportional hazards model revealed independent significance of N2-3 as an unfavorable prognostic factor in both CSS (HR = 25.51 [95% CI: 2.29–284.17] vs. N0-1, P = 0.008) and OS (HR = 4.90 [95% CI: 1.26–19.08] vs. N0-1, P = 0.022) (Table 5).

Discussion

The present study revealed that the cohort of patients with HPC and SGC who underwent TOVS as an initial treatment according to our criteria had favorable oncological outcomes, even after a long-term follow-up period. Notably, those results were achieved with fairly low incidence of surgical complication and minimal postoperative dysfunction. Thus, we regard TOVS, in

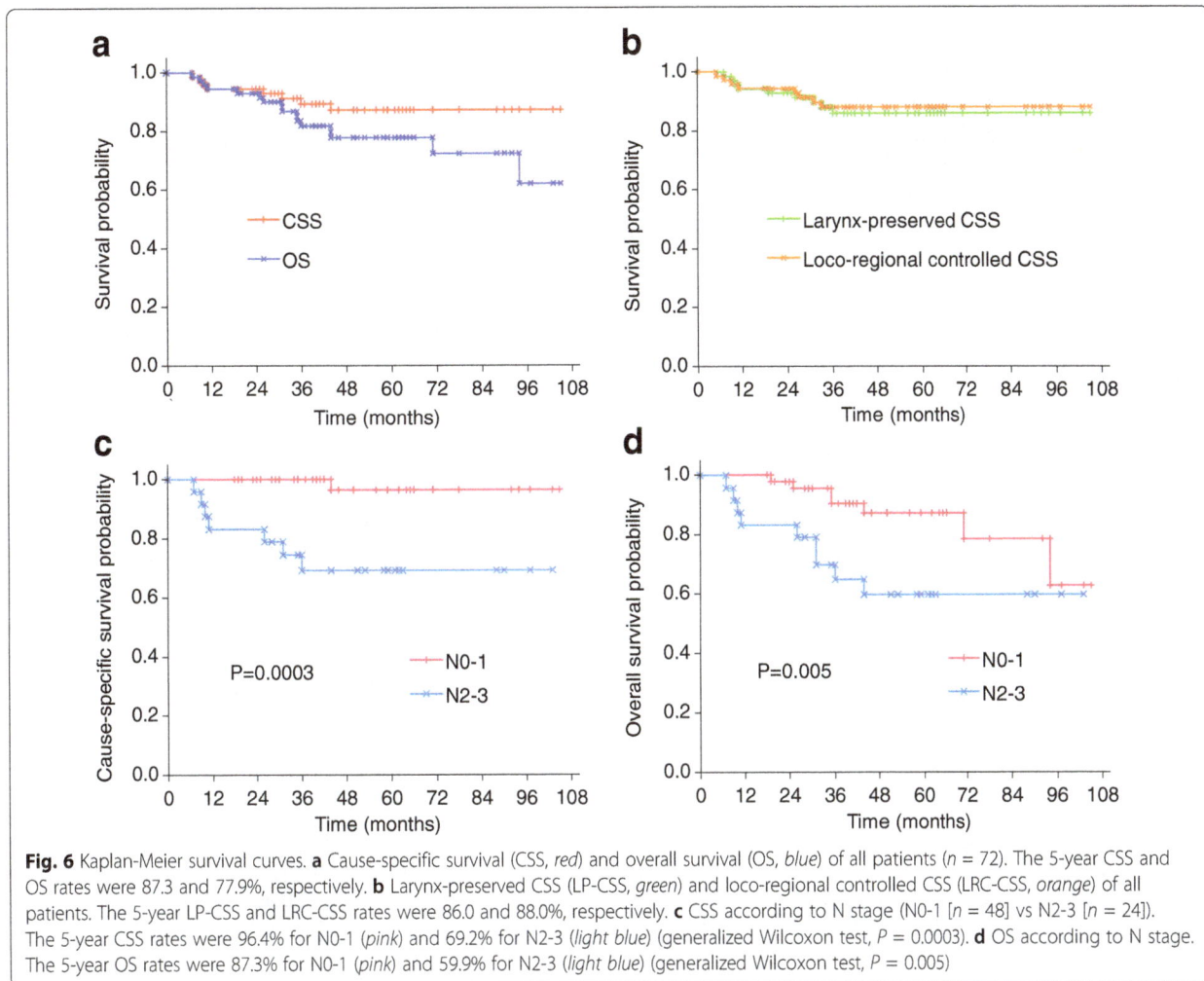

Fig. 6 Kaplan-Meier survival curves. **a** Cause-specific survival (CSS, *red*) and overall survival (OS, *blue*) of all patients (*n* = 72). The 5-year CSS and OS rates were 87.3 and 77.9%, respectively. **b** Larynx-preserved CSS (LP-CSS, *green*) and loco-regional controlled CSS (LRC-CSS, *orange*) of all patients. The 5-year LP-CSS and LRC-CSS rates were 86.0 and 88.0%, respectively. **c** CSS according to N stage (N0-1 [*n* = 48] vs N2-3 [*n* = 24]). The 5-year CSS rates were 96.4% for N0-1 (*pink*) and 69.2% for N2-3 (*light blue*) (generalized Wilcoxon test, *P* = 0.0003). **d** OS according to N stage. The 5-year OS rates were 87.3% for N0-1 (*pink*) and 59.9% for N2-3 (*light blue*) (generalized Wilcoxon test, *P* = 0.005)

combination with neck dissection and adjuvant CCRT if necessary, as one of the excellent therapeutic strategies in terms of organ-function preservation for patients with HPC and SGC.

Although several transoral approaches as less invasive surgery than conventional open PPL have been developed so far, TOVS has its own advantages over other approaches in terms of practical usefulness. When compared with TLM [16–22], TOVS has several technical advantages. First, since an endoscope lens possesses much longer depth range of focus (e.g., from 3 to 30 mm for a lens 4 mm in diameter) and wider angle of view (e.g., >110° for an above-mentioned lens) than that of a microscope, TOVS can provide a much broader surgical view in both horizontal and vertical directions compared to TLM, which helps improve recognition of anatomical orientation. Second, the field of endoscopic view is free from visual restriction due to the inner wall of the laryngeal blade that often restricts the microscopic view. Moreover, manipulation of surgical instruments is not restricted by a microscope interposed between

patient and surgeon. Third, en bloc resection of primary tumor achieved by TOVS enables accurate evaluation of pathological findings, especially about margin status, tumor depth, and horizontal diameter, which cannot be assessed in tumor specimens resected blockwise by TLM. Such pathological information, together with differentiation, vascular invasion, and lymphatic invasion, are indispensable not only for judging completeness of resection but also for assessing risk of delayed neck metastasis in clinically N0 patients [46]—this underscores the importance of en bloc resection in decision making regarding additional intervention. Fourth, the NBI mode equipped in endoscopes, including the ENDOEYE FLEX LTF-S190-5 (Olympus), is available even during surgery if necessary [33].

Although indications for use of TORS using da Vinci surgical systems have recently been extended to HPC and SGC in several countries [23–30], TORS has not been approved yet in many countries, including Japan. Instead, TOVS has been developed as a non-robotic transoral surgery in Japan. In comparison with TORS,

Table 5 Univariate and multivariate Cox regression analyses for cause-specific survival and overall survival ($n = 72$)

Variables	No.	Cause-specific survival						Overall survival					
		Univariate analysis			Multivariate analysis			Univariate analysis			Multivariate analysis		
		HR	(95% CI)	P-values	HR	(95% CI)	P-values	HR	(95% CI)	P-values	HR	(95% CI)	P-values
Age, y													
<70	45	1.00	reference		1.00	reference		1.00	reference		1.00	reference	
≧70	27	0.93	(0.22-3.89)	0.920	1.15	(0.24-5.42)	0.858	0.94	(0.34-2.60)	0.913	1.00	(0.34-2.89)	0.994
Sex													
Men	67	1.00			1.00			1.00	reference		1.00	reference	
Women	5	not calculable[a]		–	not calculable[a]		–	0.61	(0.08-4.75)	0.636	1.27	(0.13-12.38)	0.835
Tumor site													
HPC	58	1.00	reference		1.00	reference		1.00	reference		1.00	reference	
SGC	14	0.57	(0.07-4.68)	0.605	0.38	(0.04-3.43)	0.386	0.60	(0.14-2.64)	0.498	0.54	(0.11-2.69)	0.450
T stage													
Tis + T1	32	1.00	reference		1.00	reference		1.00	reference		1.00	reference	
T2-3	40	2.69	(0.54-13.34)	0.227	0.68	(0.09-5.24)	0.714	1.58	(0.57-4.35)	0.380	1.27	(0.29-5.54)	0.749
N stage													
N0-1	48	1.00	reference		1.00	reference		1.00	reference		1.00	reference	
N2-3	24	15.45	(1.90-125.69)	0.010*	25.51	(2.29-284.17)	0.008*	2.94	(1.09-7.90)	0.032*	4.90	(1.26-19.08)	0.022*
Multiple cancer													
No	18	1.00	reference		1.00	reference		1.00	reference		1.00	reference	
Yes	54	1.08	(0.22-5.36)	0.923	2.63	(0.45-15.20)	0.281	1.21	(0.39-3.82)	0.742	1.74	(0.47-6.41)	0.405
Previous RT													
No	60	1.00	reference		1.00			1.00	reference		1.00	reference	
Yes	12	0.68	(0.08-5.52)	0.717	not calculable[b]		–	1.09	(0.31-3.83)	0.894	2.23	(0.34-14.86)	0.406

HPC hypopharyngeal cancer, *SGC* supraglottic cancer, *RT* Radiotherapy, *HR* hazard ratio, *CI* confidence interval
* Statistically significant ($p < 0.05$)
[a]HR was not calculable because no woman died of the disease
[b]HR was not calculable because of strong confounding with N stage

TOVS has more practical advantages. First, since the surgeon bimanually manipulates surgical instruments directly on the real lesion, unlike TORS, the surgeon can recognize tactile sensations through those instruments; this is essential for assessing tumor invasion to the surrounding tissues and adding adequate counter-traction during the dissection procedure. Second, the cost-effectiveness of TOVS is far higher than that of TORS, because neither an extremely expensive surgical robot nor high-priced disposable equipment is required. Whereas most hospitals still cannot afford da Vinci surgical systems for TORS, the initial cost to introduce TOVS and its running costs are much lower, because most surgical instruments and devices are reusable, not originally designed for TOVS, and can be shared among other surgeries. Accordingly, TOVS can be introduced more easily than TORS in more hospitals in more countries.

Since endoscopes used in TOVS are not yet equipped with binocular vision, a three-dimensional view is not available. However, this does not really affect surgical performance because most otorhinolaryngologists/head and neck surgeons are already familiar with the two-dimensional endoscopic view. Fortunately, such a possible disadvantage compared to TLM and TORS is well compensated for by the use of high-resolution cameras. Furthermore, three-dimensional rigid endoscopes will be introduced in the near future, if necessary.

Besides TLM and TORS, a few other transoral approaches using a flexible gastrointestinal endoscope for early HPC were also reported with favorable outcomes from Japan: endoscopic mucosal resection (EMR) and endoscopic submucosal dissection (ESD) performed by gastroenterologists [47–50] and endoscopic laryngopharyngeal surgery performed by otorhinolaryngologists and gastroenterologists [43]. However, indication for use of these methods was confined to only patients with superficial lesions in the pharynx without lymph node metastasis (N0), excluding patients with SGC, invasive cancer, or lymph node metastasis (≥N1). Thus, distributions of disease stage in these patients, most of whom are at an incipient stage, are largely different from those of TOVS and others. In other words, indication for TOVS is very broad and ranges from superficial, small, or thin lesions (Tis) to invasive, exophytic, or bulky masses (up to T3 defined by size criteria). Notably, such wide-ranging lesions can be resected in the common setting with the same instruments; thus, high versatility is another advantage of TOVS.

A fair comparison of clinical outcomes between TOVS and other surgical approaches such as TLM or TORS seems difficult, because distributions of the disease stage, follow-up periods, and endpoint settings differ among them. However, oncological and functional outcomes of TOVS, including the previous report [33], are mostly comparable to those of TLM and TORS [16–30]. Considering the distribution of disease stage in the patients in our study, a half of them were stage III–IV, the long-term oncological and functional outcomes appeared to be satisfactory. These results may corroborate an overall validity of this therapeutic strategy, including the criteria of indication, the principles of surgical management, and the standards of adjuvant treatments, especially about the relatively low necessity of postoperative RT.

However, it should be noted that strict observation in the follow-up period is another crucial prerequisite to achieve high LP-CSS and LRC-CSS in this cohort, because a majority of them possessed a high risk of developing second primary cancer in the pharyngolaryngeal region, even though the primary lesion was completely resected. In our cohort, although 18 patients developed one or multiple second primary cancer in the pharyngolaryngeal region, all but one was diagnosed at an early stage. Among them, 16 patients were able to preserve the larynx by repeated TOVS alone (n = 10), by following TOVS with RT for a third primary tumor with (n = 1) or without (n = 1) cetuximab, by open PPL alone (n = 2), by following open PPL with CCRT for a close margin (n = 1), or by RT alone (n = 1); in contrast, the other two patients ultimately required total laryngectomy for unavoidable reasons. Therefore, close attention must be maintained throughout follow-up so that second or later primary lesion can be treated appropriately as early as possible.

In both CSS and OS, advanced N stage (N2-3) was found to be the only independent unfavorable prognostic factor in this cohort, probably in part because of relatively low statistical power due to small sample size. Intriguingly, in accordance with the LRC-CSS rate as high as 88.0% at 3 and 5 years, uncontrolled regional failure and related death occurred in only one of 10 patients who developed treatment failure. The remaining nine patients developed distant metastasis without locoregional failure, seven of whom died as a consequence,

suggesting that N2-3 is a strong predictor of death due to delayed distant metastasis. In agreement with these results, N2-3 was also found to be an independent unfavorable predictor of distant metastasis-free survival (data not shown). Thus, in common with many other cancers at an advanced stage, the most critical unsolved issue appears to be management of distant metastasis, irrespective of differences in therapeutic modality for locoregional lesions.

Regarding postoperative management-related issues, the incidence of temporary tracheostomy is relatively low in cohorts who underwent TOVS, including both the present (2.8%) and previous (6.7%) reports [33], while it varies largely in each of the other surgical approaches such as TLM, TORS, and ESD/EMR. Several recent studies reported a relatively high incidence of tracheostomy in TLM (12.2–16.0%) [21, 22], TORS (23.8–100%) [26, 29], and ESD/EMR (16.3%) [49]; however, these numbers seem to reflect the prophylactic use of tracheostomy to a certain extent. On the other hand, in some studies in which no patients underwent tracheostomy, instead, a high incidence of prolonged intubation of more than 24 h was reported in TLM (27.1%) [16], TORS (60.0%) [30], and ESD (30.8%) [47]. Although the necessity of tracheostomy principally depends on the extent of postoperative laryngeal edema based on depth and width of the defect after tumor resection and its location, because such estimation involved personal experience and expertise in airway management, making a decision of tracheostomy is rather subjective. In our experience, careful observation of the surgical site in view of the whole laryngopharynx under endoscope by skilled otorhinolaryngologists just after resection is sufficient to make an appropriate decision.

Fortunately, no patients experienced major postoperative hemorrhage that required return to the operation room for emergency treatment. Since we have been well aware of the potential risk of hemorrhage that can be fatal, maximum attention has always been paid to completeness of hemostasis after resection. In our practice, use of a super long bipolar forceps and/or BiClamp LAP forceps can efficiently control any active bleeding during surgery without difficulty. In case a patient has taken an anticoagulant agent, proper management of the drug during the perioperative period is also imperative to prevent increased hemorrhage.

Although aspiration pneumonia was found only in three patients, slight mucus influx into the glottis was observed temporarily in some other patients, especially at an early period after TOVS, suggesting that silent aspiration might occur more frequently. It can be assumed that such transient aspiration that could develop into pneumonia was preventively resolved in many ways, including minute endoscopic evaluation of swallowing function before and after resuming oral intake, timely removal of feeding tube without delay, thoughtful adjustment of form of meal by a dietitian, and appropriate introduction of swallowing rehabilitation if necessary. In addition, effects of preventive efforts to avoid progressive stricture, such as injection of steroid just after resection and repeated balloon dilation if necessary, also appeared to be reflected by a low incidence of persistent dysphasia. Furthermore, in some patients with advanced N stage who underwent neck dissection, reduced intensity of adjuvant CCRT, which was based on the detailed histopathological finding of lymph node metastasis, was also assumed to partly contribute to better function-preservation.

Conclusions

TOVS for patients with HPC and SGC as an initial treatment provided favorable long-term oncological outcomes with low frequency of surgical complication and minimal functional impairment, corroborating its validity as a therapeutic strategy for this cohort. While high LP-CSS and LRC-CSS reflected its excellent locoregional control, advanced N stage determined as an independent prognostic factor in both CSS and OS indirectly reflected higher risk of delayed development of distant metastasis as an unsolved issue. Considering its sound clinical outcomes and various practical advantages, TOVS can be a dependable, less invasive, and cost-effective surgical option of an organ-function preservation strategy for HPC and SGC.

Abbreviations

CCRT: Concurrent chemoradiation; CDDP: Cis-platinum; CI: Confidence interval; CIS: Carcinoma in situ; CRT: Chemoradiation; CSS: Cause-specific survival; EMR: Endoscopic mucosal resection; ESD: Endoscopic submucosal dissection; HPC: Hypopharyngeal cancer; HR: Hazard ratio; IPCL: Intra-epithelial papillary capillary loop; LP: Larynx-preserved; LRC: Loco-regional controlled; OS: Overall survival; PPL: Partial pharyngolaryngectomy; RT: Radiation; SCC: Squamous cell carcinoma; SGC: Supraglottic cancer; TLM: Transoral laser microsurgery; TORS: Transoral robotic surgery; TOVS: Transoral videolaryngoscopic surgery

Acknowledgements

We sincerely thank Akihiro Shiotani, Department of Otolaryngology-Head and Neck Surgery, National Defense Medical College, for helpful technical advice and thoughtful suggestions. We also thank Editage (https://www.edita-ge.com/new/) for English language editing.

Funding

This work was supported in part by Grants-in-Aid for Scientific Research (C) from MEXT (No.22591917 and 25462692 to Y.I.) and that from The Japan Society for the Promotion of Science (No.16K11245 to Y.I.), the research grant from Keio Gijuku Academic Development Funds (Number is not applicable), and the research grant from The Japanese Foundation For Research and Promotion of Endoscopy (Number is not applicable). Funding bodies had no role in the design of the study, or collection, analysis, or interpretation of data, or in writing the manuscript.

Authors' contributions

YI conceived and designed the study, performed and assisted surgery, collected patients' information, executed the data analysis, and drafted and finalized the manuscript. HO provided support for conducting the study, managed the patients, and contributed to the data interpretation. KS, RF, SS, NH, KOt, YS, and YW performed and assisted surgery, managed the patients, and participated in the data analysis. MS and FI managed the patients and contributed to the data analysis. TT provided general support and critical advice to the study. KOg provided comprehensive support throughout the study. All authors read and approved the final manuscript.

Competing interests

The authors declare that they have no competing interests.

Author details

[1]Department of Otorhinolaryngology–Head and Neck Surgery, Keio University School of Medicine, 35 Shinanomachi, Shinjuku, Tokyo 160-8582, Japan. [2]Department of Otorhinolaryngology, Kawasaki Municipal Kawasaki Hospital, Kawasaki, Kanagawa 210-0013, Japan. [3]Department of Otorhinolaryngology, Saiseikai Utsunomiya Hospital, Utsunomiya, Tochigi 321-0974, Japan. [4]Department of Otorhinolaryngology, Saiseikai Yokohamashi Nanbu Hospital, Yokohama, Kanagawa 234-0054, Japan. [5]Department of Otorhinolaryngology, Yokohama Municipal Citizen's Hospital, Yokohama, Kanagawa 240-8555, Japan. [6]Department of Otorhinolaryngology, Kyosai Tachikawa Hospital, Tachikawa, Tokyo 190-0022, Japan. [7]Department of Otorhinolaryngology, Saiseikai Yokohamashi Tobu Hospital, Yokohama, Kanagawa 230-8765, Japan.

References

1. Carvalho AL, Nishimoto IN, Califano JA, Kowalski LP. Trends in incidence and prognosis for head and neck cancer in the United States: a site-specific analysis of the SEER database. Int J Cancer. 2005;114:806–16.
2. Cooper JS, Porter K, Mallin K, Hoffman HT, Weber RS, Ang KK, et al. National Cancer Database report on cancer of the head and neck: 10-year update. Head Neck. 2009;31:748–58.
3. Takes RP, Strojan P, Silver CE, Bradley PJ, Haigentz M Jr, Wolf GT, et al. Current trends in initial management of hypopharyngeal cancer: the declining use of open surgery. Head Neck. 2012;34:270–81.
4. Newman JR, Connolly TM, Illing EA, Kilgore ML, Locher JL, Carroll WR. Survival trends in hypopharyngeal cancer: a population-based review. Laryngoscope. 2015;125:624–9.
5. Pointreau Y, Garaud P, Chapet S, Sire C, Tuchais C, Tortochaux J, et al. Randomized trial of induction chemotherapy with cisplatin and 5-fluorouracil with or without docetaxel for larynx preservation. J Natl Cancer Inst. 2009;101:498–506.
6. Posner MR, Norris CM, Wirth LJ, Shin DM, Cullen KJ, Winquist EW, et al. Sequential therapy for the locally advanced larynx and hypopharynx cancer subgroup in TAX 324: survival, surgery, and organ preservation. Ann Oncol. 2009;20:921–7.
7. Prades JM, Lallemant B, Garrel R, Reyt E, Righini C, Schmitt T, et al. Randomized phase III trial comparing induction chemotherapy followed by radiotherapy to concomitant chemoradiotherapy for laryngeal preservation in T3M0 pyriform sinus carcinoma. Acta Otolaryngol. 2010;130:150–5.
8. Lee WT, Akst LM, Adelstein DJ, Saxton JP, Wood BG, Strome M, et al. Risk factors for hypopharyngeal/upper esophageal stricture formation after concurrent chemoradiation. Head Neck. 2006;28:808–12.
9. Machtay M, Moughan J, Trotti A, Garden AS, Weber RS, Cooper JS, et al. Factors associated with severe late toxicity after concurrent chemoradiation for locally advanced head and neck cancer: an RTOG analysis. J Clin Oncol. 2008;26:3582–9.
10. Hutcheson KA, Lewin JS. Functional outcomes after chemoradiotherapy of laryngeal and pharyngeal cancers. Curr Oncol Rep. 2012;14:158–65.
11. Keereweer S, Kerrebijn JD, Al-Mamgani A, Sewnaik A, Baatenburg de Jong RJ, van Meerten E. Chemoradiation for advanced hypopharyngeal carcinoma: a retrospective study on efficacy, morbidity and quality of life. Eur Arch Otorhinolaryngol. 2012;269:939–46.

12. Petkar I, Rooney K, Roe JW, Patterson JM, Bernstein D, Tyler JM, et al. DARS: a phase III randomised multicentre study of dysphagia- optimised intensity-modulated radiotherapy (do-IMRT) versus standard intensity- modulated radiotherapy (S-IMRT) in head and neck cancer. BMC Cancer. 2016;16:770.

13. Gehanno P, Barry B, Guedon C, Depondt J. Lateral supraglottic pharyngolaryngectomy with arytenoidectomy. Head Neck. 1996;18:494–500.

14. Laccourreye O, Ishoo E, de Mones E, Garcia D, Kania R, Hans S. Supracricoid hemilaryngopharyngectomy in patients with invasive squamous cell carcinoma of the pyriform sinus. Part I: technique, complications, and long-term functional outcome. Ann Otol Rhinol Laryngol. 2005;114:25–34.

15. Holsinger FC, Motamed M, Garcia D, Brasnu D, Menard M, Laccourreye O. Resection of selected invasive squamous cell carcinoma of the pyriform sinus by means of the lateral pharyngotomy approach: the partial lateral pharyngectomy. Head Neck. 2006;28:705–11.

16. Ambrosch P, Kron M, Steiner W. Carbon dioxide laser microsurgery for early supraglottic carcinoma. Ann Otol Rhinol Laryngol. 1998;107:680–8.

17. Steiner W, Ambrosch P, Hess CF, Kron M. Organ preservation by transoral laser microsurgery in piriform sinus carcinoma. Otolaryngol Head Neck Surg. 2001;124:58–67.

18. Rudert HH, Hoft S. Transoral carbon-dioxide laser resection of hypopharyngeal carcinoma. Eur Arch Otorhinolaryngol. 2003;260:198–206.

19. Vilaseca I, Blanch JL, Bernal-Sprekelsen M, Moragas M. CO2 laser surgery: a larynx preservation alternative for selected hypopharyngeal carcinomas. Head Neck. 2004;26:953–9.

20. Martin A, Jackel MC, Christiansen H, Mahmoodzada M, Kron M, Steiner W. Organ preserving transoral laser microsurgery for cancer of the hypopharynx. Laryngoscope. 2008;118:398–402.

21. Karatzanis AD, Psychogios G, Waldfahrer F, Zenk J, Hornung J, Velegrakis GA, et al. T1 and T2 hypopharyngeal cancer treatment with laser microsurgery. J Surg Oncol. 2010;102:27–33.

22. Gonzalez-Marquez R, Rodrigo JP, Llorente JL, Alvarez-Marcos C, Diaz JP, Suarez C. Transoral CO(2) laser surgery for supraglottic cancer. Eur Arch Otorhinolaryngol. 2012;269:2081–6.

23. Weinstein GS, O'Malley BW Jr, Snyder W, Hockstein NG. Transoral robotic surgery: supraglottic partial laryngectomy. Ann Otol Rhinol Laryngol. 2007;116:19–23.

24. Desai SC, Sung CK, Jang DW, Genden EM. Transoral robotic surgery using a carbon dioxide flexible laser for tumors of the upper aerodigestive tract. Laryngoscope. 2008;118:2187–9.

25. Genden EM, Desai S, Sung CK. Transoral robotic surgery for the management of head and neck cancer: a preliminary experience. Head Neck. 2009;31:283–9.

26. Park YM, Kim WS, De Virgilio A, Lee SY, Seol JH, Kim SH. Transoral robotic surgery for hypopharyngeal squamous cell carcinoma: 3-year oncologic and functional analysis. Oral Oncol. 2012;48:560–6.

27. Mendelsohn AH, Remacle M, Van Der Vorst S, Bachy V, Lawson G. Outcomes following transoral robotic surgery: supraglottic laryngectomy. Laryngoscope. 2013;123:208–14.

28. Dziegielewski PT, Kang SY, Ozer E. Transoral robotic surgery (TORS) for laryngeal and hypopharyngeal cancers. J Surg Oncol. 2015;112:702–6.

29. Razafindranaly V, Lallemant B, Aubry K, Moriniere S, Vergez S, Mones ED, et al. Clinical outcomes with transoral robotic surgery for supraglottic squamous cell carcinoma: experience of a French evaluation cooperative subgroup of GETTEC. Head Neck. 2016;38(Suppl 1):E1097–101.

30. Wang CC, Liu SA, Wu SH, Wang CP, Liang KL, Jiang RS, et al. Transoral robotic surgery for early T classification hypopharyngeal cancer. Head Neck. 2016;38:857–62.

31. Shiotani A, Tomifuji M, Araki K, Yamashita T, Saito K. Videolaryngoscopic transoral en bloc resection of supraglottic and hypopharyngeal cancers using laparoscopic surgical instruments. Ann Otol Rhinol Laryngol. 2010;119:225–32.

32. Yamashita T, Tomifuji M, Araki K, Kurioka T, Shiotani A. Endoscopic transoral oropharyngectomy using laparoscopic surgical instruments. Head Neck. 2011;33:1315 21.

33. Tomifuji M, Araki K, Yamashita T, Shiotani A. Transoral videolaryngoscopic surgery for oropharyngeal, hypopharyngeal, and supraglottic cancer. Eur Arch Otorhinolaryngol. 2014;271:589–97.

34. AJCC Cancer Staging Manual. 7th ed. New York: Springer; 2010.

35. Hillel AD, Schwartz AN. Trumpet maneuver for visual and CT examination of the pyriform sinus and retrocricoid area. Head Neck. 1989;11:231–6.

36. Williams RS, Lancaster J, Karagama Y, Tandon S, Karkanevatos A. A systematic approach to the nasendoscopic examination of the larynx and pharynx. Clin Otolaryngol Allied Sci. 2004;29:175–8.

37. Freeman SR, Keith AO, Aucott W, Kazmi N, Nigam A. Comparison between two valsalva techniques for improvement of hypopharyngeal nasendoscopy: a preliminary communication. Clin Otolaryngol. 2007;32:488–91.

38. Muto M, Katada C, Sano Y, Yoshida S. Narrow band imaging: a new diagnostic approach to visualize angiogenesis in superficial neoplasia. Clin Gastroenterol Hepatol. 2005;3:S16–20.

39. Watanabe A, Taniguchi M, Tsujie H, Hosokawa M, Fujita M, Sasaki S. The value of narrow band imaging endoscope for early head and neck cancers. Otolaryngol Head Neck Surg. 2008;138:446–51.

40. Tan NC, Herd MK, Brennan PA, Puxeddu R. The role of narrow band imaging in early detection of head and neck cancer. Br J Oral Maxillofac Surg. 2012;50:132–6.

41. Nakamura H, Yano T, Fujii S, Kadota T, Tomioka T, Shinozaki T, et al. Natural history of superficial head and neck squamous cell carcinoma under scheduled follow-up endoscopic observation with narrow band imaging: retrospective cohort study. BMC Cancer. 2016;16:743.

42. Lell MM, Greess H, Hothorn T, Janka R, Bautz WA, Baum U. Multiplanar functional imaging of the larynx and hypopharynx with multislice spiral CT. Eur Radiol. 2004;14:2198–205.

43. Tateya I, Muto M, Morita S, Miyamoto S, Hayashi T, Funakoshi M, et al. Endoscopic laryngo-pharyngeal surgery for superficial laryngo-pharyngeal cancer. Surg Endosc. 2016;30:323–9.

44. Hashimoto S, Kobayashi M, Takeuchi M, Sato Y, Narisawa R, Aoyagi Y. The efficacy of endoscopic triamcinolone injection for the prevention of esophageal stricture after endoscopic submucosal dissection. Gastrointest Endosc. 2011;74:1389–93.

45. Hanaoka N, Ishihara R, Takeuchi Y, Uedo N, Higashino K, Ohta T, et al. Intralesional steroid injection to prevent stricture after endoscopic submucosal dissection for esophageal cancer: a controlled prospective study. Endoscopy. 2012;44:1007–11.

46. Tomifuji M, Imanishi Y, Araki K, Yamashita T, Yamamoto S, Kameyama K, et al. Tumor depth as a predictor of lymph node metastasis of supraglottic and hypopharyngeal cancers. Ann Surg Oncol. 2011;18:490–6.

47. Iizuka T, Kikuchi D, Hoteya S, Yahagi N, Takeda H. Endoscopic submucosal dissection for treatment of mesopharyngeal and hypopharyngeal carcinomas. Endoscopy. 2009;41:113–7.

48. Shimizu Y, Yoshida T, Kato M, Ono S, Nakagawa M, Homma A, et al. Long-term outcome after endoscopic resection in patients with hypopharyngeal carcinoma invading the subepithelium: a case series. Endoscopy. 2009;41:374–6.

49. Muto M, Satake H, Yano T, Minashi K, Hayashi R, Fujii S, et al. Long-term outcome of transoral organ-preserving pharyngeal endoscopic resection for superficial pharyngeal cancer. Gastrointest Endosc. 2011;74:477–84.

50. Hanaoka N, Ishihara R, Takeuchi Y, Suzuki M, Uemura H, Fujii T, et al. Clinical outcomes of endoscopic mucosal resection and endoscopic submucosal dissection as a transoral treatment for superficial pharyngeal cancer. Head Neck. 2013;35:1248–54.

9

The prognostic value of pretreatment tumor apparent diffusion coefficient values in nasopharyngeal carcinoma

Dan-Fang Yan[1], Wen-Bao Zhang[1], Shan-Bao Ke[4], Feng Zhao[1], Sen-Xiang Yan[1*], Qi-Dong Wang[2] and Li-Song Teng[3*]

Abstract

Background: Diffusion-weighted MR imaging (DWI) has increasingly contributed to the management of nasopharyngeal carcinoma (NPC) patients. The objective of this paper was to explore the prognostic significance of apparent diffusion coefficient (ADC) values in 93 NPC patients.

Methods: This retrospective study included 93 newly diagnosed NPC patients. Pretreatment ADC values were determined and compared with patients' age, gender, alcohol intake, smoking, tumor volume, pathological type, tumor stage, and nodal stage. Using the Kaplan-Meier method, overall survival (OS), local relapse-free survival (LRFS), and distant metastasis-free survival (DMFS) were calculated and the values compared between the low and high ADC groups. Multivariate analysis of ADC values and other 9 clinical parameters was performed using a Cox proportional hazards model to test the independent significance for OS, LRFS and DMFS.

Results: The mean ADC value for the initial nasopharyngeal tumors was 0.72×10^{-3} mm^2/s (range: 0.48–0.97×10^{-3} mm^2/s). There was no significant difference between pretreatment ADCs and patient' gender, age, smoking, alcohol intake, or tumor stage. A significant difference in the ADCs for different N stages ($P = 0.022$) and correlation with initial tumor volume ($r = -0.26$, $P = 0.012$) were observed. In comparison, the ADC value for undifferentiated carcinoma was lower than that for other 3 pathological types. With a median follow-up period of 50 months, the 3-year and 5-year OS rates were 88.2% and 83.3%, respectively, 3-year and 5-year LRFS rates were 93.5% and 93.3%, respectively, and 3-year and 5-year DMFS rates were 83.9% and 83.3%, respectively. Patients with tumor ADC values $\geq 0.72 \times 10^{-3}$ mm^2/s exhibited longer OS and LRFS periods compared with tumor ADC values $< 0.72 \times 10^{-3}$ mm^2/s, with P values 0.036 and 0.018, respectively. In addition, patients with deaths or recurrences or distant metastasis had significant lower ADC values than those without disease failures. According to a multivariate analysis using the Cox proportional hazard test, ADC values showed a significant correlation with OS ($P = 0.0004$), LRFS ($P = 0.0009$), and DMFS ($P < 0.0001$), respectively.

Conclusions: Pretreatment tumor ADC values supposed to be a noninvasive important prognostic parameter for NPC.

Keywords: Apparent diffusion coefficient value, Nasopharyngeal carcinoma, Diffusion-weighted magnetic resonance imaging

* Correspondence: yansenxiang@zju.edu.cn; Lsteng@zju.edu.cn
[1]Department of Radiation Oncology, the First Affiliated Hospital, College of Medicine, Zhejiang University, 79 Qingchun RoadHangzhou, Zhejiang 310003, People's Republic of China
[3]Department of Oncology, the First Affiliated Hospital, College of Medicine, Zhejiang University, 79 Qingchun Road, Zhejiang, Hangzhou 310003, China
Full list of author information is available at the end of the article

Background

Nasopharyngeal carcinoma (NPC) is a head and neck malignancy commonly diagnosed in southern China and southeast Asia [1]. Moreover, the World Health Organization (WHO) estimates that over 80,000 new cases of NPC are diagnosed worldwide [1]. It is important to identify factors that are useful for predicting prognosis and helping personalize therapies. Established prognostic factors include histopathological type, tumor stage, and nodal stage. Furthermore, these factors have been shown to correlate significantly with the overall survival (OS) and progress-free survival (PFS) in NPC patients [2–5].

Magnetic resonance imaging (MRI) plays an important role in managing patients with NPC. For example, it is used for tumor staging, for delineating target volumes, and for detecting recurrence [6–8]. Another valuable imaging technique is diffusion-weighted MR imaging (DWI), and for its sensitivity to the motion of water molecules, it reflects the viability and structure of tissues on a cellular level [9, 10]. DWI is increasingly applied in the head and neck patient; for example, to distinguish recurrence and post-irradiation change. Moreover, DWI can differentiate metastatic lymph nodes from benign lymphadenopathy or nodal lymphomas [11–13], and DWI can also detect nodal and distant metastases [14, 15]. Furthermore, DWI is useful for monitoring the treatment response following chemotherapy or radiation [16].

Apparent diffusion coefficient (ADC) values have recently been reported to correlate with several prognostic parameters for varied tumors [17–19], such as retinoblastoma, lung cancer, breast cancer, and head and neck cancers [20, 21]. In this study, to explore whether similar results are obtained, we correlate tumoral ADC with treatment outcomes in a homogeneous group of NPC patients who exhibit a different pathogenesis, biological behavior, and natural course from other head and neck cancer patients.

Methods

Study patients

We retrospectively analyzed pretreatment MR-images and other clinical information from 93 consecutive newly diagnosed NPC patients. Endoscopic examinations to detect a clinically suspected lesion in the nasopharynx were performed on all patients, and pathology was obtained at first diagnosis. Distant metastases were ruled out during staging workup using chest computed tomography (CT), abdominal ultrasound, and bone scintigraphy. The ethical committee of Zhejiang University approved this analysis. Patient consents were obtained from all of the studied patients.

MRI and DWI techniques

MRI was performed using a Philips 3.0 T Intera Master (Philips, Amsterdam, The Netherlands) with a standard head coil, two-channel dedicated surface neck coil, and spine coil. The transverse sequences consisted of 44 slices (5 mm each) and a 0.5 mm intersection gap. DWI was performed using a multiple section spin-echo single-shot echoplanar sequence in the transverse plane. A single-shot echoplanar sequence was also carried out before the injection of contrast agent gadolinium DTPA (Gd-DTPA), and this consisted of a 96×96 matrix, a TR/TE = 2947.1 ms/43.3 ms, b-values of 0 and 1500 s/mm^2, a field-of-view (FOV) of 260×260 mm^2, and a NSA of 6. To obtain the best image quality, an integrated phase correction was applied during DWI.

Acquisition of ADC values

DWI data was analyzed by an experienced radiologist blinded to this study. A workstation (Agfa-Gevaert, Mortsel, Belgium) was used to identify a region of interest (ROI) for each definitive solid lesion, while avoiding necrotic or cystic components that were observed to be ≤10 mm^2 with DWI. Subsequently, ADC values of ROIs were acquired from ADC maps directly, reconstructed using b values of 1500 and 0 s/mm^2. ROIs were collected on 2 to 3 slices for every lesion to quantitate the primary tumor' ADC and the tumor's final ADC value was defined as an average value for these ROIs.

Patient treatment

All 93 patients received radical intensity modulated radiation therapy (IMRT). Dose of 6540–7412 cGy/30–34F was delivered to each planned gross tumor volume (PGTV), while 5264 cGy/28F to 6016 cGy/32F was given to each planning target volume (PTV). A total of 88 patients received concurrent chemotherapy with platinum-based drugs (80 mg/m^2) intravenously every 3 weeks for 3 courses during IMRT, while the other 5 patients received IMRT alone (either because of early tumor stage or they refused to receive chemotherapy).

Clinical endpoint

Patient follow-ups were scheduled every 1 or 2 months within the first half year of a diagnosis, then every 3 months for the next 6 months, and once every 6 months thereafter. MRI with contrast enhancement and DWI were performed to evaluate locoregional recurrence. Chest CT, abdominal ultrasound, and bone scintigraphy, and less frequently positron emission tomography (PET)/CT, were also conducted to detect distant metastasis. Local relapse was established based on histologic confirmation (biopsy or surgical resection), detection of a new mass, or a serial increase in size of a residual mass. In addition, distant failure was determined with detection of any new masses in the liver, lung, bone, or brain during routine evaluations conducted during a follow-up period of at least 1 year.

Overall survival (OS) was calculated from the completion of IMRT until death. Local relapse was defined based on primary tumor or regional lymph node recurrence, while distant failure was defined as distant metastasis.

Statistical analysis

SAS v9.0 statistical software package was used for statistical analysis. In addition, mean ± standard deviation (SD) ADC values for each prognostic parameters were measured. Student's t-test was applied to independent samples to identify differences in ADC values between two groups, while one-way analysis of variance (ANOVA) was used to evaluate differences between more than two groups. Pearson correlation was performed to correlate NPC ADC values with tumor volume and to correlate primary ADC values with ADC values for the cervical lymph nodes. P-values and r values were also calculated. Using the Kaplan-Meier method, patient survival (including OS, LRFS, and DMFS) were calculated and the values compared between the low and high ADC groups; differences were compared using the log-rank test. Independent significance of different factors was tested using multivariate analysis in a Cox proportional hazards model. When testing the association with survival (including OS, LRFS, DMFS), patient age, gender, smoking, alcohol intake, tumor volume, pathological type, tumor stage, nodal stage, and pretreatment ADCs were included in multivariate analyses. A P value of less than 0.05 was considered significant.

Results

Patient characteristics

The present cohort included 69 males and 24 females with a median age of 52 years (range: 22–82 years). According to the 7th edition of the American Joint Committee on Cancer (AJCC) manual, 3 patients had stage I disease, 19 patients had stage II, 55 were stage III, and 16 were stage IV (comprising 12 with IVa disease and 4 with IVb disease). Histologically, 30 lesions were identified as well-differentiated non-keratinizing carcinomas, 39 as poorly differentiated non-keratinizing, 8 as keratinizing squamous cell, and 16 as undifferentiated carcinomas (Table 1).

Tumor ADC values and prognostic parameters

The mean ADC value for the primary tumors analyzed was 0.72×10^{-3} mm²/s, range: 0.48–0.97×10^{-3} mm²/s. In addition, Table 1 lists the minimum, maximum, and mean ADC values in correlation to patient age, gender, smoking and drinking status, tumor pathological type, tumor grade, and metastatic cervical lymph nodes. The most common histopathological type of NPC for this cohort was poorly differentiated non-keratinizing carcinoma

Table 1 Mean, minimum, and maximum ADC values for the NPC cases analyzed according to various clinical characteristics

Factors	N (Total = 93)	ADC values			P-value
		Minimum	Maximum	Mean ± SD	
Age					0.83
< 50 y	37	0.52	0.92	0.73 ± 0.11	
≥ 50 y	56	0.48	0.97	0.72 ± 0.10	
Gender					0.28
Male	69	0.48	0.97	0.72 ± 0.10	
Female	24	0.57	0.92	0.74 ± 0.10	
Smoking status					0.30
Yes	46	0.57	0.92	0.73 ± 0.09	
No	47	0.48	0.97	0.71 ± 0.11	
Alcohol intake					0.75
Yes	58	0.48	0.92	0.73 ± 0.09	
No	35	0.58	0.97	0.72 ± 0.11	
Pathological type*					0.51
1	8	0.61	0.97	0.79 ± 0.13	
2	39	0.57	0.96	0.72 ± 0.10	
3	30	0.48	0.97	0.72 ± 0.10	
4	16	0.59	0.83	0.70 ± 0.06	
Tumor stage					0.53
T1	15	0.48	0.92	0.71 ± 0.14	
T2	48	0.57	0.97	0.73 ± 0.09	
T3	17	0.59	0.95	0.74 ± 0.10	
T4	13	0.59	0.85	0.69 ± 0.07	
Nodal stage					0.022
N0	10	0.52	0.84	0.66 ± 0.08	
N1	16	0.47	0.97	0.72 ± 0.12	
N2	63	0.57	0.95	0.73 ± 0.09	
N3	4	0.64	0.97	0.81 ± 0.13	

ADC: apparent diffusion coefficient; NPC: nasopharyngeal carcinoma; SD: standard deviation
*Type1: keratinizing squamous cell carcinoma; Type 2: poorly differentiated non-keratinizing carcinoma; Type 3: well differentiated non-keratinizing carcinoma; Type 4: undifferentiated carcinoma

(type 2, $n = 39$), followed by well differentiated non-keratinizing carcinoma (type 3, $n = 30$). The ADC values for keratinizing squamous cell carcinoma (type 1), poorly differentiated non-keratinizing carcinoma(type 2), and well differentiated non-keratinizing carcinoma (type 3) NPC were $0.79 \pm 0.13 \times 10^{-3}$ mm²/s, $0.72 \pm 0.10 \times 10^{-3}$ mm²/s, and $0.72 \pm 0.10 \times 10^{-3}$ mm²/s, respectively. In comparison, the ADC value for type 4 (undifferentiated carcinoma) was $0.70 \pm 0.06 \times 10^{-3}$ mm²/s, which was lower than that for types 1–3. However, between type 1 and type 4, there was a significant difference with a P value 0.024.

The most common tumor stage was T2 (n = 48), and the ADC values for T2 and T3 tumors ($0.73 \pm 0.09 \times 10^{-3}$ mm^2/s and $0.74 \pm 0.10 \times 10^{-3}$ mm^2/s, respectively) were higher than those for T1 and T4 tumors ($0.71 \pm 0.14 \times 10^{-3}$ mm^2/s and $0.69 \pm 0.07 \times 10^{-3}$ mm^2/s, respectively). However, no significant difference between the four groups were observed (P = 0.53).

According to metastatic cervical lymph node status, the mean ADC values for the primary tumors were $0.66 \pm 0.08 \times 10^{-3}$ mm^2/s for patients with N0 (n = 10), $0.72 \pm 0.12 \times 10^{-3}$ mm^2/s for N1 (n = 16), $0.73 \pm 0.09 \times 10^{-3}$ mm^2/s for N2 (n = 63), and $0.81 \pm 0.13 \times 10^{-3}$ mm^2/s for N3 (n = 4). Furthermore, the ADC values did significantly differ between these N staging groups (P = 0.022) (Table 1).

The mean ADC value for the metastatic cervical lymph nodes was $0.70 \pm 0.095 \times 10^{-3}$ mm^2/s, and an obvious positive correlation was observed between the ADC values for primary tumors and the ADC values for metastatic cervical lymph nodes (r = 0.42, P < 0.001) (Fig. 1). The median tumor volume (including both primary nasopharyngeal tumors and metastatic cervical lymph nodes) was 85.5 ml (range, 21.8–306 ml), and the primary tumor ADC values were found to negatively correlate with tumor volume (r = −0.26, P = 0.012). Consequently, lower ADC values were found to represent larger tumor volumes (Fig. 1).

Tumor ADC values and survival outcomes

The median duration of the follow-up period following the completion of radiotherapy was 50 months (range, 36–68 months). During this time, 20/93 patients died, 3 due to fatal nasopharyngeal bleeding (caused by tumor invasion) and the remaining 17 due to distant tumor failure. The 3- and 5-year OS rates were 88.2% (88/93) and 83.3% (25/30) and the median OS period was 46 months (range, 5–68 months). 9 patients experienced

local relapse, which included 5 with nasopharyngeal primary tumor relapse, 2 with retropharyngeal lymph node (RLN) recurrence, and 2 with cervical regional lymph node relapse.

The 3- and 5-year LRFS rates were 93.5% (87/93) and 93.3% (28/30), and the median recurrence time was 44 months. Distant metastasis developed in 23/93 patients, including 8 cases with hepatic metastasis, 3 with pulmonary metastasis, 5 with bone metastasis, 1 with retroperitoneal metastasis, and 6 with poly-organ metastasis. Moreover, the 3- and 5-year DMFS rates in the present study were 83.9% (78/93) and 83.3% (25/30), respectively; the median distant failure time was 8 months. For patients with tumor ADC values <0.72×10^{-3} mm^2/s (e.g., the low ADC group, lower than mean tumor ADC values): the 3-year OS rate was 84% (42/50), the median OS period was 45 months, the 3-year LRFS rate was 88% (44/50), and the 3-year DMFS rate was 82% (41/50). For patients with tumor ADC values ≥0.72×10^{-3} mm^2/s (e.g., the high ADC group): the 3-year OS rate was 93% (40/43), the median OS period was 60 months, the 3-year LRFS rate was 97.7% (42/43), and the 3-year DMFS rate was 86% (37/43).

Most deaths (14/20) and recurrences (9/10), as well as most of the distant metastasis events (15/23), occurred in the low ADC group. Kaplan-Meier survival data are presented in Fig. 2. Patients in the low ADC group exhibited a significant difference in OS and LRFS compared with the high ADC group (P = 0.036, P = 0.018). Moreover, while DMFS periods for the high ADC group appeared to be longer than those for the low ADC group, but the difference was not indicated significant (P = 0.12) (Fig. 2).

ADC showed a significant correlation with OS (P = 0.0004), LRFS (P = 0.0009), DMFS (P < 0.0001), respectively, according to the multivariate analysis using the Cox proportional hazard test (Table 2). Results demonstrated that pretreatment ADC was an independent prognostic parameter for survival. In addition, clinical

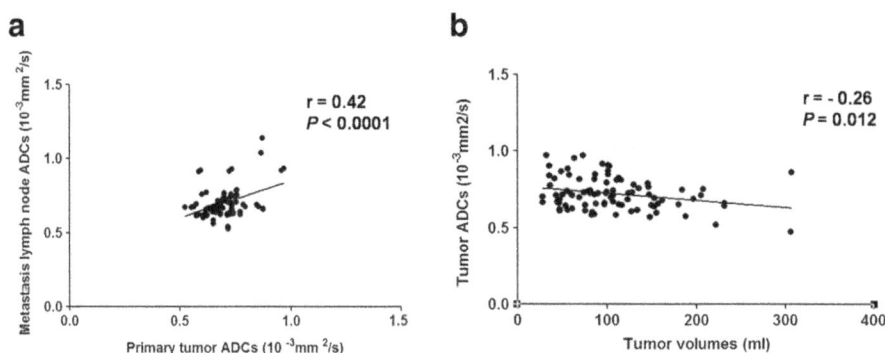

Fig. 1 Pearson correlations between pretreatment tumor apparent diffusion coefficient (ADC) values and lymph node ADC values (**a**), and between tumor volume and pretreatment tumor ADC values (**b**). ADC: apparent diffusion coefficient

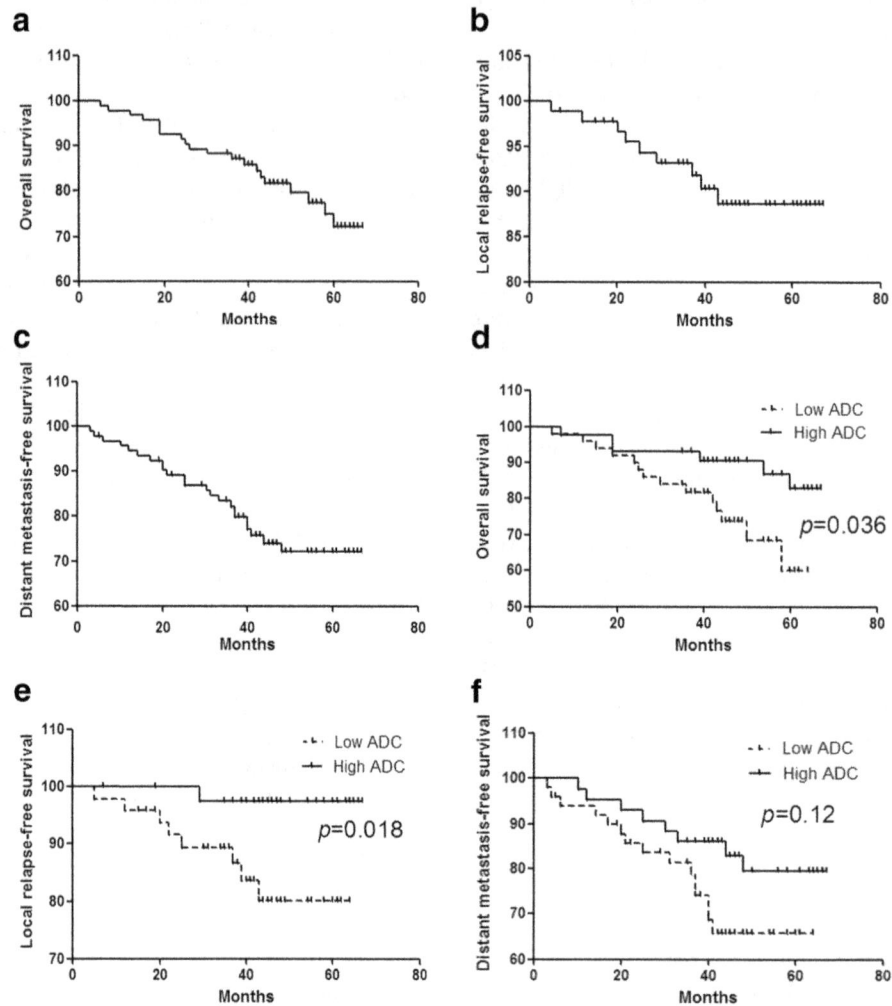

Fig. 2 Kaplan-Meier (**a**) OS curves, (**b**) LRFS curves, and (**c**) DMFS curves. In addition, (**d**) OS, (**e**) LRFS, and (**f**) DMFS curves were compared for the low ADC group (*dashed line*) and the high ADC group (*solid line*). OS: overall survival; LRFS: local relapse-free survival; DMFS: distant metastasis-free survival; ADC: apparent diffusion coefficient

Table 2 Multivariate analyses of prognostic factors in the 93 NPC patients

	OS		LRFS		DMFS	
	P value	95% CI	P value	95% CI	P value	95% CI
ADC	*0.0004*	0.001–0.13	*0.0009*	0–0.095	*0.0001*	0–0.023
Sex	0.17	0.34–1.21	0.45	0.38–1.54	0.20	0.35–1.25
Age	0.72	0.97–1.02	0.85	0.97–1.02	0.13	0.96–1.005
Clinical stage	*0.006*	1.25–3.95	0.19	0.81–3.02	*0.006*	1.26–4.01
T stage	0.076	0.49–1.04	0.61	0.59–1.36	0.11	0.93–1.93
N stage	*0.02*	0.35–0.92	0.11	0.36–1.10	*0.034*	0.36–0.96
Pathological type	0.61	0.73–1.20	0.30	0.62–1.16	0.36	0.67–1.16
Tumor volume	0.69	0.996–1.007	0.38	0.99–1.01	0.15	0.99–1.01
Smoking	0.60	0.46–1.56	0.95	0.50–2.10	0.80	0.50–1.69
Drinking	0.57	0.66–2.13	0.74	0.44–1.78	0.10	0.31–1.11

ADC: apparent diffusion coefficient; *CI*: confident index; *NPC*: nasopharyngeal carcinoma; *OS*: overall survival; *LRFS*: local relapse-free survival; *DMFS*: distant metastasis-free survival; $p < 0.05$ as statistically significant

stage and N stage were independent prognostic parameters for OS ($P = 0.0066$ and 0.0203, respectively), and DMFS ($P = 0.006$ and 0.0337, respectively) (Table 2).

Discussion

In this study, patient characteristics (such as age, gender, smoking, and drinking) showed no relationship with ADC values. But the results were similar to those of previous reports in which ADC values were found to correlate with different histologic types of carcinomas [22]. Moreover, Razek et al. reported a significant association between ADC values and the degree of tumor differentiation for retinoblastomas [19]. NPC includes nonkeratinizing carcinomas (both differentiated and undifferentiated), keratinizing squamous cell carcinoma (SCC), and basaloid SCC. Furthermore, the most common histologic type of NPC is nonkeratinizing carcinomas, consist of 75–99%. The characteristic of this type tumor is comprised tableted of concentrated carcinoma cells separated by an infiltrating of plasma cells and lymphocytes [23].

In this research, the highest mean ADC value was associated with type 1 NPC (e.g., keratinizing squamous cell carcinoma). Conversely, the lowest ADC value was associated with type 4 NPC (e.g., undifferentiated carcinomas). However, while there was a significant difference between these two types ($P = 0.024$), no significant difference was found among the other two histopathological types. Driessen et al., in a prospective study of 17 head and neck SCC [20], reported similar results-they found no obvious correlation between tumor ADC and tumor histologic grade, however a trend was found that poorly differentiated tumors had lower ADC values in comparison with moderately or well differentiated tumors.

Insufficient sample size may have limited our ability to obtain more significant results, or this result may suggest that ADC values partly reflect the differentiation of NPCs. However, a significant correlation with the histological type and mean ADC value was found among 27 cases of breast cancer in a study by Yoshikawa et al. [24]. Undifferentiated carcinomas reportedly predict the worst prognosis [3]. Results in the present study suggest that low pretreatment tumor ADC was a poor prognostic factor. In addition, necrosis should be considered a critical parameter. Even when we delineated ROI in this study as little as possible to avoid containing obvious necrosis, micronecrosis would still exist in minor ROI. Furthermore, it is known that necrosis leads to high ADC values [25]. Squamous cell carcinoma or well differentiated tumors may contain much more necrosis than undifferentiated carcinomas and thus favor high ADC values.

In the present study, we hypothesized a negative relevance between ADC values and prognostic factors reflecting mitosis (such as tumor stage, lymph node stage, and tumor volume). Interestingly, for both tumor

and regional lymph node grading, only the latter was found to significantly correlate with the mean ADC values obtained. This may be due to tumor staging in relation to the patterns of spread for NPC. For example, in some patients, the tumor may invade bony structures or intracranial tissues and/or cranial nerves by superior spread, even though the tumor volume may be small and a low lymph node staging is obtained. Furthermore, these patients are diagnosed high T stage.

When the relationship between different N stage was investigated, similar results to those reported by Razek et al. were obtained, with the ADC values being significantly lower for positive metastatic cervical lymph nodes compared with negative metastatic cervical lymph nodes [26]. In another study by Razek et al. [18], significant differences were observed in the ADC values for lung cancer cases involving N0 and N3 lymph nodes ($P = 0.043$). Similarly, a positive relation was observed between primary tumor ADC values and ADC values for metastatic cervical lymph nodes ($r = 0.17, P < 0.001$).

Taken together, these results suggest that primary tumors and metastatic cervical lymph nodes are homogeneous and may exhibit similar biological behaviors. Furthermore, this study suggests that ADC can reflect N stage more sensitive than T stage. Recent studies increasingly have raised proposals for revisions in the following edition of TNM staging system in NPC [27–30]. Some even suggested take new biomarkers such as epstein-barr virus (EBV) DNA or miRNA into account in the staging system since these biomarkers reportedly have prognostic value as well [29, 30]. Thus, as another prognostic value, ADC value should be taken into account in the new TNM staging system.

Primary NPC tumor volume reportedly is an important independent prognostic factor in NPC patients [31, 32]. For instance, in the 2011 study by Chen et al. [32], patient had a poor 5-year OS in the group with tumor volume > 50 ml, indicated that large tumor volume is almost equivalent to the T4 stage. A large tumor volume usually exhibits a greater metastatic potentiality, and therefore, is correlated with a poorer prognosis. Previously, a negative correlation between ADC values according to tumor size was identified for breast cancers ($r = -0.504, P = 0.001$), retinoblastomas ($r = -0.680, P = 0.015$), and NPCs ($r = -0.799, P = 0.03$) [17, 19, 26]. Similarly, a reversed correlation was observed between tumor volumes and ADC values in the present study ($r = -0.26, P = 0.012$). This may be explained by the observation that larger tumors are generally more restricted in their diffusion, are usually poorly differentiated, or represent an undifferentiated malignancy.

Performance status associated with local control, disease-free, and overall survival was reported in head and neck SCC and NPC in studies performed in Japan and China [33, 34]. In the present study, we defined the mean ADC value (0.72×10^{-3} mm^2/s) as the threshold level. Hence the high ADC group was higher than or equal to the mean level and the low ADC group was lower than the mean level. Results demonstrated the high ADC group was correlated with a longer OS period and LRFS period in NPC, and with a significant difference ($P = 0.036$ and 0.018, respectively). Different threshold options would likely give different results. Furthermore, a significant correlation between ADC with long-term outcomes was also observed, with the P values for OS, LRFS, and DMFS being 0.0004, 0.0009, and <0.0001, respectively. Thus, the pretreatment ADC value should be take into a consideration of a prognostic factor in NPC.

The present study has some limitations. First, due to the most patients are locoregionally advanced cases, patient selection bias may exist. Second, only two b values were used in this study for ADC measurement, so the ADC measurement may be insufficiently reliable. Third, this study was only performed at one center and was comparatively homogeneous, further multicenter and large-scale studies are required to strengthen the findings.

Conclusions

This study revealed that ADC values correlated with prognostic parameters of NPC. Specifically, a low ADC value was demonstrated to have correlation with undifferentiated tumors, a larger tumor volume, and metastatic lymph node stage. Incorporating the pretreatment ADC value in the future clinical staging system is challenging. Moreover, further studies, especially multicenter and prospective studies, are required to confirm the observation of the present study that low pretreatment tumor ADC values predict a poor prognosis for NPC patients.

Abbreviations
ADC: Apparent diffusion coefficient; AJCC: American Joint Committee on Cancer; ANOVA: One-way analysis of variance; CT: Computed tomography; DMFS: Distant metastasis-free survival; DWI: Diffusion-weighted MR imaging; EBV: Epstein-barr virus; LRFS: Local relapse-free survival; MRI: Magnetic resonance imaging; NPC: Nasopharyngeal carcinoma; OS: Overall survival; PET: Positron emission tomography; PFS: Progress-free survival; PGTV: Planned gross volume; PTV: Planning target volume; RLN: Retropharyngeal lymph node; ROI: Region of interest; SCC: Squamous cell carcinoma; SIB-IMRT: Simultaneous integrated boost intensity modulated radiation therapy; WHO: World Health Organization

Acknowledgments
None.

Funding
This study was supported possible in part by Natural Science Foundation of Zhejiang Province of China (Grant No. LY16H160013) and foundation of Zhejiang Educational Committee (Grant No. Y201534668). The funding bodies had no role in the design of the study, collection, analysis, and interpretation of data and in writing of the manuscript.

Authors'contributions
YDF obtained funding, contributed to the study concept, the design, acquisition of data, statistical analysis, analysis and interpretation of data, critical revision of the manuscript for important intellectual content, drafting the manuscript, and the decision to submit the article for publication. TLS and YSX designed and supervised the study and helped draft the manuscript, and made substantial contributions to statistical analysis, interpretation of data, critical revision of the manuscript for important intellectual content, and the decision to submit the article for publication. KSB and ZWB contributed to the clinical data collection, analysis and interpretation of data, drafting the manuscript, critical revision of the manuscript for important intellectual content, and the decision to submit the article for publication. ZF contributed to the study concept and design, acquirement and interpretation of data, critical revision of the manuscript for important intellectual content, and the decision to submit the article for publication. WQD contributed to the study design, interpretation of data, critical revision of the manuscript for important intellectual content, and the decision to submit the article for publication. In addition, each author has participated sufficiently in the work to take public responsibility for appropriate portions of the content; and has agreed to be accountable for all aspects of the work in ensuring that questions related to the accuracy or integrity of any part of the work are appropriately investigated and resolved. All authors read and approved the final manuscript.

Authors' information
TLS: Professor & Director, Department of Oncology, the First Affiliated Hospital, College of Medicine, Zhejiang University, Zhejiang, China. YSX: Professor & Director, Department of Radiation Oncology, the First Affiliated Hospital, College of Medicine, Zhejiang University, Zhejiang, China.

Competing interests
The authors declare that they have no competing interests.

Author details
[1]Department of Radiation Oncology, the First Affiliated Hospital, College of Medicine, Zhejiang University, 79 Qingchun RoadHangzhou, Zhejiang 310003, People's Republic of China. [2]Department of Radiology, the First Affiliated Hospital, College of Medicine, Zhejiang University, Zhejiang, Hangzhou 310003, China. [3]Department of Oncology, the First Affiliated Hospital, College of Medicine, Zhejiang University, 79 Qingchun Road, Zhejiang, Hangzhou 310003, China. [4]Department of Radiation Oncology, Henan Province People's Hospital, Zhengzhou, Henan 450000, China.

References

1. Parkin DM, Bray F, Ferlay J, Pisani P. Global cancer statistics. 2002. CA Cancer J Clin. 2005;55:74–108.
2. King A, Bhatia KS. Magnetic resonance imaging staging of nasopharyngeal carcinoma in the head and neck. World J Radiol. 2010;2:159–65.
3. Chong V, Ong C. Nasopharyngeal carcinoma. Eur J Radiol. 2008;66:437–47.
4. Farias TP, Dias FL, Lima RA, Kligerman J, de Sá GM, Barbosa MM, et al. Prognostic factors and outcome for nasopharyngeal carcinoma. Arch Otolaryngol Head Neck Surg. 2003;129:794–9.
5. Brandwein-Gensler M, Smith R. Prognostic indicators in head and neck oncology including the new 7th edition of the AJCC staging system. Head and Neck Pathol. 2010;4:53–61.
6. Lin GW, Wang LX, Ji M, Qian HZ. The use of MR imaging to detect residual versus recurrent nasopharyngeal carcinoma following treatment with radiation therapy. Eur J Radiol. 2013;82:2240–6.
7. Zhang SX, Han PH, Zhang GQ, Wang RH, Ge YB, Ren ZG, et al. Comparison of SPECT/CT, MRI and CT in diagnosis of skull base bone invasion in nasopharyngeal carcinoma. Biomed Mater Eng. 2014;24:1117–24.
8. Sun Y, Yu XL, Luo W, Lee AW, Wee JT, Lee N, et al. Recommendation for a contouring method and atlas of organs at risk in nasopharyngeal carcinoma patients receiving intensity-modulated radiotherapy. Radiother Oncol. 2014; 110:390–7.

9. Hein PA, Eskey CJ, Dunn JF, Hug EB. Diffusion-weighted imaging in the followup of treated high-grade gliomas: tumor recurrence versus radiation injury. AJNR Am J Neuroradiol. 2004;25:201–9.

10. Calli C, Kitis O, Yunten N, Yurtseven T, Islekel S, Akalin T. Perfusion and diffusion MR imaging in enhancing malignant cerebral tumors. Eur J Radiol. 2006;58:394–403.

11. Holzapfel K, Duetsch S, Fauser C, Maier SE, Takeda K. Value of diffusion-weighted MR imaging in the differentiation between benign and malignant cervical lymph nodes. Eur J Radiol. 2009;72:381–7.

12. Maeda M, Kato H, Sakuma H, Maier SE, Takeda K. Usefulness of the apparent diffusion coefficient in line scan diffusion-weighted imaging for distinguishing between squamous cell carcinomas and malignant lymphomas of the head and neck. AJNR Am J Neuroradiol. 2005;26:1186–92.

13. Razek AA, Kandeel AY, El-shenshawy HM, El-shenshawy HM, Kamel Y, Nada N, et al. Role of diffusion-weighted echo-planar MR imaging in differentiation of residual or recurrent head and neck tumors and posttreatment changes. AJNR Am J Neuroradiol. 2007;28:1146–52.

14. Sumi M, Sakihama N, Sumi T, Morikawa M, Uetani M, Kabasawa H, et al. Discrimination of metastatic cervical lymph nodes with diffusion-weighted MR imaging in patients with head and neck cancer. AJNR Am J Neuroradiol. 2003;24:1627–34.

15. King AD, Ahuja AT, Yeung DKW, Fong DK, Lee YY, Lei KI, et al. Malignant cervical lymphadenopathy: diagnostic accuracy of diffusion-weighted MR imaging. Radiology. 2007;245:806–13.

16. Vandecaveye V, Dirix P, De Keyzer F, de Beeck KO, Vander Poorten V, Roebben I, et al. Predictive value of diffusion-weighted magnetic resonance imaging during chemoradiotherapy for head and neck squamous cell carcinoma. Eur Radiol. 2010;20:1703–14.

17. Razek AA, Gaballa G, Denewer A, Nada N. Invasive ductal carcinoma: correlation of apparent diffusion coefficient value with pathological prognostic factors. NMR Biomed. 2010;23:619–23.

18. Razek AA, Fathy A, Gawad TA. Correlation of apparent diffusion coefficient value with prognostic parameters of lung cancer. J Comput Assist Tomogr. 2011;35:248–52.

19. Razek AA, Elkhamary S, Al-Mesfer S, Alkatan HM. Correlation of apparent diffusion coefficient at 3 tesla with prognostic parameters of retinoblastoma. AJNR Am J Neuroradiol. 2012;33:944–8.

20. Driessen JP, Caldas-Magalhaes J, Janssen LM, Pameijer FA, Kooij N, Terhaard CH, et al. Diffusion-weighted MR imaging in laryngeal and hypopharyngeal carcinoma: association between apparent diffusion coefficient and histologic findings. Radiology. 2014;272:456–63.

21. Gődény M, Léránt G. New opportunities, MRI biomarkers in the evaluation of head and neck cancer. Magy Onkol. 2014;58:269–80.

22. Ichikawa Y, Sumi M, Sasaki M, Nakamura T. Efficacy of diffusion-weighted imaging for the differentiation between lymphomas and carcinomas of the nasopharynx and oropharynx: correlations of apparent diffusion coefficients and histologic features. AJNR Am J Neuroradiol. 2012;33:761–6.

23. Barnes L, Eveson JW, Reichart P, et al. Pathology and Genetics of Head and Neck Tumors; IARC WHO Classification of Tumours. 1st ed. In: Lyon: IARC Press; 2005.

24. Yoshikawa MI, Ohsumi S, Sugata S, Kataoka M, Takashima S, Mochizuki T, et al. Relation between cancer cellularity and apparent diffusion coefficient values using diffusion-weighted magnetic resonance imaging in breast cancer. Radiat Med. 2008;26:222–6.

25. Dzik-Jurasz A, Domenig C, George M, Wolber J, Padhani A, Brown G, et al. Diffusion MRI for prediction of response of rectal cancer to chemoradiation. Lancet. 2002;360:307–8.

26. Razek AA, Kamal E. Nasopharyngeal carcinoma: correlation of apparent diffusion coefficient value with prognostic parameters. Radiol Med. 2013; 118:534–9.

27. Sze H, Chan LL, Ng WT, Hung AW, Lee MC, Chang AT, et al. Should all nasopharyngeal carcinoma with masticator space involvement be staged as T4? Oral Oncol. 2014;50:1188–95.

28. Zong J, Lin S, Lin J. Tang L1, Chen B1, Zhang M, et al. Impact of intensity-modulated radiotherapy on nasopharyngeal carcinoma: Validation of the 7th edition AJCC staging system. Oral Oncol. 2015;51:254–9.

29. Liu N, Cui RX, Sun Y, Guo R, Mao YP, Tang LL, et al. A four-miRNA signature identified from genome-wide serum miRNA profiling predicts survival in patients with nasopharyngeal carcinoma. Int J Cancer J Int Du. Cancer. 2014;134:1359–568.

30. Hsu CL, Chang KP, Lin CY, Chang HK, Wang CH, Lin TL, et al. Plasma Epstein-Barr virus DNA concentration and clearance rate as novel prognostic factors for metastatic nasopharyngeal carcinoma. Head Neck. 2012;34:1064–70.

31. Sze WM, Lee AW, Yau TK, Yeung RM, Lau KY, Leung SK, et al. Primary tumor volume of nasopharyngeal carcinoma: prognostic significance for local control. Int J Radiat Oncol Biol Phys. 2004;59:21–7.

32. Chen C, Fei Z, Pan J, Bai P, Chen L. Significance of primary tumor volume and T-stage on prognosis in nasopharyngeal carcinoma treated with intensity modulated radiation therapy. Jpn J Clin Oncol. 2011;41:537–42.

33. Hatakenaka M, Nakamura K, Yabuuchi H, Yonezawa M, Yoshiura T, Nakashima T, et al. Apparent diffusion coefficient is a prognostic factor of head and neck squamous cell carcinoma treated with radiotherapy. Jpn J Radiol. 2014;32:80–9.

34. Zhang Y, Liu X, Zhang Y, Li WF, Chen L, Mao YP, et al. Prognostic value of the primary lesion apparent diffusion coefficient (ADC) in nasopharyngeal carcinoma: a retrospective study of 541 cases. Sci Rep. 2015;5:12242.

10

Expression of von Hippel–Lindau tumor suppressor protein (pVHL) characteristic of tongue cancer and proliferative lesions in tongue epithelium

Hisashi Hasegawa[1], Yoshiaki Kusumi[2], Takeshi Asakawa[1], Miyoko Maeda[1], Toshinori Oinuma[2], Tohru Furusaka[1], Takeshi Oshima[1] and Mariko Esumi[2*]

Abstract

Background: Patients with tongue cancer frequently show loss of heterozygosity (LOH) of the von Hippel–Lindau (*VHL*) tumor suppressor gene. However, expression of VHL protein (pVHL) in tongue cancer has rarely been investigated and remains largely unknown. We performed immunohistochemical staining of pVHL in tongue tissues and dysplasia, and examined the association with LOH and its clinical significance.

Methods: Immunohistochemical staining of pVHL in formalin-fixed, paraffin-embedded sections of cancerous and other tissues from 19 tongue cancer patients showed positivity for LOH of *VHL* in four samples, negativity in four samples, and was non-informative in 11 samples. The staining pattern of pVHL was also compared with those of cytokeratin (CK) 13 and CK17.

Results: In normal tongue tissues, pVHL staining was localized to the cytoplasm of cells in the basal layer and the area of the spinous layer adjacent to the basal layer of stratified squamous epithelium. Positive staining for pVHL was observed in the cytoplasm of cancer cells from all 19 tongue cancer patients. No differences as a result of the presence or absence of LOH were found. Notably, cytoplasm of poorly differentiated invasive cancer cells was less intensely stained than that of well and moderately differentiated invasive cancer cells. pVHL staining was also evident in epithelial dysplasia lesions with pVHL-positive cells expanding from the basal layer to the middle of the spinous layer. However, no CK13 staining was noted in regions of the epithelium, which were positive for pVHL. In contrast, regions with positive staining for CK17 closely coincided with those positive for pVHL.

Conclusions: Positive staining for pVHL was observed in cancerous areas but not in normal tissues. pVHL expression was also detected in lesions of epithelial dysplasia. These findings suggest that pVHL may be a useful marker for proliferative lesions.

Keywords: Tongue cancer, pVHL, Diagnostic marker, Cytokeratin 13, Cytokeratin 17, Dysplasia

* Correspondence: esumi.mariko@nihon-u.ac.jp
[2]Department of Pathology, Nihon University School of Medicine, 30-1 Ohyaguchikami-cho, Itabashi-ku, Tokyo 173-8610, Japan
Full list of author information is available at the end of the article

Background

Tongue cancer remains a difficult disease to overcome. Despite the availability of a number of therapeutic modalities and marked advances in techniques to diagnose head and neck cancer, the 5-year survival rate of patients with tongue cancer is approximately 50% [1]. Multimodality therapy combining surgery, radiotherapy, and chemotherapy is generally indicated for advanced tongue cancer. However, in the past few decades, little improvement has been noted in its prognosis.

In general, tongue cancer is more common in older people, but even in the young, the incidence is higher than that of other types of head and neck squamous cell carcinomas (HNSCCs). In addition to chronic stimulation by contact with the teeth and certain environmental factors, alcohol intake and smoking are risk factors for tongue cancer [2], while genetic background also appears to be a strong determinant of risk, particularly in the young [3]. A previous study of genetic abnormalities in HNSCC revealed more frequent loss of heterozygosity (LOH) at loci on chromosomes 3p, 9p, and 17p [4]. Tumor suppressor genes p16 and p53 are located at loci on chromosomes 9p and 17p, respectively, and both are reported to show genetic alterations, such as mutations and methylation, in approximately 50% of tumor specimens from HNSCC patients [5, 6]. Recently, whole exome sequencing of HNSCC revealed that dysregulation of NOTCH1, IRF6, and TP63, which regulate squamous differentiation, is a driver of HNSCC carcinogenesis, similar to mutations of TP53, CDKN2A, PTEN, PIK3CA, and HRAS [7, 8]. Gross et el. found that a TP53 mutation is frequently accompanied by loss of chromosome 3p, and that the combination of both events is associated with poor outcomes [9]. Although 3p loss was determined by evaluating 12 genes located in 3p14.2, it remains unclear which factor encoded on 3p is responsible for the interaction with TP53. Asakawa et al. previously demonstrated that LOH of VHL (3p25.3), a tumor suppressor gene, occurs at a high frequency in tongue cancer, similar to that of 3p14.2 [10]. However, the biological effect of VHL loss on tongue cancer remains unclear.

The VHL gene, which is responsible for VHL disease, was identified at loci on chromosome 3p as a tumor suppressor gene in clear cell renal cell carcinoma (RCC) [11–16]. pVHL forms a multimeric complex with Elongin B and C, Culine2, and Rbx1 proteins, which then binds to the α-subunit of hypoxia-inducible factor-1 (HIF-1α) in cytoplasm to induce the ubiquitination and further degradation of HIF-1 [17–22]. HIF-1 induces vascular endothelial growth factor and other angiogenic factors, thereby promoting angiogenesis. Therefore, pVHL serves to negatively regulate angiogenesis. In addition, pVHL is reported to play a role in control of the cell cycle [23].

Here, to clarify the relationship between pVHL expression and the pathology of tongue cancer, we conducted immunohistochemical staining to detect the expression of pVHL in cancer tissues and other lesions from patients with tongue cancer.

Methods

Tissue samples

The present study involved 19 patients (eight men and 11 women) with primary tongue cancer, who were treated at Nihon University Itabashi Hospital [10]. Clinicopathological classification of carcinoma and histopathological grading of tumor tissues were based on the Cancer Staging Classification (6th edition) of the International Union Against Cancer [24]. Histological findings of dysplasia included intraepithelial neoplasia lesions lacking infiltration, which were categorized as mild, moderate, and severe dysplasia based on current World Health Organization classifications [25]. Carcinoma in situ was not included in the present analysis. For normal tongue epithelium, areas of normal epithelium contained in tissue specimens from patients with invasive tongue cancer were used for investigation. This study was approved by the Ethics Committee of Nihon University School of Medicine (Approval number 118–1). Informed consent was obtained from each patient prior to the start of the study.

Immunohistochemistry (IHC)

IHC staining was performed using anti-pVHL (556347; BD Biosciences, San Jose, CA, USA), anti-CK13 (NCL-CK13; Leica Biosystems, Nussloch GmbH, Germany), and anti-CK17 (clone E3 IR620; DAKO, Glostrup, Denmark) monoclonal antibodies. Formalin-fixed, paraffin-embedded (FFPE) sections (4-μm thick) of the tissue specimens were deparaffinized in xylene and incubated for 15 min in 5% hydrogen peroxide to inactivate endogenous peroxidases. The treated sections were immersed in 0.01 M citrate buffer (pH 6.0; Muto Pure Chemicals, Tokyo, Japan) and heated for 5 min in an autoclave for antigen retrieval. Each tissue section was then immersed in blocking solution (5% dry skim milk) at 37 °C for 30 min. After removal from the blocking solution, the tissue section was reacted with the primary antibody (anti-pVHL antibody) at a 100-fold dilution in phosphate-buffered saline (PBS) at 37 °C for 60 min. After removal from the primary antibody solution, the tissue section was washed three times (5 min per wash) with PBS.

Chromogenic detection of pVHL was achieved using Histofine Simple Stain MAX-PO (Nichirei Bioscience, Tokyo, Japan) in accordance with the manufacturer's protocol. For CK13 and CK17, the primary antibody reaction was performed as described above. The subsequent chromogenic detection was performed in two steps: each tissue section was first treated with the Envision Plus kit (EnVision™ FLEX Mini Kit, DAKO) and then with the chromogenic substrate diaminobenzidine (Histofine DAB, Nichirei Bioscience) for 5 min. Each tissue section was counterstained using hematoxylin.

Results

Clinicopathological features of tongue cancer

The mean age of the study population was 57.1 (range, 22–79) years. Four subjects were classified as stage I, nine as stage II, three as stage III, and three as stage IV. Fourteen subjects were classified as grade 1, four as grade 2, and one as grade 3. Four specimens were normal epithelium, nine were dysplasia, 16 were well-differentiated carcinoma, six were moderately differentiated carcinoma, and three were poorly differentiated carcinoma. Multiple specimens were obtained from each patient. No somatic mutations of *VHL* were detected in any patient, while four were

positive for LOH, four were negative for LOH, and 11 were not informative (Table 1) [10].

IHC staining of pVHL in tongue tissue samples

Upon examination of antigen retrieval conditions using FFPE non-cancerous tissues from clear cell RCC, we detected no staining of pVHL without antigen retrieval (Additional file 1: Figure S1A). Furthermore, trypsin treatment was ineffective for antigen retrieval. Although microwaving was effective, it resulted in strong non-specific positivity. Antigen retrieval by autoclaving facilitated the most intense staining. No pVHL staining was observed using negative control mouse monoclonal antibodies. Proximal tubule staining resembled that obtained with identical antibodies using frozen tissues [26]. Thus, staining for pVHL was performed after heat treatment with pressure. In normal renal tissues, positivity for pVHL was distributed over the entire cytoplasm of cells in the proximal tubule (Additional file 1: Figure S1A). Conversely, in clear cell RCC, the periphery of the cytoplasm was intensely positive with

Table 1 Clinicopathological features of 19 tongue squamous cell carcinomas and immunohistochemistry of pVHL

Case No.	Stage	*VHL* LOH[a]	Grade[b]	pVHL[c] Normal	Dysplasia	Tumor (differentiation) Well	Moderate	Poor
1	II	P	1		A	++	++	
2	II	P	1			++		
3	II	P	1			++		
4	II	P	2			++	++	
5	II	N	1		A	++		
6	IV	N	1			++		
7	IV	N	1	++		++		
8	I	N	1	++	B	++		
9	II	ni	1			++		
10	III	ni	1	++	C	++		+
11	I	ni	1		A	++		
12	I	ni	1	++		++		
13	II	ni	1		A	++	++	
14	I	ni	1			++		
15	II	ni	1		A	++		
16	II	ni	2			++	++	+
17	IV	ni	2		A		++	
18	III	ni	2		A		++	
19	III	ni	3					+
Total				4	9	16	6	3

[a] LOH, loss of heterozygosity, determined by single nucleotide polymorphism of the *VHL* gene (10). P, positive; N, negative; ni, non-informative
[b] Grade 1, well-differentiated; grade 2, moderately differentiated; grade 3, poorly differentiated
[c] All FFPE specimens from 19 cases were examined for histological features and immunohistochemistry of pVHL. All specimens examined were positive for pVHL: ++, strongly positive; +, weakly positive; patterns A, B and C are classifications of dysplasia determined by immunohistochemistry of pVHL together with CK13 and CK17, as shown in Fig. 2b

similar findings in frozen tissues of RCC (Additional file 1: Figure S1B).

In all specimens of normal tongue epithelium, pVHL staining was localized in the cytoplasm of cells in the basal layer and in parts of the cytoplasm in the spinous layer adjacent to the basal layer (Fig. 1b) (Table 1). No pVHL staining was observed in the stratum corneum or granular layer. In all lesions of tongue dysplasia, pVHL staining was distributed from the basal layer to the middle region of the spinous layer (Fig. 1d). All lesions of invasive tongue cancer were positive for pVHL. The cytoplasm of well-differentiated cancer cells was intensely positive for pVHL in all specimens (Fig. 1f). The peripheral regions of cancerous lesions were more strongly positive for pVHL than the central regions (Fig. 1g). The cytoplasm of moderately differentiated cancer cells was more intensely positive for pVHL than that of well-differentiated cancer cells in all specimens (Fig. 1i, j), whereas the cytoplasm of poorly differentiated cancer cells was more faintly positive for pVHL than that of well-differentiated cancer cells in all specimens (Fig. 1l, m). When the invasion mode and pVHL intensity were compared in cancerous lesions, well-defined cancer tended to be positive for pVHL, and poorly defined cancer was weakly positive for pVHL. However, the relationship was not statistically significant ($p = 0.059$, Pearson's chi-square test). Staining patterns of pVHL were

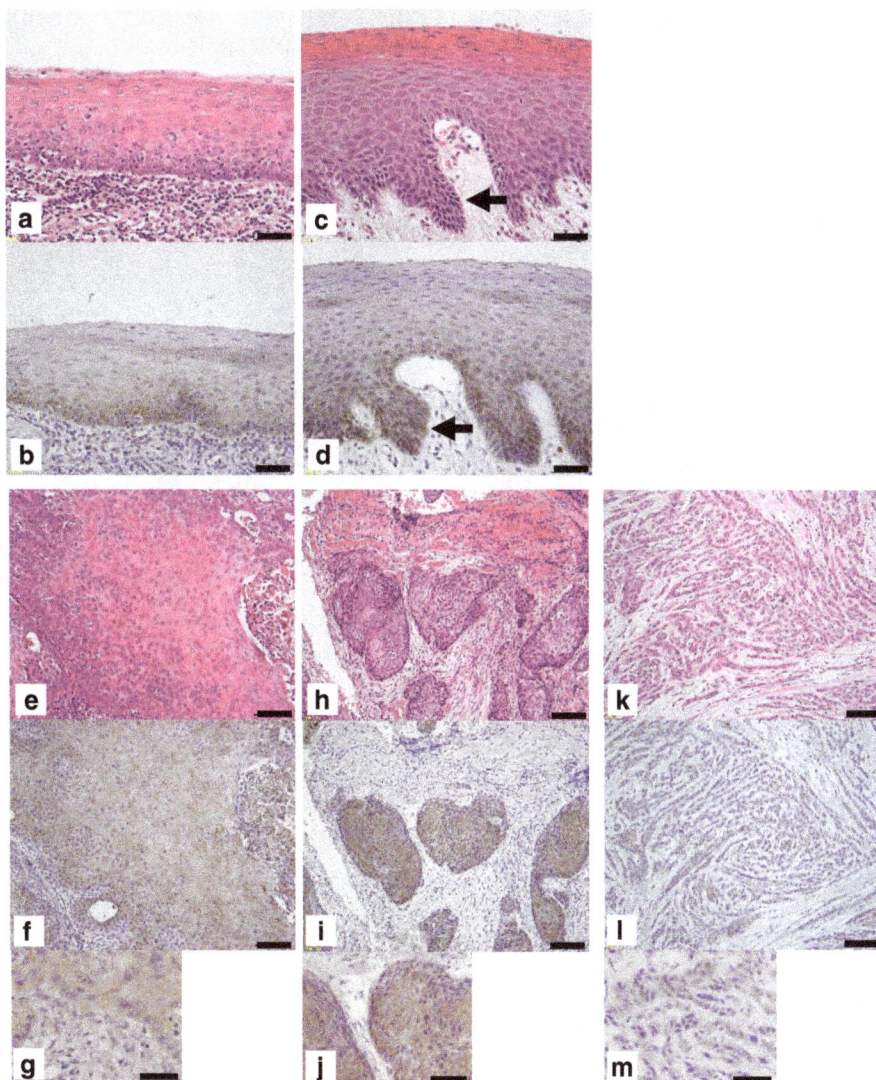

Fig. 1 Immunohistochemical staining of pVHL in tongue tissues. Tissues were stained with hematoxylin and eosin (**a**, **c**, **e**, **h**, and **k**), and serial sections were immunohistologically stained for pVHL (**b**, **d**, **f**, **g**, **i**, **j**, **l**, and **m**). **a** and **b**, normal tongue epithelium; **c** and **d**, epithelial dysplasia lesions (*arrows*). Bars indicate 25 μm. **e**, **f**, and **g**, well-differentiated invasive tongue squamous cell carcinoma; **h**, **i**, and **j**, moderately differentiated invasive tongue squamous cell carcinoma; **k**, **l**, and **m**, poorly differentiated invasive tongue squamous cell carcinoma. Bars indicate 50 μm (**e**, **f**, **h**, **i**, **k**, **l**) and 25 μm (**g**, **j**, **m**)

compared between LOH-positive and -negative cancers for the *VHL* gene. No apparent differences in staining patterns were noted between the positive and negative cases (Additional file 2: Figure. S2).

Comparison of staining patterns in epithelial dysplasia lesions: pVHL vs. CK13 and CK17

The expression patterns of CK13 and CK17 are associated with the development of squamous cell carcinoma and oral epithelial dysplasia. Therefore, these cytokeratins have been suggested to be candidate adjunctive diagnostic markers for oral lesions [27]. In normal tongue epithelium, CK13 staining was observed in the regions that were negatively stained for pVHL (Fig. 2c), but no staining of CK17 was observed in any of the layers (Fig. 2d). Various staining patterns of pVHL, CK13, and CK17 were observed in

lesions of tongue dysplasia. We classified the combinations into three categories. Pattern A was characterized by no staining for CK13 and positive staining for CK17 (Fig. 2 g, h) with staining for pVHL largely identical to that for CK17 (Fig. 2f). Pattern A was the typical type and observed in seven of the nine specimens with tongue dysplasia. Pattern B (one of nine specimens) was characterized by no staining of CK13, staining of CK17 distributed throughout all layers (Fig. 2 k, l), and pVHL staining confined to the middle region of the spinous layer (Fig. 2j), which was positive for dysplastic cells. In pattern C (one of nine specimens), CK13 staining was reduced greatly, and CK17 was slightly positive. Although assessment of the atypical grade was difficult for this staining pattern (Fig. 2 o, p), pVHL staining was positive in dysplastic cells (Fig. 2n).

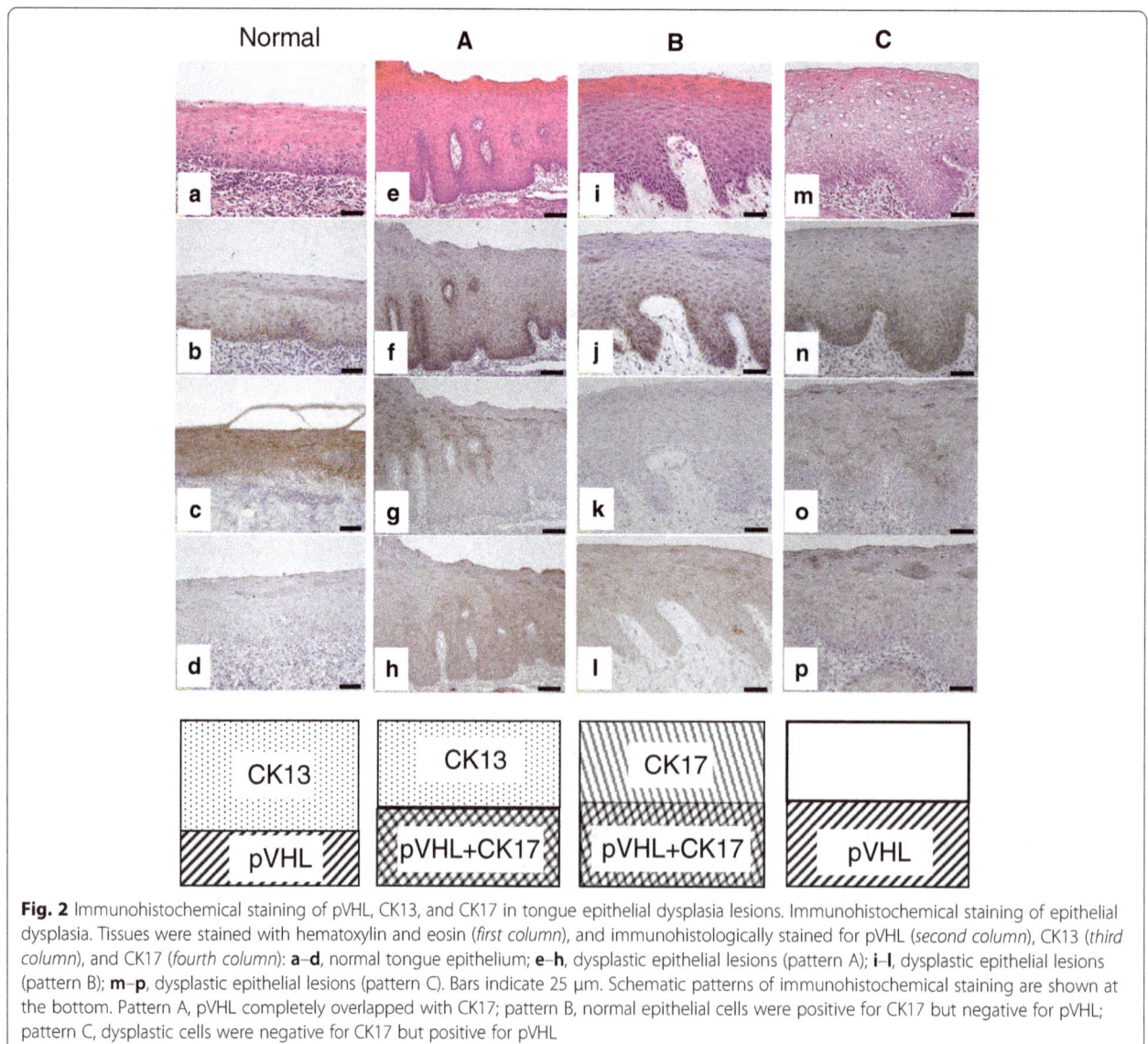

Fig. 2 Immunohistochemical staining of pVHL, CK13, and CK17 in tongue epithelial dysplasia lesions. Immunohistochemical staining of epithelial dysplasia. Tissues were stained with hematoxylin and eosin (*first column*), and immunohistologically stained for pVHL (*second column*), CK13 (*third column*), and CK17 (*fourth column*): **a–d**, normal tongue epithelium; **e–h**, dysplastic epithelial lesions (pattern A); **i–l**, dysplastic epithelial lesions (pattern B); **m–p**, dysplastic epithelial lesions (pattern C). Bars indicate 25 μm. Schematic patterns of immunohistochemical staining are shown at the bottom. Pattern A, pVHL completely overlapped with CK17; pattern B, normal epithelial cells were positive for CK17 but negative for pVHL; pattern C, dysplastic cells were negative for CK17 but positive for pVHL

In invasive tongue cancer, we observed no CK13 staining in any of the specimens, and CK17 and pVHL shared positively and negatively stained regions. However, detailed observation revealed that the keratinized regions of well-differentiated invasive cancer were intensely stained for CK17, with no staining for pVHL (Additional file 3: Figure S3).

Discussion

In this study, we characterized pVHL staining in tongue tissues and cancer as follows. (1) In normal stratified squamous epithelium, pVHL staining was localized to the cytoplasm of cells in the basal layer and parts of the cytoplasm in the spinous layer adjacent to the basal layer. (2) In dysplasia, a precancerous condition, expansion of the range of positivity was observed mainly in dysplastic cells. (3) In invasive cancer, pVHL staining was observed in all specimens, regardless of the differentiation stage. These findings suggest that pVHL will be useful as an adjunctive marker in the histopathological diagnosis of dysplasia.

Here, using our method for pVHL staining, we demonstrated that FFPE sections can be stained with mouse monoclonal antibodies (Ig32) using antigen retrieval procedures. Staining patterns of pVHL in normal renal tissues and clear cell RCC corresponded well with the results of staining using frozen tissue specimens reported by Corless et al. [26]. Claudio et al. [28] stained FFPE sections of clear cell RCC using the same antibody (Ig32) but a different method to ours. A similar staining pattern has been reported using microwaving for antigen retrieval. The present results may be considered as highly reliable. To date, only one other study has reported staining of tongue cancer specimens for pVHL. In that study, 10 of the 27 (37%) tongue cancers were positive for pVHL. Details of this previous study were not well described, but the reason for the substantial difference in the positive rate in our present study remains unclear [29]. However, it is likely a result of the different antibodies used and staining conditions.

To our knowledge, this is the first report of pVHL staining in the basal layer and the spinous layer adjacent to the basal layer of normal squamous epithelium. These results suggest that both stem cells and undifferentiated cells may be positive for pVHL because these cells exist in the same region. pVHL staining has been observed in the cytoplasm of normal epithelial cells in other tissues [26]. In particular, intense staining was noted in renal proximal tubular cells that are considered to be the origin of clear cell RCC [26]. Similarly, tongue cancer appears to develop from abnormal proliferation of stem cells in basal or parabasal cell layers of normal epithelium, which were positive for pVHL.

The clinical condition leukoplakia includes a wide range of lesions, from "reactive" to "precancerous". Differentiation between reactive and neoplastic tissues is often difficult, particularly in biopsy diagnosis where the observation target is limited to small tissue sections. Our present comparison of IHC staining for CK13/CK17 and pVHL suggests that pVHL staining may be a useful procedure in the evaluation and diagnosis of dysplasia. CK13 and CK17 are useful to evaluate dysplastic grades of certain specimens, such as those with pattern A staining. In pattern B, however, the staining patterns of CK13 and CK17 were typically observed in malignant lesions such as invasive cancer. In contrast, pVHL was stained positively in dysplasia following hematoxylin and eosin (HE) staining. In pattern C, CK13 staining was reduced greatly, while CK17 staining remained slightly positive, a pattern that hampers determination of the dysplastic grade. Nevertheless, pVHL staining was observed in the same dysplastic regions as those stained with HE, and may have superior sensitivity to stain CK13 and CK17 as adjunctive markers to detect dysplastic regions. The present report is the first to investigate the utility of pVHL staining for the diagnosis of tongue dysplasia. However, the small number of specimens examined is a limitation in this study, particularly with regard to dysplasia patterns B and C. An increased number of specimens and another large cohort study are necessary to validate the utility of pVHL in the conclusive diagnosis of preneoplastic lesions and tongue cancer. It would also be helpful to confirm IHC staining of other proliferative markers such as Ki-67 in pVHL-positive dysplasia. Because Ki-67 staining is well correlated with CK17 staining in tongue dysplasia [30], pVHL- and CK17-positive dysplastic regions, at least, may be positive for Ki-67.

Our unexpected finding is that all tongue cancers were positive for pVHL. Because no tongue cancers had nonsynonymous mutations in the present study [10], wild-type pVHL tended to be produced in more differentiated and well-defined cancers. In a HIF-1α-independent pathway, pVHL interacts directly with fibronectin and collagen IV, resulting in their assembly into the extracellular matrix (ECM) and suppression of tumorigenesis, angiogenesis, and cell invasion [31]. Therefore, even in invasive tongue cancer, it is possible that pVHL plays a role in regulation of the ECM and decrease of the invasive ability. Roland et al. demonstrated that poorly differentiated tongue cancers have a poor prognosis [32], and poorly differentiated tongue cancers were weakly stained for pVHL in the present study. In clear cell RCC, pVHL expression is also associated with a low histological grade and better prognosis [33]. Thus, pVHL in cancer possibly functions in the suppression of tumor progression. In the present study, we noted no clear relationship between LOH of the *VHL* gene and the staining pattern of pVHL in tongue cancer. Schraml et al. similarly reported the lack of a relationship between these variables in clear cell RCC [33]. These findings suggest that LOH of the *VHL* gene does not affect expression of pVHL, regardless of the cancer type. Considering the small number of specimens, these results should be considered as preliminary, particularly with regard to dysplasia and poorly differentiated tongue cancers. Therefore, further studies are needed on the topic.

Conclusions

Regardless of LOH of the *VHL* gene, pVHL was expressed in cancerous and dysplastic tissue in all patients with tongue cancer. These results suggest that pVHL may be a useful adjunctive marker in the histopathological diagnosis of dysplasia.

Additional files

Additional file 1: Figure S1. Staining of pVHL in clear cell renal cell carcinoma (RCC). (A) Staining of pVHL in normal renal tissues subjected to antigen retrieval. (a) Hematoxylin and eosin (HE) staining, (b–e) pVHL staining, (b) without antigen retrieval, (c) trypsinization, (d) microwaving treatment, (e) heating in an autoclave (arrow indicates proximal tubules), (f) heating in an autoclave (negative control staining with an unrelated monoclonal antibody). Bar indicates 50 μm. (B) Immunohistochemical staining of pVHL in clear cell RCC. (a) HE staining and (b) pVHL staining in clear cell RCC. Bar indicates 50 μm.

Additional file 2: Figure S2. Comparison of immunohistochemical staining for pVHL between LOH-positive and -negative cases of invasive tongue cancer (well differentiated). (A) Staining of pVHL in an LOH-positive case. (B) Staining of pVHL in an LOH-negative case. Bar indicates 25 μm.

Additional file 3: Figure S3. Immunohistochemical staining of keratinized regions in well-differentiated squamous cell carcinoma. Tissues stained with hematoxylin and eosin (upper), tissues immunohistologically stained for pVHL (middle), and tissues immunohistologically stained for CK17 (lower). Keratinized regions of squamous cell carcinoma were intensely stained for CK17 (arrows), while the same regions were not stained for pVHL.

Abbreviations

CK: Cytokeratin; FFPE: Formalin-fixed paraffin-embedded; HIF-1α: Alpha subunit of hypoxia-inducible factor-1; HNSCC: Head and neck squamous cell carcinoma; IHC: Immunohistochemistry; LOH: Loss of heterozygosity; pVHL: von Hippel–Lindau protein; RCC: Renal cell carcinoma; *VHL*: von Hippel–Lindau gene

Acknowledgements

We thank the late Dr. Sohei Endo for his initial conception of the study. We also thank Dr. Tomohiro Igarashi for providing clinical samples and data of clear cell RCC.

Funding

The authors have nothing to declare.

Authors' contributions

HH carried out the IHC staining, interpreted the data, and drafted the manuscript. YK participated in IHC experiments and diagnosed histopathological features. TA collected the clinical samples and performed the LOH analysis. MM determined the optimum condition for IHC and carried out the staining. TOi diagnosed histopathological features. TF and TOs participated in the clinical diagnosis and study coordination. ME designed the study and helped draft the manuscript. All authors have read and approved the final manuscript.

Competing interests

The authors declare that they have no competing interests.

Author details

[1]Deparment of Otorhinolaryngology, Head and Neck Surgery, Nihon University School of Medicine, 30-1 Ohyaguchikami-cho, Itabashi-ku, Tokyo 173-8610, Japan. [2]Department of Pathology, Nihon University School of Medicine, 30-1 Ohyaguchikami-cho, Itabashi-ku, Tokyo 173-8610, Japan.

References

1. Leemans CR, Braakhuis BJ, Brakenhoff RH. The molecular biology of head and neck cancer. Nat Rev Cancer. 2011;11(1):9–22.
2. Blot WJ, McLaughlin JK, Winn DM, Austin DF, Greenberg RS, Preston-Martin S, Bernstein L, Schoenberg JB, Stemhagen A, Fraumeni Jr JF. Smoking and drinking in relation to oral and pharyngeal cancer. Cancer Res. 1988;48(11):3282–7.
3. Vargas H, Pitman KT, Johnson JT, Galati LT. More aggressive behavior of squamous cell carcinoma of the anterior tongue in young women. Laryngoscope. 2000;110(10 Pt 1):1623–6.
4. Scully C, Field J, Tanzawa H. Genetic aberrations in oral or head and neck squamous cell carcinoma 3: clinico-pathological applications. Oral Oncol. 2000;36(5):404–13.
5. El-Naggar AK, Lai S, Clayman G, Lee J, Luna MA, Goepfert H, Batsakis JG. Methylation, a major mechanism of p16/CDKN2 gene inactivation in head and neck squamous carcinoma. Am J Pathol. 1997;151(6):1767.
6. Nagai MA, Miracca EC, Yamamoto L, Moura RP, Simpson AJ, Kowalski LP, Brentani RR. TP53 genetic alterations in head-and-neck carcinomas from Brazil. Int J Cancer. 1998;76(1):13–8.
7. Agrawal N, Frederick MJ, Pickering CR, Bettegowda C, Chang K, Li RJ, Fakhry C, Xie T-X, Zhang J, Wang J. Exome sequencing of head and neck squamous cell carcinoma reveals inactivating mutations in NOTCH1. Science. 2011;333(6046):1154–7.
8. Stransky N, Egloff AM, Tward AD, Kostic AD, Cibulskis K, Sivachenko A, Kryukov GV, Lawrence MS, Sougnez C, McKenna A. The mutational landscape of head and neck squamous cell carcinoma. Science. 2011;333(6046):1157–60.
9. Gross AM, Orosco RK, Shen JP, Egloff AM, Carter H, Hofree M, Choueiri M, Coffey CS, Lippman SM, Hayes DN. Multi-tiered genomic analysis of head and neck cancer ties TP53 mutation to 3p loss. Nat Genet. 2014;46(9):939–43.
10. Asakawa T, Esumi M, Endo S, Kida A, Ikeda M. Tongue cancer patients have a high frequency of allelic loss at the von Hippel-Lindau gene and other loci on 3p. Cancer. 2008;112(3):527–34.
11. Latif F, Tory K, Gnarra J, Yao M, Duh FM, Orcutt ML, Stackhouse T, Kuzmin I, Modi W, Geil L, et al. Identification of the von Hippel-Lindau disease tumor suppressor gene. Science. 1993;260(5112):1317–20.
12. Crossey PA, Foster K, Richards FM, Phipps ME, Latif F, Tory K, Jones MH, Bentley E, Kumar R, Lerman MI, et al. Molecular genetic investigations of the mechanism of tumourigenesis in von Hippel-Lindau disease: analysis of allele loss in VHL tumours. Hum Genet. 1994;93(1):53–8.
13. Seizinger BR, Rouleau GA, Ozelius LJ, Lane AH, Farmer GE, Lamiell JM, Haines J, Yuen JW, Collins D, Majoor-Krakauer D, et al. Von Hippel-Lindau disease maps to the region of chromosome 3 associated with renal cell carcinoma. Nature. 1988;332(6161):268–9.
14. Chino K, Esumi M, Ishida H, Okada K. Characteristic loss of heterozygosity in chromosome 3P and low frequency of replication errors in sporadic renal cell carcinoma. J Urol. 1999;162(2):614–8.
15. Phillips JL, Pavlovich CP, Walther M, Ried T, Linehan WM. The genetic basis of renal epithelial tumors: advances in research and its impact on prognosis and therapy. Curr Opin Urol. 2001;11(5):463–9.

16. Zbar B, Klausner R, Linehan WM. Studying cancer families to identify kidney cancer genes. Annu Rev Med. 2003;54:217–33.

17. Duan DR, Pause A, Burgess WH, Aso T, Chen D, Garrett KP, Conaway RC, Conaway JW, Linehan WM, Klausner RD. Inhibition of transcription elongation by the VHL tumor suppressor protein. Science. 1995;269(5229):1402–6.

18. Kibel A, Iliopoulos O, DeCaprio JA, Kaelin W. Binding of the von Hippel-Lindau tumor suppressor protein to Elongin B and C. Science. 1995;269(5229):1444–6.

19. Kishida T, Stackhouse TM, Chen F, Lerman MI, Zbar B. Cellular proteins that bind the von Hippel-Lindau disease gene product: mapping of binding domains and the effect of missense mutations. Cancer Res. 1995;55(20):4544–8.

20. Aso T, Lane WS, Conaway JW, Conaway RC. Elongin (SIII): a multisubunit regulator of elongation by RNA polymerase II. Science. 1995;269(5229):1439–43.

21. Maxwell PH, Wiesener MS, Chang GW, Clifford SC, Vaux EC, Cockman ME, Wykoff CC, Pugh CW, Maher ER, Ratcliffe PJ. The tumour suppressor protein VHL targets hypoxia-inducible factors for oxygen-dependent proteolysis. Nature. 1999;399(6733):271–5.

22. Kaelin Jr WG. The von Hippel-Lindau tumor suppressor protein and clear cell renal carcinoma. Clin Cancer Res. 2007;13(2 Pt 2):680s–4s.

23. Pause A, Lee S, Lonergan KM, Klausner RD. The von Hippel–Lindau tumor suppressor gene is required for cell cycle exit upon serum withdrawal. Proc Natl Acad Sci. 1998;95(3):993–8.

24. Sobin L, Wittekind C. International Union Against Cancer (UICC): TNM classification of malignant tumors. 6th ed. New York: Willey–Liss; 2002.

25. Barnes L, Eveson J, Recichart P, Sidransky D. Pathology and genetics of head and neck tumours. vol. 9. Lyon: IARC; 2005.

26. Corless CL, Kibel AS, Iliopoulos O, Kaelin WG. Immunostaining of the von Hippel-Lindau gene product in normal and neoplastic human tissues. Hum Pathol. 1997;28(4):459–64.

27. Mikami T, Cheng J, Maruyama S, Kobayashi T, Funayama A, Yamazaki M, Adeola HA, Wu L, Shingaki S, Saito C, et al. Emergence of keratin 17 vs. loss of keratin 13: their reciprocal immunochemical profiles in oral carcinoma in situ. Oral Oncol. 2011;47(6):497–503.

28. Di Cristofano C, Minervini A, Menicagli M, Salinitri G, Bertacca G, Pefanis G, Masieri L, Lessi F, Collecchi P, Minervini R. Nuclear expression of hypoxia-inducible factor-1α in clear cell renal cell carcinoma is involved in tumor progression. Am J Surg Pathol. 2007;31(12):1875–81.

29. Zhang S, Zhou X, Wang B, Zhang K, Liu S, Yue K, Zhang L, Wang X. Loss of VHL expression contributes to epithelial-mesenchymal transition in oral squamous cell carcinoma. Oral Oncol. 2014;50(9):809–17.

30. Nobusawa A, Sano T, Negishi A, Yokoo S, Oyama T. Immunohistochemical staining patterns of cytokeratins 13, 14, and 17 in oral epithelial dysplasia including orthokeratotic dysplasia. Pathol Int. 2014;64(1):20–7.

31. Jonasch E, Futreal PA, Davis IJ, Bailey ST, Kim WY, Brugarolas J, Giaccia AJ, Kurban G, Pause A, Frydman J. State of the science: an update on renal cell carcinoma. Mol Cancer Res. 2012;10(7):859–80.

32. Roland NJ, Caslin AW, Nash J, Stell PM. Value of grading squamous cell carcinoma of the head and neck. Head Neck. 1992;14(3):224–9.

33. Schraml P, Hergovitz A, Hatz F, Amin MB, Lim SD, Krek W, Mihatsch MJ, Moch H. Relevance of nuclear and cytoplasmic von hippel lindau protein expression for renal carcinoma progression. Am J Pathol. 2003;163(3):1013–20.

Risk factors for aspiration pneumonia after definitive chemoradiotherapy or bio-radiotherapy for locally advanced head and neck cancer: a monocentric case control study

Sadayuki Kawai[1], Tomoya Yokota[1*], Yusuke Onozawa[2], Satoshi Hamauchi[1], Akira Fukutomi[1], Hirofumi Ogawa[3], Tsuyoshi Onoe[3], Tetsuro Onitsuka[4], Takashi Yurikusa[5], Akiko Todaka[1], Takahiro Tsushima[1], Yukio Yoshida[1], Yosuke Kito[1], Keita Mori[6] and Hirofumi Yasui[1]

Abstract

Background: Chemoradiotherapy (CRT) and bio-radiotherapy (BRT) are recognized as standard therapies for head and neck cancer (HNC). Aspiration pneumonia after CRT or BRT is a common late adverse event. Our aim in this study was to evaluate the cause-specific incidence of aspiration pneumonia after CRT or BRT and to identify its clinical risk factors.

Methods: We performed a retrospective analysis of 305 patients with locally advanced HNC treated by CRT or BRT between August 2006 and April 2015.

Results: Of these 305 patients, 65 (21.3%) developed aspiration pneumonia after treatment. The median onset was 161 days after treatment. The two-year cause-specific cumulative incidence by CRT or BRT was 21.0%. Multivariate analysis revealed five independent risk factors for aspiration pneumonia, namely, habitual alcoholic consumption, use of sleeping pills at the end of treatment, poor oral hygiene, hypoalbuminemia before treatment, and the coexistence of other malignancies. A predictive model using these risk factors and treatment efficacy was constructed, dividing patients into low- (0–2 predictive factors), moderate- (3–4 factors), and high-risk groups (5–6 factors), the two-year cumulative incidences of aspiration pneumonia of which were 3.0, 41.6, and 77.3%, respectively. Aspiration pneumonia tended to be associated with increased risk of death, although this was not statistically significant (multivariate-adjusted hazard ratio 1.39, $P = 0.18$).

Conclusion: The cause-specific incidence and clinical risk factors for aspiration pneumonia after definitive CRT or BRT were investigated in patients with locally advanced HNC. Our predictive model may be useful for identifying patients at high risk for aspiration pneumonia.

Keywords: Head and neck cancer, Aspiration pneumonia, Risk factor, Chemoradiotherapy, Case–control study

* Correspondence: t.yokota@scchr.jp
[1]Division of Gastrointestinal Oncology, Shizuoka Cancer Center, 1007 Shimonagakubo, Nagaizumi, Sunto-gun, Shizuoka 411-8777, Japan
Full list of author information is available at the end of the article

Background

Chemoradiotherapy (CRT) is a standard treatment for locally advanced head and neck cancer (HNC) [1]. Radiotherapy (RT) with cetuximab, defined as bio-radiotherapy (BRT), is also considered as a treatment option for patients with locally advanced HNC [2]. Compared with radical surgery, CRT and BRT have an advantage of preserving organ function and patients' quality of life; however, their toxicities are not less harmful than the risks associated with surgery. In the previous clinical trial RTOG 91–11 [3], non-cancer-related death was more common among patients treated with CRT than with RT alone in a further follow-up, despite the higher rates of laryngeal preservation [4]. This suggests that patients cured by CRT need appropriate management against late toxicity.

Aspiration pneumonia is recognized as pneumonia secondary to the inhalation of food particles, saliva, or gastric acid. Patients with HNC who have undergone definitive CRT tend to have swallowing dysfunction due to mucositis during the treatment period or due to radiation-induced fibrosis of the oropharyngeal musculature after completion of the treatment [5]. Szczesniak et al. [6]. reported that approximately 52% of patients who received RT and 69% who received CRT suffered from dysphasia after treatment, and aspiration pneumonia accounted for 19% of non-cancer-related deaths. Additionally, Xu et al. [7]. suggested that aspiration pneumonia was a poor prognostic factor for patients with HNC who received CRT. Therefore, clinicians should assess the risk of aspiration pneumonia in order to identify patients for whom efforts to prevent it should be implemented.

The purpose of this study was to identify clinical risk factors for aspiration pneumonia after definitive CRT or BRT for patients with advanced HNC. In particular, we focused on the cause-specific incidence of aspiration pneumonia, taking competing events of death and resection of the primary lesion into account.

Methods

Study population

Three hundred and forty patients with HNC who received definitive concurrent CRT or BRT at Shizuoka Cancer Center between August 2006 and April 2015 were identified from medical records. Of these, 35 patients with a recurrent or metastatic lesion or resection of the primary lesion before CRT were excluded. Patients with other malignancies were included only if HNC was considered to be the factor most strongly determining their prognosis. Finally, 305 patients were included in this analysis. This study was approved by the Institutional Review Committee of Shizuoka Cancer Center (Shizuoka, Japan) and met the standards set forth in the Declaration of Helsinki.

Study covariates

We retrospectively collected data on the occurrence of aspiration pneumonia, time to onset of aspiration pneumonia, and overall survival (OS) from the end of treatment. Background covariate candidates for factors predictive of aspiration pneumonia included the following: tumor site, age, gender, Eastern Cooperative Oncology Group (ECOG) performance status, body mass index, TNM staging according to the AJCC/UICC TNM classification, tumor histology, smoking status, habitual alcoholic consumption, distance between the patients' home and the hospital, family members in the same household, use of proton pump inhibitors (PPIs) or H_2 blockers, use of angiotensin-converting enzyme (ACE) inhibitors or angiotensin II receptor blockers (ARBs), use of sleeping pills and main feeding at the end of the treatment, presence of gastrostomy during the treatment, oral hygiene, serum albumin (ALB) and hemoglobin (Hb) levels before treatment, coexistence of other malignancies before treatment, and Charlson comorbidity index. We defined habitual alcoholic consumption as the drinking of alcohol four or more days a week, and poor oral hygiene as the presence of moderate or more severe dental plaque assessed by a dentist and/or a dental hygienist. Charlson comorbidity index is a tool for predicting mortality by classifying or weighting comorbidities [8].

We also collected the following treatment-related covariate data: presence or absence of induction chemotherapy, chemotherapy regimen, irradiation technique [conventional three-dimensional conformal radiation therapy (3D-CRT) or intensity-modulated radiation therapy (IMRT)], irradiation field, treatment efficacy evaluated according to Response Evaluation Criteria in Solid Tumors ver. 1.1 [complete response (CR) or non-CR], mucositis and dysphagia during treatment evaluated by Common Terminology Criteria for Adverse Events ver. 4.0, and decreases of ALB, Hb, and body weight after treatment.

Aspiration pneumonia

Because it is sometimes difficult to clearly distinguish aspiration pneumonia from other types of pneumonia, different definitions of aspiration pneumonia were used in previous studies [9–11]. Therefore, in this study, we defined aspiration pneumonia as a clinical condition that met all of the following criteria: (i) Patients had both subjective and objective symptoms suggesting pneumonia. Subjective symptoms included wet cough, sputum, and fever. Objective symptoms included the presence of coarse crackles in the chest, elevated inflammatory markers (e.g. white blood cell count or C-reactive protein), or image findings (e.g. infiltration on a chest X-ray or consolidation in chest computed tomography). (ii) The presence of aspiration was suspected clinically (choking or delayed swallowing) or by endoscopic or video-fluorographic examinations. (iii) No evidence of micro-organisms that cause atypical pneumonia, such as *Legionella* and *Mycoplasma*.

Statistical analysis

The cause-specific cumulative incidence of aspiration pneumonia was estimated with nonparametric cumulative incidence functions, taking competing events of death and resection of the primary lesion into account. To investigate potential risk factors for aspiration pneumonia, univariate analysis was carried out for all covariates using Fisher's exact test, and covariates showing statistical significance were further analyzed using a multivariate logistic regression model. To construct a predictive model, we automatically selected covariates extracted from univariate analysis, and compared the goodness-of-fit among many models on the basis of the stepwise Akaike information criterion (AIC) method [12]. The minimum value from the AIC procedure allows us to select appropriate predictive factors to construct an optimal predictive model objectively. The concordance index to evaluate the discriminatory ability of the model was calculated using the final regression model [13].

The OS time was calculated from the date of treatment end to the date of death due to any cause or to the last date of confirmed survival. Survival rates were estimated using the Kaplan–Meier method. To estimate the association of covariates with overall survival, univariate analysis was carried out using the log-rank test. All statistically significant covariates in univariate analysis were analyzed in multivariate analysis using the Cox regression model.

All statistical tests were two-sided, and $P \leq 0.05$ was considered significant. Statistical analyses were performed using EZR software (Saitama Medical Center, Jichi Medical University, Saitama, Japan) [14].

Results

Among the 305 patients, 65 (21.3%) developed aspiration pneumonia after CRT or BRT. Patients' baseline and treatment-related characteristics are summarized in Table 1. The median age of the patients was 65 years (range 19–83) and 95.1% of them had ECOG PS of 0 to 1. Cisplatin, carboplatin, and cetuximab were concurrently used in 77.1, 13.7, and 9.2% of patients, respectively. Seventy-six (24.9%) of the patients received induction chemotherapy, and 87.5% of them were treated with the combination of docetaxel, cisplatin, and fluorouracil. Additionally, 96.0% of all patients had received systematic oral care [15] since initiation of the treatment. Thirty-six (11.8%) patients had coexisting malignancies included multiple primary HNC, esophageal cancer, gastric cancer, prostate cancer, lung cancer, and renal cancer. All of these cancers were found at an early stage by routine endoscopic or computed tomography

screening. After definitive CRT or BRT, 30 (9.8%) patients underwent resection of the primary lesion and 45 (14.7%) underwent neck dissection for a residual lesion or recurrence.

The median time from the end of treatment to aspiration pneumonia events was 161 days (range 3–1623). The median follow-up time was 892 days. The two-year cumulative incidences of aspiration pneumonia and competing events of death and resection of the primary lesion were 21.0% [95% confidence interval (CI) 16.4–26.0%], 12.9% (9.2–17.4%), and 6.2% (3.7–9.5%), respectively (Fig. 1).

Univariate and multivariate analyses identified five independent risk factors for aspiration pneumonia, namely, habitual alcoholic consumption, poor oral hygiene, coexistence of other malignancies, hypoalbuminemia before treatment, and the use of sleeping pills at the end of treatment (Table 2). A difference in the types of sleeping pills (benzodiazepines or others) used was not associated with the onset of aspiration pneumonia (odds ratio 0.95, 95% CI, 0.37–2.39, $P = 1.00$). Of 193 patients with poor oral hygiene before treatment, 135 had been followed up by dentists three months after the treatment. In total, 87 of 135 patients in whom oral hygiene had improved three months after the treatment had a significantly lower frequency of aspiration pneumonia than 48 patients who had poor oral hygiene (18.3% vs. 54.1%, $P = 0.00003$).

Next, we attempted to construct a predictive risk model of aspiration pneumonia from the results of univariate analysis. As a result of AIC stepwise selection, six predictive factors, consisting of the five risk factors extracted from the multivariate analysis and treatment efficacy (non-CR), were selected. Although treatment efficacy was not identified as a statistically significant risk factor, AIC stepwise selection revealed that it was a good predictive factor for the model. This predictive model well divided patients into low- (0–2 factors, $n = 180$), moderate- (3–4 factors, $n = 103$), and high-risk groups (5–6 factors, $n = 22$) by the number of predictive factors, for which the estimated two-year cumulative incidences of aspiration pneumonia were 3.0% (95% CI, 1.1–6.5%), 41.6% (31.0–51.8%), and 77.3% (51.4–90.5%), respectively (Fig. 2). The concordance index was 0.797.

Finally, we investigated the correlation between OS and the occurrence of aspiration pneumonia. Survival curves adjusted for the covariates from a Cox proportional hazard model indicated that the occurrence of aspiration pneumonia tended to be associated with the risk of death, but this was not statistically significant (hazard ratio, 1.39; 95% CI, 0.85–2.27; $P = 0.18$) (Fig. 3).

Discussion

The important goals of treatment in patients with HNC are not only a cure but also the preservation of quality

Table 1 Patients' characteristics

Background	n (%)
Age	
< 65 years	149 (49)
≥ 65 years	156 (51)
Gender	
Male	266 (87)
Female	39 (13)
ECOG performance status	
0	181 (59)
1	109 (36)
2	12 (4)
3	3 (1)
Body mass index	
< 18.5	46 (15)
18.5–25	199 (65)
≥ 25	60 (20)
Primary site	
Larynx	45 (15)
Nasopharynx	38 (12)
Hypopharynx	112 (37)
Nasal sinus	17 (6)
Oropharynx	79 (26)
Oral cavity	14 (5)
T-classification	
1	28 (9)
2	110 (36)
3	66 (66)
4	101 (33)
N-classification	
0	63 (21)
1	39 (13)
2a	3 (1)
2b	126 (41)
2c	60 (20)
3	14 (5)
Tumor histology	
SCC	287 (94)
Others	18 (6)
Smoking status	
Never	36 (12)
Past	200 (66)
Current	69 (23)
Habitual alcoholic consumption	
Yes	121 (40)
No	184 (60)

Table 1 Patients' characteristics *(Continued)*

Distance from the hospital	
< 10 km	92 (30)
≥ 10 km	213 (70)
Family members in the same household	
Yes	258 (85)
No	47 (15)
Use of ACEi or ARB	
ARB	53 (17)
ACEi	2 (1)
No	250 (82)
Use of PPI or H_2 blocker	
Yes	163 (53)
No	142 (47)
Oral hygiene before treatment	
Good	100 (33)
Poor	193 (63)
Unknown	12 (4)
Coexistence of other malignancies	
Yes	36 (12)
No	269 (88)
Comorbidity index	
0	233 (76)
≥ 1	72 (24)
Serum albumin before treatment	
Within normal limits	259 (85)
Less than normal range	46 (15)
Hemoglobin before treatment	
Within normal limits	212 (70)
Less than normal range	93 (30)
Use of sleeping pills at the end of treatment	
Yes	210 (69)
No	95 (31)
Main feeding at the end of treatment	
Oral	127 (42)
Non-oral	178 (58)
Presence of gastrostomy during the treatment	
Yes	173 (57)
No	132 (43)
Induction chemotherapy	
Yes	76 (25)
No	229 (75)
Concurrent chemotherapy regimen	
CDDP-based	235 (77)
CBDCA-based	42 (14)
Cetuximab	28 (9)

Table 1 Patients' characteristics *(Continued)*

Radiation technique	
Conventional 3D-CRT	241 (79)
IMRT	64 (21)
Irradiation field	
Primary lesion alone	40 (13)
Hemi neck	19 (6)
Whole neck	246 (81)
Treatment efficacy	
CR	199 (65)
Non-CR	106 (35)
Body weight loss after treatment	
< 10%	178 (58)
≥ 10%	127 (42)
Serum albumin decreasing post-treatment	
< 20%	114 (37)
≥ 20%	191 (63)
Hemoglobin decreasing post-treatment	
< 30%	138 (45)
≥ 30%	167 (55)
The worst mucositis grade during treatment	
0	3 (1)
1	16 (5)
2	102 (33)
3	182 (60)
4	2 (1)
The worst dysphagia grade during treatment	
0	12 (4)
1	84 (28)
2	76 (25)
3	133 (44)
4	0
Resection of primary lesion post-CRT or -BRT	
Yes	30 (10)
No	275 (90)
Neck dissection post-CRT or -BRT	
Radical neck dissection	0
Modified radical neck dissection	1 (1)
Selective neck dissection	44 (14)

Abbreviations: ECOG Eastern Cooperative Oncology Group, *SCC* Squamous cell carcinoma, *ACEi* Angiotensin-converting enzyme inhibitor, *ARB* Angiotensin II receptor blocker, *PPI* Proton pump inhibitor, *3D-CRT* Three-dimensional conformal radiation therapy, *IMRT* Intensity-modulated radiation therapy, *CR* Complete response, *CRT* Chemoradiotherapy, *BRT* Bio-radiotherapy
The normal range of laboratory data at our institution: Serum albumin (3.8–5.2 g/dl), hemoglobin (male: 13.5–17.6 g/dl, female: 11.3–15.2 g/dl)

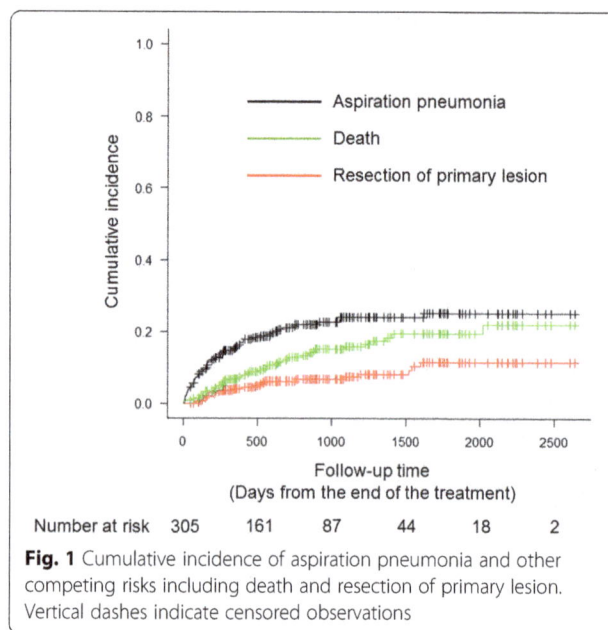

Fig. 1 Cumulative incidence of aspiration pneumonia and other competing risks including death and resection of primary lesion. Vertical dashes indicate censored observations

of life post-treatment. Although approximately 60–70% of patients with HNC treated with CRT suffer from dysphagia or aspiration as a late toxicity [16, 17], in previous studies, the incidence of aspiration pneumonia within a year after CRT was found to differ, ranging from 5.4 to 23% [9, 17, 18]. Furthermore, no differences in the frequency of aspiration pneumonia were seen between the different observation periods, despite the improvement of radiation techniques and general management of CRT over the time. This suggests that various factors other than aspiration are associated with the occurrence of aspiration pneumonia.

To clarify the population at high risk of aspiration pneumonia after CRT or BRT, we investigated the factors predictive of aspiration pneumonia. Several risk factors for aspiration pneumonia in patients with HNC after CRT were reported in previous studies [7, 9, 17]. However, evaluation of the long-term risk factors was often difficult in patients with HNC because these patients' characteristics varied according to the multimodal therapies that they had received, including surgery, CRT, and RT. In particular, previous studies did not take salvage surgery after CRT into account. Therefore, in these studies, there might not have been accurate estimates of the treatment-specific incidence of aspiration pneumonia after CRT. To our knowledge, the current study is the first regarding specific risk factors and predictive models for aspiration pneumonia as a late toxicity in patients with HNC undergoing definitive CRT or BRT.

We intended to determine risk factors for aspiration pneumonia after CRT or BRT by estimating the cause-specific cumulative incidence. To do this, we first performed cumulative incidence analysis, and regarded

Table 2 Univariate and multivariate logistic regression analyses for risk factors of aspiration pneumonia

	Univariate analysis		Multivariate analysis	
	Odds ratio (95% CI)	P-value	Odds ratio (95% CI)	P-value
Age				
< 65 years old	Ref.			
≥ 65 years old	1.71 (0.97–2.99)	0.06		
Gender				
Male	1.06 (0.46–2.43)	0.89		
Female	Ref.			
ECOG performance status				
0–1	Ref.			
2–3	2.61 (0.89–7.62)	0.07		
Body mass index				
< 18.5	Ref.			
18.5–25	0.87 (0.41–1.87)	0.73		
≥ 25	0.71 (0.27–1.83)	0.48		
Primary site				
Larynx	Ref.			
Nasopharynx	1.21 (0.32–4.55)	0.77		
Hypopharynx	2.07 (0.73–5.83)	0.17		
Nasal sinus	1.71 (0.36–8.12)	0.49		
Oropharynx	3.49 (1.23–9.94)	0.02	1.69 (0.50–5.67)	0.39
Oral cavity	4.44 (1.06–18.7)	0.04	1.95 (0.38-9.98)	0.42
T-classification				
1–2	Ref.			
3–4	2.38 (1.32–4.30)	0.004	1.75 (0.85–3.59)	0.12
N-classification				
0–2b	Ref.			
2c–3	1.39 (0.75–2.57)	0.29		
Tumor histology				
SCC	Ref.			
Others	0.20 (0.02–1.57)	0.12		
Smoking status				
Never	Ref.			
Past	0.87 (0.37–2.07)	0.76		
Current	1.14 (0.43–2.98)	0.78		
Habitual alcoholic consumption				
Yes	1.79 (1.00–3.24)	0.05	2.11 (1.01–4.38)	0.04
No	Ref.			
Distance from the hospital				
< 10 km	Ref.			
≥ 10 km	0.88 (0.48–1.59)	0.67		
Family members in the same household				
Yes	Ref.			
No	1.33 (0.64–2.73)	0.44		

Table 2 Univariate and multivariate logistic regression analyses for risk factors of aspiration pneumonia *(Continued)*

Use of ACEi or ARB				
Yes	1.50 (0.76–2.93)	0.23		
No	Ref.			
Use of PPI or H_2 blocker				
Yes	1.02 (0.58–1.77)	0.94		
No	Ref.			
Oral hygiene before treatment				
Good	Ref.			
Poor	2.63 (1.33–5.21)	0.005	2.81 (1.28–6.16)	0.01
Coexistence of other malignancies				
Yes	2.72 (1.30–5.68)	0.007	3.51 (1.46–8.42)	0.005
No	Ref.			
Comorbidity index				
0	Ref.			
≥ 1	0.59 (0.29–1.22)	0.15		
Serum albumin before treatment				
Within normal limits	Ref.			
Less than normal range	4.60 (2.37–8.95)	0.000006	2.70 (1.12–6.53)	0.02
Hemoglobin before treatment				
Within normal limits	Ref.			
Less than normal range	2.62 (1.49–4.61)	0.0008	1.08 (0.51–2.28)	0.84
Use of sleeping pills at the end of treatment				
Yes	3.22 (1.83–5.67)	0.00005	4.39 (2.21–8.74)	0.00002
No	Ref.			
Main feeding at the end of treatment				
Oral	Ref.			
Non-oral	1.66 (0.93-2.96)	0.09		
Presence of gastrostomy during the treatment				
Yes	2.6 (1.41-4.77)	0.0018	1.58 (0.754-3.31)	0.22
No	Ref.			
Induction chemotherapy				
Yes	1.20 (0.64–2.23)	0.56		
No	Ref.			
Concurrent chemotherapy regimen				
CDDP-based	Ref.			
CBDCA-based	1.01 (0.45–2.25)	0.98		
Cetuximab	1.01 (0.38–2.62)	0.98		
Radiation technique				
Conventional 3D-CRT	1.60 (0.76–3.34)	0.21		
IMRT	Ref.			
Irradiation field				
Primary alone	Ref.			
Hemi neck	3.82 (0.43–33.5)	0.22		

Table 2 Univariate and multivariate logistic regression analyses for risk factors of aspiration pneumonia *(Continued)*

Whole neck	5.43 (0.71–41.6)	0.10		
Treatment efficacy				
CR	Ref.			
non-CR	2.56 (1.46–4.48)	0.0009	1.60 (0.81–3.14)	0.17
Body weight loss after treatment				
< 10%	Ref.			
≥ 10%	1.26 (0.72–2.19)	0.41		
Serum albumin decreasing post-treatment				
< 20%	Ref.			
≥ 20%	1.12 (0.63–1.97)	0.71		
Hemoglobin decreasing post-treatment				
< 30%	Ref.			
≥ 30%	1.31 (0.75–2.29)	0.33		
The worst mucositis grade during treatment				
0–2	Ref.			
3–4	0.91 (0.51–1.58)	0.72		
The worst dysphagia grade during treatment				
0–2	Ref.			
3–4	0.59 (0.33–1.05)	0.07		

Abbreviations: *ECOG* Eastern Cooperative Oncology Group, *SCC* Squamous cell carcinoma, *ACEi* Angiotensin-converting enzyme inhibitor, *ARB* Angiotensin II receptor blocker, *PPI* Proton pump inhibitor, *3D-CRT* Three-dimensional conformal radiation therapy, *IMRT* Intensity-modulated radiation therapy, *CR* Complete response
The normal range of laboratory data at our institution: Serum albumin (3.8–5.2 g/dl), hemoglobin (male: 13.5–17.6 g/dl, female: 11.3–15.2 g/dl)

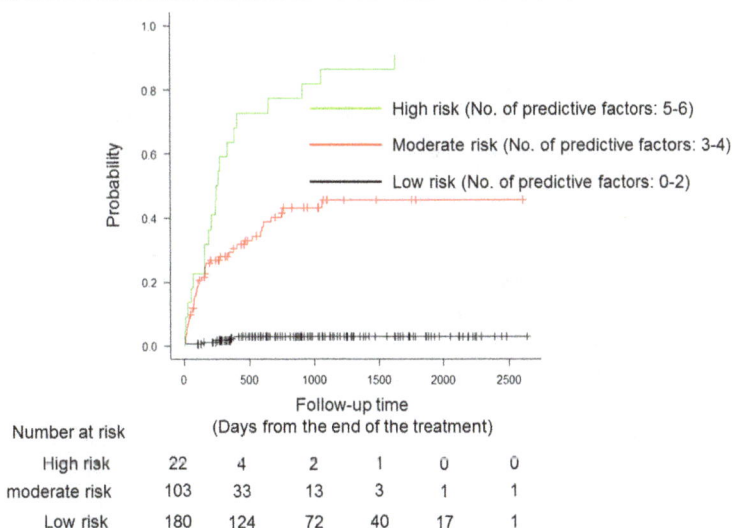

Fig. 2 The estimated cumulative incidence of aspiration pneumonia according to the number of predictive factors. Vertical dashes indicate censored observations

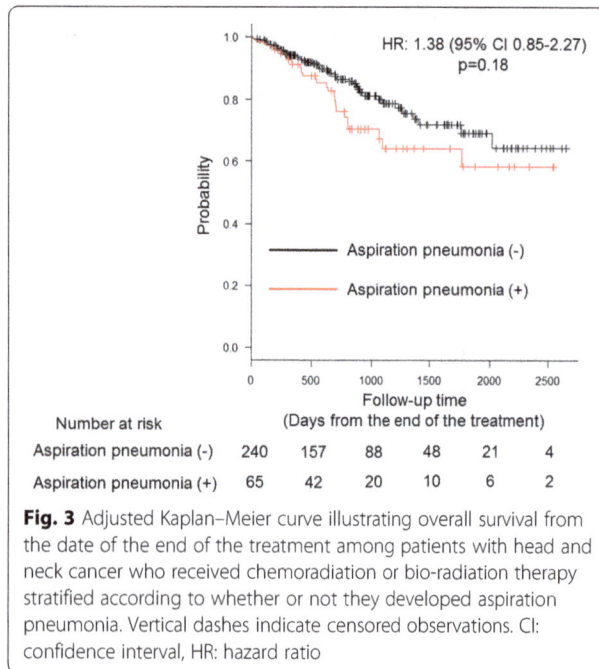

Fig. 3 Adjusted Kaplan–Meier curve illustrating overall survival from the date of the end of the treatment among patients with head and neck cancer who received chemoradiation or bio-radiation therapy stratified according to whether or not they developed aspiration pneumonia. Vertical dashes indicate censored observations. CI: confidence interval, HR: hazard ratio

resection of the primary lesion as a competing event. Surgical procedures clearly affect swallowing function. For example, total laryngectomy reduces the risk of aspiration and head and neck reconstruction changes patients' ability to swallow [19, 20]. Therefore, surgical intervention after CRT/BRT may obscure the association of aspiration with CRT or BRT. On the other hand, the effect of neck dissection on aspiration pneumonia has been controversial. For instance, Lango et al. [21]. reported that radical neck dissection (RND) increased the risk of feeding tube dependence in patients with HNC who underwent RT or CRT. On the other hand, Chapuy et al. [22]. reported that types of neck dissection including RND, modified RND, and selective neck dissection (SND) did not aggravate swallowing function. In this study, 45 patients underwent neck dissection, 44 (97%) of which underwent SND. Our analysis suggested no significant association between neck dissection and the occurrence of aspiration pneumonia ($P = 0.23$). Therefore, we did not consider neck dissection as a competing event in cumulative incidence analysis.

Consistent with previous reports [23], hypoalbuminemia was again identified as a factor predictive of aspiration pneumonia after CRT and BRT in our study. The novel predictive factors identified here were poor oral hygiene, use of sleeping pills, coexistence of other malignancies, and habitual alcohol consumption.

Several studies have demonstrated that careful oral management could reduce the risk of aspiration pneumonia in elderly people and patients with a history of cerebral infarction [24, 25]. However, few studies have focused on the correlation between oral hygiene and the

risk of aspiration pneumonia in patients with HNC. At our institution, patients with HNC undergoing RT have been routinely referred to dentists and received systematic oral care during the treatment [15]. Indeed, 96.0% of patients received oral evaluation before treatment in this cohort. However, 35.6% of patients initially evaluated as having poor oral hygiene were still assessed as having this same status after the treatment. This suggested that continuous oral management is required in high-risk patients, even after treatment.

Previous studies suggested that sleeping pills increased the risk of aspiration pneumonia [26, 27]. Among these, benzodiazepines were especially associated with the induction of aspiration through gamma-amino-butyric acid type A (GABA-A) signaling in the lesser esophageal sphincter, in addition to inhibition of the central nervous system [28]. However, in our study, benzodiazepines did not specifically increase the risk of aspiration pneumonia more than other sleeping pills. Notably, 83 out of 94 (88.3%) patients who used sleeping pills at the end of the treatment continued to use them even after the treatment. Al-Mamgani et al. [29]. demonstrated that 30.7% of patients with nasopharyngeal cancer who received RT or CRT had the complaint of insomnia during the treatment; however, approximately half of them recovered after the treatment. These findings suggest that the unnecessary administration of sleeping pills might increase the risk of aspiration pneumonia for our patients.

Our data demonstrated that the coexistence of other malignancies was a risk factor for aspiration pneumonia. Of 11 patients who had multiple primary HNC or cervical esophageal cancers simultaneously treated by CRT with main HNC, 7 (63.6%) developed aspiration pneumonia. A previous report suggested that enlargement of the irradiation field increased the risk of aspiration pneumonia [30]. Furthermore, 18 patients underwent surgical or endoscopic resection for esophageal and gastric cancer. Of these, six (33.3%) developed aspiration pneumonia, three of whom developed it within one week post-resection. Therefore, we speculated that post-surgical immunosuppression and anesthesia or sedation before endoscopy might deteriorate swallowing function.

Previous reports indicated that alcohol suppressed the cough reflex, reduced consciousness, and promoted gastro-esophageal reflux [31–33]. Therefore, such complex factors induced by habitual alcohol consumption may be involved in the occurrence of aspiration pneumonia.

Scheld et al. [34]. and Xu et al. [7]. reported that aspiration pneumonia was a significant prognostic factor. Furthermore, Szczesniak et al. [6]. reported that aspiration pneumonia accounted for 19% of non-cancer-related deaths of patients with HNC who received CRT. Therefore, we expected that aspiration pneumonia would be strongly associated with patient survival. However, our study did not show a statistically significant difference in survival between patients who developed aspiration pneumonia and those who did not, probably because of the relatively small number of deaths within the short follow-up period.

Our study had several limitations. First, it involved a retrospective analysis at a single institution. Second, differential diagnosis between aspiration pneumonia and other types of pneumonia was often difficult because the definitions of aspiration pneumonia varied among previous reports [9–11]. Third, the median follow-up of 2.4 years was shorter than in previous studies [4, 7]. The ability of our predictive model might change upon a long-term follow-up. For example, because submucosal remodeling and neurological disturbance slowly progress after irradiation [35], irradiation might have a stronger impact on the occurrence of aspiration pneumonia at a later phase.

Further studies are warranted to validate our predictive model because of the retrospective nature of this study. However, the strength of our study is that almost all patients received standard chemotherapeutic regimens containing platinum or cetuximab, with systematic supportive care such as oral care. Therefore, our predictive model may be more useful for identifying patients at high risk for aspiration pneumonia in recent clinical practice than previous evidences. For example, we propose that clinicians consider swallowing exercises for high- or moderate-risk groups to improve their swallowing function and subsequently prevent aspiration pneumonia [35].

Conclusions
We investigated the cause-specific incidence and identified risk factors for aspiration pneumonia following definitive CRT or BRT for patients with locally advanced HNC. The prediction of aspiration pneumonia may be necessary to preserve the quality of life and extend life expectancy for patients. Long-term follow-up and further prospective studies are needed to validate the usefulness of our predictive model.

Abbreviations
3D-CRT: Three-dimensional conformal radiation therapy; ACE: Angiotensin-converting enzyme; AIC: Akaike information criterion; ALB: Serum albumin; ARBs: Angiotensin II receptor blockers; BRT: Bio-radiotherapy; CR: Complete response; CRT: Chemoradiotherapy; ECOG: Eastern Cooperative Oncology Group; GABA-A: Gamma-amino-butyric acid type A; Hb: Hemoglobin; HNC: Head and neck cancer; IMRT: Intensity-modulated radiation therapy; OS: Overall survival; PPIs: Proton pump inhibitors; RND: Radical neck dissection; RT: Radiotherapy; SND: Selective neck dissection

Acknowledgements
Not applicable.

Funding
None.

Authors' contributions
Conceptualization: SK, Writing an original draft: SK, Project administration: TY, Review and editing: TY, YO, AF, Formal analysis: KM, Supervision: HY, Investigation of data: SK, TY, SH, HO, TO, TO, TY, AT, TT, YY, YK, and All authors read and approved the final manuscript.

Competing interests
The authors declare that they have no competing interests.

Author details
[1]Division of Gastrointestinal Oncology, Shizuoka Cancer Center, 1007 Shimonagakubo, Nagaizumi, Sunto-gun, Shizuoka 411-8777, Japan. [2]Division of Medical Oncology, Shizuoka Cancer Center, Sunto-gun, Shizuoka, Japan. [3]Division of Radiation Oncology and Proton Therapy, Shizuoka Cancer Center, Sunto-gun, Shizuoka, Japan. [4]Division of Head and Neck Surgery, Shizuoka Cancer Center, Sunto-gun, Shizuoka, Japan. [5]Division of Dental and Oral Surgery, Shizuoka Cancer Center, Sunto-gun, Shizuoka, Japan. [6]Clinical Research Center, Shizuoka Cancer Center, Sunto-gun, Shizuoka, Japan.

References
1. Adelstein DJ, Li Y, Adams GL, Wagner Jr H, Kish JA, Ensley JF, et al. An intergroup phase III comparison of standard radiation therapy and two schedules of concurrent chemoradiotherapy in patients with unresectable squamous cell head and neck cancer. J Clin Oncol. 2003;21:92–8.
2. Bonner JA, Harari PM, Giralt J, Azarnia N, Shin DM, Cohen RB, et al. Radiotherapy plus cetuximab for squamous-cell carcinoma of the head and neck. N Engl J Med. 2006;354:567–78.
3. Forastiere AA, Goepfert H, Maor M, Pajak TF, Weber R, Morrison W, et al. Concurrent chemotherapy and radiotherapy for organ preservation in advanced laryngeal cancer. N Engl J Med. 2003;349:2091–8.
4. Forastiere AA, Zhang Q, Weber RS, Maor MH, Goepfert H, Pajak TF, et al. Long-term results of RTOG 91–11: a comparison of three nonsurgical treatment strategies to preserve the larynx in patients with locally advanced larynx cancer. J Clin Oncol. 2013;31:845–52.
5. Russi EG, Corvo R, Merlotti A, Alterio D, Franco P, Pergolizzi S, et al. Swallowing dysfunction in head and neck cancer patients treated by radiotherapy: review and recommendations of the supportive task group of the Italian Association of Radiation Oncology. Cancer Treat Rev. 2012;38:1033–49.
6. Szczesniak MM, Maclean J, Zhang T, Graham PH, Cook IJ. Persistent dysphagia after head and neck radiotherapy: a common and under-reported complication with significant effect on non-cancer-related mortality. Clin Oncol. 2014;26:697–703.
7. Xu B, Boero IJ, Hwang L, Le QT, Moiseenko V, Sanghvi PR, et al. Aspiration pneumonia after concurrent chemoradiotherapy for head and neck cancer. Cancer. 2015;121:1303–11.
8. Charlson ME, Pompei P, Ales KL, MacKenzie CR. A new method of classifying prognostic comorbidity in longitudinal studies: development and validation. J Chronic Dis. 1987;40:373–83.
9. Mortensen HR, Jensen K, Grau C. Aspiration pneumonia in patients treated with radiotherapy for head and neck cancer. Acta Oncol. 2013;52:270–6.
10. Chen SW, Yang SN, Liang JA, Lin FJ. The outcome and prognostic factors in patients with aspiration pneumonia during concurrent chemoradiotherapy for head and neck cancer. Eur J Cancer Care. 2010;19:631–5.
11. Nguyen NP, Smith HJ, Dutta S, Alfieri A, North D, Nguyen PD, et al. Aspiration occurrence during chemoradiation for head and neck cancer. Anticancer Res. 2007;27:1669–72.
12. Akaike H. A new look at the statistical model identification. IEEE T Automat Contr. 1974;19:716–23.
13. Harrell Jr FE, Lee KL, Mark DB. Multivariable prognostic models: issues in developing models, evaluating assumptions and adequacy, and measuring and reducing errors. Stat Med. 1996;15:361–87.
14. Kanda Y. Investigation of the freely available easy-to-use software 'EZR' for medical statistics. Bone Marrow Transplant. 2013;48:452–8.
15. Yokota T, Tachibana H, Konishi T, Yurikusa T, Hamauchi S, Sakai K, et al. Multicenter phase II study of an oral care program for patients with head and neck cancer receiving chemoradiotherapy. Support Care Cancer. 2016;24:3029–36.

16. Langerman A, Maccracken E, Kasza K, Haraf DJ, Vokes EE, Stenson KM. Aspiration in chemoradiated patients with head and neck cancer. Arch Otolaryngol Head Neck Surg. 2007;133:1289–95.

17. Eisbruch A, Lyden T, Bradford CR, Dawson LA, Haxer MJ, Miller AE, et al. Objective assessment of swallowing dysfunction and aspiration after radiation concurrent with chemotherapy for head-and-neck cancer. Int J Radiat Oncol Biol Phys. 2002;53:23–8.

18. Hunter KU, Lee OE, Lyden TH, Haxer MJ, Feng FY, Schipper M, et al. Aspiration pneumonia after chemo-intensity-modulated radiation therapy of oropharyngeal carcinoma and its clinical and dysphagia-related predictors. Head Neck. 2014;36:120–5.

19. Rathod S, Livergant J, Klein J, Witterick I, Ringash J. A systematic review of quality of life in head and neck cancer treated with surgery with or without adjuvant treatment. Oral Oncol. 2015;51:888–900.

20. Kao SS, Peters MD, Krishnan SG, Ooi EH. Swallowing outcomes following primary surgical resection and primary free flap reconstruction for oral and oropharyngeal squamous cell carcinomas: A systematic review. Laryngoscope. 2016 [Epub ahead of print].

21. Lango MN, Egleston B, Ende K, Feigenberg S, D'Ambrosio DJ, Cohen RB, et al. Impact of neck dissection on long-term feeding tube dependence in patients with head and neck cancer treated with primary radiation or chemoradiation. Head Neck. 2010;32:341–7.

22. Cl C, Annino DJ, Snavely A, Li Y, Tishler RB, Norris CM, et al. Swallowing function following postchemoradiotherapy neck dissection: review of findings and analysis of contributing factors. Otolaryngol Head Neck Surg. 2011;145:428–34.

23. Purkey MT, Levine MS, Prendes B, Norman MF, Mirza N. Predictors of aspiration pneumonia following radiotherapy for head and neck cancer. Ann Otol Rhinol Laryngol. 2009;118:811–6.

24. van der Maarel-Wierink CD, Vanobbergen JN, Bronkhorst EM, Schols JM, de Baat C. Oral health care and aspiration pneumonia in frail older people: a systematic literature review. Gerodontology. 2013;30:3–9.

25. Wagner C, Marchina S, Deveau JA, Frayne C, Sulmonte K, Kumar S. Risk of stroke-associated pneumonia and oral hygiene. Cerebrovasc Dis. 2016;41:35–9.

26. Knol W, van Marum RJ, Jansen PA, Souverein PC, Schobben AF, Egberts AC. Antipsychotic drug use and risk of pneumonia in elderly people. J Am Geriatr Soc. 2008;56:661–6.

27. Obiora E, Hubbard R, Sanders RD, Myles PR. The impact of benzodiazepines on occurrence of pneumonia and mortality from pneumonia: a nested case–control and survival analysis in a population-based cohort. Thorax. 2013;68:163–70.

28. Rushnak MJ, Leevy CM. Effect of diazepam on the lower esophageal sphincter. A double-blind controlled study. Am J Gastroenterol. 1980; 73:127–30.

29. Al-Mamgani A, van Rooij P, Tans L, Verduijn GM, Sewnaik A, de Jong RJ B. A prospective evaluation of patient-reported quality-of-life after (chemo) radiation for oropharyngeal cancer: which patients are at risk of significant quality-of-life deterioration? Radiother Oncol. 2013;106:359–63.

30. Langendijk JA, Doornaert P, Rietveld DH, Verdonck-de Leeuw IM, Leemans CR, Slotman BJ. A predictive model for swallowing dysfunction after curative radiotherapy in head and neck cancer. Radiother Oncol. 2009;90:189–95.

31. Berkowitz H, Reichel J, Shim C. The effect of ethanol on the cough reflex. Clin Sci Mol Med. 1973;45:527–31.

32. Lee A, Festic E, Park PK, Raghavendran K, Dabbagh O, Adesanya A, et al. Characteristics and outcomes of patients hospitalized following pulmonary aspiration. Chest. 2014;146:899–907.

33. Matsuki N, Fujita T, Watanabe N, Sugahara A, Watanabe A, Ishida T, et al. Lifestyle factors associated with gastroesophageal reflux disease in the Japanese population. J Gastroenterol. 2013;48:340–9.

34. Scheld WM, Mandell GL. Nosocomial pneumonia: pathogenesis and recent advances in diagnosis and therapy. Rev Infect Dis. 1991;13:S743–51.

35. DI R, Lewin JS, Eisbruch A. Prevention and treatment of dysphagia and aspiration after chemoradiation for head and neck cancer. J Clin Oncol. 2006;24:2636–43.

12

Chemokine CCL27 is a novel plasma biomarker for identification the nasopharyngeal carcinoma patients from the Epstein-Barr virus capsid antigen-specific IgA seropositive population

Min-jie Mao[1^], Ning Xue[2^], Xue-ping Wang[1^], Pei-dong Chi[1], Yi-jun Liu[1], Qi Huang[3], Shu-qin Dai[1*] and Wan-li Liu[1*] (iD)

Abstract

Background: To investigate the predictive value of chemokine CCL27 for identifying early stage nasopharyngeal carcinoma (NPC) patients within a population seropositive for Epstein-Barr virus (EBV) capsid antigen-specific IgA (VCA-IgA).

Methods: CCL27 in plasma samples from 104 NPC patients, 112 VCA-IgA–positive healthy donors, and 140 VCA-IgA–negative normal subjects was measured by ELISA. Expression of CCL27 in nasopharyngeal tissue from 20 VCA-IgA–positive healthy donors and 20 NPC patients was examined by immunohistochemical staining.

Results: Levels of CCL27 in the plasma of VCA-IgA–positive healthy donors (607.33 ± 218.81 pg/ml) were significantly higher than the levels in all NPC patients (437.09 ± 217.74, $P = < 0.0001$) and in the subset of patients with early stage NPC (463.85 ± 226.17, $P = 0.0126$). Plasma CCL27 levels were significantly lower in the VCA-IgA–negative normal subjects (358.22 ± 133.15 pg/ml) than in either the VCA-IgA–positive healthy donors ($P < 0.0001$) or the NPC patients ($P = 0.0113$). CCL27 protein was detected in 16 of 20 (80%) nasopharyngeal tissue samples from VCA-IgA–positive healthy donors and in 3 of 20 (15%) tumor tissue samples from NPC patients. There was no relationship between CCL27 levels and VCA-IgA titers or plasma EBV DNA content. Receiver operating characteristic (ROC) curves demonstrated that plasma CCL27 levels had a sensitivity of 67.00%, a specificity of 73.10%, and an area under the ROC of 0.725 (95% confidence interval [CI]: 0.657–0.793) for distinguishing between NPC patients and VCA-IgA–positive healthy donors. Further analysis showed that CCL27 levels could distinguish between early stage NPC patients and VCA-IgA–positive healthy donors with an area under the ROC of 0.712 (95% CI: 0.560–0.865), a sensitivity of 59.80%, and a specificity of 84.60%.

Conclusions: Chemokine CCL27 could successfully identify NPC patients within a VCA-IgA–positive population.

Keywords: CCL27, VCA-IgA, Nasopharyngeal carcinoma, Early screening

* Correspondence: daishq@sysucc.org.cn; liuwanli126@126.com
^Deceased
[1]Department of Laboratory Medicine, State Key Laboratory of Oncology in South China, Collaborative Innovation Center for Cancer Medicine, Sun Yat-sen University Cancer Center, Guangzhou 510060, China
Full list of author information is available at the end of the article

Background

Nasopharyngeal carcinoma (NPC) is one of the most common malignant neoplasms in South China and Southeast Asia. The etiology of NPC includes Epstein-Barr virus (EBV) infection, environmental and genetic factors, and dietary habits [1, 2]. Because EBV infection is closely associated with the occurrence of NPC, EBV-related biomarkers, such as EBV viral capsid antigen-specific IgA (VCA-IgA), have been widely used in NPC screening.

VCA-IgA shows good sensitivity but the false-positive rate in primary screening is high and the specificity for identification of NPC within EBV antibody-positive diseases is poor [3] (Lin et al., 1977) [4] reported that VCA-IgA has been measured during NPC screening of 413,164 subjects, of whom 12,629 cases were VCA-IgA positive (positive rate of 3.06%). After the last follow-up, only 174 of the 12,629 subjects were confirmed to have NPC (positive predictive value of 1.4%). In large population screens in Taiwan [5] and Hong Kong [6], the VCA-IgA–positive rate was 3–6% and the NPC-positive rate was 1.5–4.4% [7]. In our previous study, we used nasopharyngoscopy and serology to screen 28,688 individuals in Guangdong Sihui and Zhongshan from 2008 to 2010. Of the 3046 subjects who were VCA-IgA and/or EBNA1-IgA positive, NPC was diagnosed in 10.6%. After 6 years of follow-up, only 41 cases of NPC were verified, to give a positive predictive rate of only 1.3%. Thus, VCA-IgA and EBNA1-IgA can be used effectively to screen for NPC, but the positive predictive value for NPC is low [8]. Therefore, it is crucial to find new biomarkers that can identify NPC patients in the VCA-IgA–positive population.

Chemokines are small structurally related multifunctional proteins that play important roles in T cell development, differentiation, maturation, and trafficking, and other aspects of immune function [9]. Recent studies have shown that chemokines play an important role in the regulation of tumor progression, including proliferation and metastasis [10, 11]. CCL27 is a C-C motif chemokine also known as cutaneous T cell-attracting chemokine (CTACK). The only known receptor for CCL27 is CCR10, which is expressed in normal skin, which can make a small amount of CCR10+/CLA+ memory T cells homing to the inflammation microenvironment to maintain immune surveillance. However, the predictive value of CCL27 in NPC remains unclear [12, 13].

To shed light on the association between CCL27 and NPC, we measure plasma CCL27 levels in NPC patients, VCA-IgA–positive healthy donors, and VCA-IgA–negative normal subjects, and evaluated the diagnostic performance of CCL27 for NPC detection in a VCA-IgA–positive population.

Methods

Patients

Between September 2015 and December 2015, 104 NPC patients (median age 45 years, range 23–69 years; 79 men and 25 women) at the Sun Yat-Sen University Cancer Center were enrolled in this study. The inclusion criteria for NPC were as follows: all of the patients met the diagnostic criteria for NPC (TNM staging defined by the 2009 Union for International Cancer Control/American Joint Committee on Cancer staging system for NPC), and all 104 NPC patients were seropositive for EBV VCA-IgA. Exclusion criteria were as follows: (1) patients who received chemoradiotherapy or surgery before enrolling in this study; (2) patients who with concomitant diseases, such as skin disease or another type of malignancy. We also enrolled 112 VCA-IgA–positive cancer-free healthy donors (median age 41 years, range 27–65 years, 64 men and 48 women), who were followed up for 6 months to exclude cancer and inflammation-related diseases. A VCA-IgA–negative control population consisted of 140 normal subjects who were free of detectable infection, cancer, or other known disease. Samples from the healthy donors and normal subjects were collected from the physical examination department at the Sun Yat-Sen University Cancer Center. Venous blood samples (2–4 ml) obtained from the NPC patients at the time of diagnosis (before treatment) were mixed with EDTA-K$_2$ anticoagulant, centrifuged at 3000 rpm for 10 min, and stored at –80 °C until use. Written informed consent for the use of plasma and tissue samples was obtained from all patients and healthy participants. This study was approved by the Institute Research Ethics Committee of the Sun Yat-Sen University Cancer Center, Guangzhou, China.

Tissue specimens

For immunochemistry, formalin-fixed and paraffin-embedded nasopharyngeal tissue from 20 NPC patients and 20 VCA-IgA–positive healthy donors were obtained from the Sun Yat-Sen University Cancer Center. All NPC samples were collected immediately after surgical resection and the diagnosis were confirmed by pathological review.

ELISA assay

Plasma CCL27 concentrations were measured using a double-antibody sandwich ELISA according to the manufacturer's instructions (R&D Systems, Minneapolis, MN, USA). In brief, 100 μl/well of the capture antibody (mouse anti-human CCL27, 4.0 μg/ml) was added to 96-well microplates overnight at room temperature. Test samples or CCL27 standard (100 μl/well) were added to the wells and the plates were incubated for 2 h. Detection antibody (biotinylated goat anti-human CCL27, 75 ng/ml) was added at 100 μl/well and the plate was incubated for 2 h. Finally, 100 μl/well of horseradish peroxidase-conjugated streptavidin was added to each well. After addition of a colorimetric reagent for 0.5 h, the reaction was stopped by the addition of 2 N sulfuric acid and the absorbance was measured at 450 nm. Each test included a standard control (coefficient of variation = 12%).

Immunohistochemical staining

Nasopharyngeal tissue sections were incubated with a goat anti-CCL27 antibody (1:20, R&D Systems) overnight at 4 ° C. The samples were washed and the chromogenic reaction step was performed using a PV-9001 Polymer Detection System kit for immunohistochemical staining (Beijing Golden Bridge Biotechnology, China).

Statistical analysis

Statistical analysis was performed with SPSS 16.0 for Windows software (SPSS, Chicago, IL, USA). Relationships between CCL27 protein expression and clinicopathologic features were analyzed by the Mann–Whitney U test. Comparison of CCL27 concentrations and EBV DNA copies between groups was assessed using the Kruskal–Wallis test. The diagnostic value of CCL27 was assessed by area under the receiver operating characteristic (ROC) curve (AUC). The cut-off value for CCL27 discrimination was defined by maximization of the Youden index. P values <0.05 were considered statistically significant. All reported P values are two sided.

Results

Relationship between plasma CCL27 levels and patient clinicopathological characteristics

The associations between the median plasma CCL27 concentrations and clinical variables for the 104 NPC patients are presented in Table 1.

Plasma levels of CCL27 in NPC patients, VCA-IgA–positive healthy donors, and VCA-IgA–negative normal subjects

As shown in Fig. 1, the plasma levels of CCL27 in VCA-IgA–positive healthy donors (607.33 ± 218.81 pg/ml) were significantly higher than the pre-treatment levels in all NPC patients (437.09 ± 217.74 pg/ml, P < 0.0001) and the subset of patients with early stage NPC (Stage I + II, 463.85 ± 226.17, P = 0.0126). Furthermore, plasma CCL27 levels in VCA-IgA–negative normal subjects (358.22 ± 133.15 pg/ml) were significantly lower than the levels in either the VCA-IgA–positive healthy donors (P < 0.0001) or the NPC patients (P = 0.0113).

Expression of CCL27 in nasopharyngeal epithelial tissue from NPC patients and VCA-IgA–positive healthy donors

We investigated the expression of CCL27 protein in nasopharyngeal tissue from healthy donors and NPC patients by immunohistochemical staining. High expression of CCL27 protein was observed in 16 of 20 (80%) in nasopharyngeal epithelium from VCA-IgA–positive healthy donors, and no expression of CCL27 protein was observed in 17 of 20 (85%) tumor tissues from NPC

Table 1 Associations between plasma CCL27 levels and clinical characteristics of the patients with NPC

Characteristics	No.	Median(range)	P value
Age			0.8556
≤45	52	405.35(107.33-1296.94)	
>45	52	383.76(84.03-872.33)	
Sex			0.5555
Female	25	375.12(107.33-917.17)	
Male	79	403.27(84.03-1296.94)	
pT stage			0.8991
PT1-pT2	25	403.27(217.84-1067.05)	
pT3	47	403.96(84.03-1296.94)	
pT4	32	395.68(108.98-872.26)	
pN stage			0.1946
pN 0/1	53	373.05(84.03-1067.05)	
pN 2/3	51	420.32(109.05-1296.94)	
Stage			0.9685
I + II	13	376.25(227.77-1067.05)	
III	50	397.70(84.03-1296.94)	
IV	41	403.27(108.98-872.26)	

patients. CCL27 was located mainly in the cytoplasm of the nasopharyngeal epithelial cells (Fig 2).

Relationship between CCL27 level, VCA-IgA titer, and EBV DNA content

To assess the relationship between CCL27 levels and VCA-IgA titer, the NPC patients were assigned to four

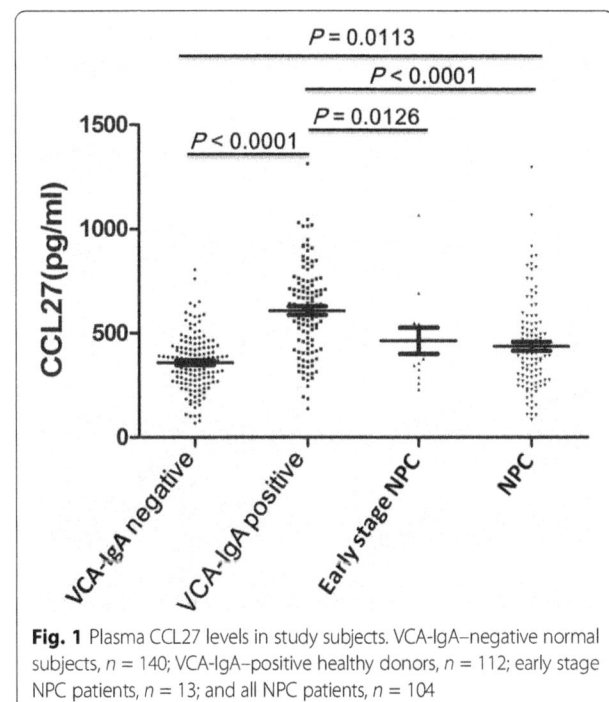

Fig. 1 Plasma CCL27 levels in study subjects. VCA-IgA–negative normal subjects, n = 140; VCA-IgA–positive healthy donors, n = 112; early stage NPC patients, n = 13; and all NPC patients, n = 104

groups based on VCA-IgA titers: ≤1:40, 1:80, 1:160, and ≥1:320. There were no significant differences in plasma CCL27 levels among the four groups ($P > 0.05$), suggesting that CCL27 levels are unlikely to be directly related to the VCA-IgA titer (Fig 3). Similar results were obtained when the NPC patients were assigned to four groups based on plasma EBV DNA copy number: $≥10^5$ ($n = 11$), $10^4–10^5$ ($n = 26$), $10^2–10^4$ ($n = 16$), and $<10^2$ ($n = 36$). Here, too, we observed no significant differences in plasma CCL27 levels among the four groups ($P > 0.05$), suggesting that CCL27 levels are unlikely to be directly related to EBV DNA copy numbers (Fig 4).

Diagnostic performance of plasma CCL27 levels in identifying NPC patients in a VCA-IgA–positive population

ROC curves were plotted to identify a cut-off value that could distinguish the NPC patients from the VCA-IgA–positive healthy donors. As shown in Fig. 5a, the optimal cut-off value was 516.98 pg/ml CCL27 (AUC = 0.725, 95% CI: 0.657–0.793), with a sensitivity of 67.00% and a specificity of 73.10%. Further analysis showed that CCL27 levels could also distinguish between the early stage NPC patients and the VCA-IgA–positive healthy donors, with a cut-off value of 552.71 pg/ml (AUC = 0.712, 95% CI: 0.560–0.865), a sensitivity of 59.80%, and a specificity of 84.60% (Fig 5b).

Discussion

NPC is a nasopharyngeal epithelial cell malignancy. In southern China, it is the most common form of head and neck cancer. The incidence of the disease is closely associated with infection with EBV, a herpes virus [14]. After infection, viral products can influence cell proliferation, apoptosis and gene mutation, which might contribute to malignant transformation [15]. EBV DNA copy numbers

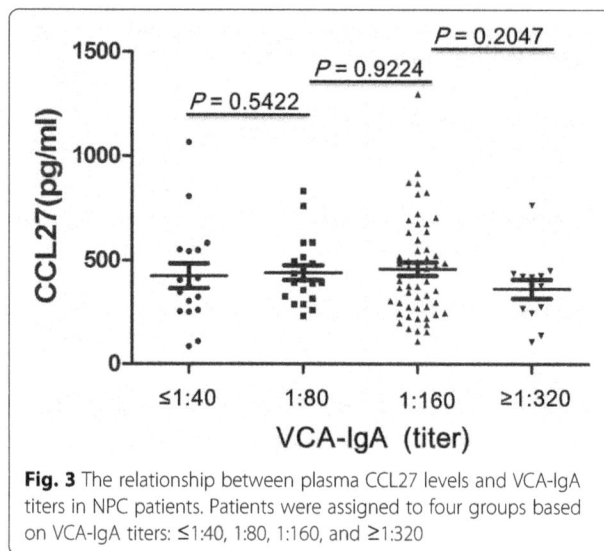

Fig. 3 The relationship between plasma CCL27 levels and VCA-IgA titers in NPC patients. Patients were assigned to four groups based on VCA-IgA titers: ≤1:40, 1:80, 1:160, and ≥1:320

and VCA-IgA antibody titers can indirectly reflect the activation state of EBV in the body [16–18]. CCL27 is a C-C motif chemokine, and the rationales to pick up CCL27 are as follows: Firstly, we have done gene chip detection between 8 NPC patients and 8 VCA-positive healthy donors, and found that CCL27 is down regulated in NPC patients; Secondly, we have tried our best to consult the reference: CCL27 is increased in inflammatory skin diseases, such as psoriasis, atopic dermatitis, and contact dermatitis, as well as other types of skin inflammation associated with T lymphocyte infiltration. Classic CCL27 contains secreting peptide,which has chemotaxis to the activation of CD4 + T cells, and plays a major role on skin inflammation, mainly produced by the skin keratinocyte cell. CCL27 has also been reported to be highly expressed

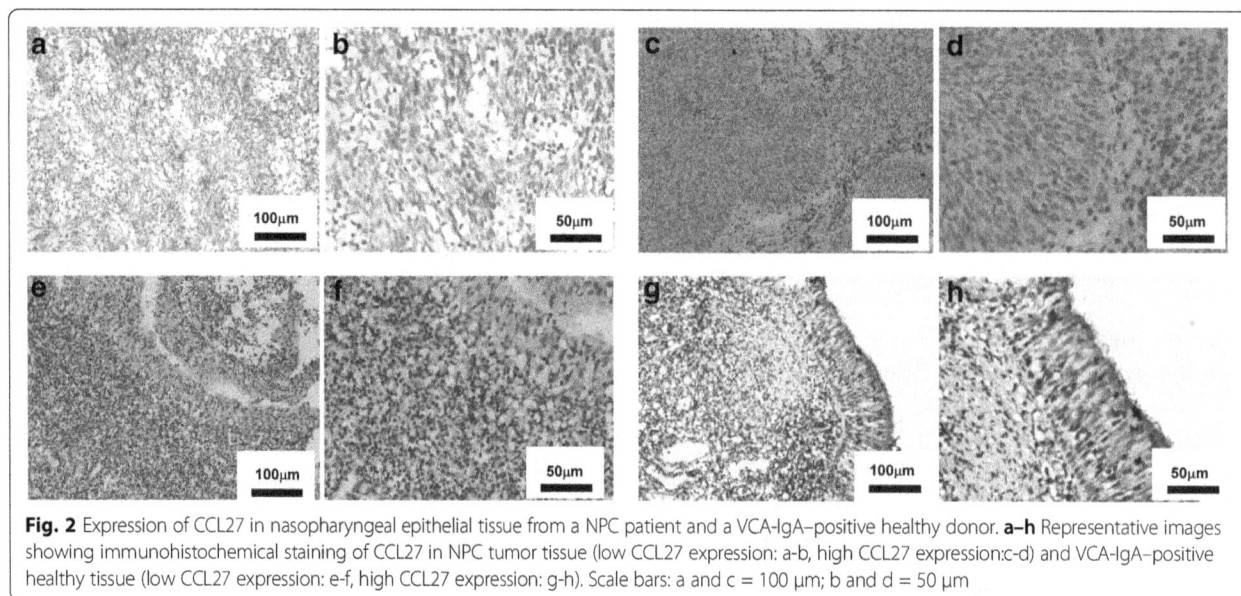

Fig. 2 Expression of CCL27 in nasopharyngeal epithelial tissue from a NPC patient and a VCA-IgA–positive healthy donor. **a–h** Representative images showing immunohistochemical staining of CCL27 in NPC tumor tissue (low CCL27 expression: a-b, high CCL27 expression:c-d) and VCA-IgA–positive healthy tissue (low CCL27 expression: e-f, high CCL27 expression: g-h). Scale bars: a and c = 100 μm; b and d = 50 μm

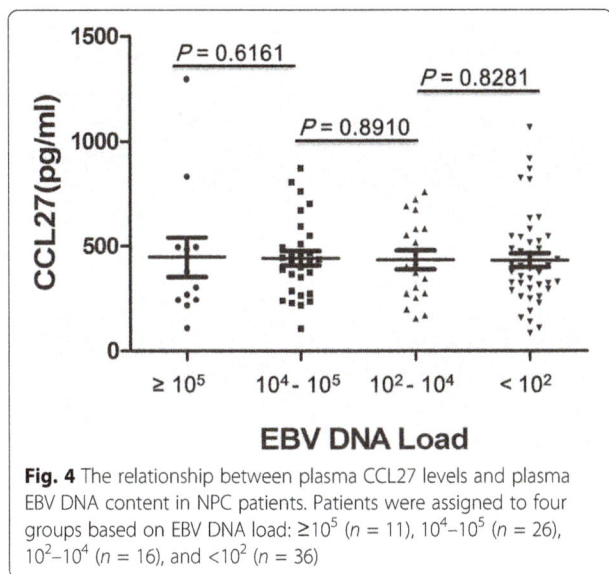

Fig. 4 The relationship between plasma CCL27 levels and plasma EBV DNA content in NPC patients. Patients were assigned to four groups based on EBV DNA load: $\geq 10^5$ ($n = 11$), 10^4–10^5 ($n = 26$), 10^2–10^4 ($n = 16$), and $< 10^2$ ($n = 36$)

in squamous cell epithelial cells and melanoma cells, and NPC is non- squamous type; in the latter, it may be involved in invasion and metastasis [19].

This study is the first to investigate CCL27 as a potential biomarker for use in primary screening for NPC, especially in VCA-IgA–positive individuals. The results show that CCL27 levels were significantly higher in EBV-infected individuals (i.e., NPC patients and VCA-IgA–positive healthy donors) than in uninfected normal subjects. The main mechanisms were that CCL27 will be increased

according to the high expressed of CCR10, which is upregulated on T cells immortalized by EBV infection. We also found that plasma CCL27 concentrations were higher in the VCA-IgA–positive healthy donors than in the NPC patients, for which there are several potential explanations. First, EBV infection induces an immune response that, in a normal situation, would increase CCL27 levels for recruitment of T cells [20]; however, CCL27 concentrations may be lower in subjects with abnormal immune function [21]. Second, Pivarcsi et al. [22] reported that reduced levels of cytokines and chemokines, such as CCL27, could allow tumors to evade the immune system. Compared with normal skin, keratinocyte-derived cutaneous tumor cells may downregulate the expression of CCL27 via the epidermal growth factor receptor–Ras–MARK signaling pathway, thereby evading the T cell-dependent antitumor immune response [23].

In recent years, several methods have been routinely used to diagnose NPC, such as nasopharyngoscopy, imaging modalities, anti-EBV antibody detection, and EBV DNA quantification [24]. However, these methods have limited sensitivity and specificity and are not entirely reliable, and the gold standard for diagnosis is nasopharyngeal lesion biopsy. VCA, the capsid antigen, and EA, the early antigen, are released soon after EBV infection. VCA is strongly immunogenic, more than 90% of NPC patients are VCA-IgA positive, and the levels can be reduced by treatment. Therefore, VCA-IgA could function as an NPC screening marker, an independent

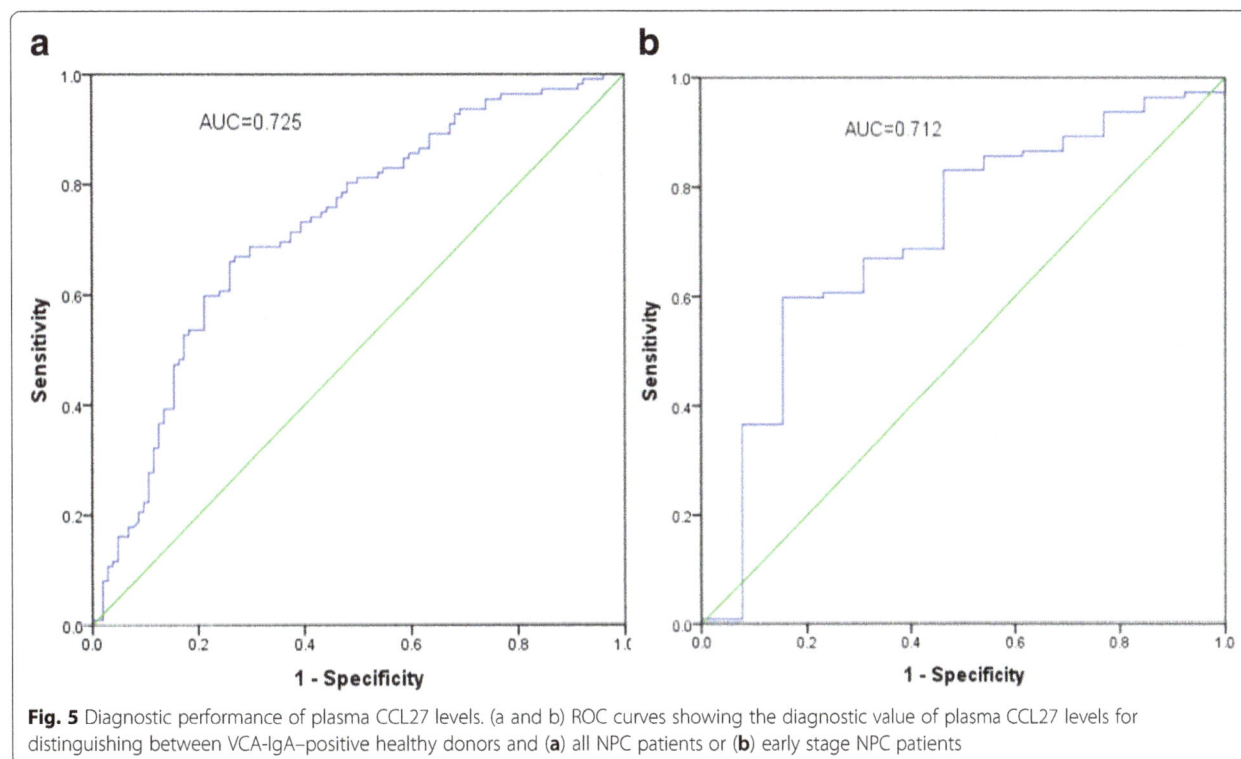

Fig. 5 Diagnostic performance of plasma CCL27 levels. (a and b) ROC curves showing the diagnostic value of plasma CCL27 levels for distinguishing between VCA-IgA–positive healthy donors and (**a**) all NPC patients or (**b**) early stage NPC patients

prognostic factor, and a predictive index in NPC therapy. EA-specific IgA, which is produced when EBV begins to replicate, has high specificity but limited sensitivity for the detection of early NPC and it is mismatched with the severity of NPC [25]. EBV DNA is integrated into the lymphocyte genome and is also present in the cytoplasm in the form of circular DNA. Thus, EBV DNA copy number in the plasma is a direct reflection of the EBV load in the patient [26, 27]. However, Han et al. [1] systematically reviewed 18 studies from China and elsewhere and found a positive predictive value of VCA-IgA for NPC of only 8.84%. Collectively, the combination of the poor specificity of VCA-IgA, the limited sensitivity of EA-IgA, the low diagnostic rate of EBV DNA content, and invasion of pathological biopsies means that there is no suitable method for screening of the general population for NPC. Therefore, it is critical to find a biomarker able to identify NPC patients in the VCA-IgA–positive population.

In our study, ROC curves showed that plasma CCL27 concentrations could effectively differentiate NPC patients from the VCA-IgA–positive healthy donors (AUC = 0.725, 95% CI: 0.657–0.793) with a sensitivity of 67.00% and a specificity of 73.10%. Moreover, CCL27 could also distinguish between early stage NPC patients and the VCA-IgA–positive healthy donors (AUC = 0.712, 95% CI: 0.560–0.865) with a sensitivity of 59.80% and a specificity of 84.60%. These results indicate that CCL27 could be used as a biomarker to identify NPC patients, and served as the complement of *VCA-IgA titers*.

However, there were no significant correlations between plasma CCL27 levels and either VCA-IgA titer or EBV DNA copy number. This may be because EBV VCA-IgA is produced in the early stage of infection and has a longer half-life than CCL27; indeed, VCA-IgA is present at high concentrations even after EBV is cleared from the body. CCL27 is involved in the general immune response and is a dominant player in tumor immunity; thus, its level might not be associated with a change in EBV VCA-IgA [28]. As a cellular marker, CCL27 differs from the traditional EBV markers. The combination of viral markers and cellular markers could provide a new and effective method to diagnose NPC, with CCL27 complementing the more traditional biomarkers such as VCA-IgA and EA-IgA. Detection of VCA-IgA and EA-IgA is complex, objective, which have less precision and accuracy. In contrast, detection of CCL27 in plasma can be achieved with good accuracy and reproducibility and it does not require specialized equipment. Thus, it could be a convenient monitoring biomarker in routine examinations.

Conclusions

The major limitations of this study are as follows: First, Our study is a single-center analysis in our hospital, and

need to be validated in large prospective trials of multicenter; Second, our study is a prospective analysis, we plan to collect complete patient data pre- and post-treatment to further evaluate the prognostic value and biological function of CCL27 in NPC; Third, although our study found that CCL27 could be a useful biomarker for identifying NPC patients within a VCA-IgA–positive population, but the mechanisms of how CCL27 influences NPC patients is not clear, further studies aim at investigating the role of CCL27 in NPC. Our study is the first to investigate CCL27 as a potential complement biomarker for use in primary screening for NPC, especially in VCA-IgA–positive individuals, which was used to identify NPC and VCA-IgA–positive healthy donors and improve the positive predictive value of VCA-IgA in NPC.

Abbreviations

CCL27: C-C Motif Chemokine Ligand 27; CTACK: Cutaneous T cell-attracting chemokine; EBV: Epstein-Barr virus; NPC: Nasopharyngeal carcinoma; VCA-IgA: Viral capsid antigen-specific IgA

Acknowledgments

We would like to thank all of our colleagues for their contribution to this study.

Funding

This work was financially supported by the NSFC (No. 81472008). The funding body have no role in the design of the study, collection, analysis, and interpretation of data nor in writing the manuscript.

Authors' contributions

WLL is the overall project lead and the grant holder with responsibility for the conception and design the protocol. All authors contributed to the development of the protocol. MJM provided expertise on patients recruitment, data collection, data analysis and interpretation. NX and QH provided expertise on immunostaining evaluation and data analysis. XPW and PDC provided expertise on ELISA evaluation and data analysis. SQD and YJL wrote the manuscript. MJM and XPW revised the manuscript. All authors have read and approved the final version of this manuscript.

Competing interests

The authors declare that they have no competing interest.

Author details

Department of Laboratory Medicine, State Key Laboratory of Oncology in South China, Collaborative Innovation Center for Cancer Medicine, Sun Yat-sen University Cancer Center, Guangzhou 510060, China. 2Department of Laboratory Medicine, Affiliated Tumor Hospital of Zhengzhou University, Henan Tumor Hospital, Zhengzhou 450100, China. 3Guangdong Medical University, Guangzhou 523808, China.

References

1. Han BL, XY X, Zhang CZ, JJ W, Han CF, Wang H, Wang X, Wang GS, Yang SJ, Xie Y. Systematic review on Epstein-Barr virus (EBV) DNA in diagnosis of nasopharyngeal carcinoma in Asian populations. Asian Pac J Cancer Prev. 2012;13(6):2577–81.

2. ZJ X, Zheng RS, Zhang SW, Zou XN, Chen WQ. Nasopharyngeal carcinoma incidence and mortality in China in 2009. Chin J Cancer. 2013;32(8):453–60.

3. Lin TM, Yang CS, Chiou JF, SM T, Chen TY, YC T, Lin PJ, Kawamura AJ, Hirayama T. Antibodies to Epstein-Barr virus capsid antigen and early antigen in nasopharyngeal carcinoma and comparison groups. Am J Epidemiol. 1977;106(4):336–9.

4. Zeng Y, Zhang LG, Li HY, Jan MG, Zhang Q, YC W, Wang YS, GR S. Serological mass survey for early detection of nasopharyngeal carcinoma in Wuzhou City, China. Int J Cancer. 1982;29(2):139–41.

5. Pickard A, Chen CJ, Diehl SR, Liu MY, Cheng YJ, Hsu WL, Sun B, Hsu MM, Chen IH, Chen JY, et al. Epstein-Barr virus seroreactivity among unaffected individuals within high-risk nasopharyngeal carcinoma families in Taiwan. Int J Cancer. 2004;111(1):117–23.

6. Liu Z, Ji MF, Huang QH, Fang F, Liu Q, Jia WH, Guo X, Xie SH, Chen F, Liu Y, et al. Two Epstein-Barr virus-related serologic antibody tests in nasopharyngeal carcinoma screening: results from the initial phase of a cluster randomized controlled trial in southern China. Am J Epidemiol. 2013; 177(3):242–50.

7. Luo J, Chia KS, Chia SE, Reilly M, Tan CS, Ye W. Secular trends of nasopharyngeal carcinoma incidence in Singapore, Hong Kong and Los Angeles Chinese populations, 1973-1997. Eur J Epidemiol. 2007;22(8):513–21.

8. Liu Y, Huang Q, Liu W, Liu Q, Jia W, Chang E, Chen F, Liu Z, Guo X, Mo H, et al. Establishment of VCA and EBNA1 IgA-based combination by enzyme-linked immunosorbent assay as preferred screening method for nasopharyngeal carcinoma: a two-stage design with a preliminary performance study and a mass screening in southern China. Int J Cancer. 2012;131(2):406–16.

9. Monlish DA, Bhatt ST, Schuettpelz LG. The role of toll-like receptors in hematopoietic malignancies. Front Immunol. 2016;7:390.

10. Vicari AP, Caux C. Chemokines in cancer. Cytokine Growth Factor Rev. 2002; 13(2):143–54.

11. Zlotnik A. Chemokines in neoplastic progression. Semin Cancer Biol. 2004; 14(3):181–5.

12. Thangavadivel S, Zelle-Rieser C, Olivier A, Postert B, Untergasser G, Kern J, Brunner A, Gunsilius E, Biedermann R, Hajek R, et al. CCR10/CCL27 crosstalk contributes to failure of proteasome-inhibitors in multiple myeloma. Oncotarget. 2016;7(48):78605–18.

13. Huang V, Lonsdorf AS, Fang L, Kakinuma T, Lee VC, Cha E, Zhang H, Nagao K, Zaleska M, Olszewski WL, et al. Cutting edge: rapid accumulation of epidermal CCL27 in skin-draining lymph nodes following topical application of a contact sensitizer recruits CCR10-expressing T cells. J Immunol. 2008; 180(10):6462–6.

14. Wani SQ, Khan T, Wani SY, Mir LR, Lone MM, Malik TR, Najmi AM, Afroz F, Teli MA, Khan NA. Nasopharyngeal carcinoma: a 15 year study with respect to Clinicodemography and survival analysis. Indian J Otolaryngol Head Neck Surg. 2016;68(4):511–21.

15. Zhang J, Shu C, Song Y, Li Q, Huang J, Ma X. Epstein-Barr virus DNA level as a novel prognostic factor in nasopharyngeal carcinoma: a meta-analysis. Medicine (Baltimore). 2016;95(40):e5130.

16. Tang LQ, Chen QY, Fan W, Liu H, Zhang L, Guo L, Luo DH, Huang PY, Zhang X, Lin XP, et al. Prospective study of tailoring whole-body dual-modality [18F]fluorodeoxyglucose positron emission tomography/computed tomography with plasma Epstein-Barr virus DNA for detecting distant metastasis in endemic nasopharyngeal carcinoma at initial staging. J Clin Oncol. 2013;31(23):2861–9.

17. Le QT, Zhang Q, Cao H, Cheng AJ, Pinsky BA, Hong RL, Chang JT, Wang CW, Tsao KC, Lo YD, et al. An international collaboration to harmonize the quantitative plasma Epstein-Barr virus DNA assay for future biomarker-guided trials in nasopharyngeal carcinoma. Clin Cancer Res. 2013;19(8): 2208–15.

18. KJ Y, Hsu WL, Pfeiffer RM, Chiang CJ, Wang CP, Lou PJ, Cheng YJ, Gravitt P, Diehl SR, Goldstein AM, et al. Prognostic utility of anti-EBV antibody testing for defining NPC risk among individuals from high-risk NPC families. Clin Cancer Res. 2011;17(7):1906–14.

19. Simonetti O, Goteri G, Lucarini G, Filosa A, Pieramici T, Rubini C, Biagini G, Offidani A. Potential role of CCL27 and CCR10 expression in melanoma progression and immune escape. Eur J Cancer. 2006;42(8):1181–7.

20. Kagami S, Sugaya M, Minatani Y, Ohmatsu H, Kakinuma T, Fujita H, Tamaki K. Elevated serum CTACK/CCL27 levels in CTCL. J INVEST DERMATOL. 2006; 126(5):1189–91.

21. Martinez-Rodriguez M, Thompson AK, Monteagudo C. High CCL27 immunoreactivity in 'supratumoral' epidermis correlates with better prognosis in patients with cutaneous malignant melanoma. J Clin Pathol. 2017;70(1):15–19.

22. Pivarcsi A, Muller A, Hippe A, Rieker J, van Lierop A, Steinhoff M, Seeliger S, Kubitza R, Pippirs U, Meller S, et al. Tumor immune escape by the loss of homeostatic chemokine expression. Proc Natl Acad Sci U S A. 2007;104(48): 19055–60.

23. Khaiboullina SF, Gumerova AR, Khafizova IF, Martynova EV, Lombardi VC, Bellusci S, Rizvanov AA. CCL27: novel cytokine with potential role in pathogenesis of multiple sclerosis. Biomed Res Int. 2015;2015:189638.

24. Chen Y, Xin X, Cui Z, Zheng Y, Guo J, Chen Y, Lin Y, Su G. Diagnostic value of serum Epstein-Barr virus Capsid antigen-IgA for nasopharyngeal carcinoma: a meta-analysis based on 21 studies. Clin Lab. 2016;62(6): 1155–66.

25. Shao JY, Li YH, Gao HY, QL W, Cui NJ, Zhang L, Cheng G, LF H, Ernberg I, Zeng YX. Comparison of plasma Epstein-Barr virus (EBV) DNA levels and serum EBV immunoglobulin a/virus capsid antigen antibody titers in patients with nasopharyngeal carcinoma. CANCER-AM CANCER SOC. 2004; 100(6):1162–70.

26. Henle G, Henle W. Epstein-Barr virus-specific IgA serum antibodies as an outstanding feature of nasopharyngeal carcinoma. Int J Cancer. 1976;17(1):1–7.

27. Lo YM, Chan LY, Chan AT, Leung SF, Lo KW, Zhang J, Lee JC, Hjelm NM, Johnson PJ, Huang DP. Quantitative and temporal correlation between circulating cell-free Epstein-Barr virus DNA and tumor recurrence in nasopharyngeal carcinoma. Cancer Res. 1999;59(21):5452–5.

28. Zhang C, Zong Y, Huang B, Sun Y, Ye Y, Feng K, Li J, Zhang F. Enhancing the efficiency of Epstein-Barr viral serologic test in the diagnosis of nasopharyngeal carcinoma. Zhonghua Zhong Liu Za Zhi. 2002;24(4):356–9.

13

Progressive resistance training in head and neck cancer patients during concomitant chemoradiotherapy – design of the DAHANCA 31 randomized trial

Camilla K. Lonkvist[1], Simon Lønbro[2,3], Anders Vinther[4], Bo Zerahn[5], Eva Rosenbom[6], Hanne Primdahl[7], Pernille Hojman[8] and Julie Gehl[1*] (iD)

Abstract

Background: Head and neck cancer patients undergoing concomitant chemoradiotherapy (CCRT) frequently experience loss of muscle mass and reduced functional performance. Positive effects of exercise training are reported for many cancer types but biological mechanisms need further elucidation. This randomized study investigates whether progressive resistance training (PRT) may attenuate loss of muscle mass and functional performance. Furthermore, biochemical markers and muscle biopsies will be investigated trying to link biological mechanisms to training effects.

Methods: At the Departments of Oncology at Herlev and Aarhus University Hospitals, patients with stage III/IV squamous cell carcinoma of the head and neck, scheduled for CCRT are randomized 1:1 to either a 12-week PRT program or control group, both with 1 year follow-up. Planned enrollment is 72 patients, and stratification variables are study site, sex, p16-status, and body mass index. Primary endpoint is difference in change in lean body mass (LBM) after 12 weeks of PRT, assessed by dual-energy X-ray absorptiometry (DXA). The hypothesis is that 12 weeks of PRT can attenuate the loss of LBM by at least 25%. Secondary endpoints include training adherence, changes in body composition, muscle strength, functional performance, weight, adverse events, dietary intake, self-reported physical activity, quality of life, labor market affiliation, blood biochemistry, plasma cytokine concentrations, NK-cell frequency in blood, sarcomeric protein content in muscles, as well as muscle fiber type and fiber size in muscle biopsies. Muscle biopsies are optional.

Discussion: This randomized study investigates the impact of a 12-week progressive resistance training program on lean body mass and several other physiological endpoints, as well as impact on adverse events and quality of life. Furthermore, a translational approach is integrated with extensive biological sampling and exploration into cytokines and mechanisms involved. The current paper discusses decisions and methods behind exercise in head and neck cancer patients undergoing concomitant chemoradiotherapy.

Keywords: Head and neck cancer, Head and neck squamous cell carcinoma, Chemoradiotherapy, Progressive resistance training, Exercise, Physical activity, Body composition, Lean body mass, Body weight, Weight

* Correspondence: karen.julie.gehl@regionh.dk
[1]Department of Oncology, Herlev and Gentofte Hospital, University of Copenhagen, Herlev, Denmark
Full list of author information is available at the end of the article

Background

Patients with locally advanced head and neck squamous cell carcinoma (HNSCC) undergoing concomitant chemoradiotherapy (CCRT) are often subjected to severe treatment side effects which may lead to weight loss, including loss of lean body mass, negatively impacting physical function and maybe even treatment outcome [1–7]. The loss of lean body mass (LBM) during treatment is likely to be multifactorial and HNSCC patients are particularly susceptible for several reasons: Cancer disease per se can cause muscle wasting [8, 9]; along with cisplatin chemotherapy [10, 11] and prednisolone [12, 13], which is often used as antiemetic treatment. Furthermore, many HNSCC patients fail to maintain sufficient energy and protein intake for a period of time [14, 15] due to treatment side effects, e.g. mucositis, dry mouth, pain, and fatigue. This may render patients in a catabolic state, a condition that inevitably will lead to further loss of muscle mass [16] as muscles are the largest and primary protein and energy reserve of the body. Interestingly, it has been shown that patients fail to maintain weight and LBM despite sufficient dietary intake [14], hence other interventions with potential to attenuate muscle wasting in HNSCC patients during treatment are needed.

In a preclinical study voluntary exercise efficiently mitigated cisplatin-induced muscle wasting [17]. Specifically, progressive resistance training (PRT) induces muscle hypertrophy in both healthy adults and cancer patients and definitely holds the potential to counteract cancer-related muscle wasting, too [8, 18, 19]. Twelve weeks of PRT after radiotherapy has been shown to rebuild LBM in HNSCC patients [20, 21], hence, PRT could be a meaningful approach for LBM preservation during treatment.

In a pilot study of a 12-week supervised PRT program during CCRT at our facility, we found that the intervention was feasible and appreciated by patients (Lonkvist et al., manuscript submitted). Knowing this, the present randomized trial is launched to investigate whether PRT during CCRT has a clinically relevant advantage, in terms of attenuated loss of LBM, compared with a control group not offered any structured training. In addition, extensive biological sampling is incorporated in this study adopting a translational approach, with the aim of exploring not only *if* it works, but also contributing to questions of *how* and *why*.

There is an echoing lack in clinical studies investigating the biological mechanisms. Preclinical studies demonstrate a direct inhibitory effect on cancer growth through different mechanisms [22–26]. One very plausible mechanism being exercise-mediated induction of intratumoral natural killer cells (NK cells) [27], unequivocally linking exercise to attenuation of tumor growth in mice [28, 29]. Exercise in its broadest sense is a very heterogeneous activity making the description of exercise interventions

in clinical trials critical [30]. This article describes the study design of a 12-week progressive resistance training program in head and neck cancer patients undergoing concomitant chemoradiotherapy, sharing thoughts behind the decision making.

Methods/design

Design

In this prospective phase II multi-center randomized study in patients with HNSCC scheduled for radiotherapy concomitant with chemotherapy (cisplatin), the effects of 12-week PRT are investigated. The study is planned to include 72 patients from the departments of oncology at Aarhus and Herlev Hospitals in Denmark, see study flow in Fig. 1. Also, a third center was opted to participate but this site will not be including patients due to capacity issues.

Ethics approval has been obtained from the regional Ethics Committee for the Capital Region of Denmark (H-15003725) and the Danish Data Protection Agency (HGH-2015-003; 2005–41-4802; 2014–41-3510). The study is registered at clinicaltrials.gov (NCT02557529) September 11th 2015. This article describes protocol version 4.0 from April 1st 2016.

The manuscript applies to the SPIRIT guidelines of randomized trials. The SPIRIT checklist, appendix for the SPIRIT checklist, as well as the World Health Organization (WHO) Trial Registration Data Set can be found in additional files 1, 2 and 3.

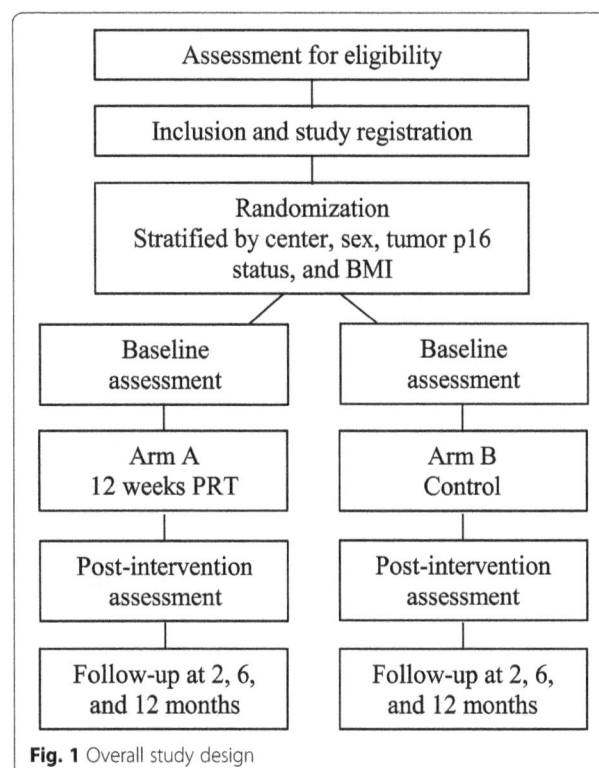

Fig. 1 Overall study design

Participants

Patients are eligible if the following inclusion criteria are fulfilled: 1) Histologically verified primary head and neck squamous cell carcinoma (HNSCC) of the oral cavity, oropharynx, hypopharynx, larynx, or in lymph nodes of the neck from an unknown primary tumor; 2) candidate for curatively intended CCRT (weekly cisplatin during radiotherapy, 66–68 Gy) according to Danish Head and Neck Cancer (DAHANCA) group (i.e. patients with stage III-IV disease, www.dahanca.dk) [31]; 3) performance status (PS) 0–1 (Eastern Cooperative Oncology Group Performance (ECOG); 4) age ≥ 18 years; 5) signed informed consent.

Exclusion criteria are: 1) Body Mass Index (BMI) < 20.5; 2) comorbidity potentially interfering with attendance or test results, e.g. other cancers, diabetes, prednisolone treatment); 3) tonsillectomy within 1 week before inclusion; 4) psychological, social or geographical conditions that could influence protocol adherence; 5) insufficient bone marrow function (hemoglobin <6 mmol/L, leucocytes <2.5 × 10^9/L, or thrombocytes <50 × 10^9/L; 6) diastolic blood pressure < 45 or >95, resting heart rate > 100; 7) signs of ischemia on electrocardiogram; 8) pregnancy.

Randomization

Patients will be stratified by site (Herlev/Aarhus), sex (male/female), p16-status of the tumor (positive/negative) and BMI (<30/≥30) and randomized 1:1 to either a training group performing a 12-week PRT program or control group. If a patient leaves the study within the first week, the number of patients randomized will be increased by one. Patient inclusion form is faxed to The Danish Head and Neck Cancer (DAHANCA, Aarhus, Denmark) group administration, that performs the randomization using a software randomization file (developed and used by the DAHANCA group) that automatically and randomly allocates each patient in either group. The personnel conducting the randomization are independent of clinical personnel and are not otherwise involved in the study.

Treatment

All patients will receive curatively intended CCRT, 66 to 68 Gy, in 2 Gy fractions, 6 fractions/week, with concurrent nimorazole perorally (1200 mg/m^2) [32] before each fraction (1000 mg/m^2 for same day second fraction), and weekly cisplatin (40 mg/m^2, max. 70 mg). Prophylactic antiemetics are administered according to institutional guidelines (Additional file 4: Table S1).

Intervention

The PRT program comprises seven conventional resistance training exercises targeting the large muscle groups of the body (chest press, low row (Herlev site)/lateral

pull down (Aarhus site), hamstring curls, knee extension, leg press, abdominal crunches (Herlev site)/sit ups (Aarhus site), back extensions) (Additional file 5: Figure S1). The latter two included primarily to ensure a full body workout. The training protocol (Table 1) was tested in our pilot study (Lonkvist et al., manuscript submitted) and is almost identical to the protocol developed and used in the DAHANCA 25 trials [20, 21]. The first week is an introductory week with high repetition number and low load, as many HNSCC patients are resistance training naïve. The intensity and volume progressed throughout the program from two to three sets with a load corresponding to 15 to 8 repetition maximum (RM), i.e. the load that can be lifted respectively 15 to 8 times using proper technique (See Tables 1 and 2). This progression model is in accordance with the guidelines from the American College of Sports Medicine (ACSM) [33]. Due to the focus on muscular hypertrophy, patients are urged to perform all sets in all exercises to exhaustion within the given RM target, thereby ensuring local muscular fatigue. In accordance, patients are instructed to perform all sets of each exercise before moving on to the next exercise and also to perform the lower body exercises after each other before moving to upper body exercises. Each exercise is executed in full range of motion and with rest periods of no more than 60 s between sets (Table 2). If more repetitions than planned can be performed, the training load will be increased to match the specific RM target. Training sessions are planned three times a week every other day ensuring optimal recovery time for maximal hypertrophic response. In case of temporary discontinuation, patients will proceed with the same weight as when they paused, but will be adjusted to ensure the proper RM target is reached.

The PRT program starts concurrently with CCRT. 36 training sessions are planned, i.e. thrice weekly for 12 weeks, thus continuing approximately 6 weeks further than CCRT. If a session is cancelled due to treatment related interventions, radiotherapy, scans, or due to public holidays, the session will be replaced at the end of the training program. Sessions missed for personal reasons or incapacitation will not be substituted. It will be ensured that the PRT program and tests never compromise treatment schedule.

At the Herlev site conventional exercise equipment is used for all exercises but due to different equipment

Table 1 Exercise progression model

Training session	Repetitions	Sets
1–3	15	2
4–6	12	2
7–18	12	3
19–31	10	3
32–36	8	3

Table 2 Description of the PRT program

Load	15 RM (week 1), 12 RM (week 2–6), 10 RM (week 7–10), 8 RM (week 11–12)
Repetitions	15 (week 1), 12 (week 2–6), 10 (week 7–10), 8 (week 11–12)
Sets per sessions	2 (week 1–2), 3 (week 3–12)
Sessions per week	3
Duration of training period	12 weeks
Rest between sets	45–60 s
Rest between repetitions	0 s
Range of motion	Maximum possible
Rest between training sessions	Training every other day

Abbreviations: *PRT* progressive resistance training, *RM* repetition maximum, e.g. 15 RM is the heaviest load that can be lifted 15 times using proper technique. Sec, seconds

available at the involved sites, three specific exercises differ but with only minimal difference in target muscle groups or progression options. Thus, at the Aarhus site sit-ups will be performed as traditional floor exercises with free weights ensuring possible progression in intensity. Hamstring curls will be performed using elastic bands (TheraBand, The Hygenic Corporation, Ohio, USA) with varying resistance and lateral pull down replaces low seated row in Aarhus. Conventional resistance training machines (Technogym, Gambettola, Italy) are used at both sites.

During the first 6 weeks all training sessions are supervised by physiotherapist or educated training instructors. When possible the same supervised training modality at the hospital training facility will continue for the remaining 6 weeks. If a patient is unable to attend training sessions at the hospital, e.g. due to prolonged transport time, the remaining training sessions will be tailored individually at commercial training facilities near the patients' own home. However, patients must attend at least one session per week supervised at the hospital training facility.

If patients, due to treatment side effects, are unable to attend at least one weekly training session, they will be given a leaflet describing two simple exercises (backward lunges and push-ups), and they will be encouraged to do the exercises (3 sets, 12 repetitions) every day until they are able to attend the supervised training again. Patients will fill in training logs during every session from which training adherence, changes in training volume, and intensity are reported.

No direct criteria for discontinuing the training program are provided, but if a patient feels incapable of training or if the physician, physiotherapist or training instructor deems the patient's general condition not compatible with training, the program will be paused.

To support energy intake and mitigate negative energy balance on training days, patients are offered a meal and/or a protein supplement (e.g. Nutridrink compact (Nutricia), 125 mL, 1260 kJ, 12 g protein) immediately after training sessions. Patients in both groups are continuously screened (i.e. body weight assessments) by trained nurses ensuring the best possible energy intake to limit the risk of catabolic state during the CCRT and the approximately 6-week follow-up period immediately after.

Controls

No restrictions on physical activity (PA) or other concomitant care are made for the control patients but no organized training will be offered to them. PA is reported in training logs. Except for blood sampling which, obviously, will not be drawn after any training session (see below) in the control group, there are no differences in tests and assessments between the groups.

Study objectives and assessments

The primary endpoint is change in lean body mass (LBM). Secondary endpoints are training adherence and changes in and difference between groups in body composition, muscle strength, functional performance, weight, adverse events, dietary intake, self-reported PA, quality of life (QoL), labor market affiliation, blood biochemistry, cytokines in plasma, NK-cells in peripheral blood, sarcomeric protein content in muscles, as well as muscle fiber type and fiber size in muscle biopsies. See Table 3 for all assessment time points.

Clinical outcomes
Body composition

The primary endpoint is change in lean body mass (LBM) which will be assessed after 12 weeks of PRT or control using Dual Energy X-ray Absorptiometry (DXA) (Herlev site: GE lunar iDXA, GE Healthcare Technologies; Aarhus site: Hologic QDR-series, Hologic Inc., Bedford, MA, USA). The hypothesis is that 12 weeks of progressive resistance training can attenuate the loss of LBM by at least 25%. This time span was chosen since 12 weeks are considered a sufficient period of PRT needed to affect LBM. Furthermore, this time point is a usual evaluating point for head and neck cancer as it coincide with the 2-month post-radiotherapy follow-up. Changes in total body mass and fat mass will also be assessed. Total body weight, with patients in light clothing and no shoes, will be measured weekly by the same digital scale at each site during therapy and bi-weekly thereafter.

Adherence

Adherence to the PRT program is registered by the physiotherapist or educated training instructors. Adherence to the study in general is encouraged by highlighting the importance of both groups in order for the trial to produce valid results. Furthermore, most appointments are planned when patients already have an appointment at

Table 3 Time schedule for study assessments

Time point (week no.)	0	1	2	3	4	5	6	7	8	9	10	11	12	13/14	15 Approx.	32 Approx.	58 Approx.
Time point (follow-up)															2 months follow-up	6 months follow-up	12 months follow-up
Enrollment:																	
Eligibility screen	X																
Informed consent	X																
Allocation	X																
Intervention:																	
Progressive resistance training / Control	◆—————————————————◆ - ◆ (weeks 0 to 13/14)																
Adverse events:																	
Adverse events	X		X	X	X	X	X		X						X	X	X
Blood samples:																	
Hemoglobin. leucocytes. platelets	X		X	X	X	X	X		X		X	X	X		X	X	X
Creatinine, carbamide, sodium, potassium, magnesium, calcium, e-GFR, albumin, glucose, ALT, ALP, LDH, bilirubin, triglycerid, cholesterols, HS-CRP	X		X	X	X	X	X		X		X	X	X		X	X	X
Phosphate, zinc	X		X	X	X	X	X		X						X		
TSH	X								X						X	X	X
INR	X					X					X	X					
Cytokine analyses	X		xx			xx	xx		xx		xx		xx		X	X	X
NK-cells			X						X								
Examinations:																	
Weight	X	X	X	X	X	X	X	X	X		X	X	X		X	X	X
DXA scan	X						X						X			X	X
Physical test	X						X						X			X	X
Muscle biopsy	X						X						X				X
Questionnaires:																	
Training diary		X	X	X	X	X	X	X	X	X	X	X	X	X			
Diet diary		X	X	X	X	X	X	X	X						X	X	X
Quality of life	X														X	X	X
Physical activity	X														X	X	X
Questionnaire about contentment with the program														X			
Affiliation to work market															X	X	X

X marks when an examination is planned. XX marks at which time points blood samples are drawn both before and after a training session in the training group. Regarding week 13/14: Due to public holidays training can extend beyond 12 weeks, training continues until 36 sessions have been offered. Blood samples are drawn, weight registered and other examinations are performed after the 36 sessions. Abbreviations: ALT, alanine aminotransferase. ALP, alkaline phosphatase. e-GFR, estimated glomerular filtration rate. LDH, lactate dehydrogenase. HS-CRP, high-sensitive c-reactive protein. TSH, thyroid stimulating hormone. INR, international normalized ratio. DXA, dual-energy X-ray absorptiometry. Approx., approximately

the hospital, making it as convenient as possible for the patients.

Maximal muscle strength

All physical tests are conducted by the physiotherapist or the training instructors. Muscle strength will be evaluated by 1RM test of unilateral leg press (dominant leg) and bi-lateral chest press performed in the conventional equipment used in training. One RM tests are widely used when evaluating changes in maximal muscle strength in cancer patients [34, 35]. Following an exercise specific warm up, the patient will have one attempt with a given load, which will gradually be increased until the patient is unable to lift the load throughout a standardized range of motion using proper technique. As few attempts as possible will be used and a two-minute rest is ensured between all attempts to limit the risk of muscular fatigue.

Functional performance

Functional performance resembling activities of daily living will be evaluated using the 30 s chair stand test, 30 s arm curl test, and maximal stair climbing performance, best of two attempts. These are frequently used in cancer patients, including patients with HNSCC [20].

Treatment side-effects

Adverse events will be monitored according to Common Terminology Criteria for Adverse Events (CTCAE) version 4.0 [36], performance status will be registered according to ECOG scale, and pain using the Numeric Rating Scale (NRS) for pain, consisting of 11 points from 0 (no pain) to 10 (worst pain imaginable) [37].

Cytokine analyses, standard blood samples, and NK-cells

Standard blood samples will be taken according to schedule (Table 3). Blood samples for cytokine analyses will be taken before and after training sessions according to schedule (Table 3). Based on comprehensive explorative analyses with samples from a primary cohort of patients (Lonkvist et al., manuscript submitted), we have identified a list of particularly interesting cytokines and other molecules for further analyses, including 6Ckine/chemokine (C-C motif) ligand 21 (CCL21), cutaneous T cell-attracting chemokine (CTACK)/CCL27, interleukin 6 (IL-6), IL-8/CXCL8, IL-15, IL-16, monocyte chemoattractant protein 1 (MCP-1)/CCL2, MCP-2/CCL8, macrophage-derived chemokine (MDC)/CCL22, macrophage migration inhibitory factor (MIF), macrophage inflammatory protein-1α (MIP-1α)//CCL3, thymus-expressed chemokine (TECK)/CCL25, tumor necrosis factor α (TNF-α), soluble epidermal growth factor receptor (sEGFR), basic fibroblast growth factor (FGF-basic), follistatin, hepatocyte growth factor (HGF), leptin, platelet-derived growth factor AB/BB (PDGF-AB/BB), prolactin, stem cell factor (SCF), soluble vascular endothelial growth factor-1 (sVEGFR-1), and sVEGFR-2. In initial analyses some of these cytokines increased during CCRT whilst others decreased, and the interesting point would be to investigate if PRT may affect these changes in either direction. Furthermore, the mobilization of NK-cells during PRT will be evaluated in week 3 and 12. The frequency and cytotoxic profile of the NK-cells will be analyzed by flow cytometry by staining for the surface receptors CD3, CD16 and CD56, as well as intracellular expression of Granzyme B and Ki-67.

Muscle biopsies

Muscle biopsies are optional for patients, but if accepted, they will be collected under sterile conditions from the middle lateral part of the vastus lateralis muscle using a 5 mm Bergstrom biopsy cannula preceded by local anesthesia (lidocaine 10 mg/ml). Both satisfactory thrombocyte count ($\geq 40 \times 10^9$/L) and International Standard Ratio (≤ 1.5) will be confirmed. Biopsies are taken from the mid-thigh of the same leg but a few centimeters from the previous biopsy at each time point to avoid variation between legs in the analyses. The samples will be dissected to be free of visible fat and connective tissue. A well-aligned portion of the biopsy for muscle fiber morphology analyses will immediately mounted in Tissue-Tek (Qiagen, Valencia, CA) and frozen in isopentane precooled in liquid nitrogen. The rest of the biopsy for later proteomics analyses will be frozen directly in liquid nitrogen. All samples will be stored at −80 °C until analysis.

The muscle biopsies are planned to be used for investigating differences in changes in muscle fiber types, protein expression, and metabolic pathways between the two groups.

Questionnaires
Physical activity

To register PA in addition to the supervised training of the PRT group as well as all PA in the control group, patients will fill in a weekly trial specific questionnaire on PA. Thus, type of activity (running, resistance training, walking etc.) and the daily duration of the activity will be registered every week from baseline to the end of the training period. Also, patients will fill in a physical activity scale (PAS) questionnaire for measuring average weekly PA of sleep, work, and leisure time [38].

Energy intake

Patients will receive dietary counseling by clinical dietician before or immediately after start of treatment as well as by educated nurses during the treatment period. If patients are admitted due to nutritional issues during the treatment period, they will be seen by a clinical dietician. Resting metabolic rate (RMR) will be estimated using the Mifflin-St. Jeor formula described elsewhere [39]. Energy expenditure (kilojoules per day) is measured as: Energy need (kJ) = RMR x activity factor × 4.184. Activity factor will be based on self-reported PA at the different time points. Protein need will be estimated as 18% of total energy need: Protein need (gram) = (total energy need (kJ) × 18)/17. A clinical dietician will calculate total daily energy intake based on patient reported information from a questionnaire filled in weekly during treatment (Table 3). The number of patients needing tube feeding and the duration of the tube feeding will also be registered.

Quality of Life (QoL)

Changes in QoL will be evaluated using the European Organisation for Research and Treatment of Cancer (EORTC) quality of life questionnaires, QLQ-C30 and QLQ-H&N-35, which have previously been used in exercise studies in cancer survivors [40] and in Danish HNSCC patients [41].

Satisfaction with the program

A semi-structured questionnaire was developed asking patients to grade the effect the program have had on their physical, psychological, and social well-being on a scale from 1 to 10, 1 being "very positively"; 10 being "very negatively". Furthermore, patients are asked if scheduling was convenient and whether the PRT program was appropriate, too hard or too light (training group only). In addition, they can make free text on all questions.

Work

Affiliation to work market will be registered as a measure of convalescence, measuring how soon patients return to work and to what extent. At 2, 6, and 12 months follow-up patients fill in a questionnaire with information about current work status, date when work was resumed, and at 2 months follow-up, also, educational status, occupation, and work hours prior to diagnosis will be registered.

Blinding procedures

Assessment of the primary endpoint (LBM) will be blinded since the personnel performing DXA scans will not be aware of randomization status of the patients. Due to practicalities physical tests cannot be blinded. However, tests are standardized and performed by the same personnel regardless of randomization. Personnel analyzing blood samples and muscle biopsies are blinded to patient identity and group allocation.

Statistical considerations

The primary endpoint is difference in mean change of LBM between the training and the control group, specifically, whether attending this particular PRT program can significantly attenuate the loss of LBM after 12 weeks of PRT, which approximately aligns with the time where the treatment is evaluated (2 months after end of radiotherapy). Thus, the time at which the primary endpoint is evaluated is at 12 weeks after initiation of PRT.

The second important decision was to define a clinically meaningful endpoint in terms of difference in change in LBM loss. Of course, the 12 week period in which it was possible to train was included as a parameter since the short training period would influence the possible outcome, and even more so as patients were expected to lose LBM as a result of side effects to treatment. Limited clinical data were available on the possible effect of a 12-week PRT program on LBM change during concomitant chemoradiotherapy, though Lonbro et al. did find that head and neck cancer patients attending a 12-week PRT program initiated after radiotherapy gained an average of 2.3 kg (95% CI 1.7–3.0) [20]. A similar effect can probably not be expected when PRT is performed during chemoradiotherapy as the patients during this time are in a catabolic state. This was seen in our pilot study where patients despite PRT had a mean LBM loss of 3.6 kg (Lonkvist et al., manuscript submitted).

Based on these deliberations we concluded that a difference of 25% in LBM loss between the exercise group and the control group (which, estimated from data in the pilot study, would be 1.2 kg of LBM in absolute difference) would be a clinically meaningful difference, and yet, an obtainable goal in the circumstance of undergoing CCRT.

Thus, the sample size calculation is based on changes in LBM in our one-armed pilot study where a 3.6 kg reduction (corresponding to 6.8%) in LBM was detected after 12 weeks of PRT (Lonkvist et al., manuscript submitted). A priori, a sample size of 34 in each group will have 80% power to detect a difference in means of 25%

((9.06%–6.8%)/9.06%) between the two groups (corresponding to an estimated mean LBM loss of 6.80% from baseline in the training group and an estimated LBM loss of 9.06% in the control group with a standard deviation of 3.27). A two group t-test with a 0.05 two-sided significance level was used.

An anticipated drop-out rate of 5% is included in the calculations to ameliorate the risk of inadequate patient number for analyses, hence 36 patients are planned to be enrolled in each group (total $n = 72$). Patients dropping out before or during the first week of treatment will be replaced by another patient.

Analyses will include descriptive analyses as well as mixed model repeated measures analyses examining differences between groups and over time. The α-level of statistical significance will be set to 0.05.

Discussion

An increasing body of evidence underlines the numerous benefits of physical exercise in terms of improving patient wellbeing and rehabilitation after cancer therapy, and very interestingly a tumor-inhibiting effect of exercise is being unraveled [27, 42–47].

In particular head and neck cancer patients experience perturbing loss of lean body mass and are severely affected by treatment for weeks and months after completion [1, 48]. Thus, there is ample reason to investigate a possible beneficial role of exercise during head and neck cancer treatment but at the same time exercise studies require careful attention to a number of issues. In particular, when investigating exercise in patients undergoing CCRT a number of specific challenges must be addressed. We designed a randomized trial on exercise for head and neck cancer patients undergoing concomitant CCRT and decided to describe the strategy in this article about the protocol.

The choice of primary endpoint, as well as the assessment hereof, should be cautiously chosen. We chose difference in change in LBM at the 12-week assessment, as it has been shown that weight loss, especially loss of LBM, may negatively affect physical function, morbidity and mortality in patients undergoing CCRT [5, 7]. Thus, it would be interesting to investigate if PRT may ameliorate LBM loss, and 12 weeks are often considered a minimum amount of time for an effect on LBM by PRT. Furthermore, a standard evaluation time point in head and neck cancer patients is at this time as it almost coincides with the 2-month post CCRT assessment. At this time evaluation of the effect of treatment is performed and side-effects have often diminished substantially.

The chosen assessment method is conventional DXA scan based on several factors: Compared to other methods it is a low risk, precise measurement of whole body composition [49–52] where data may be retrieved and reevaluated at a later time point, if needed. Furthermore, it is fast and relatively inexpensive.

In this study we are only including patients receiving an intense treatment with concomitant chemoradiotherapy. The patients have the most intense treatment schedule, hence, if it possible for them to attend and benefit from the program, there is no reason to assume that the findings may not be relevant for head and neck cancer patients receiving other radiotherapy regimens.

Prescribing exercise in a training intervention study could be thought of as prescribing medicine, where it is indisputable that specifications such as type, dose, interval, and duration of treatment are essential information in reporting. In this trial, PRT is the obvious choice of training modality, with the primary endpoint being change in LBM. Exercise intensity, volume and frequency are chosen to ensure optimal progression throughout the program and are based on previous studies in HNSCC patients [20, 21] as well as guidelines from the American College of Sports Medicine (ACSM) [33]. Training days and number of sessions per week are chosen to ensure adequate rest between sessions for optimal hypertrophy response in the muscles. Likewise, patients are instructed to exercise to exhaustion for maximal hypertrophic response. In general, all training sessions are supervised by physiotherapists or educated training instructors. However, for practical reasons, an exception is allowed, i.e. it will be possible for the last 6 weeks to train at a public center closer to home, and only attend supervised training once a week to ensure progression. Unsupervised training holds the advantage of flexibility for both patient and caregiver team, while on the other hand, supervised sessions are a necessity to ensure that prescribed dose is executed and reported correctly.

To ensure faster enrollment the study is conducted at two institutions which can compromise standardization of the PRT program. Three specific exercises differ, but cautions are taken so that it should not influence primary outcome notably.

An essential aspect to consider is the fact that these patients have a very busy schedule in regards to treatment. Radiotherapy six times a week, combined with chemotherapy treatment once a week, as well as appointments with doctors and nurses make planning a challenge. Treatment delays are deleterious to outcome [53], thus, planning training sessions, tests, and scans conveniently so they do not interfere with treatment is crucial. Furthermore, seeing to that patients do not have too strenuous days and that meals are offered are also significant factors for attendance and thus effect of the intervention. The patients often suffer from side effects, e.g. fatigue, nausea, and xerostomia, which are likely to be limiting factors in any intention to exercise. Hence, optimizing schedule is crucial for several reasons and should be carefully managed.

Sufficient protein and energy supply is vital for muscle growth or preservation. Hence, reporting on the effect of any training modality in HNSCC patients must include reporting of dietary intake, too. In this study customized diet diaries are completed regularly by patients. These diaries also form a basis for starting a conversation about diet and advised strategy for the patient, e.g. about tube feeding when necessary.

Anemia during radiotherapy is associated with response to treatment [54–56] which is an important factor to consider when planning blood sampling. Patients receive weekly cisplatin, hence blood sampling is done weekly, evaluating hematology. If hemoglobin is low blood sampling for research purposes will be paused. Furthermore, blood sampling for cytokine analyses are planned so that only a maximum of 42 mL of extra blood is drawn during the entire treatment period, while more frequent sampling is done in the approximately 6 weeks after treatment.

Blood samples will be used for explorative analyses of the differences between the groups in regards to cytokines and cancer markers over time. Furthermore, the PRT group will have samples taken before and after training sessions to investigate whether a bout of resistance training will release myokines and NK-cells as it is known from endurance exercise [27, 57, 58]. Doing this is important to contribute to the investigation of the biological mechanisms behind a possible effect. Muscle biopsies are optional in order for it not to be a limiting factor for patient recruitment. When performing samples on a part of patients, bias can be a concern, however, in our pilot study 2/3 of patients accepted muscle biopsies (Lonkvist et al., manuscript submitted).

It is planned to investigate the effect of resistance training on changes in muscle fiber types, protein expression, and metabolic pathways between the two groups.

Several patient-reported outcome measures are also evaluated in this study, including QoL and PA. Exercise has been shown to increase QoL in cancer patients [59, 60], and exercise studies in HNSCC patients confirm the positive effect [61–64]. Still, it is relevant to include QoL measures in new intervention studies, if the type of intervention or program differs from prior programs. EORTC QLQ-30 and H&N-35 questionnaires have been chosen to evaluate QoL, these questionnaires are validated and often used in cancer research [2, 59]. PA is evaluated using the validated PAS questionnaire [38] to assess level of PA in both groups since an apparent bias is that patients in the control group might start to exercise regularly, thereby affecting the between group differences.

To evaluate patients' satisfaction with the program, we developed a semi-structured questionnaire asking patients about the effect of the program on their physical, psychological, and social well-being. We have added this to set a direct reaction on what patients felt about the program.

An inherent bias in all exercise trials is that patients who have less comorbidity and are in better performance status may be more inclined to accept participation. In our pilot study all patients had p16-positive (HPV-associated) tumors (Lonkvist et al., manuscript submitted). Patients with p16-positive tumors have been shown to have larger disease stages, averagely less tobacco and alcohol consumption, fewer comorbidities, and be in better performance status [65]. Further studies will be needed to look at the effects of exercise programs in patients with poor performance status, comorbidities, or with a history of tobacco or alcohol consumption.

Designing and performing exercise trials in cancer patients requires careful consideration to optimal modality, dose, duration, and many other parameters depending on desired outcome measures. Also, and at least as important, is a detailed description in order to ensure clarity and reproducibility. Finally, interpretation of biological sampling for mechanistic investigations must be recommended and these samples, in connection with the clinical data, may help to generate important knowledge. With this study, we hope to contribute with influential results regarding progressive resistance training in head and neck cancer patients undergoing concomitant chemoradiotherapy.

Additional files

Additional file 1: SPIRIT checklist. The SPIRIT checklist.

Additional file 2: Appendix A for SPIRIT checklist. Appendix A for SPIRIT checklist.

Additional file 3: Appendix B for SPIRIT checklist. WHO Trial Registration Data Set.

Additional file 4: Table S1. Antiemetic regimens. Antiemetics are given according to institutional guidelines. At Herlev site the regimen changed May 23rd 2016 due to standardization in the Capital Region. Day 1 is the day cisplatin is given. In addition, Domperidon 20–30 mg PRN is administered P.O. a maximum of thrice daily. Abbreviations: p.o., per os. PRN, pro re nata (when necessary).

Additional file 5: Figure S1. Illustrations of the exercises. Illustrations of the exercises.

Abbreviations
ALP: Alkaline Phosphatase; ALT: Alanine Aminotransferase; BMI: Body Mass Index; CCRT: Concomitant Chemoradiotherapy; DAHANCA: Danish Head and Neck Cancer; DXA: Dual-energy X-ray Absorptiometry; e-GFR: Estimated Glomerular Filtration Rate; EORTC: European Organisation for Research and Treatment of Cancer; FM: Fat Mass; HNSCC: Head and Neck Squamous Cell Carcinoma; HPV: Human Papillomavirus; HS-CRP: High-Sensitive C-Reactive Protein; INR: International Normalized Ratio; KJ: Kilojoules; LBM: Lean Body Mass; LDH: Lactate Dehydrogenase; P.O.: Perorally; PA: Physical Activity; PAS: Physical Activity Scale; PRN: Pro Re Nata (when necessary); PROM: Patient Reported Outcome Measure; PRT: Progressive Resistance Training; QLQ: Quality of Life Questionnaire; QoL: Quality of Life; RM: Repetition Maximum; RMR: Resting Metabolic Rate; TBM: Total Body Mass; TSH: Thyroid Stimulating Hormone

Acknowledgements
Not applicable.

Funding
The study is investigator initiated and sponsored study. The investigators are solely responsible for the study and reporting hereof. The study is supported by grants from The Danish Cancer Society (R90-A5865–14-S2, awarded after a peer-review process), and TrygFonden. The funding parties have had no influence on study design and will have no influence on data collection, analysis, or interpretation.

Authors' contributions
Study concept was conceived by JG, PH, and CKL and design devised by CKL, SL, AV, BZ, ER, HP, PH, and JG. CKL was primary author of the protocol but all authors contributed to some parts. CKL, SL, PH, and JG wrote the manuscript; all authors read and approved the final manuscript.

Authors' information
No additional information about the authors' is relevant for this article.

Competing interests
The authors declare that they have no competing interests.

Study status
The study is ongoing, patients are currently being enrolled.

Author details
[1]Department of Oncology, Herlev and Gentofte Hospital, University of Copenhagen, Herlev, Denmark. [2]Department of Experimental Clinical Oncology, Aarhus University Hospital, Aarhus, Denmark. [3]Department of Public Health, Section for Sports Science, Aarhus University, Aarhus, Denmark. [4]Department of Rehabilitation, Herlev and Gentofte Hospital, University of Copenhagen, Herlev, Denmark. [5]Department of Clinical Physiology and Nuclear Medicine, Herlev and Gentofte Hospital, University of Copenhagen, Herlev, Denmark. [6]Nutritional Research Unit, Herlev and Gentofte Hospital, University of Copenhagen, Herlev, Denmark. [7]Department of Oncology, Aarhus University Hospital, Aarhus, Denmark. [8]Centre of Inflammation and Metabolism (CIM) and Centre for Physical Activity Research (CFAS), Department of Infectious Diseases, Rigshospitalet, University of Copenhagen, Copenhagen, Denmark.

References
1. Jackson W, Alexander N, Schipper M, Fig L, Feng F, Jolly S. Characterization of changes in total body composition for patients with head and neck cancer undergoing chemoradiotherapy using dual-energy x-ray absorptiometry. Head Neck. 2014;36(9):1356–62.
2. Langius JE, Van Dijk AM, Doornaert P, Kruizenga HM, Langendijk JA, Leemans CR, et al. More than 10% weight loss in head and neck cancer patients during radiotherapy is independently associated with deterioration in quality of life. Nutr Cancer. 2013;65(1):76–83.
3. Lonbro S, Dalgas U, Primdahl H, Johansen J, Nielsen JL, Overgaard J, et al. Lean body mass and muscle function in head and neck cancer patients and healthy individuals–results from the DAHANCA 25 study. Acta Oncol. 2013; 52(7):1543–51.
4. Platek ME, Myrick E, Mccloskey SA, Gupta V, Reid ME, Wilding GE, et al. Pretreatment weight status and weight loss among head and neck cancer patients receiving definitive concurrent chemoradiation therapy: implications for nutrition integrated treatment pathways. Support Care Cancer. 2013;21(10):2825–33.
5. Capuano G, Grosso A, Gentile PC, Battista M, Bianciardi F, Di Palma A, et al. Influence of weight loss on outcomes in patients with head and neck cancer undergoing concomitant chemoradiotherapy. Head Neck. 2008;30(4):503–8.
6. Wang C, Vainshtein JM, Veksler M, Rabban PE, Sullivan JA, Wang SC, et al. Investigating the clinical significance of body composition changes in patients undergoing chemoradiation for oropharyngeal cancer using analytic morphomics. Spring. 2016;5:429.

7. Grossberg AJ, Chamchod S, Fuller CD, Mohamed AS, Heukelom J, Eichelberger H, et al. Association of Body Composition with Survival and Locoregional Control of radiotherapy-treated head and neck Squamous cell carcinoma. JAMA Oncol. 2016;2(6):782–9.

8. Al-Majid S, Waters H. The biological mechanisms of cancer-related skeletal muscle wasting: the role of progressive resistance exercise. Biol Res Nurs. 2008;10(1):7–20.

9. Der-Torossian H, Couch ME, Dittus K, Toth MJ. Skeletal muscle adaptations to cancer and its treatment: their fundamental basis and contribution to functional disability. Crit rev Eukaryot Gene Expr. 2013;23(4):283–97.

10. Chen JA, Splenser A, Guillory B, Luo J, Mendiratta M, Belinova B, et al. Ghrelin prevents tumour- and cisplatin-induced muscle wasting: characterization of multiple mechanisms involved. J Cachexia Sarcopenia Muscle. 2015;6(2):132–43.

11. Sakai H, Sagara A, Arakawa K, Sugiyama R, Hirosaki A, Takase K, et al. Mechanisms of cisplatin-induced muscle atrophy. Toxicol Appl Pharmacol. 2014;278(2):190–9.

12. Lofberg E, Gutierrez A, Wernerman J, Anderstam B, Mitch WE, Price SR, et al. Effects of high doses of glucocorticoids on free amino acids, ribosomes and protein turnover in human muscle. Eur J Clin Investig. 2002;32(5):345–53.

13. Schakman O, Kalista S, Barbe C, Loumaye A, Thissen JP. Glucocorticoid-induced skeletal muscle atrophy. Int J Biochem Cell Biol. 2013;45(10):2163–72.

14. Jager-Wittenaar H, Dijkstra PU, Vissink A, Langendijk JA, Der Laan BFaM V, Pruim J, et al. Changes in nutritional status and dietary intake during and after head and neck cancer treatment. Head Neck. 2011;33(6):863–70.

15. Van Den Berg MG, Rasmussen-Conrad EL, Gwasara GM, Krabbe PF, Naber AH, Merkx MA. A prospective study on weight loss and energy intake in patients with head and neck cancer, during diagnosis, treatment and revalidation. Clin Nutr. 2006;25(5):765–72.

16. Deutz NE, Bauer JM, Barazzoni R, Biolo G, Boirie Y, Bosy-Westphal A, et al. Protein intake and exercise for optimal muscle function with aging: recommendations from the ESPEN expert group. Clin Nutr. 2014;33(6): 929–36.

17. Hojman P, Fjelbye J, Zerahn B, Christensen JF, Dethlefsen C, Lonkvist CK, et al. Voluntary exercise prevents cisplatin-induced muscle wasting during chemotherapy in mice. PLoS One. 2014;9(9):e109030.

18. Stene GB, Helbostad JL, Balstad TR, Riphagen II, Kaasa S, Oldervoll LM. Effect of physical exercise on muscle mass and strength in cancer patients during treatment–a systematic review. Crit rev Oncol Hematol. 2013;88(3):573–93.

19. Borst SE. Interventions for sarcopenia and muscle weakness in older people. Age Ageing. 2004;33(6):548–55.

20. Lonbro S, Dalgas U, Primdahl H, Johansen J, Nielsen JL, Aagaard P, et al. Progressive resistance training rebuilds lean body mass in head and neck cancer patients after radiotherapy–results from the randomized DAHANCA 25B trial. Radiother Oncol. 2013;108(2):314–9.

21. Lonbro S, Dalgas U, Primdahl H, Overgaard J, Overgaard K. Feasibility and efficacy of progressive resistance training and dietary supplements in radiotherapy treated head and neck cancer patients–the DAHANCA 25A study. Acta Oncol. 2013;52(2):310–8.

22. Murphy EA, Davis JM, Barrilleaux TL, Mcclellan JL, Steiner JL, Carmichael MD, et al. Benefits of exercise training on breast cancer progression and inflammation in C3(1)SV40Tag mice. Cytokine. 2011;55(2):274–9.

23. Abdalla DR, Aleixo AA, Murta EF, Michelin MA. Innate immune response adaptation in mice subjected to administration of DMBA and physical activity. Oncol Lett. 2014;7(3):886–90.

24. Esser KA, Harpole CE, Prins GS, Diamond AM. Physical activity reduces prostate carcinogenesis in a transgenic model. Prostate. 2009;69(13):1372–7.

25. Aoi W, Naito Y, Takagi T, Tanimura Y, Takanami Y, Kawai Y, et al. A novel myokine, secreted protein acidic and rich in cysteine (SPARC), suppresses colon tumorigenesis via regular exercise. Gut. 2013;62(6):882–9.

26. Rundqvist H, Augsten M, Stromberg A, Rullman E, Mijwel S, Kharaziha P, et al. Effect of acute exercise on prostate cancer cell growth. PLoS One. 2013; 8(7):e67579.

27. Pedersen L, Idorn M, Olofsson GH, Lauenborg B, Nookaew I, Hansen RH, et al. Voluntary running suppresses tumor growth through epinephrine- and IL-6-dependent NK cell mobilization and redistribution. Cell Metab. 2016;23(3):554–62.

28. Pedersen L, Christensen JF, Hojman P. Effects of exercise on tumor physiology and metabolism. Cancer J. 2015;21(2):111–6.

29. Idorn M, Hojman P. Exercise-dependent regulation of NK cells in cancer protection. Trends Mol med. 2016;22(7):565 77.

30. Jones LW. Precision oncology framework for investigation of exercise as treatment for cancer. J Clin Oncol. 2015;33(35):4134–7.

31. Sobin LHG, Gospodarowicz MK, Wittekind C. TNM classification of malignant tumours, Seventh edition edn. Chichester: Wiley-Blackwell; 2009.

32. Overgaard J, Hansen HS, Overgaard M, Bastholt L, Berthelsen A, Specht L, et al. A randomized double-blind phase III study of nimorazole as a hypoxic radiosensitizer of primary radiotherapy in supraglottic larynx and pharynx carcinoma. Results of the Danish head and neck cancer study (DAHANCA) protocol 5-85. Radiother Oncol. 1998;46(2):135–46.

33. American College of Sports Medicine position stand. Progression models in resistance training for healthy adults. Med Sci Sports Exerc. 2009;41(3):687–708.

34. Adamsen L, Quist M, Andersen C, Moller T, Herrstedt J, Kronborg D, et al. Effect of a multimodal high intensity exercise intervention in cancer patients undergoing chemotherapy: randomised controlled trial. BMJ. 2009;339:b3410.

35. Galvão DA, Nosaka K, Taaffe DR, Spry N, Kristjanson LJ, Mcguigan MR, et al. Resistance training and reduction of treatment side effects in prostate cancer patients. Med Sci Sports Exerc. 2006;38(12):2045–52.

36. National Cancer Institute. Common Terminology Criteria for Adverse Events v4.0 http://ctep.cancer.gov/protocolDevelopment/electronic_applications/ ctc.htm.

37. Hawker GA, Mian S, Kendzerska T, French M. Measures of adult pain: visual analog scale for pain (VAS pain), numeric rating scale for pain (NRS pain), McGill pain questionnaire (MPQ), short-form McGill pain questionnaire (SF-MPQ), chronic pain grade scale (CPGS), short form-36 bodily pain scale (SF-36 BPS), and measure of intermittent and constant osteoarthritis pain (ICOAP). Arthritis Care res (Hoboken). 2011;63(Suppl 11):S240–52.

38. Andersen LG, Groenvold M, Jorgensen T, Aadahl M. Construct validity of a revised physical activity scale and testing by cognitive interviewing. Scand J Public Health. 2010;38(7):707–14.

39. Frankenfield D, Roth-Yousey L, Compher C. Comparison of predictive equations for resting metabolic rate in healthy nonobese and obese adults: a systematic review. J am Diet Assoc. 2005;105(5):775–89.

40. Ferrari P, Friedenreich C, Matthews CE. The role of measurement error in estimating levels of physical activity. Am J Epidemiol. 2007;166(7):832–40.

41. Jensen K, Jensen AB, Grau C. A cross sectional quality of life study of 116 recurrence free head and neck cancer patients. The first use of EORTC H&N35 in Danish. Acta Oncol. 2006;45(1):28–37.

42. Fong DYT, Ho JWC, Hui BPH, Lee AM, Macfarlane DJ, Leung SSK, et al. Physical activity for cancer survivors: meta-analysis of randomised controlled trials. Bmj. 2012;344:e70.

43. Speck RM, Courneya KS, Masse LC, Duval S, Schmitz KH. An update of controlled physical activity trials in cancer survivors: a systematic review and meta-analysis. J Cancer Surviv. 2010;4(2):87–100.

44. Bouillet T, Bigard X, Brami C, Chouahnia K, Copel L, Dauchy S, et al. Role of physical activity and sport in oncology: scientific commission of the National Federation Sport and cancer CAMI. Crit Rev Oncol Hematol. 2015;94(1):74–86.

45. Brown JC, Winters-Stone K, Lee A, Schmitz KH. Cancer, physical activity, and exercise. Compr Physiol. 2012;2(4):2775–809.

46. Ibrahim EM, Al-Homaidh A. Physical activity and survival after breast cancer diagnosis: meta-analysis of published studies. Med Oncol. 2011;28(3):753–65.

47. Je Y, Jeon JY, Giovannucci EL, Meyerhardt JA. Association between physical activity and mortality in colorectal cancer: a meta-analysis of prospective cohort studies. Int J Cancer. 2013;133(8):1905–13.

48. Ottosson S, Zackrisson B, Kjellén E, Nilsson P, Laurell G. Weight loss in patients with head and neck cancer during and after conventional and accelerated radiotherapy. Acta Oncol. 2013;52(4):711–8.

49. Brodie DA, Stewart AD. Body composition measurement: a hierarchy of methods. J Pediatr Endocrinol Metab. 1999;12(6):801–16.

50. Jebb SA, Elia M. Techniques for the measurement of body composition: a practical guide. Int J Obes Relat Metab Disord. 1993;17(11):611–21.

51. Lee SY, Gallagher D. Assessment methods in human body composition. Curr Opin Clin Nutr Metab Care. 2008;11(5):566–72.

52. Visser M, Fuerst T, Lang T, Salamone L, Harris TB. Validity of fan-beam dual-energy X-ray absorptiometry for measuring fat-free mass and leg muscle mass. Health, aging, and body composition study–dual-energy X-ray Absorptiometry and body composition working group. J Appl Physiol (1985) 1999, 87(4):1513-1520.

53. Gonzalez Ferreira JA, Jaen Olasolo J, Azinovic I, Jeremic B. Effect of radiotherapy delay in overall treatment time on local control and survival in

head and neck cancer: review of the literature. Rep Pract Oncol Radiother. 2015;20(5):328–39.

54. Lee WR, Berkey B, Marcial V, Fu KK, Cooper JS, Vikram B, et al. Anemia is associated with decreased survival and increased locoregional failure in patients with locally advanced head and neck carcinoma: a secondary analysis of RTOG 85-27. Int J Radiat Oncol Biol Phys. 1998;42(5):1069–75.

55. Fortin A, Wang CS, Vigneault E. Effect of pretreatment anemia on treatment outcome of concurrent radiochemotherapy in patients with head and neck cancer. Int J Radiat Oncol Biol Phys. 2008;72(1):255–60.

56. Overgaard J, Hansen HS, Jorgensen K, Hjelm Hansen M. Primary radiotherapy of larynx and pharynx carcinoma–an analysis of some factors influencing local control and survival. Int J Radiat Oncol Biol Phys. 1986; 12(4):515–21.

57. Hojman P, Dethlefsen C, Brandt C, Hansen J, Pedersen L, Pedersen BK. Exercise-induced muscle-derived cytokines inhibit mammary cancer cell growth. Am J Physiol Endocrinol Metab. 2011;301(3):E504–E10.

58. Pedersen BK. Muscles and their myokines. J exp Biol. 2011;214(Pt 2):337–46.

59. Gerritsen JK, Vincent AJ. Exercise improves quality of life in patients with cancer: a systematic review and meta-analysis of randomised controlled trials. Br J Sports med. 2016;50(13):796–803.

60. Mishra SI, Scherer RW, Snyder C, Geigle PM, Berlanstein DR, Topaloglu O. Exercise interventions on health-related quality of life for people with cancer during active treatment. Cochrane Database Syst rev. 2012;8: CD008465.

61. Capozzi LC, Mcneely ML, Lau HY, Reimer RA, Giese-Davis J, Fung TS, et al. Patient-reported outcomes, body composition, and nutrition status in patients with head and neck cancer: results from an exploratory randomized controlled exercise trial. Cancer. 2016;122(8):1185–200.

62. Rogers LQ, Anton PM, Fogleman A, Hopkins-Price P, Verhulst S, Rao K, et al. Pilot, randomized trial of resistance exercise during radiation therapy for head and neck cancer. Head Neck. 2013;35(8):1178–88.

63. Samuel SR, Maiya GA, Babu AS, Vidyasagar MS. Effect of exercise training on functional capacity & quality of life in head & neck cancer patients receiving chemoradiotherapy. Indian J med res. 2013;137(3):515–20.

64. Zhao SG, Alexander NB, Djuric Z, Zhou J, Tao Y, Schipper M, et al. Maintaining physical activity during head and neck cancer treatment: results of a pilot controlled trial. Head Neck. 2016;38(Suppl 1):E1086–96.

65. Deschler DG, Richmon JD, Khariwala SS, Ferris RL, Wang MB. The "new" head and neck cancer patient-young, nonsmoker, nondrinker, and HPV positive: evaluation. Otolaryngol Head Neck Surg. 2014;151(3):375–80.

14

HSP90 inhibition sensitizes head and neck cancer to platin-based chemoradiotherapy by modulation of the DNA damage response resulting in chromosomal fragmentation

Martin McLaughlin[1]*, Holly E. Barker[1], Aadil A. Khan[1], Malin Pedersen[1], Magnus Dillon[1], David C. Mansfield[1], Radhika Patel[1], Joan N. Kyula[1], Shreerang A. Bhide[2,3], Kate L. Newbold[2,3], Christopher M. Nutting[2,3] and Kevin J. Harrington[1,2,3]

Abstract

Background: Concurrent cisplatin radiotherapy (CCRT) is a current standard-of-care for locally advanced head and neck squamous cell carcinoma (HNSCC). However, CCRT is frequently ineffective in patients with advanced disease. It has previously been shown that HSP90 inhibitors act as radiosensitizers, but these studies have not focused on CCRT in HNSCC. Here, we evaluated the HSP90 inhibitor, AUY922, combined with CCRT.

Methods: The ability of AUY922 to sensitize to CCRT was assessed in p53 mutant head and neck cell lines by clonogenic assay. Modulation of the CCRT induced DNA damage response (DDR) by AUY922 was characterized by confocal image analysis of RAD51, BRCA1, 53BP1, ATM and mutant p53 signaling. The role of FANCA depletion by AUY922 was examined using shRNA. Cell cycle checkpoint abrogation and chromosomal fragmentation was assessed by western blot, FACS and confocal. The role of ATM was also assessed by shRNA. AUY922 in combination with CCRT was assessed in vivo.

Results: The combination of AUY922 with cisplatin, radiation and CCRT was found to be synergistic in p53 mutant HNSCC. AUY922 leads to significant alterations to the DDR induced by CCRT. This comprises inhibition of homologous recombination through decreased RAD51 and pS1524 BRCA1 with a corresponding increase in 53BP1 foci, activation of ATM and signaling into mutant p53. A shift to more error prone repair combined with a loss of checkpoint function leads to fragmentation of chromosomal material. The degree of disruption to DDR signalling correlated to chromosomal fragmentation and loss of clonogenicity. ATM shRNA indicated a possible rationale for the combination of AUY922 and CCRT in cells lacking ATM function.

Conclusions: This study supports future clinical studies combining AUY922 and CCRT in p53 mutant HNSCC. Modulation of the DDR and chromosomal fragmentation are likely to be analytical points of interest in such trials.

Keywords: RAD51, FANCA, ATM, AUY922, HNSCC, DDR

* Correspondence: martin.mclaughlin@icr.ac.uk
[1]Targeted Therapy Team, The Institute of Cancer Research, Chester Beatty Laboratories, 237 Fulham Road, London SW3 6JB, UK
Full list of author information is available at the end of the article

Background

Concurrent cisplatin radiotherapy (CCRT) is a standard-of-care for patients with locally advanced head and neck squamous cell carcinoma (HNSCC). Despite improving outcomes with CCRT, patients with locally-advanced HNSCC have a poor prognosis. Novel tumor-selective therapies are urgently needed, with efficacy in conjunction with existing CCRT being the most likely route to clinical development [1, 2].

HSP90 is a molecular chaperone involved in the initial folding and continued conformational maintenance of a pool of client proteins. Many of these have been identified as oncoproteins or key components in repair and cell cycle arrest following exposure to DNA damaging agents [3–5]. HSP90 inhibitors mediate sensitization through multifaceted effects and radiosensitize a broad range of genetically diverse tumor types [6–12].

HSP90 inhibition has been shown to have a significant direct impact on cell cycle and DNA repair mechanisms. HSP90 client proteins include cell cycle regulators such as CHK1, WEE1, CDK1 and CDK4 [13, 14], as well as DNA repair proteins such as ATR, FANCA, RAD51 and BRCA2 [4, 15–17]. HSP90 inhibition does not alter Ku70, Ku80 or DNA-PK total protein levels but can reduce phosphorylation of DNA-PKcs. This has been shown to be due to disruption of EGFR activity via HER2 depletion in cells lacking HER3 [17, 18]. Together with the observation that HSP90 co-localizes with γH2Ax repair foci [19], these previous findings suggest HSP90 inhibition as a promising target for radio- and chemo-sensitization studies.

AUY922 [20] is a small molecule HSP90 inhibitor (HSP90i) that is currently recruiting in Phase II trials for NSCLC and gastrointestinal stromal tumours. Previous studies reported AUY922 as a radiosensitizer and that other HSP90 inhibitors can sensitize to cisplatin alone [21–25]. Since meaningful clinical utility for HSP90i in HNSCC is most likely to be in the context of CCRT, we sought to assess the combinations of AUY922 with CCRT in p53 mutant (p53mt) HNSCC cell lines. TCGA data has shown 85% of HPV negative HNSCC harbour mutations in p53. Our goal was to thoroughly profile the impact of AUY922 on DNA damage response (DDR) signalling due to CCRT. A greater understanding of how AUY922 modulates the DDR is crucial to establishing future planning and assessment of clinical trials in p53mt HNSCC.

Methods

Cell culture conditions

Cal27 (CRL-2095) and FaDu (HTB-43) cells were obtained from ATCC. LICR-LON-HN5 were a kind gift from Suzanne Eccles (The Institute of Cancer Research, Sutton, London, UK). All three cell lines were HPV negative and p53 mutant. Cells were cultured in DMEM (Invitrogen, Paisley, UK) supplemented with 10% FCS, 2 mM L-glutamine and 1% penicillin/streptomycin in a humidified incubator at 37 °C with 5% CO_2. Cells were tested for mycoplasma using the eMyco PCR kit from IntroBio (Seongnam-Si, South Korea) and authenticated by STR profiling (Bio-Synthesis Inc, Texas, US).

Drugs and irradiation

AUY922 was kindly donated by Novartis in the form of the mesylated salt. Cisplatin was from Teva Hospitals (Castleford, UK). In western blot, confocal and FACS analysis 10 nM AUY922 or 10 μM cisplatin was used unless otherwise indicted. AUY922 was added 16 h before cisplatin or irradiation. Irradiation was carried out using an AGO 250 kV X-ray machine (AGO, Reading, UK).

Clonogenic assay

Long-term survival in response to radiation was measured by colony formation assay. Cells were trypsinized, diluted and counted before seeding in 6-well dishes or 10 cm dishes at appropriate seeding densities. Cells were allowed to attach before addition of 5 nM AUY922 or DMSO only control for 16 h. Cells were exposed to 5 μM cisplatin for 3 h with cells subject to concurrent-cisplatin radiotherapy being irradiated immediately after cisplatin addition. After 3 h exposure to cisplatin, both cisplatin and AUY922 were replaced by drug-free medium. Colonies were fixed and stained in 5% gluteraldehyde, 0.5% crystal violet, with colonies containing more than 50 cells counted. Colony counting was performed both manually and by automated quantification using CellProfiler 2.0 (Broad Institute, MA, USA). Surviving fraction was calculated by normalization to untreated controls.

Western blotting

Medium and cells were harvested in PBS-containing 1 mM Na_3VO_4 and 1 mM NaF. Cells were pelleted before lysis in 50 mM Tris.HCl pH 7.5, 150 mM NaCl, 1% NP-40, 0.5% deoxycholate and 0.1% SDS. Samples were thawed on ice, centrifuged at 14,000 rpm for 20 min at 4 °C and supernatants quantified by BCA assay from Pierce (Leicestershire, UK). 30 μg total protein lysate was separated by reducing SDS-PAGE, transferred to PVDF (GE Healthcare, Bucks, UK) and blocked with 5% non-fat dry milk in TBS. The following primary antibodies were used: rabbit anti-HSP72 from Stressgen (Exeter, UK); rabbit anti-GAPDH, rabbit anti-ATR, rabbit anti-phospho-ATR (S428), rabbit anti-CHK1, rabbit anti-phospho-CHK1 (S345), rabbit anti-RAD51, rabbit anti-ATM, rabbit anti-phospho-ATM (S1981), rabbit anti-phospho-BRCA1 (S1524), rabbit anti-phospho-p53 (S15) and rabbit anti-phospho-H2Ax (S139) were purchased from Cell Signaling (MA, USA); rabbit anti-FANCA was purchased from Bethyl Laboratories (TX, USA). Secondary antibodies used were sheep anti-mouse IgG and donkey anti-rabbit IgG HRP from GE Healthcare (Buckinghamshire, UK). Chemiluminescent detection was carried out using immobilon western substrate from Millipore (East Midlands, UK). In vivo samples were processed using a Precellys®24 homogenizer from Bertin Technologies (Montigny, France).

Lentiviral shRNA production and infection

Short hairpin sequences were cloned into the lentiviral shRNA plasmid pHIVSiren [26]. The plasmid pHIVSiren was kindly donated by Professor Greg Towers, University College London and was derived from a parent plasmid, CSGW (Prof Adrian Thrasher, University College London). FANCA and ATM short hairpin target sequences were 5'-GTGGCATCTTCACGTACAA-3' and 5'-GTGGCATCTTCACGTACAA-3', respectively. Scrambled short hairpin target sequence was 5'-GTTATAGGCTCGCAAAAGG-3'. Short hairpin containing pHIVSiren was co-transfected with the packaging plasmids psPAX2, pMD2.G into HEK293T cells using lipofectamine 2000 (Life Technologies, Paisley, UK). Viral supernatants were collected and target cells infected in the presence of 1 µg per mL polybrene.

Flow cytometry

Cells were stained for mitosis or DNA double-stranded breaks with rabbit anti-phospho-histone H3 S10 (DD2C8) AlexaFluor647 or anti-phospho-histone H2Ax S139 (20E3) AlexaFluor488 (Cell Signaling, MA, USA) using the manufacturer's protocol. Cells were analyzed on an LSR II from BD Biosciences (Oxford, UK).

DDR confocal image based analysis

Cells were plated in 35 mm glass-bottomed dishes (Mattek, MA, USA). Samples were fixed in 4% PFA, permeabilized in 0.2% Triton X-100 and treated with DNaseI (Roche, West Sussex, UK). Cells were blocked in 1% BSA, 2% FCS in PBS before staining with rabbit anti-phospho-H2Ax S139 (γH2Ax), rabbit anti-RAD51, rabbit anti-53BP1, anti-phospho-BRCA1 (S1524), rabbit anti-phospho-p53 (S15) or mouse anti-phospho-ATM (S1981) (Cell Signaling, MA, USA) with goat anti-rabbit Alexafluor488 or goat anti-mouse Alexfluor546 as secondary antibodies (Invitrogen, Paisley, UK). Nuclei were counterstained with DAPI. Samples were imaged using a Zeiss LSM710 inverted confocal microscope (Zeiss, Jena, Germany). Automated quantification of foci in 100-300 nuclei per experiment was carried out using CellProfiler 2.0 (Broad Institute, MA, USA). Formalin-fixed paraffin embedded (FFPE) in vivo blocks were sectioned and

antigen retrieved for RAD51 (pH9 Tris-EDTA) or 53BP1 (pH6 citrate buffer). Antigen retrieved slides were blocked, stained, imaged and quantified as outlined for in vitro samples above.

In vivo human xenograft model

Female 5-6 week-old athymic BALBc nude mice (Charles River, UK) were used with all experiments, complying with NCRI guidelines. 2×10^6 FaDu cells were injected subcutaneously. Developing tumors were distributed into groups containing a minimum of n = 8 per group, with matching average tumor volumes. AUY922 40 mg/kg in 5% dextrose was administered in three doses by i.p. injection on days one, three and five. Fractionated radiation treatment of the tumor consisted of a total dose of 6 Gy in 2 Gy fractions on day two, four and six. Cisplatin was administered as a single dose of 5 mg/kg on day four immediately before irradiation. Tumor volume was calculated as volume = (width × length × depth)/2 and was plotted as mean tumor volume for each group.

Statistical analysis

Statistical analysis was carried out using Graphpad prism (version 6.0f). Unpaired two-tailed student t-test was utilized for parametric analysis. Synergy was determined by Bliss independence analysis using the equation $E_{exp} = E_x + E_y - (E_xE_y)$ [27]. E_{exp} is the expected effect if two treatments are additive with E_x and E_y corresponding to the effect of each treatment individually. $\Delta E = E_{observed} - E_{exp}$. Synergy is represented by ΔE and 95% confidence intervals (CI) from observed data all above zero; addition to values above and below zero; antagonism where all values are below zero.

Results

AUY922 sensitizes p53mt HNSCC to cisplatin, radiation and concurrent-cisplatin radiotherapy (CCRT)

The ability of AUY922 to sensitize to cisplatin, radiation and CCRT was assessed in a panel of cell lines by clonogenic assay using the scheduling outlined (Fig. 1a). We focused our studies on p53mt since p53 pathway abnormalities exist in 85% of HPV-negative HNSCC (TCGA).

Clonogenic data are presented as surviving fractions, normalised to drug free control wells (Fig. 1b). Qualitative images of colonies for each cell line and condition are also shown with numbers indicating the number of cells plated in each well shown (Fig. 1c). Bliss independence analysis (Fig. 1d) indicated synergy for the combination of AUY922 and cisplatin, except HN5 in which the interaction was additive. Synergy for the combination of AUY922 with both radiation and CCRT was observed in all cell lines tested. Values for synergy between 0 and 0.2 are in keeping with those observed in recent

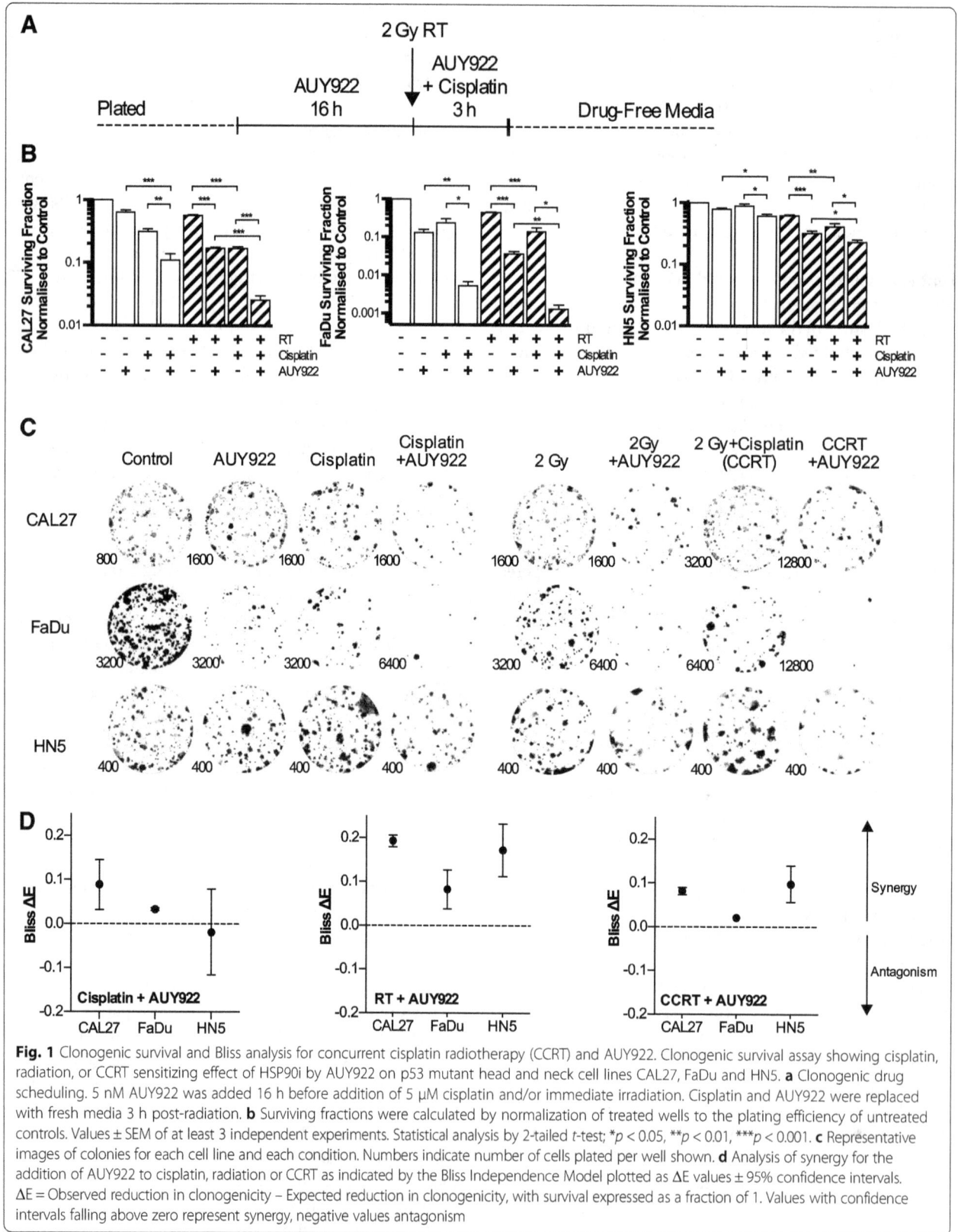

Fig. 1 Clonogenic survival and Bliss analysis for concurrent cisplatin radiotherapy (CCRT) and AUY922. Clonogenic survival assay showing cisplatin, radiation, or CCRT sensitizing effect of HSP90i by AUY922 on p53 mutant head and neck cell lines CAL27, FaDu and HN5. **a** Clonogenic drug scheduling. 5 nM AUY922 was added 16 h before addition of 5 µM cisplatin and/or immediate irradiation. Cisplatin and AUY922 were replaced with fresh media 3 h post-radiation. **b** Surviving fractions were calculated by normalization of treated wells to the plating efficiency of untreated controls. Values ± SEM of at least 3 independent experiments. Statistical analysis by 2-tailed t-test; *p < 0.05, **p < 0.01, ***p < 0.001. **c** Representative images of colonies for each cell line and each condition. Numbers indicate number of cells plated per well shown. **d** Analysis of synergy for the addition of AUY922 to cisplatin, radiation or CCRT as indicated by the Bliss Independence Model plotted as ΔE values ± 95% confidence intervals. ΔE = Observed reduction in clonogenicity – Expected reduction in clonogenicity, with survival expressed as a fraction of 1. Values with confidence intervals falling above zero represent synergy, negative values antagonism

radiosensitization studies for CHK1 and ATR inhibition [28, 29]. FaDu cells were substantially more sensitive to AUY922 and cisplatin monotherapies as well as AUY922 and cisplatin or CCRT combinations. HN5 cells were more resistant to monotherapies and were one to two orders of magnitude more resistant to the combination of AUY922 and CCRT compared to other cell lines.

Inhibition of HR via RAD51 and BRCA1 corresponds to increased 53BP1 foci and signalling into mutant p53

We investigated the impact of AUY922 on CCRT-induced RAD51 focus formation. CCRT induced an increase in early RAD51 focus formation which was significantly reduced by AUY922 (Fig. 2a, b). Western blots looking at DDR signalling with radiation and cisplatin

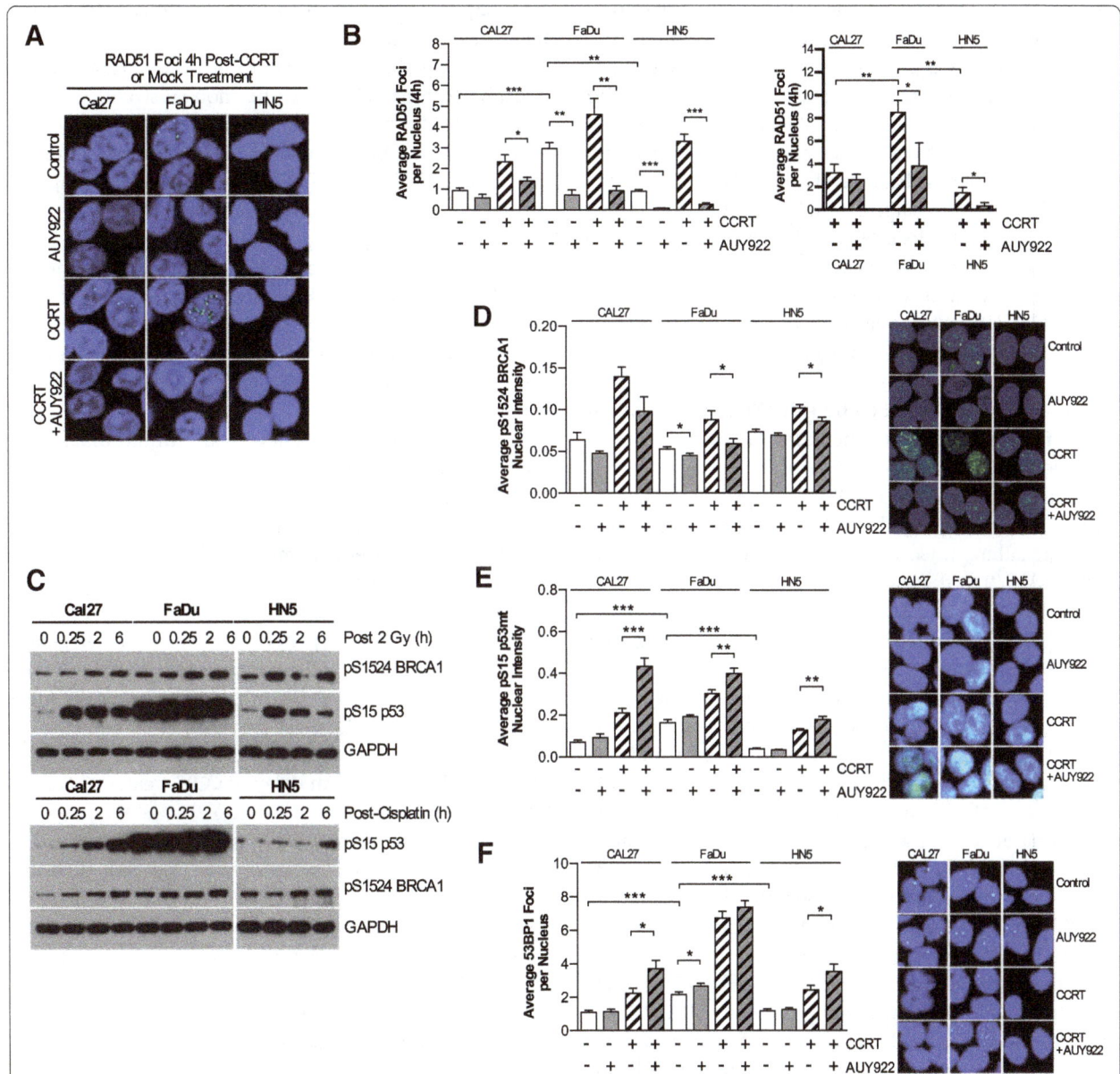

Fig. 2 AUY922 reduces HR in response to CCRT but increases 53BP1 focal formation and mutant p53 signaling. **a** Representative images of RAD51 foci in the HNSCC cell lines CAL27, FaDu and HN5. Nuclear localization indicated by DAPI staining. AUY922 refers to 10 nM added 16 h pre-DNA damage. 2 Gy radiation plus 10 µM cisplatin for brevity is referred to as concurrent-cisplatin radiotherapy (CCRT). **b** Quantitation of the average RAD51 foci per nucleus at 4 h and for CCRT and CCRT + AUY922 conditions at 24 h also. Values shown are means ± SEM of a minimum of three independent experiments. **c** Western blot analysis of pS1524 BRCA1 and pS15 p53 signaling post irradiation or cisplatin treatment. **d**, **e**, **f** Automated image based quantification of average nuclear pS1524 BRCA1 intensity, average pS15 p53mt nuclear intensity, and average 53BP1 foci per nucleus with treatment schedule as outlined in panel **b**. Representative nuclear staining for each cell line and condition are shown. Values shown are means ± SEM from a minimum quantification of 12 fields of view across two independent experiments, except for pS1524 BRCA1 in CAL27 cells which represent 8-10 fields of view from a single experiment. Statistical analysis by 2-tailed t-test; *p < 0.05, **p < 0.01, ***p < 0.001

alone revealed similar levels of S1524 BRCA1 in all cell lines, but diverse phosphorylation of mutant p53 S15. FaDu cells were constitutively high for pS15 p53 with levels in HN5 cells rapidly decreasing after an early radiation induced spike (Fig. 2c).

To more conclusively investigate this difference we looked at nuclear staining of pS1524 BRCA1, pS15 p53 and 53BP1 focus formation. Nuclear intensity of pS1524 BRCA1 signalling increased due to CCRT and was statistically lower due to AUY922 (Fig. 2d). Nuclear intensity of CCRT induced pS15 p53 increased in all cell lines due to the addition of AUY922 (Fig. 2e). CCRT induced 53BP1 foci increased in all cell lines due to the addition of AUY922 (Fig. 2f). Overall it was observed that FaDu cells exhibited the highest basal levels of RAD51, 53BP1 and pS15 p53 with the largest number of CCRT induced RAD51 and 53BP1 foci. HN5 cell displayed the lowest basal DDR signalling pattern and low levels of RAD51 foci persisting at 24 h as well as low levels of pS15 mutant p53. Cal27s fell in between, with this pattern correlating to the results observed in clonogenic assays (Fig. 1b).

FANCA and RAD51 depletion by AUY922 perturbs normal RAD51 focus formation and increases ATM focus formation in response to CCRT

Previously reported as a HSP90 client protein, we investigated how FANCA and RAD51 depletion may impact ATM signalling (measured by autophosphorylation on S1981). AUY922 depleted both RAD51 and FANCA to similar levels in CAL27, FaDu and HN5 cells with canonical drug-on-target induction of HSP72 (Fig. 3a). Stable knockdown in CAL27 cells of FANCA and ATM by lentiviral shRNA is shown by western blot (Fig. 3b).

As expected, FANCA knockdown increased sensitivity to cisplatin and CCRT with no statistically significant difference between control and scrambled shRNA conditions (Fig. 3c). FANCA knockdown significantly increased basal RAD51 and pS1981 ATM focus formation in response to CCRT (Fig. 3d, e). CCRT-induced pS1981 ATM foci were further increased by the addition of AUY922 in all cell lines (Fig. 3e, f) coinciding with a reduction in RAD51 foci (Fig. 2b, Fig. 3d).

We then generated ATM knockdown cells to investigate the role of ATM in compensating for loss of RAD51 and FANCA due to AUY922. Knockdown of ATM in CAL27 cells resulted in increased sensitivity to cisplatin, radiation and CCRT (Fig. 3g). AUY922 was able to further sensitize to cisplatin, radiation or CCRT. Overall survival was profoundly decreased in all combinations vs scrambled.

AUY922 abrogates ATR-CHK1 signaling and induces chromosomal fragmentation

Following on from evidence of increased ATM foci induced by AUY922, we looked at ATR-CHK1 signaling.

In all cell lines, moderate decreases in phospho-ATR, total-ATR and total-CHK1 combined to give a substantial reduction in phospho-CHK1 signaling (Fig. 4b). In studying the impact of this inhibition on mitotic entry by phospho-histone H3 staining (Fig. 4c), AUY922 was found to induce a profound increase in the mitotic population. This was much less pronounced in CAL27 cells, while HN5 cells exhibited an increase in the mitotic population from 2.9 to 8.1% due to AUY922 treatment (data not shown).

Co-staining FACS analysis of both the mitotic marker phospho-histone H3 and the double-stranded break marker γH2Ax revealed that this AUY922-induced mitotic population became highly γH2Ax positive immediately after CCRT (Fig. 4d). Confocal microscopy (Fig. 4e) further confirmed the presence of high levels of γH2Ax foci in nuclei displaying a mitotic morphology post-CCRT, as well as chromosome fragments or missegregation. We quantified the presence of micronuclei at 24 h post CCRT (Fig. 4f). AUY922 alone increased micronuclei compared to basal and significantly increased micronuclei when combined with CCRT vs CCRT alone in all cell lines.

FaDu cells showed high levels of chromosomal fragmentation both basally and in response to AUY922 plus CCRT. HN5 cells showed low basal levels and the lowest number of micronuclei in response to CCRT plus AUY922. This pattern of micronuclei formation closely aligned to that observed for RAD51, 53BP1 repair foci formation and signalling into mutant p53 (Fig. 2b, e, f). This DNA repair foci pattern and micronuclei generation correlated to the differences in sensitivity observed in clonogenic assays (Fig. 1b) with FaDus being the most sensitive and HN5s the most resistant.

AUY922 enhances growth delay of CCRT treated FaDu HNSCC xenograft tumors

DNA damage signaling basally and in response to radiation was assessed in FaDus in vivo (Fig. 5a). Cisplatin treatment of FaDu xenografts was confirmed to increase DNA damage signaling 24 h after 5 mg/kg cisplatin injection (Fig. 5b, c). Depletion of HSP90 client proteins by AUY922 in FaDu xenografts was assessed at both 40 mg/kg and 80 mg/kg with three IP injections on days 1, 3 and 5. Tumor lysates were collected 24 h after final injection. HER2 as a known and highly sensitive HSP90 client protein was also assessed. Reductions in RAD51 and HER2 were observed at 40 mg/kg with increased S15 phospho-p53 signaling also detected (Fig. 5b, c).

The lowest dose of 40 mg/kg AUY922 was selected to look for sensitization effects in tumor volume experiments (Fig. 5d). Mice were treated when tumors reached 5-7 mm in width with groups composed of mice with equal average tumor volume. AUY922 40 mg/kg was

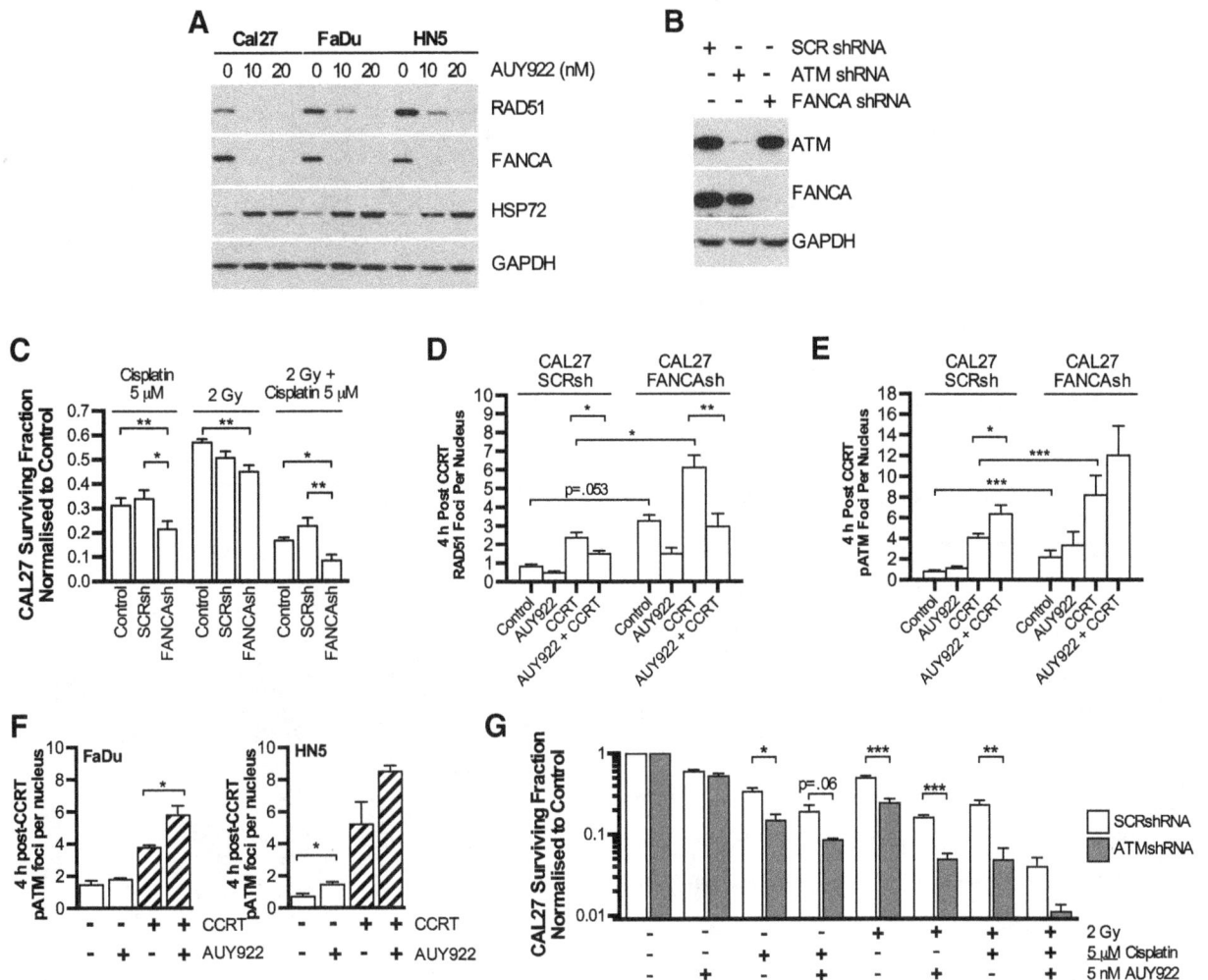

Fig. 3 AUY922 disruption of FANCA leads to increased dependency on ATM in response to CCRT. **a** Western blot analysis of RAD51 and FANCA depletion by AUY922 in the p53mt HNSCC cell lines CAL27, FaDu and HN5. **b** Confirmation of FANCA and ATM knockdown using lentiviral shRNA by western blot in the p53 mutant HNSCC cell line CAL27 vs scrambled shRNA. **c** Clonogenic survival assay showing cisplatin; radiation; or CCRT toxicity to CAL27 cells expressing scrambled (SCR) or FANCA shRNA vs control cells with no lentiviral infection. **d, e** Quantification of RAD51 or S1981 phospho-ATM foci by confocal microscopy in SCRsh or ATMsh CAL27 cells. CCRT and AUY922 doses as outlined in Fig. 2. **f** S1981 phospho-ATM foci in FaDu and HN5 cells in response to CCRT and AUY922. **g** Clonogenic survival assay showing cisplatin, radiation, or CCRT sensitizing effect of HSP90i by AUY922 in scrambled of ATM shRNA expressing CAL27 cells. All values mean ± SEM of at least 3 independent experiments. Statistical analysis by 2-tailed t-test; *$p < 0.05$, **$p < 0.01$, ***$p < 0.001$

administered by IP injection on days 1, 3 and 5. Radiation was delivered in 3×2 Gy fractions on days 2, 4 and 6 with 5 mg/kg cisplatin administered by IP injection before irradiation on day 4. CCRT combined with AUY922 was tolerable with average weight loss of <10% (data not shown). The addition of AUY922 successfully delayed time to reach 800 mm^3 from 27 days for CCRT only to 34 days from CCRT plus AUY922.

To assess DDR signalling at the level of repair foci formation in vivo, staining for RAD51 and 53BP1 was carried out on sections from FFPE tumour blocks which were all fixed 16 h after the final radiation fraction. Cisplatin and radiation combined to increase RAD51 foci in vivo, with AUY922 at the 40 mg/kg dose used in therapy

experiments able to reduce RAD51 focus formation (Fig 5e). 53BP1 focus formation as a result of radiation decreased due to the addition of cisplatin. AUY922 addition to CCRT in increased the number of 53BP1 foci detected. These findings are in line with those shown in vitro (Fig. 2b, f).

Discussion

The standard-of-care for locally advanced HNSCC is CCRT, yet almost 50% of patients do not survive past 5 years [30]. The anti-EGFR-targeting monoclonal antibody cetuximab is the only targeted therapy approved for HNSCC treatment. However, the RTOG 0522 phase III study showed there was no benefit from adding

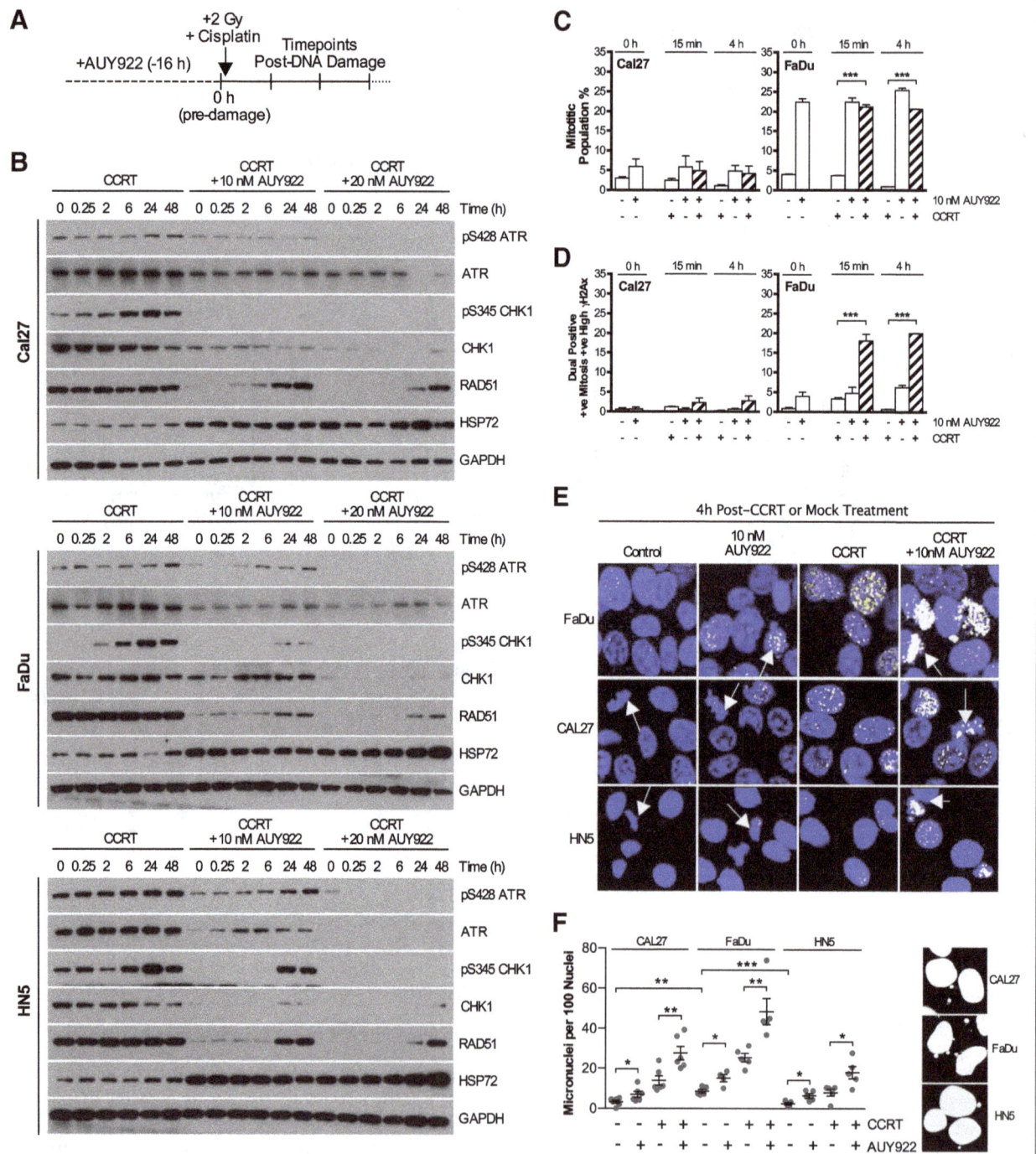

Fig. 4 AUY922 abrogates ATR-CHK1 signaling allowing increased chromosomal fragmentation in response to CCRT. **a** Scheduling showing 0 h time point post 16 h AUY922 addition but pre-RT, cisplatin or combined CCRT addition and subsequent time point analysis post as used in panels **b-f**. **b** AUY922 disruption of ATR-CHK1 signaling in response to CCRT alongside depletion of total RAD51. **c** Mitotic accumulation as measured by FACS analysis of phospho-histone H3 positive cells. **d** Co-staining for phospho-histone H3 and γH2Ax was analyzed by FACS. Population plotted is the percentage of the total cell number positive for both high γH2Ax levels and the mitotic marker phospho-histone H3. **e** γH2Ax staining in mitotic cells was confirmed in HNSCC cell lines by confocal microscopy, DAPI as nuclear stain. Nuclei with mitotic morphology indicated by arrows. **f** Micronuclei quantification of DAPI stained confocal images at 24 h in response to CCRT and AUY922. Values are mean ± SEM of at least three independent experiments. Statistical analysis by 2-tailed *t*-test; *$p < 0.05$, **$p < 0.01$, ***$p < 0.001$

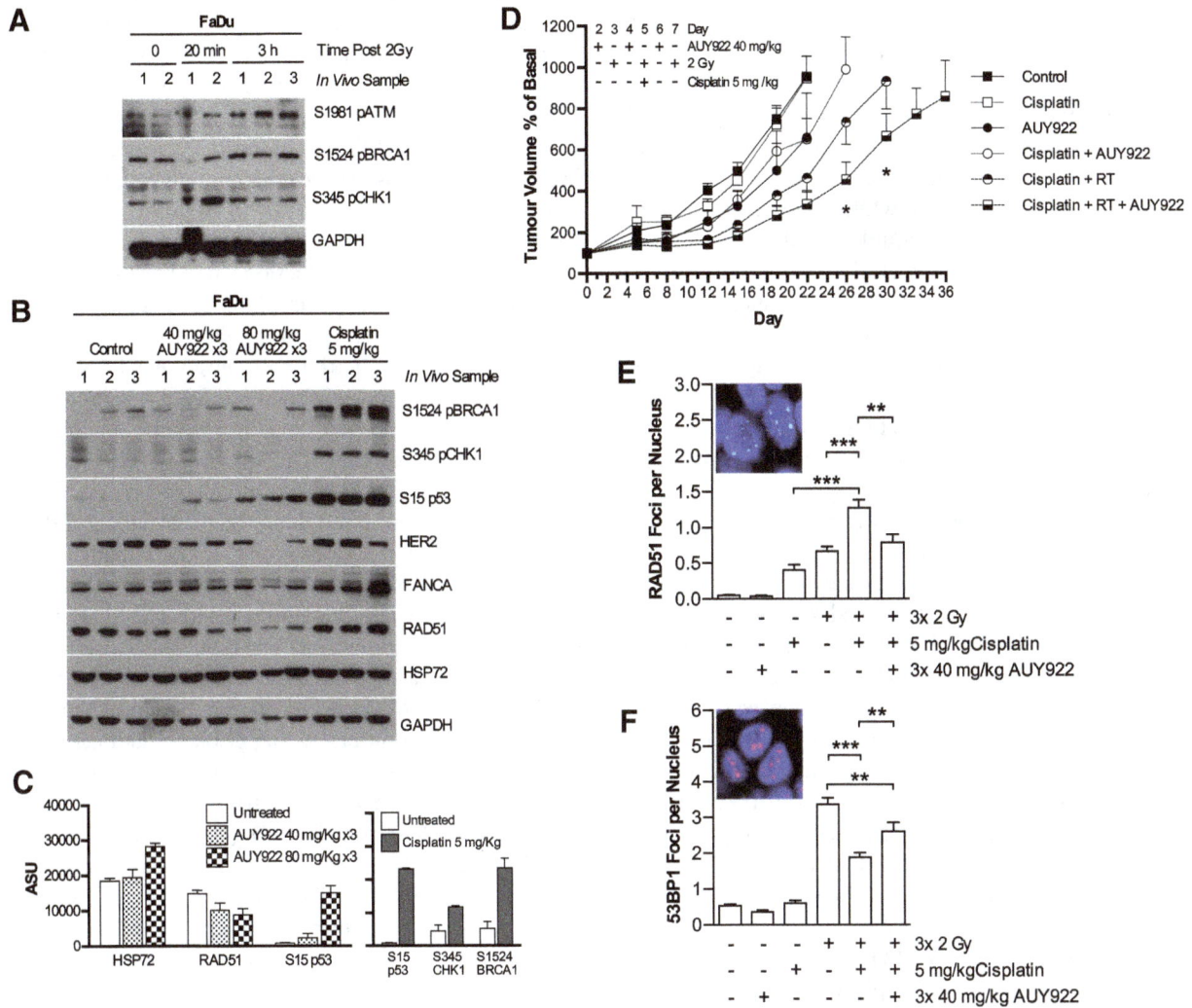

Fig. 5 AUY922 delays tumor growth in conjunction with CCRT. **a** FaDu cells were implanted subcutaneously in BALB/c nude mice. After reaching 5-7 mm, tumors were treated with 2 Gy radiation. Tumors harvested at the times post radiation as indicated and probed for DNA damage signaling by western blot. **b** FaDu cells implanted as in A before treatment with cisplatin 5 mg/kg or three doses of AUY922 40 mg/kg on alternate days. Tumors treated with AUY922 were collected 16 h post final injection, cisplatin 24 h post injection. Western blot analysis performed for DNA damage signaling in response to cisplatin or reduction in HSP90 client proteins by AUY922. **c** Densitometry of changes due to HSP90 inhibition and response to cisplatin as shown in panel **b**, expressed as arbitrary scanning units adjusted for changes in GAPDH levels.
d FaDu cells implanted as in A. Tumors were distributed into the following treatment groups with matching average tumor volumes; control; Cisplatin 5 mg/kg; AUY922 40 mg/kg × 3; cisplatin 5 mg/kg plus AUY922 40 mg/kg × 3; cisplatin 5 mg/kg plus three fractions of 2Gy; cisplatin 5 mg/kg plus three fractions of 2 Gy plus AUY922 40 mg/kg × 3. Exact scheduling as outlined in methods. Tumor volume expressed as percentage increase over basal volume at start of treatment. **e, f** FFPE blocks were sectioned and stained for RAD51 and 53BP1 foci. Automated quantification shown represents a minimum of 36 randomly distributed fields of view for RAD51 across 2 tumor blocks, 16-24 fields of view across for 53BP1 foci. Values ± SEM, statistical analysis by 2-tailed t-test; $*p < 0.05$, $**p < 0.01$, $***p < 0.001$

cetuximab to cisplatin-based CCRT [31]. Cetuximab illustrates that success in clinical trials is likely to be measured by the capability to improve survival as an addition to CCRT rather than with radiation alone.

Our goal in this study was to iterate on the already established ability of HSP90 inhibition to radiosensitize. We set out to determine if HSP90 inhibition in combination with CCRT was likely to offer a significant stepwise improvement or if the addition of cisplatin had the

potential to interfere with radiation sensitization by AUY922. The addition of AUY922 to cisplatin, radiation and CCRT combinations was shown to be synergistic across a panel of p53mt. AUY922. and was capable of enhancing the efficacy of CCRT in vivo.

Sensitization to CCRT by HSP90i has previously been published in both NSCLC [21] and bladder cancer [25]. Wang et al. examined the ability of HSP90i by ganetespib to sensitize a panel of NSCLC KRAS mt p53 wt and

KRAS wt p53 mt/null cell lines [21]. Ganetespib radio-sensitized all cell lines but they showed HSP90i produced variable results both in vitro and in vivo to carboplatin-paclitaxel and concomitant carboplatin-paclitaxel and radiation. The use of paclitaxel-carboplatin rather than carboplatin alone complicates interpretation of these results relative to our study. We see broad sensitization to CCRT while they see cases of antagonism by HSP90i. This could be cell line specific or related to paclitaxel. Yoshida et al. assessed cisplatin and radiation in bladder cancer cell lines showing sensitization by 17-DMAG to radiation and CCRT [25]. While a number of studies have looking at HSP90i sensitization to radiation or cisplatin individually in head and neck [12, 24, 32], none extensively address the ability of HSP90i to sensitize p53mt HNSCC to concurrent-cisplatin radiotherapy.

We concentrated on investigating the ability of AUY922 to disrupt HR induced by CCRT and other DDR signalling pathways by extensive confocal image based analysis. RAD51, BRCA1 and BRCA2 have previously been identified as HSP90 client proteins, with depletion of RAD51 and RAD52 occurring upon loss or inhibition of HSP90 isoforms in budding yeast [17, 23, 33]. Previous mechanistic studies on HSP90i have not focused extensively on DDR signalling. In the HSP90i and platinum-radiotherapy combinations mentioned above, 53BP1 foci alone were analysed but only for ganetespib and radiation [21]. For HSP90i and CCRT in bladder cancer, mechanistic studies focused on HER2 and AKT signalling with no investigation of the impact of HSP90i on DDR signalling [25]. Likewise studies into sensitization to radiation or cisplatin alone often focused on cell cycle, growth and apoptotic signalling pathways [22, 24, 32, 34–36]. Choi et al. identified HSP90i by bioinformatics as a means to convert HR proficient to HR deficient tumours [23] but DDR analysis was restricted to γH2Ax and RAD51 foci formation as has been the case in other studies [17, 22, 35].

In this study we comprehensively profiled HSP90i modulation of the DDR to CCRT. Reduction in HR by HSP90i occurs due to decreased RAD51 focus formation and nuclear pS1524 BRCA1. This corresponds to HSP90i induced increases in 53BP1 foci. This may be in part a separate inhibitory event on the resolution of 53BP1 repair sites or a switch from HR to NHEJ. 53BP1 has been identified to antagonise DSB end resection promoting NHEJ over HR. It has been proposed that 53BP1 is displaced in S-phase in a BRCA1 dependent manner. The role of BRCA1 in promoting HR over NHEJ through 53BP1 has been recently reviewed [37, 38]. This suggests HSP90i via a reduction in nuclear BRCA1 signalling may also shift HR to more error prone NHEJ repair rather than a delay in existing 53BP1 foci resolution

alone. Modulation of DDR at the repair foci level in vivo has also been demonstrated for the first time in FFPE blocks. This may be a beneficial for analysis of future clinical trials where FFPE biopsies are more routinely used for analysis.

HSP90i increased CCRT induced nuclear pS15 p53mt levels. The role this increased p53mt signalling may play is not known. The early HSP90 inhibitor 17-AAG has been shown to stabilise wild type p53 in head and neck cell lines through a reduction in MDMX increasing apoptosis in response to cisplatin [24]. Parallel studies were not performed on mutant p53.

In exploring the role the HR component FANCA may play in HSP90 chemosensitization, we discovered a profound increase in ATM foci in response to AUY922. FANCA is part of the Fanconi Anemia core complex that ubiquitinates FANCD2 at interstrand crosslink sites, leading to crosslink unhooking, lesion bypass and downstream completion of repair by RAD51-mediated HR [39]. FANCA depletion alone by shRNA revealed an increase in RAD51 alongside increased ATM focus formation. It is not known if FANCA loss results in a numerical increase in the incidence of damage requiring RAD51 and ATM focus formation or simply prevents the timely resolution of existing cisplatin adducts leading to accumulation. The exact cause of this increased ATM signal due to AUY922 is hard to pinpoint. ATM is autophosphorylated on Ser1981 [40]. FANCA mutation and ATR loss have both been shown to increase phosphorylation of S1981 ATM and S15 p53 [41, 42] with ATM known to phosphorylate S15 of p53 in response to DNA damage [43]. This suggests decreased levels of ATR and FANCA by HSP90i lead to compensatory signalling via ATM and p53 in response to CCRT. An illustration of the hypothesised changes in CCRT induced DDR signalling triggered by HSP90i and downstream consequences is summarised in Fig. 6.

Decreased RAD51, FANCA and ATR function by HSP90 inhibition may lead to increased dependence on ATM for repair. Cells subject to ATM knockdown by shRNA were substantially more sensitive to cisplatin, RT and CCRT alone and in combination with HSP90i. Loss of ATM has been shown to occur in head and neck due to loss of the distal region of chromosome 11q [44]. Much discussion has occurred around the potential to target ATM loss as a synthetic lethal strategy [45]. ATR inhibition alone is being investigated as a radiosensitizer with some studies showing ATR inhibition leading to increased dependency on ATM [46, 47].

The ultimate consequence of a shift to more error prone repair and loss of S-phase and G2/M checkpoint fidelity was missegregation of chromosomal material and micronucleus formation. We observed that the most sensitive cell line in clonogenic assays (FaDu) displayed

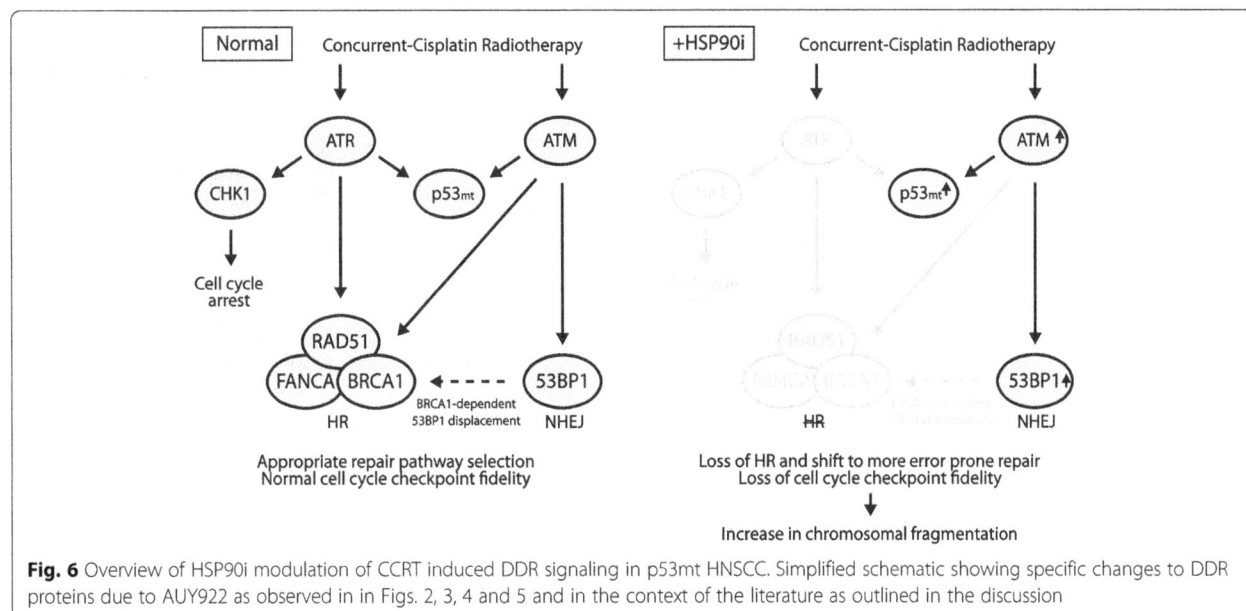

Fig. 6 Overview of HSP90i modulation of CCRT induced DDR signaling in p53mt HNSCC. Simplified schematic showing specific changes to DDR proteins due to AUY922 as observed in in Figs. 2, 3, 4 and 5 and in the context of the literature as outlined in the discussion

the highest levels of DDR signalling due to CCRT and the highest levels of chromosomal fragmentation with the addition of HSP90i. The least sensitive cell line in clonogenic assays (HN5) displayed the lowest levels of both DDR signalling and chromosomal fragmentation. Micronuclei deficient in nuclear import, prone to rupturing and incomplete replication [48, 49] are putatively the major toxic event induced by AUY922 inhibition in combination with CCRT.

Conclusions

In summary, this study demonstrated inhibition of HSP90 by AUY922 had a synergistic interaction with CCRT in a panel of p53 mutant cell lines. HSP90i leads to significant alterations to the DDR induced by CCRT. This comprises inhibition of HR, a shift to more error prone repair and loss of checkpoint function leading to fragmentation of chromosomal material. Additionally, these results indicate there may be a rationale for the combination of AUY922 and CCRT in cells lacking ATM function. In conclusion, these data show that HSP90 inhibition can improve upon CCRT standard-of-care and support further preclinical and clinical studies in HNSCC.

Abbreviations
CCRT: Concurrent-cisplatin radiation; CI: Confidence interval; DDR: DNA damage response; HNSCC: Head and neck squamous cell carcinoma; HR: Homologous recombination; HSP: Heat shock protein; p53mt: p53 mutant

Acknowledgements
We would like to thank Clare Gregory for technical assistance in in vivo studies.

Funding
MM, HEB, SAB, KLN, CMN and KJH were funded by Cancer Research UK Programme Grant A13407. AAK was funded by the Wellcome Trust. MM and MP were funded by the Oracle Cancer Trust. MD was funded by CRUK and The Rosetrees Trust. KJH received support from The Rosetrees Trust, The Anthony Long Charitable Trust and the Mark Donegan Foundation. Authors acknowledge support from the RM/ICR NIHR Biomedical Research Centre. Funding bodies played no role in the design of the study, data collection, analysis, interpretation or the writing the manuscript.

Authors' contributions
MM, HEB, AAK, MP, MD, DCM, RP and JNK contributed to experimental design, procedure and data acquisition. MM, SAB, KLN, CMN and KJH contributed to data interpretation as well as manuscript drafting or revision. All authors read and approved the final manuscript.

Competing interests
Intellectual property from the research collaboration with Vernalis Ltd. on HSP90 inhibitors was licensed from The Institute of Cancer Research London to Vernalis Ltd. and Novartis. The Institute of Cancer Research London has benefited from this and requires its employees to declare this potential conflict of interest.

Author details
[1]Targeted Therapy Team, The Institute of Cancer Research, Chester Beatty Laboratories, 237 Fulham Road, London SW3 6JB, UK. [2]The Royal Marsden Hospital, 203 Fulham Road, London SW3 6JJ, UK. [3]Division of Radiotherapy and Imaging, The Institute of Cancer Research, 237 Fulham Road, London, UK.

References
1. Harrington KJ, Billingham LJ, Brunner TB, Burnet NG, Chan CS, Hoskin P, Mackay RI, Maughan IS, Macdougall J, McKenna WG, Nutting CM, Oliver A, Plummer R, Stratford IJ, Illidge T. Guidelines for preclinical and early phase clinical assessment of novel radiosensitisers. Br J Cancer. 2011;105:628–39.
2. Dillon MT, Harrington KJ. Human papillomavirus-negative pharyngeal cancer. J Clin Oncol. 2015;33:3251–61.
3. Trepel J, Mollapour M, Giaccone G, Neckers L. Targeting the dynamic HSP90 complex in cancer. Nat Rev Cancer. 2010;10:537–49.

4. Oda T, Hayano T, Miyaso H, Takahashi N, Yamashita T. Hsp90 regulates the Fanconi anemia DNA damage response pathway. Blood. 2007;109:5016–26.

5. Arlander SJH, Felts SJ, Wagner JM, Stensgard B, Toft DO, Karnitz LM. Chaperoning checkpoint kinase 1 (Chk1), an Hsp90 client, with purified chaperones. J Biol Chem. 2006;281:2989–98.

6. Camphausen K, Tofilon PJ. Inhibition of Hsp90: a multitarget approach to radiosensitization. Clin Cancer Res. 2007;13:4326–30.

7. Russell JS, Burgan WE, Oswald KA, Camphausen K, Tofilon PJ. Enhanced cell killing induced by the combination of radiation and the heat shock protein 90 inhibitor 17-allylamino-17- demethoxygeldanamycin: a multitarget approach to radiosensitization. Clin Cancer Res. 2003;9:3749–55.

8. Machida H, Matsumoto Y, Shirai M, Kubota N. Geldanamycin, an inhibitor of Hsp90, sensitizes human tumour cells to radiation. Int J Radiat Biol. 2003;79: 973–80. http://dx.doi.org/10.1080/09553000310001626135.

9. Zaidi SH, Huddart RA, Harrington KJ. Novel targeted radiosensitisers in cancer treatment. Curr Drug Discov Technol. 2009;6:103–34.

10. Bisht KS, Bradbury CM, Mattson D, Kaushal A, Sowers A, Markovina S, Ortiz KL, Sieck LK, Isaacs JS, Brechbiel MW, Mitchell JB, Neckers LM, Gius D. Geldanamycin and 17-allylamino-17-demethoxygeldanamycin potentiate the in vitro and in vivo radiation response of cervical tumor cells via the heat shock protein 90-mediated intracellular signaling and cytotoxicity. Cancer Res. 2003;63:8984–95.

11. Dote H, Cerna D, Burgan WE, Camphausen K, Tofilon PJ. ErbB3 expression predicts tumor cell radiosensitization induced by Hsp90 inhibition. Cancer Res. 2005;65:6967–75.

12. Zaidi S, McLaughlin M, Bhide SA, Eccles SA, Workman P, Nutting CM, Huddart RA, Harrington KJ. The HSP90 inhibitor NVP-AUY922 radiosensitizes by abrogation of homologous recombination resulting in mitotic entry with unresolved DNA damage. PLoS One. 2012;7:e35436.

13. Arlander SJH, Eapen AK, Vroman BT, McDonald RJ, Toft DO, Karnitz LM. Hsp90 inhibition depletes Chk1 and sensitizes tumor cells to replication stress. J Biol Chem. 2003;278:52572–7.

14. Moran DM, Gawlak G, Jayaprakash MS, Mayar S, Maki CG. Geldanamycin promotes premature mitotic entry and micronucleation in irradiated p53/p21 deficient colon carcinoma cells. Oncogene. 2008;27:5567–77.

15. Ha K, Fiskus W, Rao R, Balusu R, Venkannagari S, Nalabothula NR, Bhalla KN. Hsp90 inhibitor-mediated disruption of chaperone association of ATR with hsp90 sensitizes cancer cells to DNA damage. Mol Cancer Ther. 2011;10: 1194–206.

16. Dungey FA, Caldecott KW, Chalmers AJ. Enhanced radiosensitization of human glioma cells by combining inhibition of poly(ADP-ribose) polymerase with inhibition of heat shock protein 90. Mol Cancer Ther. 2009; 8:2243–54.

17. Noguchi M, Yu D, Hirayama R, Ninomiya Y, Sekine E, Kubota N, Ando K, Okayasu R. Inhibition of homologous recombination repair in irradiated tumor cells pretreated with Hsp90 inhibitor 17-allylamino-17-demethoxygeldanamycin. Biochem Biophys Res Commun. 2006;351:658–63.

18. Dote H, Burgan WE, Camphausen K, Tofilon PJ. Inhibition of hsp90 compromises the DNA damage response to radiation. Cancer Res. 2006;66: 9211–20.

19. Quanz M, Herbette A, Sayarath M, de Koning L, Dubois T, Sun J-S, Dutreix M. Heat shock protein 90α (Hsp90α) is phosphorylated in response to DNA damage and accumulates in repair foci. J Biol Chem. 2012;287:8803–15.

20. Eccles SA, Massey A, Raynaud FI, Sharp SY, Box G, Valenti M, Patterson L, de Haven BA, Gowan S, Boxall F, Aherne W, Rowlands M, Hayes A, Martins V, Urban F, Boxall K, Prodromou C, Pearl L, James K, Matthews TP, Cheung K-M, Kalusa A, Jones K, McDonald E, Barril X, Brough PA, Cansfield JE, Dymock B, Drysdale MJ, Finch H, et al. NVP-AUY922: a novel heat shock protein 90 inhibitor active against xenograft tumor growth, angiogenesis, and metastasis. Cancer Res. 2008;68:2850–60.

21. Wang Y, Liu H, Diao L, Potter A, Zhang J, Qiao Y, Wang J, Proia DA, Tailor R, Komaki R, Lin SH. Hsp90 inhibitor ganetespib sensitizes non-small cell lung cancer to radiation but has variable effects with chemoradiation. Clin Cancer Res. 2016;22:5876–86.

22. Hashida S, Yamamoto H, Shien K, Ohtsuka T, Suzawa K, Maki Y, Furukawa M, Soh J, Asano H, Tsukuda K, Miyoshi S, Kanazawa S, Toyooka S. Hsp90 inhibitor NVP-AUY922 enhances the radiation sensitivity of lung cancer cell lines with acquired resistance to EGFR-tyrosine kinase inhibitors. Oncol Rep. 2015;33:1499–504.

23. Choi YE, Battelli C, Watson J, Liu J, Curtis J, Morse AN, Matulonis UA, Chowdhury D, Konstantinopoulos PA. Sublethal concentrations of 17-AAG suppress homologous recombination DNA repair and enhance sensitivity to carboplatin and olaparib in HR proficient ovarian cancer cells. Oncotarget. 2014;5:2678–87.

24. Roh J-L, Kim EH, Park HB, Park JY. The Hsp90 inhibitor 17-(allylamino)-17-demethoxygeldanamycin increases cisplatin antitumor activity by inducing p53-mediated apoptosis in head and neck cancer. Cell Death Dis. 2013;4: e956.

25. Yoshida S, Koga F, Tatokoro M, Kawakami S, Fujii Y, Kumagai J, Neckers L, Kihara K. Low-dose Hsp90 inhibitors tumor-selectively sensitize bladder cancer cells to chemoradiotherapy. Cell Cycle. 2011;10:4291–9.

26. Rasaiyaah J, Tan CP, Fletcher AJ, Price AJ, Blondeau C, Hilditch L, Jacques DA, Selwood DL, James LC, Noursadeghi M, Towers GJ. HIV-1 evades innate immune recognition through specific cofactor recruitment. Nature. 2013; 503:402–5.

27. Greco WR, Bravo G, Parsons JC. The search for synergy: a critical review from a response surface perspective. Pharmacol Rev. 1995;47:331–85.

28. Barker HE, Patel R, McLaughlin M, Schick U, Zaidi S, Nutting CM, Newbold KL, Bhide S, Harrington KJ. CHK1 inhibition radiosensitises head and neck cancers to paclitaxel-based chemoradiotherapy. Mol Cancer Ther. 2016;15(9): 2042–54.

29. Dillon MT, Barker HE, Pedersen M, Hafsi H, Bhide S, Newbold KL, Nutting CM, McLaughlin M, Harrington KJ. Radiosensitization by the ATR inhibitor AZD6738 through generation of acentric micronuclei. Mol Cancer Ther. 2017;16(1):25–34.

30. Pignon J-P, le Maître A, Maillard E, Bourhis J, MACH-NC Collaborative Group. Meta-analysis of chemotherapy in head and neck cancer (MACH-NC): an update on 93 randomised trials and 17,346 patients. Radiother Oncol. 2009; 92:4–14.

31. Ang KK, Zhang Q, Rosenthal DI, Nguyen-Tan PF, Sherman EJ, Weber RS, Galvin JM, Bonner JA, Harris J, El-Naggar AK, Gillison ML, Jordan RC, Konski AA, Thorstad WL, Trotti A, Beitler JJ, Garden AS, Spanos WJ, Yom SS, Axelrod RS. Randomized phase III trial of concurrent accelerated radiation plus cisplatin with or without cetuximab for stage III to IV head and neck carcinoma: RTOG 0522. J Clin Oncol. 2014;32:2940–50.

32. Friedman JA, Wise SC, Hu M, Gouveia C, Vander Broek R, Freudlsperger C, Kannabiran VR, Arun P, Mitchell JB, Chen Z, Van Waes C. HSP90 inhibitor SNX5422/2112 targets the dysregulated signal and transcription factor network and malignant phenotype of head and neck squamous cell carcinoma. Transl Oncol. 2013;6:429–41.

33. Suhane T, Laskar S, Advani S, Roy N, Varunan S, Bhattacharyya D, Bhattacharyya S, Bhattacharyya MK. Both the charged linker region and ATPase domain of hsp90 are essential for rad51-dependent DNA repair. Eukaryot Cell. 2015;14:64–77.

34. Yin X, Zhang H, Lundgren K, Wilson L, Burrows F, Shores CG. BIIB021, a novel Hsp90 inhibitor, sensitizes head and neck squamous cell carcinoma to radiotherapy. Int J Cancer. 2010;126:1216–25.

35. Stingl L, Stühmer T, Chatterjee M, Jensen MR, Flentje M, Djuzenova CS. Novel HSP90 inhibitors, NVP-AUY922 and NVP-BEP800, radiosensitise tumour cells through cell-cycle impairment, increased DNA damage and repair protraction. Br J Cancer. 2010;102:1578–91.

36. Djuzenova CS, Blassl C, Roloff K, Kuger S, Katzer A, Niewidok N, Günther N, Polat B, Sukhorukov VL, Flentje M. Hsp90 inhibitor NVP-AUY922 enhances radiation sensitivity of tumor cell lines under hypoxia. Cancer Biol Ther. 2012;13:425–34.

37. Panier S, Boulton SJ. Double-strand break repair: 53BP1 comes into focus. Nat Rev Mol Cell Biol. 2014;15:7–18.

38. Daley JM, Sung P. 53BP1, BRCA1, and the choice between recombination and end joining at DNA double-strand breaks. Mol Cell Biol. 2014;34:1380–8.

39. Kim H, D'Andrea AD. Regulation of DNA cross-link repair by the Fanconi anemia/BRCA pathway. Genes Dev. 2012;26:1393–408.

40. Bakkenist CJ, Kastan MB. DNA damage activates ATM through intermolecular autophosphorylation and dimer dissociation. Nature. 2003; 421:499–506.

41. Yamamoto K, Nihrane A, Aglipay J, Sironi J, Arkin S, Lipton JM, Ouchi T, Liu JM. Upregulated ATM gene expression and activated DNA crosslink-induced damage response checkpoint in Fanconi anemia: implications for carcinogenesis. Mol Med. 2008;14:167 74.

42. Cortez D. Caffeine inhibits checkpoint responses without inhibiting the ataxia-telangiectasia-mutated (ATM) and ATM- and Rad3-related (ATR) protein kinases. J Biol Chem. 2003;278:37139–45.

43. Banin S, Moyal L, Shieh S, Taya Y, Anderson CW, Chessa L, Smorodinsky NI, Prives C, Reiss Y, Shiloh Y, Ziv Y. Enhanced phosphorylation of p53 by ATM in response to DNA damage. Science. 1998;281:1674–7.

44. Parikh RA, White JS, Huang X, Schoppy DW, Baysal BE, Baskaran R, Bakkenist CJ, Saunders WS, Hsu L-C, Romkes M, Gollin SM. Loss of distal 11q is associated with DNA repair deficiency and reduced sensitivity to ionizing radiation in head and neck squamous cell carcinoma. Genes Chromosomes Cancer. 2007;46:761–75.

45. Knittel G, Liedgens P, Reinhardt HC. Targeting ATM-deficient CLL through interference with DNA repair pathways. Front Genet. 2015;6:207.

46. Dillon MT, Good JS, Harrington KJ. Selective targeting of the G2/M cell cycle checkpoint to improve the therapeutic index of radiotherapy. Clin Oncol (R Coll Radiol). 2014;26:257–65.

47. Menezes DL, Holt J, Tang Y, Feng J, Barsanti P, Pan Y, Ghoddusi M, Zhang W, Thomas G, Holash J, Lees E, Taricani L. A synthetic lethal screen reveals enhanced sensitivity to ATR inhibitor treatment in mantle cell lymphoma with ATM loss-of-function. Mol Cancer Res. 2015;13:120–9.

48. Crasta K, Ganem NJ, Dagher R, Lantermann AB, Ivanova EV, Pan Y, Nezi L, Protopopov A, Chowdhury D, Pellman D. DNA breaks and chromosome pulverization from errors in mitosis. Nature. 2012;482:53–8.

49. Zhang C-Z, Spektor A, Cornils H, Francis JM, Jackson EK, Liu S, Meyerson M, Pellman D. Chromothripsis from DNA damage in micronuclei. Nature. 2015; 522:179–84.

15

Chemoradiotherapy versus surgery followed by postoperative radiotherapy in tonsil cancer: Korean Radiation Oncology Group (KROG) study

Sanghyuk Song[1], Hong-Gyun Wu[2*], Chang Geol Lee[3], Ki Chang Keum[3], Mi Sun Kim[3], Yong Chan Ahn[4], Dongryul Oh[4], Hyo Jung Park[4], Sang-Wook Lee[5], Geumju Park[5], Sung Ho Moon[6], Kwan Ho Cho[6], Yeon-Sil Kim[7], Yongkyun Won[7], Young-Taek Oh[8], Won-Taek Kim[9] and Jae-Uk Jeong[10]

Abstract

Background: Treatment of tonsil cancer, a subset of oropahryngeal cancer, varies between surgery and radiotherapy. Well-designed studies in tonsil cancer have been rare and it is still controversial which treatment is optimal. This study aimed to assess the outcome and failure patterns in tonsil cancer patients treated with either approaches.

Methods: We retrospectively reviewed medical records of 586 patients with tonsil cancer, treated between 1998 and 2010 at 16 hospitals in Korea. Two hundred and one patients received radiotherapy and chemotherapy (CRT), while 385 patients received surgery followed by radiotherapy and/or chemotherapy (SRT). Compared with the SRT group, patients receiving CRT were older, with more advanced T stage and received higher radiotherapy dose given by intensity modulation techniques. Overall survival (OS), disease-free survival (DFS), locoregional recurrence-free survival (LRRFS), distant metastasis-free survival (DMFS), and clinicopathologic factors were analyzed.

Results: At follow-up, the 5-year OS, DFS, LRRFS and DMFS rates in the CRT group were 82, 78, 89, and 94%, respectively, and in the SRT group were 81, 73, 87, and 89%, respectively. Old age, current smoking, poor performance status, advanced T stage, nodal involvement, and induction chemotherapy were associated with poor OS. Induction chemotherapy had a negative prognostic impact on OS in both treatment groups ($p = 0.001$ and $p = 0.033$ in the CRT and SRT groups, respectively).

Conclusions: In our multicenter, retrospective study of tonsil cancer patients, the combined use of radiotherapy and chemotherapy resulted in comparable oncologic outcome to surgery followed by postoperative radiotherapy, despite higher-risk patients having been treated with the definitive radiotherapy. Induction chemotherapy approaches combined with either surgery or definitive radiotherapy were associated with unfavorable outcomes.

Keywords: Tonsil cancer, Chemoradiotherapy, Surgery, Adjuvant radiotherapy, Induction chemotherapy

* Correspondence: wuhg@snu.ac.kr
[2]Department of Radiation Oncology, Seoul National University College of Medicine, 101 Daehangno, Jongno-gu, Seoul 110-744, Republic of Korea
Full list of author information is available at the end of the article

Background

The tonsils, a subsite of the oropharynx, are the most common site of oropharyngeal neoplasm [1]. The incidence of tonsil cancer is increasing [2, 3]. Odynophagia, dysphagia, otalgia and asymptomatic mass is common presentations. Histologically, squamous cell carcinoma is most commonly observed in tonsil cancer. Regional nodal metastases are frequent in more than half of patients, while contralateral nodal diseases are found in more than one fifth of patients with tonsil cancer [4]. Management of tonsil cancer is limited to either surgery or radiotherapy, yet there is a scarcity of randomized prospective trials comparing these treatment options. However, several retrospective studies published similar oncologic outcomes with both modalities [5–7]. Therefore, current guidelines recommend both strategies based on such findings [8].

In recent decades, breakthroughs in the field have included the introduction of chemotherapy, resulting in improved survival rates after definitive radiotherapy and postoperative radiotherapy [9, 10]. Furthermore, randomized clinical trial data showed that more than half of oropharyngeal cancers were human papillomavirus (HPV) positive and responded well to definitive radiotherapy [11]. The incidence of HPV positive tumors is continuously increasing [12]. In the era of chemotherapy and endemic HPV, comparisons of the efficacy between treatment modalities is still controversial. In the present study, we conducted a large-scale retrospective multicenter study to evaluate the outcome of chemoradiotherapy and surgery followed by postoperative radiotherapy in tonsil cancer patients.

Methods

A total of 620 tonsil cancer patients who were treated with radiotherapy between 1998 and 2010 were identified in 16 institutions in Korea. Of these, we analyzed data from 586 patients who were treated with definitive radiotherapy with chemotherapy (CRT; 201 patients) or surgery followed by radiotherapy and/or chemotherapy (SRT; 385 patients). All institutional review boards of participating hospitals approved the collection of these data. The need for consent had been waived by the institutional review boards. Patient demographics, performance status, smoking history, imaging study, stage, pathology, type of surgery, radio- and chemotherapeutic information, and follow-up results were compiled.

The median age at diagnosis was 56 (range, 26–89) and patients were predominantly male (89%). The performance status of most patients was Eastern Cooperative Oncology Group (ECOG) grade 0–1 (94%). More than half of the patients (52%) had a history of smoking. Computed tomography (CT) scans of the neck were performed at diagnosis in 91% of individuals; positron emission tomography (PET) or CT scans were taken in 69% of patients, while magnetic resonance imaging of the oropharynx and neck was performed in 48%.

Patient characteristics according to the two treatment groups are summarized in Table 1. Younger patients and those with early T stage were more likely to receive surgery (p = 0.041 and 0.002, respectively). Unknown histologic differentiation was less frequent in the SRT group. Chemotherapy and intensity modulated radiotherapy (IMRT) were more commonly used in the CRT group (p < 0.001 and 0.014, respectively). Radiotherapy dose was also higher in the CRT group than in those receiving SRT (p < 0.001).

Overall survival (OS) was defined as the time from the date of treatment initiation to either death or last follow-up. Disease-free survival (DFS) was defined as the time from treatment initiation to recurrence, death, or last follow-up. Locoregional recurrence-free survival (LRRFS) and distant metastasis-free survival (DMFS) were defined as the time from treatment initiation to locoregional/distant recurrence or last follow-up, respectively. Univariate and multivariate analyses were performed using the log rank test and Cox-proportional hazard regression model, respectively.

Results

With a median follow-up duration of 54 months (range, 2–176 months), 67 (11%) patients demonstrated locoregional recurrence, while 50 (9%) patients failed with distant metastases. The 5-year OS, DFS, LRRFS, and DMFS rates of the cohort as a whole were 81, 75, 87, and 91%, respectively. When the data from the CRT and SRT groups were analyzed independently, no significant differences were observed between the two groups. The 5-year OS rates were 82 and 81% (p = 0.698) in the CRT and SRT groups, respectively; DFS, 78 and 73% (p = 0.612); LRRFS, 89 and 87% (p = 0.695); and DMFS, 94 and 89% (p = 0.157). The survival curves of each group are plotted in Fig. 1.

Older age, current smoking, advanced T and N stage, and induction chemotherapy treatment were associated with poor OS in the univariate analysis (Table 2). Furthermore, patients undergoing induction chemotherapy showed inferior survival in both treatment groups (Fig. 2); the 5-year OS rates of patients treated with and without induction chemotherapy were 71 and 83%, respectively (p < 0.001). This significant finding was also observed when the treatment groups were analyzed independently; in the CRT group, the 5-year OS rates of patients with or without induction chemotherapy were 70 and 84% (p = 0.001), respectively, and 72% vs 82% in the SRT group (p = 0.033).

The multivariate analysis (Table 3) also indicated that induction chemotherapy was a risk factor for poor OS

Table 1 Patient Characteristics

Characteristic	Number of patients (%)						
	All (n = 586)		CRT (n = 201)		SRT (n = 385)		p-value
Sex							0.913
Male	523	(89)	179	(89)	344	(89)	
Female	63	(11)	22	(11)	41	(11)	
Age (years)							0.041
< 60	395	(67)	125	(62)	270	(70)	
≥ 60	189	(32)	76	(38)	113	(29)	
Unknown	2	(0)	0	(0)	2	(1)	
Smoker							0.673
Never smoker	232	(40)	73	(36)	159	(41)	
Ex-smoker [a]	98	(17)	32	(16)	66	(17)	
Current smoker	206	(35)	73	(36)	133	(35)	
Unknown	50	(8)	23	(11)	27	(7)	
Performance							0.351
ECOG 0	197	(34)	74	(37)	123	(32)	
ECOG 1	351	(60)	117	(58)	234	(61)	
ECOG 2	21	(3)	5	(2)	16	(4)	
Unknown	17	(3)	5	(2)	12	(3)	
PET/CT							0.072
No	182	(31)	72	(36)	110	(29)	
Yes	404	(69)	129	(64)	275	(71)	
Differentiation							<0.001
WD	62	(11)	15	(7)	47	(12)	
MD	297	(51)	73	(36)	224	(58)	
PD	129	(22)	37	(18)	92	(24)	
UD	16	(3)	11	(5)	5	(1)	
Unknown	82	(14)	65	(32)	17	(4)	
T stage							0.002
T1	134	(23)	31	(15)	103	(27)	
T2	292	(50)	101	(50)	191	(50)	
T3	74	(13)	30	(15)	44	(11)	
T4a	73	(12)	30	(15)	43	(11)	
T4b	13	(2)	9	(4)	4	(1)	
N stage							0.779
N0	73	(12)	20	(10)	53	(14)	
N1	79	(13)	28	(14)	51	(13)	
N2a	45	(8)	16	(8)	29	(8)	
N2b	307	(52)	105	(52)	202	(52)	
N2c	60	(10)	23	(11)	37	(10)	
N3	22	(4)	9	(4)	13	(3)	
Stage							0.092
I	8	(1)	2	(1)	6	(2)	
II	42	(7)	23	(11)	37	(10)	

Table 1 Patient Characteristics *(Continued)*

III	82	(14)	29	(14)	53	(14)	
IVA	419	(72)	143	(71)	276	(72)	
IVB	35	(6)	18	(9)	17	(4)	
Chemotherapy							<0.001
Induction	61	(10)	33	(16)	28	(7)	
Concurrent	244	(42)	167	(83)	77	(20)	
Adjuvant	13	(2)	1	(1)	12	(3)	
No	268	(46)	0	(0)	268	(70)	
Radiotherapy technique							0.014
3D–CRT	391	(67)	121	(60)	270	(70)	
IMRT	194	(33)	80	(40)	114	(30)	
Unknown	1	(0)	0	(0)	1	(0)	
Total dose of radiotherapy	Median 66		Median 70		Median 63		<0.001
(Gy)	(range, 25.2–76)		(range, 59.4–76)		(range, 25.2–72.6)		

Abbreviations: CRT radiotherapy with chemotherapy, *SRT* surgery followed by radiotherapy, *ECOG* Eastern Cooperative Oncology Group, *PET/CT* positron emission tomography/computed tomography, *WD* well differentiated, *MD* moderate differentiation, *PD* poor differentiation, *UD* undifferentiated, *3D–CRT* three-dimensional conformal radiotherapy, *IMRT* intensity modulated radiotherapy
[a]An adult who has smoked at least 100 cigarettes in his or her lifetime but who had quit smoking at the time of diagnosis

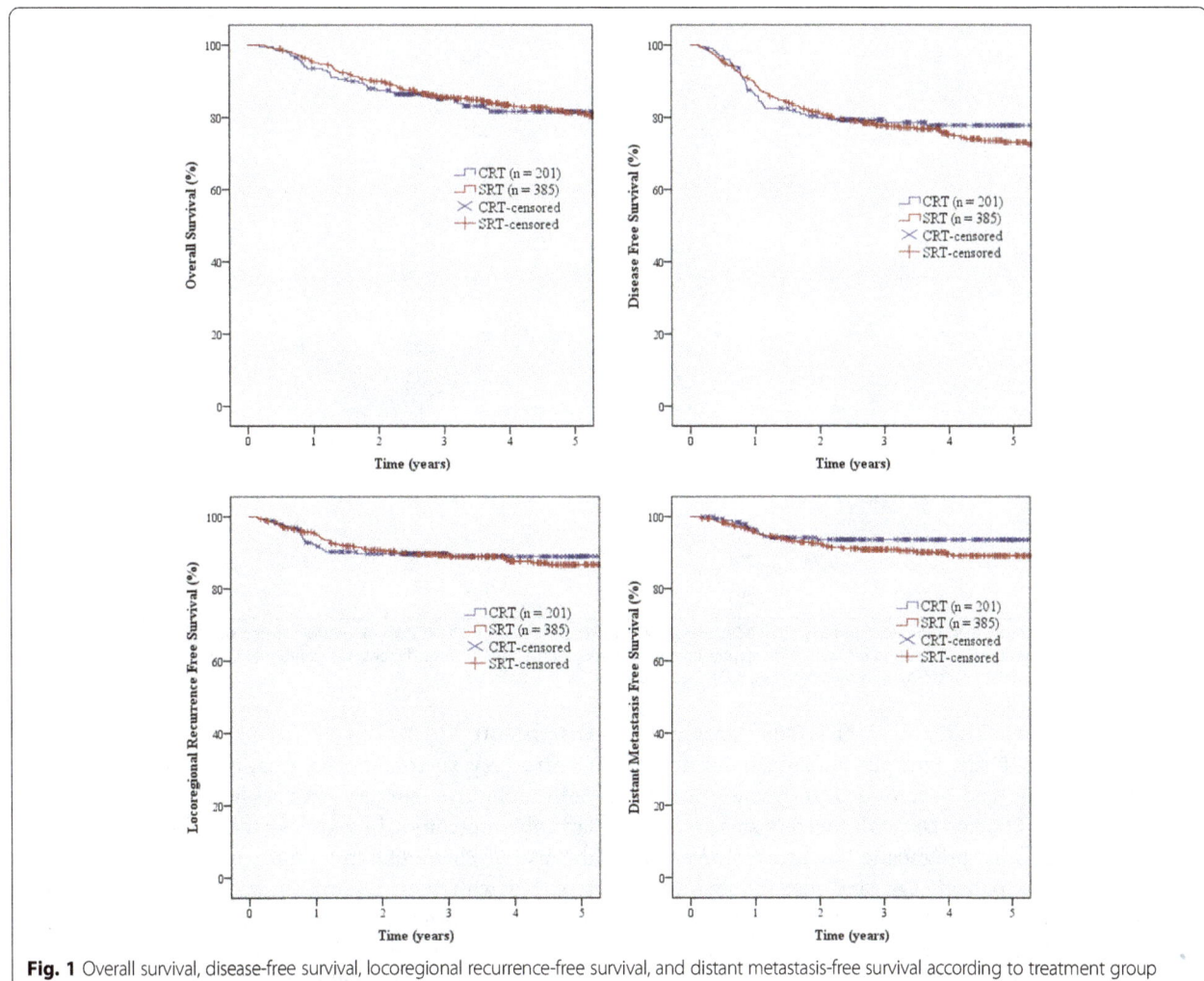

Fig. 1 Overall survival, disease-free survival, locoregional recurrence-free survival, and distant metastasis-free survival according to treatment group

Table 2 Univariate Analyses

Characteristic	OS			DFS			LRRFS			DMFS		
	No.	5Y (%)	p-value	No.	5Y (%)	p-value	No.	5Y (%)	p-value	No.	5Y (%)	p-value
Sex												
Male	523	80	0.082	521	73	0.037	525	86	0.025	522	91	0.787
Female	63	90		63	88		63	94		63	91	
Age (years)												
< 60	395	85	<0.001	393	80	<0.001	395	89	0.121	394	92	0.026
≥ 60	189	73		189	62		189	83		189	86	
Smoking history												
Never/ex-smoker	330	85	0.001	329	79	0.001	330	90	0.005	330	92	0.306
Current smoker	206	76		205	67		206	82		205	89	
Performance status												
ECOG 0	197	85	0.094	197	80	0.027	197	93	0.008	197	92	0.45
ECOG 1–2	372	79		370	72		372	85		371	90	
PET/CT												
No	182	79	0.226	181	74	0.847	182	88	0.669	182	93	0.311
Yes	404	83		403	74		404	87		403	89	
T stage												
T1–T2	426	87	<0.001	425	81	<0.001	426	90	0.003	425	94	<0.001
T3–T4	160	67		159	58		160	81		160	82	
N stage												
N0–N2b	504	84	0.005	503	78	<0.001	504	88	0.055	504	83	<0.001
N2c–N3	82	67		81	55		82	81		81	79	
Stage												
I–III	132	90	0.066	132	85	0.016	132	93	0.06	132	97	0.004
IVA–IVB	454	79		452	72		454	86		453	89	
Chemotherapy												
Concurrent/no	525	83	<0.001	523	76	0.006	525	88	0.263	524	90	0.762
Induction	61	71		61	64		61	83		61	93	
Radiotherapy technique												
3D–CRT	391	80	0.420	389	74	0.36	391	87	0.754	390	90	0.235
IMRT	194	84		194	76		194	88		194	92	
Treatment modality												
CRT	201	82	0.698	201	78	0.612	201	89	0.695	201	94	0.157
SRT	385	81		383	73		385	87		384	89	

Abbreviations: OS overall survival, *DFS* disease-free survival, *LRRFS* locoregional recurrence-free survival, *DMFS* distant metastasis-free survival, *ECOG* Eastern Cooperative Oncology Group, *PET/CT* positron emission tomography–computed tomography, *3D–CRT* three-dimensional conformal radiotherapy, *IMRT* intensity modulated radiotherapy, *CRT* radiotherapy with chemotherapy, *SRT* surgery followed by radiotherapy

and DFS, but not for LRRFS or DMFS. Other prognostic factors such as old age, current smoking, poor initial performance status and advanced T stage were associated with inferior OS. For DFS, advanced N stage was an additional significant prognostic factor. However, in terms of LRRFS, patient age and use of induction chemotherapy were not included in the Cox model. Age, and T and N stage were also identified as independent prognostic factors for DMFS.

Discussion

Controversy surrounds the treatment of tonsil cancer. Both definitive surgery and radiotherapy resulted in favorable outcomes in retrospective studies [5–7]. With the use of chemotherapy, improved survival rates were reported with both treatment modalities [9, 10]. However, no well-designed prospective study comparing radiotherapy and surgery has been completed in the era of widely used chemotherapy. The only prospective

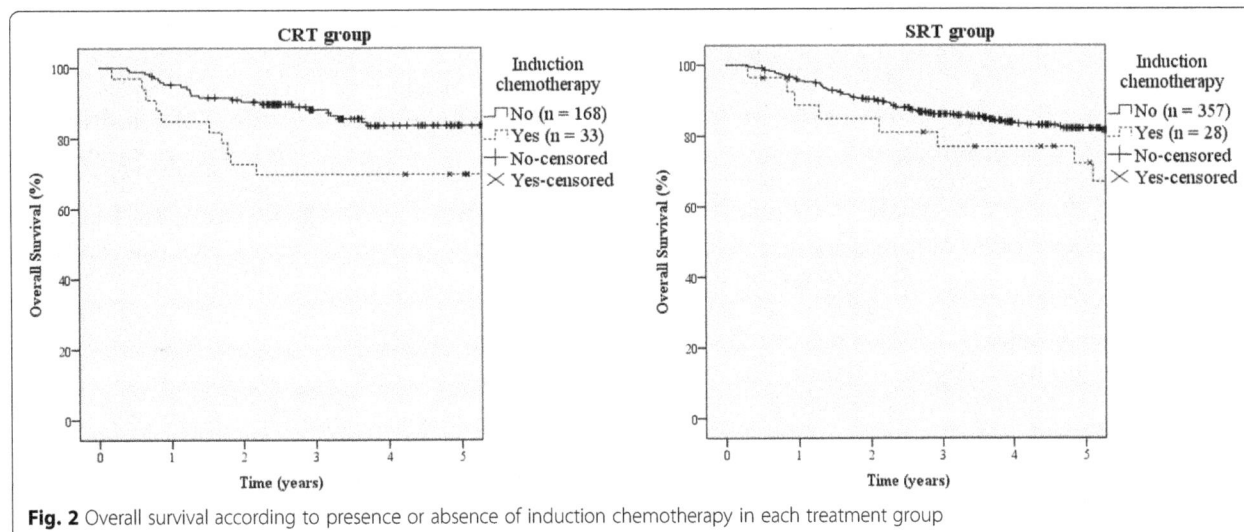

Fig. 2 Overall survival according to presence or absence of induction chemotherapy in each treatment group

randomized trial comparing chemoradiotherapy and surgery followed by radiotherapy was stopped prematurely due to slow accrual and therefore failed to detect any significant difference in DFS between treatment groups [13].

In the present study, we report the outcome of 586 patients from 16 hospitals. To the best of our knowledge, this is one of the largest tonsil cancer cohorts in the literature. We found that old age and advanced T stage which were associated with inferior survival in a multivariate analysis are more found in the CRT group. Despite these discrepancies in patient demographic and disease stage, there was no significant difference between the two treatment modalities under investigation in

terms of survival, recurrence, or failure pattern. Our findings suggest that the CRT approach is more effective than SRT; however, further studies are required to confirm this hypothesis.

If the outcome is comparable between two treatment options, morbidity associated with the treatment becomes important when choosing the treatment modality. Unfortunately, we were unable to collect extensive information regarding treatment-related toxicities. Future trials should address not only the outcomes of treatment, but also any associated complications.

The outcomes of our multicenter study are comparable with those of previously published series. Canis et al. reported the outcome of 102 tonsil cancer patients

Table 3 Multivariate Analyses

Characteristics	OS			DFS			LRRFS			DMFS		
	p-value	HR	95% CI	p-value	HR	95% CI	p-value	HR	95% CI	p-value	HR	95% CI
Age (years)												
≥ 60	<0.001	3.000	2.001–4.497	<0.001	2.516	1.779–3.560				0.009	2.227	1.217–4.077
Smoking history												
Current smoker	0.012	1.663	1.116–2.478	0.015	1.54	1.089–2.176	0.014	1.919	1.141–3.226			
Performance status												
ECOG 1–2	0.045	1.566	1.010–2.426	0.017	1.587	1.087–2.315	0.019	2.094	1.130–3.879			
T stage												
T3–T4	<0.001	2.913	1.943–4.366	<0.001	2.572	1.808–3.659	0.021	1.852	1.097–3.127	<0.001	3.312	1.804–6.082
N stage												
N2c–N3	0.069	1.542	0.966 2.462	0.008	1.735	1.155–2.007	0.075	1.747	0.946–3.226	0.007	2.435	1.271–4.664
Chemotherapy												
Induction	0.003	2.224	1.313–3.768	0.033	1.712	1.044–2.806						

Abbreviations: OS overall survival, DFS disease-free survival, LRRFS locoregional recurrence-free survival, DMFS distant metastasis-free survival, HR hazard ratio, CI confidence interval, ECOG Eastern Cooperative Oncology Group

who were treated with transoral laser microsurgery [14]. The 5-year locoregional control rates of T1–T2 and T3–T4 stage tumors were 78 and 75%, respectively. In the current study, the corresponding rates were 90 and 81%, respectively. Similarly, researchers from MD Anderson Cancer Center reported 5-year locoregional control and OS rates of 97 and 86%, respectively, in 120 patients who were treated with tonsillectomy followed by postoperative radiotherapy [15]. Poulsen et al. studied the outcomes of 148 patients who received surgery followed by radiotherapy or definitive radiotherapy [16], yielding 5-year locoregional control and OS rates of 84 and 57%, respectively. Other studies performed before the early 2000s reported lower 5-year locoregional control rates of 63–77% and OS rates of 53–60% [7, 17–19], possibly because these studies included a large proportion of patients who were treated in the pre-chemotherapy era. Although direct comparisons are not possible, our treatment outcomes are acceptable when compared with the literature.

In the present study, the induction chemotherapy approach negatively influenced both OS and DFS, but had little effect on LRRFS or DMFS in the multivariate analysis. These findings suggest that induction chemotherapy may cause non-cancer related death. Recently, randomized trials reported increased toxicities and no survival gain with induction chemotherapy [20, 21]. Despite the limitations of retrospective studies (e.g., patient selection), our findings support the proposal that the toxicity associated with routine use of induction chemotherapy might be potentially harmful to tonsil cancer patients who are highly curable without such treatment. This is further indicated by our finding that patients with tonsil cancer showed favorable prognosis and a low rate of distant metastasis, despite 86% demonstrating stage III–IVA disease.

Tobacco smoking is a well-known risk factor for head and neck cancer [22]. Indian researchers reported that prior tobacco abuse was an independent poor prognostic factor for DFS and locoregional control in oropharyngeal cancer [23]. Less than half of tumors in that study were located in the tonsils. In our study, current smokers showed significantly worse OS, DFS, and LRRFS than non- or ex-smokers in the multivariate analysis. Differing tumor biology in smokers may affect disease outcome [24]. It is well known that persistent smoking during radiation therapy adversely affects the response and survival rate of head and neck cancer patients [25]. Smoking cessation may be beneficial and should be encouraged in patients with tonsil cancer.

Age of >60 years was associated with a significant risk of death, disease recurrence, and distant metastasis in the multivariate analysis. HPV infection, which correlated with favorable prognosis, was more frequently observed in

younger patients than in the elderly; [12] therefore, smoking history and old age could be secondary surrogates of poor tumor biology which is unrelated to HPV infection. Unfortunately, because the HPV status of patients in the present study was unknown, this hypothesis could not be tested. Regarding that many recent studies for altering therapy based on HPV status are in progress, the lack of details of HPV status in this study has significant limitations [26].

Conclusion

Our large, multicenter, retrospective review of tonsil cancer patients showed favorable survival and disease control. Despite more high-risk patients being treated with definitive chemoradiotherapy than surgery followed by radiotherapy, demonstrated comparable outcomes. Furthermore, our study indicated that induction chemotherapy is correlated with significant risk of death and should not be routinely given to tonsil cancer patients.

Abbreviations
CRT: Chemoradiotherapy; CT: Computed tomography; DFS: Disease-free survival; DMFS: Distant metastasis-free survival; ECOG: Eastern Cooperative Oncology Group; HPV: Human papillomavirus; IMRT: Intensity modulated radiotherapy; KROG: Korean Radiation Oncology Group; LRRFS: Locoregional recurrence-free survival; OS: Overall survival; PET: Positron emission tomography; SRT: Surgery followed by postoperative radiotherapy

Acknowledgements
None.

Funding
This research was supported by a grant from the National Research Foundation of Korea (NRF), which is funded by the Korean government (MEST, grant no.2015M2A2A7055063); a grant of the Korean Health Technology R&D Project, Ministry of Health and Welfare, Republic of Korea (H14C3459); and the National R&D Program through the Dong-nam Institute of Radiological and Medical Sciences (DIRAMS) funded by the Ministry of Education, Science, and Technology (50595–2016). The funding bodies had no role in the design of the study and collection, analysis, and interpretation of data and in writing the manuscript.

Authors' contributions
SS, HGW, LCG, KCK, YCA, DO, SWL, KHC, YSK, YTO and WTK were involved in the study concept and design. Data acquisition was undertaken by CGL, KCK, MSK, DO, HJP, SWL, GP, SHM, YW, YTO, WTK and JUJ. Analysis and interpretation of data were performed by SS, HGW, YCA, YSK and KHC. SS, HGW, HJP, GP, MSK, SHM, YW and JUJ drafted the manuscript. All of the authors have read and approved the final manuscript.

Competing interests
The authors declare that they have no competing interests.

Author details
[1]Department of Radiation Oncology, Kangwon National University Hospital, Baengnyeong-ro 156, Chuncheon 24289, Republic of Korea. [2]Department of Radiation Oncology, Seoul National University College of Medicine, 101 Daehangno, Jongno-gu, Seoul 110-744, Republic of Korea. [3]Department of Radiation Oncology, Yonsei Cancer Center, 50-1 Yonsei-ro, Seodaemun-gu,

Seoul 03722, Republic of Korea. [4]Department of Radiation Oncology, Samsung Medical Center, Sungkyunkwan University School of Medicine, 81 Irwon-Ro Gangnam-gu, Seoul 06351, Republic of Korea. [5]Department of Radiation Oncology, Asan Medical Center, University of Ulsan College of Medicine, Seoul, South Korea. [6]Research Institute and Hospital, National Cancer Center, 323 Ilsan-ro, Ilsandong-gu, Goyang-si, Gyeonggi-do 10408, Republic of Korea. [7]Department of Radiation Oncology, Seoul St. Mary's Hospital, The Catholic University of Korea, 222 Banpo-daero, Seocho-gu, Seoul 06591, Republic of Korea. [8]Department of Radiation Oncology, Ajou University School of Medicine, Gyeonggi, South Korea. [9]Department of Radiation Oncology, Pusan National University Hospital and Pusan National University School of Medicine, 179 Gudeok-ro, Seo-gu, Busan 49241, Republic of Korea. [10]Department of Radiation Oncology, Chonnam National University Medical School, 42 Jebong-ro, Dong-gu, Gwangju 61469, Republic of Korea.

References

1. Cohan DM, Popat S, Kaplan SE, Rigual N, Loree T, Hicks WL Jr. Oropharyngeal cancer: current understanding and management. Curr Opin Otolaryngol Head Neck Surg. 2009;17:88–94.
2. Olaleye O, Moorthy R, Lyne O, Black M, Mitchell D, Wiseberg J. A 20-year retrospective study of tonsil cancer incidence and survival trends in South East England: 1987-2006. Clin Otolaryngol. 2011;36:325–35.
3. Mehta V, Yu GP, Schantz SP. Population-based analysis of oral and oropharyngeal carcinoma: changing trends of histopathologic differentiation, survival and patient demographics. Laryngoscope. 2010;120:2203–12.
4. Chung EJ, Oh JI, Choi KY, et al. Pattern of cervical lymph node metastasis in tonsil cancer: predictive factor analysis of contralateral and retropharyngeal lymph node metastasis. Oral Oncol. 2011;47:758–62.
5. Park G, Lee SW, Kim SY, et al. Can concurrent chemoradiotherapy replace surgery and postoperative radiation for locally advanced stage III/IV tonsillar squamous cell carcinoma? Anticancer Res. 2013;33:1237–43.
6. Koo TR, Wu HG, Hah JH, et al. Definitive radiotherapy versus postoperative radiotherapy for tonsil cancer. Cancer Res Treat. 2012;44:227–34.
7. Mendenhall WM, Amdur RJ, Stringer SP, Villaret DB, Cassisi NJ. Radiation therapy for squamous cell carcinoma of the tonsillar region: a preferred alternative to surgery? J Clin Oncol. 2000;18:2219–25.
8. NCCN Guidelines Panels. NCCN clinical practice guidelines in oncology: head and neck cancers. Available from URL: https://www.nccn.org/professionals/physician_gls/pdf/head-and-neck.pdf. Accessed 29 Aug 2017.
9. Calais G, Alfonsi M, Bardet E, et al. Randomized trial of radiation therapy versus concomitant chemotherapy and radiation therapy for advanced-stage oropharynx carcinoma. J Natl Cancer Inst. 1999;91:2081–6.
10. Cooper JS, Pajak TF, Forastiere AA, et al. Postoperative concurrent radiotherapy and chemotherapy for high-risk squamous-cell carcinoma of the head and neck. N Engl J Med. 2004;350:1937–44.
11. Ang KK, Harris J, Wheeler R, et al. Human papillomavirus and survival of patients with oropharyngeal cancer. N Engl J Med. 2010;363:24–35.
12. Westra WH. The changing face of head and neck cancer in the 21st century: the impact of HPV on the epidemiology and pathology of oral cancer. Head Neck Pathol. 2009;3:78–81.
13. Soo KC, Tan EH, Wee J, et al. Surgery and adjuvant radiotherapy vs concurrent chemoradiotherapy in stage III/IV nonmetastatic squamous cell head and neck cancer: a randomised comparison. Br J Cancer. 2005;93:279–86.
14. Canis M, Martin A, Kron M, et al. Results of transoral laser microsurgery in 102 patients with squamous cell carcinoma of the tonsil. Eur Arch Otorhinolaryngol. 2013;270:2299–306.
15. Yildirim G, Morrison WH, Rosenthal DI, et al. Outcomes of patients with tonsillar carcinoma treated with post-tonsillectomy radiation therapy. Head Neck. 2010;32:473–80.
16. Poulsen M, Porceddu SV, Kingsley PA, Tripcony L, Coman W. Locally advanced tonsillar squamous cell carcinoma: treatment approach revisited. Laryngoscope. 2007;117:45–50.
17. Mendenhall WM, Morris CG, Amdur RJ, et al. Definitive radiotherapy for tonsillar squamous cell carcinoma. Am J Clin Oncol. 2006;29:290–7.
18. Pernot M, Malissard L, Hoffstetter S, et al. Influence of tumoral, radiobiological, and general factors on local-control and survival of a series of 361 tumors of the velotonsillar area treated by exclusive irradiation (external-beam irradiation plus brachytherapy or brachytherapy alone). Int J Radiat Oncol Biol Phys. 1994;30:1051–7.
19. Perez CA, Patel MM, Chao KSC, et al. Carcinoma of the tonsillar fossa: prognostic factors and long-term therapy outcome. Int J Radiat Oncol BiolPhys. 1998;42:1077–84.
20. Haddad R, O'Neill A, Rabinowits G, et al. Induction chemotherapy followed by concurrent chemoradiotherapy (sequential chemoradiotherapy) versus concurrent chemoradiotherapy alone in locally advanced head and neck cancer (PARADIGM): a randomised phase 3 trial. Lancet Oncol. 2013;14:257–64.
21. Cohen EEW, Karrison T, Kocherginsky M, et al. DeCIDE: a phase III randomized trial of docetaxel (D), cisplatin (P), 5-fluorouracil (F) (TPF) induction chemotherapy (IC) in patients with N2/N3 locally advanced squamous cell carcinoma of the head and neck (SCCHN). ASCO Meeting Abstracts. 2012;30: 5500.
22. Marur S, Forastiere AA. Head and neck cancer: changing epidemiology, diagnosis, and treatment. Mayo Clin Proc. 2008;83:489–501.
23. Agarwal JP, Mallick I, Bhutani R, et al. Prognostic factors in oropharyngeal cancer–analysis of 627 cases receiving definitive radiotherapy. Acta Oncol. 2009;48:1026–33.
24. Ragin CC, Taioli E, Weissfeld JL, et al. 11q13 amplification status and human papillomavirus in relation to p16 expression defines two distinct etiologies of head and neck tumours. Br J Cancer. 2006;95:1432–8.
25. Browman GP, Wong G, Hodson I, et al. Influence of cigarette smoking on the efficacy of radiation therapy in head and neck cancer. N Engl J Med. 1993;328(3):159–63.
26. Vokes EE, Agrawal N, Seiwert TY. HPV-associated head and neck cancer. J Natl Cancer Inst. 2015;107(12):djv344.

16

Regular recreational physical activity and risk of head and neck cancer

Chen-Lin Lin[1†], Wei-Ting Lee[2†], Chun-Yen Ou[2], Jenn-Ren Hsiao[2], Cheng-Chih Huang[2], Jehn-Shyun Huang[3], Tung-Yiu Wong[3], Ken-Chung Chen[3], Sen-Tien Tsai[2], Sheen-Yie Fang[2], Tze-Ta Huang[3], Jiunn-Liang Wu[2], Yuan-Hua Wu[4], Wei-Ting Hsueh[4], Chia-Jui Yen[5], Yu-Hsuan Lai[4], Hsiao-Chen Liao[2], Shang-Yin Wu[5], Ming-Wei Yang[4], Forn-Chia Lin[4], Jang-Yang Chang[5,6], Yi-Hui Wang[6], Ya-Ling Weng[6], Han-Chien Yang[6], Yu-Shan Chen[2] and Jeffrey S. Chang[6*]

Abstract

Background: Although substantial evidence supports a 20–30% risk reduction of colon cancer, breast cancer, and endometrial cancer by physical activity (PA), the evidence for head and neck cancer (HNC) is limited. Three published studies on the association between PA and HNC have generated inconsistent results. The current study examined the association between recreational PA (RPA) and HNC risk with a more detailed assessment on the intensity, frequency, duration, and total years of RPA.

Methods: Data on RPA were collected from 623 HNC cases and 731 controls by in-person interview using a standardized questionnaire. The association between RPA and HNC risk was assessed using unconditional logistic regression, adjusted for sex, age, educational level, use of alcohol, betel quid, and cigarette, and consumption of vegetables and fruits.

Results: A significant inverse association between RPA and HNC risk was observed in a logistic regression model that adjusted for sex, age, and education (odds ratio (OR) = 0.65, 95% confidence interval (CI): 0.51-0.82). However, after further adjustment for the use of alcohol, betel quid, and cigarette, and consumption of vegetables and fruits, RPA was no longer associated with HNC risk (OR =0.97, 95% CI: 0.73-1.28). No significant inverse association between RPA and HNC risk was observed in the analysis stratified by HNC sites or by the use of alcohol, betel quid, or cigarette.

Conclusion: Results from our study did not support an inverse association between RPA and HNC risk. The major focus of HNC prevention should be on cessation of cigarette smoking and betel chewing, reduction of alcohol drinking, and promotion of healthy diet that contains plenty of fruits and vegetables.

Keywords: Physical activity, Head and neck cancer, Case–control

* Correspondence: jeffreychang@nhri.org.tw
†Equal contributors
6National Institute of Cancer Research, National Health Research Institutes, 1F No 367, Sheng-Li Road, Tainan 70456, Taiwan
Full list of author information is available at the end of the article

Background

Head and neck cancer (HNC) (cancers of the oral cavity, oropharynx, hypopharynx, and larynx) is the fifth leading cancer in the world, with approximately 600,000 annual incident cases [1]. The majority of HNC cases are due to alcohol drinking, cigarette smoking, or betel quid chewing [2]. Recently, there is an increasing trend in the incidence of human papillomavirus-associated oropharyngeal cancer [3]. Studies of HNC have focused mostly on the risk factors and less information is available regarding factors associated with a decreased HNC risk. To date, only consumption of fruits and vegetables has been consistently associated with a reduced HNC risk [4].

Physical inactivity has been identified as the fourth leading contributor to global mortality [5]. The World Health Organization recommends adults 18–64 years old to perform at least 150 min of moderate-intensity aerobic physical activity (PA) or 75 min of vigorous-intensity aerobic PA per week [5]. Many studies have investigated the benefit of PA to reduce the risk of cancer. There is substantial evidence to support a 20–30% risk reduction of colon cancer, breast cancer, and endometrial cancer by PA, while the evidence for other cancers is limited [6, 7].

PA may have the potential to influence HNC risk by modulating the level of immunoglobulin A (IgA), which is the major class of antibodies in the fluids secreted by the mucosal surface, including saliva. IgA may serve as the first-line defense against foreign agents, including environmental carcinogens. It was shown that compared to the saliva of healthy controls, saliva of oral cancer patients had 45% lower level of IgA [8, 9].

To date, only three studies have investigated the association between PA and HNC risk and the results have been inconsistent. A cohort study by Leitzmann et al. reported a null association between recreational PA (RPA) and HNC risk while another cohort study by Hashibe et al. reported a significant inverse association between PA and HNC [10, 11]. A case–control study by Nicolotti et al. observed a 22% reduction in HNC risk with moderate RPA [12]. These studies did not have complete assessment of PA. Leitzmann et al. only examined the frequency (times per week) of PA [10]. Hashibe et al. only examined hours spent in vigorous activity per week [11], and Nicolotti et al. did not have sufficient information to calculate metabolic equivalent of task (MET) for evaluating dose–response relationship [12].

The current study examined the association between RPA and HNC risk with complete information on the intensity, frequency, duration, and total years of RPA.

Methods

The institutional review boards of the National Health Research Institutes and the National Cheng Kung University Hospital approved this study. A signed informed consent was obtained from all participants of the study.

Study subject recruitment

Data for the current analysis are from an ongoing HNC case–control study that began subject recruitment on September 1, 2010. Because questions on RPA were added later, the current analysis included subjects that were recruited from March 20, 2011 to October 29, 2015. Subject recruitment was conducted in the Department of Otolaryngology and the Department of Stomatology at the National Cheng Kung University Hospital. The eligibility criteria for the cases were: 1) pathologically confirmed diagnosis of squamous cell carcinoma of the head and neck, including cancers of the oral cavity, oropharynx, hypopharynx, and larynx; 2) no history of any type of cancer diagnosis; and 3) between the age of 20 and 80. Controls were recruited for comparing the risk of HNC and were selected by frequency-matching according to the sex and age (±5 years) distributions of the cases. The eligibility criteria for the controls were: 1) subjects who underwent surgery for non-cancerous conditions that are not associated with the consumption of alcohol, betel quid, and cigarette, with the most common diagnoses being benign lesions of the head and neck (oral cavity, oropharynx, hypopharynx, and larynx), chronic otitis media, chronic sinusitis, neck lipoma, obstructive sleep apnea, sialolithiasis, and thyroglossal duct cyst; 2) no history of any type of cancer diagnosis; and 3) between the age of 20 and 80.

Data collection by interview

Each study participant was interviewed by a trained interviewer using a standardized questionnaire to collect information on demographic characteristics (sex, age, and educational level) and regular RPA (Questions on RPA in Chinese can be seen on Additional file 1: Questionnaire). Each participant was asked whether he or she had been participating in RPA for at least three days a week, which we defined as regular RPA. Those with a positive response were further asked about the type of RPA, frequency (number of days per week), duration (number of hours per day), and the total years involved in each type of RPA. Individuals who engage in RPA may have a healthier lifestyle in general with less consumption of alcohol, betel quid, and cigarette and higher intake of vegetables and fruits, which have all been shown to influence HNC risk (Fig. 1). Therefore, to account for the potential confounding effect of other lifestyle factors, we also collected information on the use of alcohol, betel quid, and cigarette, and intake of vegetables and fruits. For alcohol, betel quid, and cigarette, detailed information was collected on starting age, quitting age (for former users), and dose (number of cigarettes per day, number of betel quids per day, and

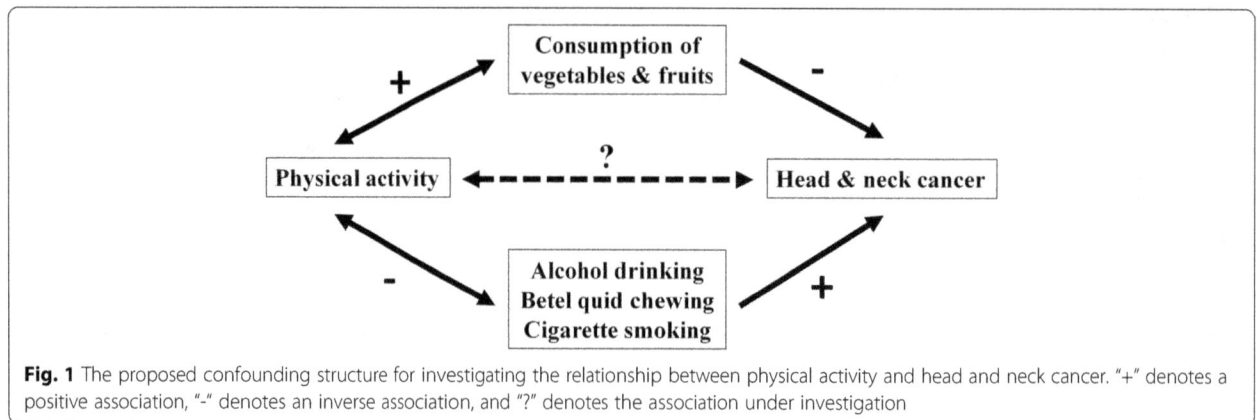

Fig. 1 The proposed confounding structure for investigating the relationship between physical activity and head and neck cancer. "+" denotes a positive association, "-" denotes an inverse association, and "?" denotes the association under investigation

drinks of alcohol per week with each drink =150 ml of alcohol). For vegetables and fruits, participants were asked about the number of days per week that they ate vegetables or fruits.

Statistical analysis

The distributions of demographic variables and lifestyle factors (alcohol drinking, betel quid chewing, cigarette smoking, and consumption of vegetables and fruits) between cases and controls were compared by performing T-tests (for continuous variables) and chi-squared tests (for categorical variables).

Odds ratio (OR) and 95% confidence interval (CI) were estimated to analyze the association between RPA and HNC risk using unconditional logistic regression, adjusted for sex, age, educational level, alcohol drinking (frequency), betel quid chewing (pack-years), cigarette smoking (pack-years), and consumption of vegetables and fruits (daily vs. non-daily). The pack-year of cigarette smoking = (number of cigarettes smoked per day/20) x number of years smoked. The pack-year of betel quid chewing = (number of betel quids chewed per day/20) x number of years chewed. We did not adjust for body mass index because we considered body mass index as an intermediate variable and not a confounder on the association between RPA and HNC risk. RPA was analyzed in several ways: 1) as a yes/no variable, with yes =3 or more days per week, no = less than 3 days per week; 2) by intensity: each type of RPA was assigned a MET value according to the 2011 Compendium of Physical Activities [13]. Each RPA was then assigned an intensity with light intensity =1.6-2.9 METs, moderate intensity =3.0-5.9 METs, and vigorous intensity =6.0 or more METs [14]. Individuals engaging in multiple RPAs with different levels of intensity were assigned the highest intensity among the multiple RPAs; 3) by frequency: no RPA (= less than 3 days per week), 3 days per week, 4–5 days per week, and 6–7 days per week; 4) by total MET-hours per week: for each individual, MET-hours

per week was calculated for each type of RPA = MET for specific RPA x hours per day x days per week. Total MET-hours were then calculated by summing the MET-hours per week of all the RPAs performed for each individual; and 5) by the total of years RPA.

The development of HNC may influence an individual's capability of performing RPA. To assess the possibility of reverse causality between RPA and HNC risk, sensitivity analysis was performed by censoring RPA at 5 years before the reference date (date of HNC diagnosis for the cases and date of interview for the controls).

Unconditional logistic regression was performed stratified by the use of alcohol, betel quid, or cigarette to examine the influence of alcohol, betel quid, or cigarette consumption on the association between RPA and HNC. Unconditional logistic regression model with the interaction term (RPA x alcohol, RPA x betel quid, or RPA x cigarette) was compared with the model without the interaction term by the log-likelihood ratio test to assess the heterogeneity between strata.

Results

This analysis included 623 HNC cases and 731 controls. Cases and controls had similar mean age (55.4 years vs. 54.6 years, $P = 0.20$) (Table 1). Because the study is still ongoing with case–control frequency matching, case group had a higher percentage of women than the control group (6.7% vs. 2.5% $P = 0.0001$). More cases were users of alcohol, betel quid, and cigarette compared to controls ($P < 0.0001$). More controls ate vegetables and fruits daily than HNC cases ($P < 0.0001$).

Among either HNC cases or controls, those who participated in regular RPA were less likely to consume alcohol, betel quid, or cigarette and more likely to eat vegetables and fruits daily (Table 2).

In the unconditional logistic regression model adjusted for sex, age, and education (Model 1), RPA was associated with a significantly decreased HNC risk (OR =0.65, 95% CI = 0.51-0.82) (Table 3). After additional adjustment for

Table 1 Demographic and lifestyle characteristics of the head and neck cancer patients and control subjects

Characteristics	Case N = 623 n (%)	Control N = 731 n (%)	P
Age (years)			
Mean (SE)	55.4 (0.4)	54.6 (0.4)	0.20
Sex			
Men	581 (93.3)	713 (97.5)	0.0001
Women	42 (6.7)	18 (2.5)	
Education			
≤ Elementary school	168 (27.0)	123 (16.8)	<0.0001
Junior high	185 (29.7)	133 (18.2)	
High school/Technical school	202 (32.4)	259 (35.4)	
Some college or more	68 (10.9)	216 (29.6)	
Alcohol drinking			
Never + occasional	196 (31.5)	385 (52.7)	<0.0001
Former regular	89 (14.3)	93 (12.7)	
Current regular	338 (54.2)	253 (34.6)	
Never	186 (29.9)	351 (48.0)	<0.0001
1 drink or less per month	10 (1.6)	34 (4.7)	
1-2 drinks per week	26 (4.2)	51 (7.0)	
3-5 drinks per week	32 (5.1)	44 (6.0)	
Daily drinkers	353 (56.6)	245 (33.5)	
Unknown	16 (2.6)	6 (0.8)	
Betel quid chewing			
Never	179 (28.7)	509 (69.7)	<0.0001
Former	235 (37.7)	141 (19.3)	
Current	209 (33.6)	80 (10.9)	
Unknown	0 (0.0)	1 (0.1)	
Never	179 (28.7)	509 (69.7)	<0.0001
0.1–9.9 pack-years	92 (14.8)	74 (10.1)	
10.0–19.9 pack-years	75 (12.0)	44 (6.0)	
20.0–29.9 pack-years	68 (10.9)	32 (4.4)	
30.0 or more pack-years	193 (31.0)	69 (9.4)	
Unknown	16 (2.6)	3 (0.4)	
Pack-years (SE)	26.8 (1.6)	8.3 (0.8)	<0.0001
Cigarette smoking			
Never	89 (14.3)	230 (31.5)	<0.0001
Former	117 (18.8)	146 (20.0)	
Current	416 (66.8)	354 (48.4)	
Unknown	1 (0.1)	1 (0.1)	
Never	89 (14.3)	230 (31.5)	<0.0001
0.1–9.9 pack-years	27 (4.3)	61 (8.3)	
10.0–19.9 pack-years	58 (9.3)	89 (12.2)	
20.0–29.9 pack-years	109 (17.5)	90 (12.3)	

Table 1 Demographic and lifestyle characteristics of the head and neck cancer patients and control subjects (Continued)

	Case	Control	P
30.0 or more pack-years	332 (53.3)	256 (35.0)	
Unknown	8 (1.3)	5 (0.7)	
Pack-years (SE)	35.8 (1.1)	23.8 (1.0)	<0.0001
Vegetable intake			
Non-daily	113 (18.1)	59 (8.1)	<0.0001
Daily	508 (81.6)	672 (91.9)	
Unknown	2 (0.3)	0 (0.0)	
Fruit intake			
Non-daily	434 (69.6)	334 (45.7)	<0.0001
Daily	186 (29.9)	396 (54.2)	
Unknown	3 (0.5)	1 (0.1)	

Abbreviations: N number, SE standard error

consumption of alcohol, betel quid, and cigarette (Model 2) the OR moved toward the null and became non-statistically significant (OR =0.83, 95%: 0.64-1.09). Further adjustment for daily intake of vegetables and fruits (Model 3) generated a null association between RPA and HNC risk (OR =0.97, 95% CI: 0.73-1.28). For the intensity of RPA, the model with adjustment for sex, age, and education showed an inverse trend between the intensity of RPA and HNC risk with moderate and vigorous intensity being associated with a significantly reduced HNC risk (moderate intensity: OR =0.72, 95% CI: 0.53-0.98; vigorous intensity: OR =0.57, 95% CI: 0.42-0.77). However, after additional adjustment for alcohol, betel quid, cigarette, vegetables, and fruits, the reduced HNC risk associated with moderate intensity RPA became null (OR =1.09, 95% CI: 0.77-1.54) and the reduced HNC risk associated with vigorous intensity RPA became non-statistically significant (OR =0.85, 95% CI: 0.60-1.22). The analyses with RPA frequency, total MET-hours per week, and total years all showed a significant inverse association with HNC risk in models adjusted for sex, age, and education, although a dose–response relationship was not apparent. After further adjustment for alcohol, betel quid, cigarette, vegetables, and fruits, no significant association was found between HNC risk and RPA frequency, total MET-hours per week, or total years.

We performed sensitivity analysis by censoring RPA at 5 years before the reference date (date of HNC diagnosis for the cases and date of interview for the controls). The result showed a null association between RPA censored at 5 years before the reference date and HNC risk (OR =1.08, 95% CI = 0.77-1.51).

No significant association was observed between RPA (yes/no, intensity, frequency, and total MET-hours per week) and HNC risk in analyses stratified by HNC sites (Table 4). No significant association between total years

Table 2 The association between regular recreational physical activity and lifestyle characteristics by head and neck cancer status

Characteristics	Case			Control		
	No regular recreational physical activity N = 414 n (%)	Regular recreational physical activity N = 209 n (%)	P	No regular recreational physical activity N = 397 n (%)	Regular recreational physical activity N = 334 n (%)	P
Alcohol drinking						
Never + occasional	117 (28.3)	79 (37.8)	0.004	197 (49.6)	188 (56.3)	0.19
Former regular	53 (12.8)	36 (17.2)		55 (13.9)	38 (11.4)	
Current regular	244 (58.9)	94 (45.0)		145 (36.5)	108 (32.3)	
Never	111 (26.8)	75 (35.9)	0.07	177 (44.6)	174 (52.1)	0.02
1 drink or less per month	6 (1.4)	4 (1.9)		20 (5.0)	14 (4.2)	
1-2 drinks per week	17 (4.1)	9 (4.3)		29 (7.3)	22 (6.6)	
3-5 drinks per week	19 (4.6)	13 (6.2)		17 (4.3)	27 (8.1)	
Daily drinkers	252 (60.9)	101 (48.3)		151 (38.0)	94 (28.1)	
Unknown	9 (2.2)	7 (3.4)		3 (0.8)	3 (0.9)	
Betel quid chewing						
Never	93 (22.5)	86 (41.2)	<0.0001	246 (61.9)	263 (78.7)	<0.0001
Former	158 (38.1)	77 (36.8)		86 (21.7)	55 (16.5)	
Current	163 (39.4)	46 (22.0)		65 (16.4)	15 (4.5)	
Unknown	0 (0.0)	0 (0.0)		0 (0.0)	1 (0.3)	
Never	93 (22.5)	86 (41.2)	<0.0001	246 (61.9)	263 (78.7)	<0.0001
0.1–9.9 pack-years	59 (14.3)	33 (15.8)		49 (12.3)	25 (7.5)	
10.0–19.9 pack-years	49 (11.8)	26 (12.4)		28 (7.1)	16 (4.8)	
20.0–29.9 pack-years	54 (13.0)	14 (6.7)		21 (5.3)	11 (3.3)	
30.0 or more pack-years	147 (35.5)	46 (22.0)		51 (12.9)	18 (5.4)	
Unknown	12 (2.9)	4 (1.9)		2 (0.5)	1 (0.3)	
Pack-years (SE)	30.5 (2.1)	19.5 (2.3)	0.0004	10.8 (1.3)	5.3 (1.0)	0.0007
Cigarette smoking						
Never	43 (10.4)	46 (22.0)	<0.0001	101 (25.4)	129 (38.6)	<0.0001
Former	65 (15.7)	52 (24.9)		60 (15.1)	86 (25.8)	
Current	305 (73.7)	111 (53.1)		236 (59.5)	118 (35.3)	
Unknown	1 (0.2)	0 (0.0)		0 (0.0)	1 (0.3)	
Never	43 (10.4)	46 (22.0)	0.004	101 (25.4)	129 (38.6)	0.0004
0.1–9.9 pack-years	18 (4.4)	9 (4.3)		29 (7.3)	32 (9.6)	
10.0–19.9 pack-years	39 (9.4)	19 (9.1)		48 (12.1)	41 (12.3)	
20.0–29.9 pack-years	72 (17.4)	37 (17.7)		54 (13.6)	36 (10.8)	
30.0 or more pack-years	234 (56.5)	98 (46.9)		162 (40.8)	94 (28.1)	
Unknown	8 (1.9)	0 (0.0)		3 (0.8)	2 (0.6)	
Pack-years (SE)	37.8 (1.3)	32.0 (2.1)	0.02	27.5 (1.4)	19.4 (1.4)	<0.0001
Vegetable intake						
Non-daily	95 (22.9)	18 (8.6)	<0.0001	44 (11.1)	15 (4.5)	0.001
Daily	317 (76.6)	191 (91.4)		353 (88.9)	319 (95.5)	
Unknown	2 (0.5)	0 (0.0)		0 (0.0)	0 (0.0)	
Fruit intake						
Non-daily	328 (79.2)	106 (50.7)	<0.0001	229 (57.7)	105 (31.4)	<0.0001
Daily	83 (20.1)	103 (49.3)		167 (42.1)	229 (68.6)	
Unknown	3 (0.7)	0 (0.0)		1 (0.2)	0 (0.0)	

Table 3 The association between regular recreational physical activity and head and neck cancer

Regular recreational physical activity	Case N = 623 n (%)	Control N = 731 n (%)	Model 1[a] OR (95% CI)	Model 2[b] OR (95% CI)	Model 3[c] OR (95% CI)
Yes/No					
No regular exercise	414 (66.5)	397 (54.3)	Reference	Reference	Reference
Regular exercise	209 (33.5)	334 (45.7)	0.65 (0.51–0.82)	0.83 (0.64–1.09)	0.97 (0.73–1.28)
Intensity					
No regular exercise	414 (66.5)	397 (54.3)	Reference	Reference	Reference
light	10 (1.6)	10 (1.4)	0.88 (0.34–2.25)	0.98 (0.36–2.65)	1.07 (0.39–2.92)
moderate	114 (18.3)	154 (21.1)	0.72 (0.53–0.98)	0.95 (0.68–1.33)	1.09 (0.77–1.54)
vigorous	85 (13.6)	170 (23.3)	0.57 (0.42–0.77)	0.72 (0.51–1.02)	0.85 (0.60–1.22)
Frequency					
No regular exercise	414 (66.5)	397 (54.3)	Reference	Reference	Reference
3 days per week	38 (6.1)	60 (8.2)	0.76 (0.49-1.19)	1.13 (0.69-1.85)	1.29 (0.78-2.14)
4–5 days per week	26 (4.2)	54 (7.4)	0.50 (0.30-0.83)	0.72 (0.41-1.27)	0.83 (0.47-1.47)
6–7 days per week	145 (23.2)	220 (30.1)	0.66 (0.50-0.86)	0.79 (0.58-1.07)	0.93 (0.68-1.27)
Total MET-hours per week					
No regular exercise	414 (66.5)	397 (54.3)	Reference	Reference	Reference
0.1–10.0	43 (6.9)	64 (8.8)	0.63 (0.41–0.98)	0.84 (0.52–1.37)	0.95 (0.58–1.55)
10.1–20.0	63 (10.1)	91 (12.4)	0.68 (0.47–0.98)	0.82 (0.55–1.24)	0.93 (0.61–1.41)
20.1–30.0	38 (6.1)	64 (8.8)	0.63 (0.40–0.98)	0.82 (0.50–1.34)	0.97 (0.59–1.59)
> 30.0	64 (10.3)	115 (15.7)	0.64 (0.45–0.91)	0.84 (0.56–1.24)	1.02 (0.68–1.54)
Unknown	1 (0.1)	0 (0.0)	–	–	–
Total years of regular exercise					
No regular exercise	414 (66.5)	397 (54.3)	Reference	Reference	Reference
0.1–5.0	114 (18.3)	165 (22.6)	0.71 (0.53–0.94)	0.80 (0.58–1.10)	0.90 (0.64–1.25)
5.1–10.0	46 (7.4)	92 (12.6)	0.51 (0.34–0.76)	0.66 (0.42–1.03)	0.82 (0.52–1.28)
> 10	49 (7.8)	77 (10.5)	0.69 (0.46–1.05)	1.28 (0.80–2.03)	1.54 (0.96–2.49)

Abbreviations: *CI* confidence interval, *N* number, *OR* odds ratio
[a]Model 1: OR and 95% CI were calculated using unconditional logistic regression, adjusted for sex, age, and education
[b]Model 2: OR and 95% CI were calculated using unconditional logistic regression, adjusted for sex, age, education, cigarette smoking (pack-year categories), betel quid chewing (pack-year categories), and alcohol drinking (frequency)
[c]Model 3: OR and 95% CI were calculated using unconditional logistic regression, adjusted for sex, age, education, cigarette smoking (pack-year categories), betel quid chewing (pack-year categories), alcohol drinking (frequency), and intake of vegetables and fruits

of RPA and risk of pharyngeal cancer or laryngeal cancer was observed. A positive association was found between >10 years of RPA and oral cancer risk (OR =1.87, 95% CI: 1.06-3.28).

In analysis stratified by the use of alcohol, betel quid, or cigarette, no significant association was found between RPA and HNC risk (Table 5).

Discussion

In the current analysis, we found a significant inverse association between RPA and HNC risk in the logistic regression model that adjusted for sex, age, and education. However, after further adjustment for the use of alcohol, betel quid, and cigarette, and consumption of vegetables and fruits, RPA was no longer associated with HNC risk. No significant inverse association between RPA and HNC

risk was observed in the analysis stratified by HNC sites or by the use of alcohol, betel quid, or cigarette.

To date, three studies have been published on the association between PA and HNC and the results have been inconsistent. Leitzmann et al. examined the association between RPA and HNC risk in a cohort of 487,732 subjects [10]. They found that individuals who engaged in RPA five or more times per week had a reduced HNC risk (relative risk (RR) = 0.62, 95% CI: 0.52-0.74) compared to those who performed RPA less than once per month in a statistical model that adjusted for age and sex only [10]. After including smoking as an additional covariate, the RR moved substantially toward the null and became non-statistically significant (RR = 0.86, 95% CI: 0.72-1.03) [10]. Further adjustment for body mass index, race/ethnicity, marital status, family history of any

Table 4 The association between regular recreational physical activity and head and neck cancer by disease site

Regular recreational physical activity	Control N = 731 n (%)	Oral Cancer Cases N = 395 n (%)	OR (95% CI)[a]	Pharyngeal Cancer Cases N = 154 n (%)	OR (95% CI)[a]	Laryngeal Cancer Cases N = 74 n (%)	OR (95% CI)[a]
Yes/No							
No regular exercise	397 (54.3)	265 (67.1)	Reference	107 (69.5)	Reference	42 (56.8)	Reference
Regular exercise	334 (45.7)	130 (32.9)	1.02 (0.74–1.41)	47 (30.5)	0.79 (0.49–1.27)	32 (43.2)	1.03 (0.58–1.85)
Intensity							
No regular exercise	397 (54.3)	265 (67.1)	Reference	107 (69.5)	Reference	42 (56.8)	Reference
light	10 (1.4)	5 (1.3)	0.91 (0.26–3.12)	1 (0.6)	0.27 (0.3–2.49)	4 (5.4)	2.45 (0.61–9.95)
moderate	154 (21.1)	71 (17.9)	1.19 (0.80–1.78)	26 (16.9)	0.89 (0.49–1.61)	17 (23.0)	0.93 (0.46–1.87)
vigorous	170 (23.3)	54 (13.7)	0.87 (0.58–1.32)	20 (13.0)	0.75 (0.41–1.38)	11 (14.8)	1.01 (0.45–2.24)
Frequency							
No regular exercise	397 (54.3)	265 (67.1)	Reference	107 (69.5)	Reference	42 (56.8)	Reference
3 days per week	60 (8.2)	23 (5.8)	1.34 (0.73–2.44)	11 (7.1)	1.44 (0.65–3.19)	4 (5.4)	1.19 (0.36–3.96)
4–5 days per week	54 (7.4)	21 (5.3)	1.02 (0.54–1.92)	4 (2.6)	0.51 (0.16–1.59)	1 (1.3)	0.32 (0.04–2.55)
6–7 days per week	220 (30.1)	86 (21.8)	0.95 (0.66–1.38)	32 (20.8)	0.70 (0.41–1.22)	27 (36.5)	1.14 (0.61–2.12)
Total MET-hours per week							
No regular exercise	397 (54.3)	265 (67.1)	Reference	107 (69.5)	Reference	42 (56.8)	Reference
0.1-10.0	64 (8.8)	29 (7.3)	1.07 (0.61–1.90)	11 (7.1)	0.90 (0.40–2.01)	3 (4.0)	0.43 (0.12–1.60)
10.1-20.0	91 (12.4)	37 (9.4)	0.94 (0.58–1.53)	13 (8.4)	0.59 (0.28–1.23)	13 (17.6)	1.14 (0.52–2.51)
20.1-30.0	64 (8.8)	22 (5.6)	0.91 (0.50–1.65)	8 (5.2)	1.03 (0.43–2.48)	8 (10.8)	1.37 (0.54–3.47)
> 30.0	115 (15.7)	42 (10.6)	1.16 (0.72–1.87)	15 (9.8)	0.84 (0.42–1.70)	7 (9.5)	1.10 (0.42–2.87)
Unknown	0 (0.0)	0 (0.0)	–	0 (0.0)	–	1 (1.3)	–
Total years of regular exercise							
No regular exercise	397 (54.3)	265 (67.1)	Reference	107 (69.5)	Reference	42 (56.8)	Reference
0.1-5.0	165 (22.6)	76 (19.2)	0.97 (0.67–1.42)	24 (15.6)	0.71 (0.41–1.25)	14 (18.9)	0.79 (0.39–1.62)
5.1-10.0	92 (12.6)	24 (6.1)	0.70 (0.40–1.24)	12 (7.8)	0.92 (0.43–1.96)	10 (13.5)	1.74 (0.73–4.14)
> 10.0	77 (10.5)	30 (7.6)	1.87 (1.06–3.28)	11 (7.1)	0.91 (0.39–2.11)	8 (10.8)	1.14 (0.41–3.14)

Abbreviations: *CI* confidence interval, *N* number, *OR* odds ratio

[a]OR and 95% CI were calculated using unconditional logistic regression, adjusted for sex, age, education, cigarette smoking (pack-year categories), betel quid chewing (pack-year categories), alcohol drinking (frequency), and intake of vegetables and fruits

cancer, education, intake of fruits and vegetables, red meat, and alcohol only had a small impact (RR = 0.89, 95% CI = 0.74-1.06) [10]. In another cohort study, Hashibe et al. evaluated the development of HNC by PA status in a cohort of 101,182 subjects [11]. With PA information available for less than half of the subjects, they observed a significantly reduced HNC risk for those who participated in 3 or more hours of vigorous activity at baseline interview compared to those who had <1 h of vigorous activity at baseline interview (RR = 0.58, 95% CI: 0.35-0.96), adjusted for age, sex, race, education, drinking frequency, and tobacco pack-years [11]. When PA was examined at age 40, those who participated in 3 or more hours of vigorous activity at age 40 had a non-significantly reduced HNC risk compared to those who had <1 h of vigorous activity at age 40 (RR = 0.69, 95% CI: 0.42-1.14), adjusted for age, sex, race, education,

drinking frequency, and tobacco pack-years [11]. In a pooled case–control study of 2289 HNC cases and 5580 controls, Nicolotti et al. reported that moderate RPA was associated with a significantly reduced HNC risk (OR =0.78, 95%: 0.66-0.91) and high RPA was associated with a non-significantly reduced HNC risk (OR =0.72, 95% CI: 0.46-1.16), adjusted for age, sex, study center, ethnicity, education, occupational PA, cigarette smoking and alcohol drinking [12].

In the investigation for the association between PA and HNC, it would be important to adjust for other life-style factors that have been strongly associated with an increased HNC risk, including use of alcohol, betel quid, and cigarette, and reduced consumption of fruits and vegetables [2, 4]. Individuals who participate in PA tend to have different health behavior patterns from individuals who live a sedentary lifestyle [15, 16]. In our

Table 5 The association between regular recreational physical activity and risk of head and neck cancer stratified by the use of alcohol, betel quid, or cigarette

	No regular recreational physical activity vs. regular recreational physical activity OR (95% CI)[a]
Alcohol drinking	
Never + occasional	0.97 (0.63–1.49)
Former regular	1.34 (0.59–3.04)
Current regular	0.99 (0.64–1.53)
Former regular + current regular	1.05 (0.72–1.52)
	P-interaction =0.83
Betel quid	
Never	0.95 (0.63–1.43)
Former	0.79 (0.49–1.28)
Current	1.96 (0.91–4.21)
Former + Current	1.04 (0.70–1.53)
	P-interaction =0.75
Cigarette	
Never	1.59 (0.81–3.10)
Former	0.73 (0.40–1.33)
Current	0.96 (0.66–1.40)
Former + Current	0.92 (0.67–1.25)
	P-interaction =0.61

Abbreviations: *CI* confidence interval, *OR* odds ratio

[a]OR and 95% CI were calculated using unconditional logistic regression, adjusted for sex, age, education, cigarette smoking (pack-year categories), betel quid chewing (pack-year categories), alcohol drinking (frequency), and intake of vegetables and fruits

analysis, we found that individuals who engaged in RPA were less likely to drink alcohol, chew betel quid, and smoke cigarette and more likely to eat fruits and vegetables everyday. When we adjusted for sex, age, and education only, we observed a significant inverse association between RPA and HNC risk. However, this inverse association became null after we further adjusted for use of alcohol, betel quid, and cigarette, and consumption of vegetables and fruits. This indicated that the inverse association between RPA and HNC was cofounded by these other lifestyle factors and RPA was not independently associated with HNC. The two studies that found a significant inverse association between PA and HNC did not adjust for intake of fruits and vegetables and there could be residual confounding for the association in these studies [11, 12].

When we examined the association between RPA and HNC risk by HNC sites, we didn't find any significant association except for the positive association between >10 years of RPA and oral cancer risk. It is unclear why higher total years of RPA would be associated an increased oral cancer risk. Because of the smaller numbers

in the stratified analysis, chance finding could not be ruled out. Leitzmann et al. did not find a significant association between RPA (5 more times of RPA per week vs. no physical activity) and any of the HNC sites (Oral cavity: RR = 0.98, 95% CI: 0.75-1.29; pharynx: RR = 0.70, 95% CI: 0.45-1.08; larynx: RR = 0.82, 95% CI: 0.59-1.13) [10]. Nicolotti et al. reported an inverse association between moderate RPA and oral cancer (OR =0.74, 95% CI: 0.56-0.97) and pharyngeal cancer (OR =0.67, 95% CI: 0.53-0.85) [12]. In addition, they found that high RPA was associated with a reduced risk of oral cancer risk (OR =0.53, 95% CI: 0.32-0.88) and pharyngeal cancer (OR =0.58, 95% CI: 0.38-0.89) but an increased risk of laryngeal cancer (OR =1.73, 95% CI: 1.04-2.88) [12]. Again, the reduced risk reported by Nicolotti could be attributed partly to the residual confounding by not adjusting for intake of fruits and vegetables. According to Nicolotti et al., the increased laryngeal cancer risk associated with high RPA levels could be due to residual confounding by cigarette smoking because of the higher percentage of cigarette smokers among laryngeal cancer patients with high PA levels [12].

We examined whether the association between RPA and HNC risk could be modified by the use of alcohol, betel quid, or cigarette. Our results did not indicate any effect modification of these lifestyle factors on the association between RPA and HNC. Leitzmann et al. showed the inverse association between RPA and HNC risk was more evident among ever alcohol drinkers than among never alcohol drinkers (P for heterogeneity between strata =0.03) [10]. Nicolotti showed that the reduced HNC risk associated with moderate RPA was more evident among ever tobacco smokers and ever alcohol drinkers, although it was not statistically significant between the strata (P for heterogeneity between strata =0.25) [12]. Given the inconsistencies among studies, further investigations are needed to determine whether RPA is beneficial for certain subgroups, in particular alcohol drinkers and cigarette smokers, for reducing HNC risk.

This study has several limitations. Because case–control studies collect exposure data by asking participants to recall their past exposures or activities, there can be recall bias and recall error. Recall bias often occurs when the case subjects ruminate on the exposure that may possibly cause their development of disease, resulting in a spurious positive association between exposure and the disease. However, this may not be a major issue for our study because we found a null association between RPA and HNC risk. Since the public is not aware of the possible association between RPA and HNC, non-differential random recall error was more likely for our study and could have biased our results toward the null. Another limitation is that we did not collect information on occupation and thus could not adjust for occupational

PA in our statistical models. Finally, although human papillomavirus is an important risk factor for oropharyngeal cancer, we did not have access to the tumor tissue to test for HPV status. For HNC occurring in the oral cavity, hypopharynx, and larynx, the contribution of HPV is likely very low [17]. We conducted an additional sensitivity analysis focusing on two HNC sites (tonsil and base of the tongue) that show the strongest association with HPV [18]. We did not see an association between RPA and cancers of the tonsil and the base of the tongue (Additional file 2: Table S1). In addition, no population-based study has been conducted in Taiwan to assess the contribution of HPV to the development of oropharyngeal cancer. A study from Taiwan with 111 samples of tonsillar squamous cell carcinoma found that only 12.6% of the samples were HPV positive [19]. Overall, we think that HPV status made minimal impact on our results showing a null association between RPA and HNC.

The major strength of the current study is the detailed assessment of RPA. We collected information on the type, intensity, frequency, and duration of RPA. This allowed us to be the first study to calculate MET-hours for evaluating the dose–response relationship between RPA and HNC risk. Another strength is that we adjusted for lifestyle factors that have been strongly associated with HNC risk, including use of alcohol, betel quid, and cigarette, and consumption of vegetables and fruits. This minimized the possibility of confounding on the association between RPA and HNC risk by other health behaviors.

Conclusions

In conclusion, results from our study did not support an inverse association between RPA and HNC risk. Although RPA is beneficial in reducing the risk of various chronic diseases and certain cancers, including colon cancer, breast cancer, and endometrial cancer [6, 7], our results suggested that RPA is unlikely to play a major role to reduce HNC risk. The major focus of HNC prevention should be on cessation of cigarette smoking and betel chewing, reduction of alcohol drinking, and promotion of healthy diet that contains plenty of fruits and vegetables.

Abbreviations
CI: Confidence interval; HNC: Head and neck cancer; HPV: Human papillomavirus; OR: Odds ratio; PA: Physical activity; RPA: Recreational physical activity

Acknowledgements
Not applicable.

Funding
This work was supported by the Establishment of Cancer Research System Excellence Program funded by the Ministry of Health and Welfare, Taiwan (MOHW106-TDU-B-211-144-004, MOHW105-TDU-B-212-134-013) and by the National Health Research Institutes (CA-106-SP-01). The funding agencies did not play any role in the design of the study, data collection, analysis and interpretation of data, and writing the manuscript.

Authors' contributions
CLL collected the data, interpreted the results, prepared the manuscript, and approved the final manuscript. WTL collected the data, interpreted the results, prepared the manuscript, and approved the final manuscript. CYO collected the data, interpreted the results, and approved the final manuscript. JRH designed the study, collected the data, interpreted the results, and approved the final manuscript. CCH collected the data, interpreted the results, and approved the final manuscript. JSH collected the data, interpreted the results, and approved the final manuscript. TYW collected the data, interpreted the results, and approved the final manuscript. KCC collected the data, interpreted the results, and approved the final manuscript. STT collected the data, interpreted the results, and approved the final manuscript. SYF collected the data, interpreted the results, and approved the final manuscript. TTH collected the data, interpreted the results, and approved the final manuscript. JLW collected the data, interpreted the results, and approved the final manuscript. YH Wu collected the data, interpreted the results, and approved the final manuscript. WTH collected the data, interpreted the results, and approved the final manuscript. CJY collected the data, interpreted the results, and approved the final manuscript. YHL collected the data, interpreted the results, and approved the final manuscript. HCL collected the data, interpreted the results, and approved the final manuscript. SYW collected the data, interpreted the results, and approved the final manuscript. MWY collected the data, interpreted the results, and approved the final manuscript. FCL collected the data, interpreted the results, and approved the final manuscript. JYC collected the data, interpreted the results, and approved the final manuscript. YH Wang collected the data, interpreted the results, and approved the final manuscript. YLW collected the data, interpreted the results, and approved the final manuscript. HCY collected the data, interpreted the results, and approved the final manuscript. YSC collected the data, interpreted the results, and approved the final manuscript. JSC designed the study, collected the data, performed data analysis, interpreted the results, prepared the manuscript, and approved the final manuscript.

Competing interests
The authors declare that they have no competing interests.

Author details
[1]Department of Nursing, National Cheng Kung University Hospital, College of Medicine, National Cheng Kung University, Tainan, Taiwan. [2]Department of Otolaryngology, National Cheng Kung University Hospital, College of Medicine, National Cheng Kung University, Tainan, Taiwan. [3]Department of Stomatology, National Cheng Kung University Hospital, College of Medicine, National Cheng Kung University, Tainan, Taiwan. [4]Department of Radiation Oncology, National Cheng Kung University Hospital, College of Medicine, National Cheng Kung University, Tainan, Taiwan. [5]Division of Hematology/ Oncology, Department of Internal Medicine, National Cheng Kung University Hospital, College of Medicine, National Cheng Kung University, Tainan, Taiwan. [6]National Institute of Cancer Research, National Health Research Institutes, 1F No 367, Sheng-Li Road, Tainan 70456, Taiwan.

References
1. Ferlay J, Soerjomataram I, Ervik M, Dikshit R, Eser S, Mathers C, Rebelo M, Parkin DM, Forman D, Bray F. GLOBOCAN 2012 v1.0, Cancer Incidence and Mortality Worldwide: IARC CancerBase No. 11 [Internet]. International Agency for Research on Cancer: Lyon, France; 2013. Available from: http:// globocan.iarc.fr, accessed on 15 Oct 2015
2. Boyle P. Levin B (eds.): World Cancer Report. International Agency for Research on Cancer: Lyon; 2008.

3. Young D, Xiao CC, Murphy B, Moore M, Fakhry C, Day TA. Increase in head and neck cancer in younger patients due to human papillomavirus (HPV). Oral Oncol. 2015;51:727–30.

4. Bravi F, Edefonti V, Randi G, Ferraroni M, La Vecchia C, Decarli A. Dietary patterns and upper aerodigestive tract cancers: an overview and review. Ann Oncol. 2012;23:3024–39.

5. The World Health Organization. Global recommendations on physical activity for health. Geneva, Switzerland: The World Health Organization; 2010.

6. Kruk J, Czerniak U. Physical activity and its relation to cancer risk: updating the evidence. Asian Pac J Cancer Prev. 2013;14:3993–4003.

7. Leitzmann M, Powers H, Anderson AS, Scoccianti C, Berrino F, Boutron-Ruault MC, Cecchini M, Espina C, Key TJ, Norat T, et al. European Code against Cancer 4th Edition: Physical activity and cancer. Cancer Epidemiol. 2015;39(Suppl 1): S46–55.

8. Shpitzer T, Bahar G, Feinmesser R, Nagler RM. A comprehensive salivary analysis for oral cancer diagnosis. J Cancer Res Clin Oncol. 2007;133:613–7.

9. Trochimiak T, Hubner-Wozniak E. Effect of exercise on the level of immunoglobulin a in saliva. Biol Sport. 2012;29:255–61.

10. Leitzmann MF, Koebnick C, Freedman ND, Park Y, Ballard-Barbash R, Hollenbeck AR, Schatzkin A, Abnet CC. Physical activity and head and neck cancer risk. Cancer Causes Control. 2008;19:1391–9.

11. Hashibe M, Hunt J, Wei M, Buys S, Gren L, Lee YC. Tobacco, alcohol, body mass index, physical activity, and the risk of head and neck cancer in the prostate, lung, colorectal, and ovarian (PLCO) cohort. Head Neck. 2013; 35:914–22.

12. Nicolotti N, Chuang SC, Cadoni G, Arzani D, Petrelli L, Bosetti C, Brenner H, Hosono S, La Vecchia C, Talamini R, et al. Recreational physical activity and risk of head and neck cancer: a pooled analysis within the international head and neck cancer epidemiology (INHANCE) Consortium. Eur J Epidemiol. 2011;26:619–28.

13. Ainsworth BE, Haskell WL, Herrmann SD, Meckes N, Bassett Jr DR, Tudor-Locke C, Greer JL, Vezina J, Whitt-Glover MC, Leon AS. 2011 Compendium of Physical Activities: a second update of codes and MET values. Med Sci Sports Exerc. 2011;43:1575–81.

14. Strath SJ, Kaminsky LA, Ainsworth BE, Ekelund U, Freedson PS, Gary RA, Richardson CR, Smith DT, Swartz AM. Guide to the assessment of physical activity: Clinical and research applications: a scientific statement from the American Heart Association. Circulation. 2013;128:2259–79.

15. Laaksonen M, Prattala R, Karisto A. Patterns of unhealthy behaviour in Finland. Eur J Pub Health. 2001;11:294–300.

16. Choi JE, Ainsworth BE. Associations of food consumption, serum vitamins and metabolic syndrome risk with physical activity level in middle-aged adults: the National Health and Nutrition Examination Survey (NHANES) 2005–2006. Public Health Nutr. 2016:1–10.

17. Castellsague X, Alemany L, Quer M, Halec G, Quiros B, Tous S, Clavero O, Alos L, Biegner T, Szafarowski T et al. HPV Involvement in Head and Neck Cancers: Comprehensive Assessment of Biomarkers in 3680 Patients. J Natl Cancer Inst. 2016; 108:djv403.

18. Ndiaye C, Mena M, Alemany L, Arbyn M, Castellsague X, Laporte L, Bosch FX, de Sanjose S, Trottier H. HPV DNA, E6/E7 mRNA, and p16INK4a detection in head and neck cancers: a systematic review and meta-analysis. Lancet Oncol 2014; 15:1319–1331.

19. Chien CY, Su CY, Fang FM, Huang HY, Chuang HC, Chen CM, Huang CC. Lower prevalence but favorable survival for human papillomavirus-related squamous cell carcinoma of tonsil in Taiwan. Oral Oncol. 2008;44:174–9.

17

Feasibility and acceptability of combining cognitive behavioural therapy techniques with swallowing therapy in head and neck cancer dysphagia

J. M. Patterson[1,2]*, M. Fay, C. Exley[3], E. McColl[1], M. Breckons[1] and V. Deary[4]

Abstract

Background: Head and neck cancer squamous cell carcinoma (HNSSC) patients report substantial rates of clinically significant depression and/or anxiety, with dysphagia being a predictor of distress and poorer quality of life. Evidence-based dysphagia interventions largely focus on the remediation of physical impairment. This feasibility study evaluates an intervention which simultaneously uses a psychological therapy approach combined with swallowing impairment rehabilitation.

Methods: This prospective single cohort mixed-methods study, recruited HNSCC patients with dysphagia, from two institutions. The intervention combined Cognitive Behavioural Therapy with swallowing therapy (CB-EST), was individually tailored, for up to 10 sessions and delivered by a speech and language therapist. Primary acceptability and feasibility measures included recruitment and retention rates, data completion, intervention fidelity and the responsiveness of candidate outcome measures. Measures included a swallowing questionnaire (MDADI), EORTC-QLQH&N35, dietary restrictions scale, fatigue and function scales and the Hospital Anxiety and Depression Scale (HADS), administered pre-, post-CB-EST with three month follow-up and analysed using repeated measures ANOVA. Qualitative interviews were conducted to evaluate intervention processes.

Results: A total of 30/43 (70%) eligible patients agreed to participate and 25 completed the intervention. 84% were male, mean age 59 yrs. Patients were between 1 and 60 months (median 4) post-cancer treatment. All patients had advanced stage disease, treated with surgery and radiotherapy (38%) or primary chemoradiotherapy (62%). Pre to post CB-EST data showed improvements in MDADI scores ($p = 0.002$), EORTC-QLQH&N35 ($p = 0.006$), dietary scale ($p < 0.0001$), fatigue ($p = 0.002$) but no change in function scales or HADS. Barriers to recruitment were the ability to attend regular appointments and patient suitability or openness to a psychological-based intervention.

Conclusions: CB-EST is a complex and novel intervention, addressing the emotional, behavioural and cognitive components of dysphagia alongside physical impairment. Preliminary results are promising. Further research is required to evaluate efficacy and effectiveness.

* Correspondence: joanne.patterson@ncl.ac.uk
[1]Institute of Health and Society, Newcastle University, The Baddiley-Clark Building, Richardson Road, Newcastle upon Tyne NE2 4AX, UK
[2]Speech & Language Therapy Department, Sunderland Royal Hospital, Sunderland, UK
Full list of author information is available at the end of the article

Background

Chronic swallowing difficulties (dysphagia) are a common and highly distressing side effect of surgery and/or (chemo)radiotherapy for the treatment of head and neck cancer (HNSCC) [1]. Dysphagia is associated with a higher risk of pneumonia, poor oral intake, malnutrition and prolonged tube feeding [2]. HNSSC patients report substantial rates of clinically significant depression and/or anxiety, with dysphagia being a predictor of distress [3, 4]. Our previous qualitative work reported on fundamental changes to eating habits, social lives and wellbeing, with some patients being better able to adjust to such changes than others [5].

Evidence based HNSCC dysphagia interventions largely centre on impairment-focused treatments delivered by speech & language therapists (SLTs) [6]. These typically include exercises to increase the range and co-ordination of swallowing function, to improve efficiency and safety. These may be administered before (as a preventative approach), during or after HNSCC treatment. The degree to which exercises prevent or reduce dysphagia is unclear due to poor patient adherence and differing exercise protocols [7]. Patients need support in coping with side effects [8], but to date, there are minimal reports of interventions addressing the psychosocial sequelae of dysphagia.

General psychosocial interventions for HNSCC patients such as psycho-education, counselling and cognitive behavioural therapy (CBT) have been reported. A Cochrane review concluded that the subsequent impact on quality of life of these interventions was uncertain due to study design limitations [9]. Whether a psychological-based treatment can be combined with impairment-based swallowing therapy to address dysphagia is an unknown. Potentially this type of intervention could improve patient engagement with rehabilitation and facilitate adjustment in living with swallowing difficulties. CBT has previously been used with HNSCC [10] and has been used by SLTs for other conditions [11].

This study aims to investigate the feasibility and acceptability of a cognitive behavioural enhanced swallowing therapy (CB-EST) for HNSCC dysphagia, using a mixed methods design.

Methods

This is a multi-centre, prospective, longitudinal non-randomised single cohort study to explore feasibility and acceptability of a CBT enhanced swallowing therapy intervention (CB-EST) in HNSCC patients. The feasibility design was informed by guidance set out by the CONSORT 2010 statement [12].

Patients and eligibility

HNSCC patients were recruited from two units in NE England. They were eligible for the study if they 1) had completed HNSCC treatment with curative intent 2) were medically stable and 3) scored <80 points on the MD Anderson Dysphagia Inventory [13] (swallowing specific quality of life questionnaire). Patients were excluded if they 1) had pre-existing major psychiatric diagnosis 2) had residual/recurrent HNSCC 3) were on a palliative care pathway 4) had significant communication difficulties rendering them unable to participate in a talking therapy 5) were currently receiving a psychological intervention 6) were awaiting an intervention for the purpose of improving swallowing performance (e.g. a dilatation) or 7) had significant ill-health precluding regular hospital attendance. Patients were screened and approached by members of the multi-disciplinary HNSCCC team and gave written consent before participation. The study aimed to recruit thirty participants, to provide data to perform a sample size calculation for a potential future effectiveness study [14].

Intervention

The main researcher (JP), a SLT trained in CBT to post graduate certificate level, delivered the intervention. CB-EST was individually tailored, but aimed to include key CBT components i.e. in-depth assessment, identification of maintaining factors within a formulation, identification of a therapy goal, Socratic questioning style, cognitive and/or behavioural therapy techniques and homework tasks. The intervention also included individualised swallowing exercises, diet modifications and food texture advice, if appropriate to the patient's therapy goal. Between 45 and 60 min were allowed for each session. Treatment was on a weekly or fortnightly basis (depending on patient preference and need for support) for up to 10 sessions by mutual agreement, with a follow up assessment at three months to monitor generalisation and maintenance. JP received supervision from an expert CBT practitioner every 2–3 weeks.

Feasibility outcomes

As this was primarily a feasibility study, primary outcomes were those that related to the acceptability of the intervention to participants and the feasibility of trialling the intervention in a larger study. The acceptability and feasibility outcomes are as follows:

1. Acceptability was measured by the proportion of patients approached and consented and the number of sessions attended. Retention rates and reasons for drop out was documented. We aimed for a 50% recruitment rate for CB-EST to be deemed an acceptable treatment.
2. Feasibility and fidelity were measured by assessing whether the intervention could be delivered as planned, by a SLT with CBT training. Session

content and treatment plans, recorded in patients' notes were evaluated by a CBT expert practitioner as part of supervision, reliability and validity checking. Content analysis of sessions including a) whether a therapy goal was identified b) whether a CBT formulation was identified c) whether cognitive and/or behaviour change techniques were used. These outcomes would also indicate the acceptability of the intervention to patients.

3. A selection of candidate measures targeting swallowing self-report, dietary restrictions, quality of life, functioning and mood were chosen to identify appropriate tools to capture CB-EST outcomes. Acceptability to patients was monitored by percentage data completion. The measures listed below and were administered pre-, immediately following CB-EST, and at three months.

i. The MDADI [13] has twenty items, each marked using a five-point scale and summarised using a total score (range 20–100). Higher scores indicate a better outcome and a change in ≥10 points is considered a clinically significant difference [15].

ii. The European Organization for Research and Treatment of Cancer questionnaires (EORTC QLQ-C30) [16] is a general quality of life questionnaire with 30 items, five functioning scales (physical, role, emotional, cognitive, and social), three symptom scales. The EORTC QLQ-H&N35 is a disease-specific module of 35 questions divided into 7 subscales about pain, swallowing, senses, speech, social eating, social contact, and sexuality. Higher scores on the functional scales refer to better health status, whereas higher scores in symptom scales and the QLQ-H&N35 represent more severe symptoms.

iii. Chalder Fatigue Questionnaire (CFQ-11) [17] measures fatigue severity. Eleven items are answered on a four-point scale (range 0–33), with high scores representing more fatigue.

iv. Work and Social Adjustment Scale(WASA) [18] measures functional and social impairment. Five questions are answered on a nine-point scale (range 0–40) with higher scores indicating more impairment.

v. Hospital Anxiety and Depression Scale (HADS) [19] has two seven item subscales measuring anxiety (HADS-A) and depression (HADS-D). Each item is scored on a four-point scale (range 0–21 for each subscale). Subscale scores 0–7 classify participants as non-cases, 8–10 indicates borderline cases, and scores ≥11 indicate clinical levels. Total HADS scores (HADS-T) ≥ 15 indicate clinically significant distress.

vi. Performance Status Scales (PSS) Normalcy of Diet [20] measures diet texture restrictions and is clinician-rated. The scale has ten ranked categories ranging from 0 (nil by mouth) to 100 (full diet without restrictions).

The presence of a feeding tube was recorded at the same time points. The sensitivity of the candidate measures was tested by making preliminary estimates of change from pre- to post CB-EST. Data were analysed using SPSS v21 (Chicago, Illinois). We used a one way within subjects repeated measures analysis of variance complete case model. The level for statistical significance was set at 0.05. Bonferroni's test was used for multiple post hoc comparisons. Means are reported with standard deviations and 95% confidence intervals.

4. The acceptability and feasibility of delivering CB-EST as-was or modifying it for a larger trial was further assessed using semi-structured interviews. Patients were purposively sampled to ensure a range of pre to post CB-EST changes in MDADI scores, a range of HNSCC treatment and time post-treatment. Patients were selected from those at the initial stages of CB-EST and at the end of CB-EST. Interviews were conducted by two independent researchers. Patients had the option of a telephone or face to face interview, at a time and place of their choice. All interviews were digitally recorded, t ranscribed verbatim and anonymised. Transcripts were read several times and in detail by the qualitative sub-team. Data were then discussed and coded using thematic analysis. Quotations relating to afore mentioned topics were independently selected and coded into key issues and themes.

Ethics

Ethical approval was granted by the UK North East Research Ethics Committee reference 14/NE/1045.

Results

Feasibility and acceptability as measured by recruitment and retention

Fifty patients were screened over 20 months. Seven patients reported that their eating and drinking issues had resolved and/or they scored >80 on the MDADI, so were ineligible. Forty-three patients were approached and 30 gave written consent (69.8%). Patient characteristics for consented patients are summarised in Table 1. There was no statistical difference in distribution of gender, age, disease site, stage, type of treatment or time since treatment ($p > 0.05$) between those that consented to participation and those that did not.

Table 1 Patient baseline characteristics and demographics for consented CB-EST patients

Characteristics	Number (%)
Gender	
Male	26 (87)
Female	4 (13)
Age	59 (range 49–79)
Disease site	
Oropharynx	18 (60)
Oral	5 (17)
Nasopharynx	3 (10)
Larynx	2 (7)
Hypopharynx	1 (3)
Unknown primary	1 (3)
Stage	
0	1 (3)
1	2 (6)
2	13 (43)
3	7 (24)
4	7 (24)
Nodes	
0	3 (10)
1	7 (24)
2	20 (66)
Treatment	
Chemoradiotherapy	19 (63)
Surgery and radiotherapy +/– chemotherapy	9 (30)
Surgery	1 (3.5)
Radiotherapy	1 (3.5)
Time post-treatment (months)	Median 4 (IQR, Range 3,13; 1–60)
Partner	Yes (23)
	No (7)

Reasons for non-participation included difficulties with regular hospital attendance (5), did not think CB-EST would help (3), did not attend (2), currently receiving CBT (1), and too much to take on (2). Twenty five patients were retained (83%) in the intervention. Three patients dropped out at sessions 3, 4 and 5 due to disease (2 local disease, 1 lung cancer). Two patients opted not to continue with CB-EST at session 2 and 5; one found it difficult to envisage how CB-EST might be of benefit and the other felt he was making insufficient progress. No outcome data were available for drop-outs. The number of CB-EST sessions for the retained patients ranged from 3 to 10 sessions, median 6. At three month follow up, one patient was too unwell to complete questionnaires.

Feasibility and acceptability as measured by intervention fidelity

All retained patients were able to identify a goal specific to their eating and drinking problem. Goals fell into six main areas (see Table 2). A formulation for all but one drop-out patient was developed and verified during supervision. Examples of formulations are provided in Fig. 1. A range of cognitive and behavioural techniques were utilised during CB-EST and are recorded in Table 2.

Acceptability and utility of candidate outcome measures

Data completeness ranged from 76 to 100%, the PSS Normalcy of diet scale having the highest compliance, QLQ-C30 having the lowest compliance (see Table 3). Post CB-EST improvements were observed in several measures. Although not powered for effectiveness, a statistically significant improvement was observed in MDADI scores ($p = 0.002$, mean difference 8.1); three domains of QLQ-C30 function scales ($p = 0.004-0.03$ mean difference 10.4–21.3); seven domains on QLQ-HN35 symptoms scales ($p < 0.0001-0.01$ mean difference 10.8–14.7); CFS ($p = 0.002$ mean difference 4.1) and PSS Normalcy of diet scale ($p < 0.0001$ mean difference 15.8). These improvements were maintained at three months. No statistical improvement was observed for two domains on QLQ-C30 functioning scales; two domains on QLQ-HN35 symptom scales; WASA scales or the HADS (see Table 3).

Feasibility and acceptability as measured by participant interviews

Sixteen patients were approached for interview and 15 consented. The interviewer was unable to arrange a convenient time for three patients. There were ten telephone and two face to face interviews. One patient opted to be interviewed with her partner present. The sample reflected baseline characteristics for gender, age, site and stage of disease (see Table 4).

Three main CB-EST process themes were identified.

Duration and frequency

Participants were referred to CB-EST either by a specialist nurse or a SLT and all felt this was an appropriate pathway. Overall, patients were happy with the duration of sessions. Session length of approximately one hour was deemed sufficient to explore issues and to decide on homework until the following session. Generally, patients felt that between 8 and 10 sessions was an appropriate set of meetings. Some felt that regular intervals (weekly/fortnightly) were beneficial whilst others would have preferred them to be more frequent in the early stages of CB-EST.

Table 2 Therapy goals and associated CB-EST interventions for participants

Therapy goal	CB-EST Interventions												
	Swallowing exercises	Swallowing posture recommendation	Texture modification advice	Food selection/preparation advice	Size and positioning of bolus advice	Education on eating	Education on management of choking	Sleep/fatigue management	Graded behavioural experiments	Activity scheduling	Exposure/graded tasks	Thought records	Identifying unhelpful thinking habits
To get feeding tube out (n = 11)	×	×	×	×	×	×	×	×	×	×	×	×	×
To increase eating amount (n = 8)	×									×	×		×
To increase confidence in socialising (n = 4)									×		×	×	×
Become more confident about eating (n = 4)			×	×			×	×	×				×
Feel better about changes to eating and drinking (n = 2)			×	×		×	×	×		×	×	×	×
To adjust to life without eating and drinking (n = 1)							×	×	×	×		×	×

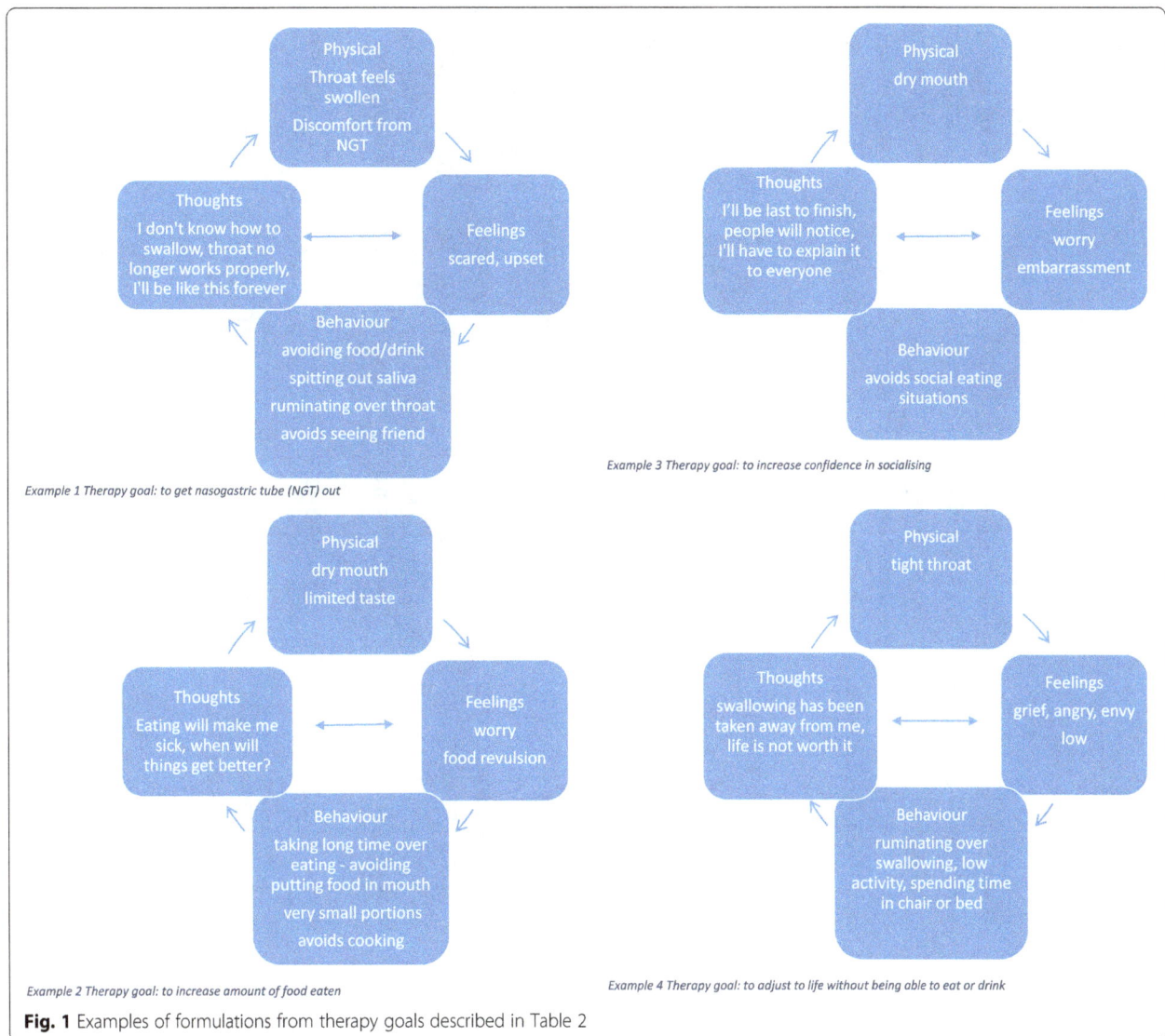

Example 1 Therapy goal: to get nasogastric tube (NGT) out

Example 2 Therapy goal: to increase amount of food eaten

Example 3 Therapy goal: to increase confidence in socialising

Example 4 Therapy goal: to adjust to life without being able to eat or drink

Fig. 1 Examples of formulations from therapy goals described in Table 2

'The timeframe between that was just balanced nicely and allowed me to kind of make those plans and have an experience to then come back and talk about it, so yeah it worked well' (S3 aged 51 yrs).

Participants understood that sessions were a finite resource and moving on was an inevitable and necessary part of the intervention. Several participants stated that they would have happily continued as they discovered an overall benefit on recovery and well-being. Patients liked the combination of talking, visualising issues using a whiteboard and other applied techniques, and concrete goal setting.

Timing
Most participants felt that the timing of their participation in CB-EST worked well, with some expressing that they wished they had earlier access.

'Maybe it should be part of the initial journey and treatment ... not everybody might take it but at least it is there isn't it' (S7 aged 61 years).

There was variation about whether there is an ideal time point to start sessions. Timing seemed to be related to individual preferences and symptom severity. Participants seem to fall roughly into two groups: those who would prefer the sessions to accompany their treatment (i.e. start soon after diagnosis) and those who thought sessions are more beneficial following (but not too long after) treatment.

Suitability
Some participants described themselves as being suited to an intervention such as CB-EST, i.e. either being open to talk about emotions and/or relatively open to help and change. Others described themselves as being more

Table 3 Questionnaire and feeding tube results for CB-EST

Measure	Pre-CB-EST	Post CB-EST	3 months	ANOVA, Effect size (ES)	Pre to post [95% CI]	Pre to 3 m [95% CI]	Post to 3 m [95% CI]
MDADI	n = 25 (100%)	n = 23 (92%)	n = 24 (96%)	p = 0.002 (2,42) F = 8.8 ES = 0.29*	p = 0.03 [0.7–15.5]	p = 0.003 [2.6–14.6]	p = 1.0 [3.6–4.7]
	53.1 (15.1)	61.2 (15.6)	61.8 (16.0)				
QLQ-C30	n = 25 (100%)	n = 22 (88%)	n = 19 (76%)				
Physical	63.7 (21.8)	74.1 (21.9)	74.4 (21.8)	p = 0.006 (2,34) F = 5.9 ES = 0.26	p = 0.05 [0.1–28.8]	p = 0.03 [0.7–20.8]	p = 1.0 [–8.1–7.2]
Role	48.1(38.3)	61.1(34.7)	72.2(34.3)	p = 0.03 (1,20) F = 4.8 ES = 0.22*	p = 0.5 [10.9–36.8]	p = 0.06 [1.2–49.4]	p = 0.01 [2.3–19.9]
Emotional	67.6 (31.0)	75.9 (31.7)	75.4 (24.8)	p = 0.15 (1,17) F = 2.3 ES = 0.11	p = 0.06 [0.4–17.1]	p = 0.4 [5.9–21.7]	p = 1.0 [11.9–12.9]
Cognitive	70.4 (34.6)	75.9 (34.9)	87.0 (19.4)	p = 0.06 (2,21) F = 3.8 ES = 0.18*	p = 0.2 [2.4–13.5]	p = 0.1 [2.6–35.9]	p = 0.4 [7.8–30.0]
Social	44.4 (37.0)	65.7 (36.8)	62.9 (36.8)	p = 0.004 (2,34) F = 6.5 ES = 0.28	p = 0.03 [1.1–41.4]	p = 0.01 [3.8–33.2]	p = 1.0 [12.9–18.5]
Symptoms							
Fatigue	40.7(24.9)	33.9 (26.8)	26.5(25.6)	p = 0.02 (2,34) F = 4.2 ES = 0.2	p = 0.79 [8.8–22.4]	p = 0.02 [1.4–27.0]	p = 0.2 [2.7–17.5]
Nausea	12.9 (25.9)	5.5 (9.9)	8.3 (17.4)	p = 0.2 (2,34) F = 1.6 ES = 0.1	p = 0.41 [5.1–19.9]	p = 0.86 [–6.5–15.8]	p = 1.0 [–11.7–6.2]
Pain	31.5 (32.3)	29.9 (34.8)	26.8 (30.3)	p = 0.71 (2,34) F = 0.3 ES = 0.02	p = 1.0 [14.4–25.5]	p = 1.0 [18.5–27.7]	p = 1.0 [12.7–14.5]
QLQ-H&N35	n = 25 (100%)	n = 22 (88%)	n = 22 (88%)				
Oral pain	32.2 (19.8)	23.3 (22.7)	27.1 (21.9)	p = 0.29 (2,38) F = 1.3, ES = 0.06	p = 0.29 [–4.0–19.8]	p = 1.0 [–9.8–17.5]	p = 1.0 [–17.3–9.8]
Swallow	45.8 (31.2)	35.0 (26.0)	28.3 (18.2)	p = 0.006 (2,38) F = 5.9, ES = 0.24	p = 0.2 [–4.1–25.7]	p = 0.01 [3.8–31.1]	p = 0.46 [–5.1–18.4]
Senses	45.5 (29.4)	32.5 (21.2)	22.5 (26.6)	p < 0.0001 (2,38) F = 10.7, ES = 0.36	p = 0.09 [–1.8–21.2]	p = 0.003 [6.3–33.7]	p = 0.02 [1.4–18.6]
Speech	40.8 (35.6)	28.3 (35.9)	20.8 (22.8)	p = 0.01 (2,38) F = 5.1, ES = 0.21	p = 0.02 [1.1–28.9]	p = 0.04 [0.8–39.2]	p = 0.89 [–10.9–25.8]
Social eating	58.7 (37.8)	36.1(27.0)	38.3 (35.1)	p = 0.006 (2,38) F = 5.9, ES = 0.24	p = 0.03 [1.2–44.1]	p = 0.05 [–0.5–41.4]	p = 1.0 [–16.0–11.6]
Social context	31.0 (25.9)	16.3 (22.7)	15.7 (17.5)	p = 0.001 (2,38) F = 9.0, ES = 0.32	p = 0.01 [2.7–26.6]	p = 0.004 [4.5–26.1]	p = 1.0 [–8.6–9.9]
Sexuality	53.3 (44.1)	48.3 (46.2)	35.0 (46.1)	p = 0.12 (2,38) F = 0.23, ES = 0.11	p = 1.0 [–21.8–31.8]	p = 0.06 [–0.7–37.4]	p = 0.47 [–10.3–37.0]
CFS	n = 25 (100%)	n = 24 (96%)	n = 22 (88%)				
	20.3 (5.0)	16.2 (6.8)	15.9 (5.9)	p = 0.002 (2,42) F = 7.3, ES = 0.39	p = 0.04 [0.1–8.1]	p = 0.04 [0.1–8.1]	p = 1.0 [2.5–2.9]
WASA	n = 25 (100%)	n = 23 (92%)	n = 22 (88%)				
	20.0 (9.2)	13.9(11.6)	16.9 (22.5)	p = 0.34(2,40) F = 1.1, ES = 0.05*	p = 0.07 [0.5–12.7]	p = 1.0 [9.2–15.3]	p = 1.0 [9.2–15.3]
HADS	n = 25 (100%)	n = 23 (92%)	n = 22 (88%)				
Anxiety	6.9 (4.9)	6.6 (5.9)	5.9 (4.1)	p = 0.54 (2,38) F = 0.6, ES = 0.03	p = 1.0 [–1.8–2.7]	p = 0.8 [–1.4–3.3]	p = 1.0 [–1.6–2.6]
Depression	6.0 (3.4)	5.6 (4.1)	4.9(4.1)	p = 0.49 (2,38) F = 0.7, ES = 0.37	p = 1.0 [–2.0–2.8]	p = 0.78 [–1.4–3.6]	p = 1.0 [–1.6–3.0]
Total	12.8 (7.1)	12.0 (9.6)	10.8 (3.4)	p = 0.38 (2,38) F = 1.0, ES = 0.05	p = 1.0 [–2.9–4.6]	p = 0.58 [–1.9–6.0]	p = 1.0 [–2.7–5.1]
PSS Diet	n = 25 (100%)	n = 25 (100%)	n = 24 (96%)				

Table 3 Questionnaire and feeding tube results for CB-EST *(Continued)*

Measure	Pre-CB-EST	Post CB-EST	3 months	ANOVA, Effect size (ES)	Pre to post [95% CI]	Pre to 3 m [95% CI]	Post to 3 m [95% CI]
	39.2 (19.9)	55.0 (14.4)	61.3 (18.5)	*p < 0.0001 (2,46) F = 15.0, ES = 0.4**	*p = 0.002 [5.3–26.4]*	*p = 0.001 [8.3–35.8]*	*p = 0.8 [0.4–12.9]*
Feeding tube	*n = 30*	*n = 25*	*n = 25*				
None	14 (56%)	22 (88%)	22 (88%)				
Nasogastric	9 (30%)	1 (4%)	0				
Gastrostomy	7 (24%)	2 (8%)	3 (12%)				

QLQ-C30, MDADI, CFS, WASA, HADS, PSS Diet higher score is better patient reported outcome. QLQ-H&N35 and HADS lower score indicates better patient reported outcome *sphericity violated for repeated measures ANOVA and adjusted using epsilon correction

Table 4 Characteristics of interview participants

Gender	
Male	9
Female	3
Age	61 (range 49–70)
Disease site	
Oropharynx	8
Oral	1
Nasopharynx	2
Larynx	1
T Stage	
2	5
3	5
4	2
Node stage	
0	2
1	3
2	7
Treatment	
Chemoradiotherapy	9
Surgery and radiotherapy +/– chemotherapy	3
Time post-treatment (months)	Median 5 range 1–60
MDADI pre to post CB-EST	
Decreased (4–19 points)	3
Similar (0–4 points)	3
Increased (5–36 points)	6

reluctant, not used to discussing emotional issues, and not the type to require psychological support.

'It will not fit everybody. Some people probably won't want to sit there and say about their life and say how your wife was in tears and say how you were in tears and talk about things like that'(S10 aged 54 years).

However, even those unaccustomed to this approach felt techniques and tasks were tailored to their requirements. In part, due to the ability to tailor the intervention, all participants agreed that there is potential for anyone to benefit from CB-EST. Some said that they didn't know what to expect but either approached sessions with an open mind or simply a 'nothing to lose' attitude. Even those who thought they were less likely to get much out of the sessions reported benefit in interviews, which was not always reflected in their MDADI scores.

Discussion

CB-EST is a novel treatment and had good rates of patient uptake and retention; formulations and goals were possible for most, candidate measures had good uptake and completeness providing some evidence of effect, and patients reported that they liked the intervention. CB-EST was delivered by a CBT trained SLT and was completed within ten sessions. Results need to be interpreted with caution as patients were self-selecting and not consecutively screened and therefore it is likely that more willing patients volunteered for the intervention. Recruitment rates were marginally lower than those reported in other general HNSCC psychosocial interventions [10]. Early indications are that CB-EST is an acceptable intervention for a range of HNSCC patients not confined to treatment type, time post-treatment, or site of disease. The sample was weighted towards patients with advanced staged disease, the majority having combined modality treatment. This was likely due to the predominance of self-reported dysphagia by patients treated with chemoradiotherapy or surgery plus adjuvant radiotherapy [1, 21]. Interview data suggest that people had individual preferences as to how soon CB-EST might be offered following their treatment. Barriers to recruitment were identified. Practicalities of regular out-patient attendance needs to be taken into consideration following intensive HNSCC treatment regimens as well as additional financial costs to the patient [22]. Not all HNSCC patients wish to receive psychological support and may be unsuitable for such an intervention [23]. Drop-out rates due to disease or ill-health are expected but unavoidable in the HNSCC population.

Our previous qualitative work showed that patients view their eating and drinking problems more broadly than just physical impairment [5]. CB-EST was able to respond to individual need, addressing the psychosocial issues of dysphagia by integrating core features of CBT alongside swallowing therapy, with some reporting general improvement in their quality of life. The most common patient goal was removal of feeding tube, which involved a range of physical, cognitive and behavioural techniques. Addressing unhelpful thinking habits was a technique used across all goals. Goals for improving confidence in social eating or adjustment to permanent non-oral feeding did not require impairment based swallowing therapy.

This study employed a selection of candidate measures to assess patient acceptability and sensitivity to change. All achieved a completion rate of ≥88%. Outcomes specifically related to eating and drinking (MDADI, EORTC HN35 Swallow and Social Eating and PSS Diet score) were responsive to change, although lack of follow up data from drop outs may positively skew results. Elsewhere, a comparable longitudinal cohort study reported a MDADI mean difference of 4.7 points in the first year post-treatment [24], suggesting some spontaneous adjustment occurs. Under trial conditions for a prophylactic swallow exercise intervention, minimal change was seen in EORTC HN35 Swallow and Social Eating scores (mean difference 0 and 5) [25]. The current study found no change on the HADS, despite CBT being an effective intervention for anxiety and depression. This may be due to the sample size, although approximately two thirds of pre-CB-EST patients were either non-cases or had borderline mood issues according to cut-off criteria.

Future work

This preliminary study directs several areas for further investigation. Future work on refining the selection criteria is required, with early results suggesting that some patients may be more suitable for CB-EST than others. CB-EST was delivered by a single SLT; whether SLTs are willing to be trained, the extent of training and access to regular supervision is unknown. In order to assess effectiveness, CB-EST would need to be protocoled, while allowing for an individually tailored approach, with fidelity checks. A proportion of patients declined participation, citing difficulties with regular attendance. It is uncertain as to whether CB-EST requires face to face intervention or if components could be administered via other mediums such as telemedicine, self-help booklets or web-based programmes. However, patients often express a preference for individual, face to face help, preferably at home [23]. It is unknown as to whether patients would be willing to be randomised in the context of a trial. Using MDADI scores, a sample size for a future trial would require 84 patients, providing 80% probability of detecting a difference at two sided significance level of 0.05. Accounting for an intervention completion rate of 58% from the available sample, 145 patients would be required to conduct such a study.

Conclusion

The addition of cognitive behavioural techniques to swallowing therapy delivered by a trained SLT, is a feasible and acceptable treatment, addressing the physical and psychosocial components of HNSCC dysphagia. Further work is needed to establish efficacy, effectiveness and cost-effectiveness of the intervention, in the context of a randomised controlled trial.

Abbreviations

CB-EST: Cognitive Behavioural-Enhanced Swallow Therapy; CBT: Cognitive Behaviour Therapy; CFQ: Chalder Fatigue Questionnaire; EORTC-HN: European Organization for Research and Treatment of Cancer – Head and Neck module; EORTC-QLQ: European Organization for Research and Treatment of Cancer- Quality of Life Questionnaire; HADS: Hospital Anxiety and Depression Scale; HNSCC: Head and neck squamous cell carcinoma; MDADI: MD Anderson Dysphagia Inventory; NGT: Nasogastric tube; PSS: Performance Status Scale; SLT: Speech and Language therapist; WASA: Work and Social Adjustment Scale

Acknowledgments

There are no other acknowledgments.

Funding

Dr. J Patterson is funded by a National Institute for Health Research award (Clinical Lecturer). This paper presents independent research funded by the National Institute for Health Research. The views expressed are those of the authors and not necessarily those of the NHS, the NIHR or the Department of Health. The funding body peer reviewed the study, but had no role in the design, data collection and analysis, interpretation of data or writing of the manuscript. The authors declare no conflicts of interest.

Authors' contributions

All authors made substantial contributions to the conception and design of this study. JP, EMc, CE and VD conceived the research design and developed the study protocol. JP delivered the intervention and VD provided supervision. JP acquired and analysed the quantitative data. MF and MB acquired and analysed the qualitative data. All authors were involved in the interpretation of data and preparation of the manuscript. They have revised the content, are accountable and have given approval for the current submission to be considered for publication.

Competing interests

The authors declare that they have no competing interests.

Author details

[1]Institute of Health and Society, Newcastle University, The Baddiley-Clark Building, Richardson Road, Newcastle upon Tyne NE2 4AX, UK. [2]Speech & Language Therapy Department, Sunderland Royal Hospital, Sunderland, UK. [3]Faculty of Health and Life Sciences, Northumbria University, Newcastle upon Tyne, UK. [4]Psychology Department, Northumbria University, Newcastle upon Tyne, UK.

References

1. Wilson JA, Carding PN, Patterson JM. Dysphagia after nonsurgical head and neck cancer treatment: patients' perspectives. Otolaryngology - Head & Neck Surgery. 2011;145(5):767–71.
2. Semenov YR, Starmer HM, Gourin CG. The effect of pneumonia on short-term outcomes and cost of care after head and neck cancer surgery. Laryngoscope. 2012;122(9):1994–2004.
3. Ichikura K, Yamashita A, Sugimoto T, Kishimoto S, Matsushima E. Persistence of psychological distress and correlated factors among patients with head and neck cancer. Palliative & Supportive Care. 2016;14(1):42–51.
4. Lin BM, Starmer HM, Gourin CG. The relationship between depressive symptoms, quality of life, and swallowing function in head and neck cancer patients 1 year after definitive therapy. Laryngoscope. 2012;122(7):1518–25.
5. Patterson JM, McColl E, Wilson J, Carding P, Rapley T. Head and neck cancer patients' perceptions of swallowing following chemoradiotherapy. Support Care Cancer. 2015;
6. Cousins N, MacAulay F, Lang H, MacGillivray S, Wells M. A systematic review of interventions for eating and drinking problems following treatment for head and neck cancer suggests a need to look beyond swallowing and trismus. Oral Oncol. 2013;49(5):387–400.
7. Perry A, Lee SH, Cotton S, Kennedy C. Therapeutic exercises for affecting post-treatment swallowing in people treated for advanced-stage head and neck cancers. Cochrane Database Syst Rev. 2016;16(8):CD011112.
8. Reich M, Leemans CR, Vermorken JB, Bernier J, Licitra L, Parmar S, Golusinski W, Lefebvre JL. Best practices in the management of the psycho-oncologic aspects of head and neck cancer patients: recommendations from the European head and neck cancer society make sense campaign. Ann Oncol. 2014;25(11):2115–24.
9. Semple C, Parahoo K, Norman A, McCaughan E, Humphris G, Mills M. Psychosocial interventions for patients with head and neck cancer. Cochrane Database Syst Rev. 2013;7

10. Semple CJ, Dunwoody L, Kernohan WG, McCaughan E. Development and evaluation of a problem-focused psychosocial intervention for patients with head and neck cancer. Support Care Cancer. 2009;17(4):379–88.

11. Miller T, Deary V, Patterson J. Improving access to psychological therapies in voice disorders: a cognitive behavioural therapy model. Current Opinion in Otolaryngology and Head and Neck Surgery. 2014;22(3):201–5.

12. Eldridge SM, Chan CL, Campbell MJ, Bond CM, Hopewell S, Thabane L, Lancaster GA. CONSORT 2010 statement: extension to randomised pilot and feasibility trials. BMJ. 2016;355

13. Chen AY, Frankowshi R, Bishop-Leone J, Hebert T, Leyk S, Lewin J, Goepfert H. The development and validation of a dysphagia-specific quality-of-life questionnaire for patients with head and neck cancer: the M. D. Anderson dysphagia inventory. Archives of Otolaryngol Head Neck Surg. 2001;127(7):870–6.

14. Lancaster GA, Dodd S, Williamson PR. Design and analysis of pilot studies: recommendations for good practice. J Eval Clin Pract. 2004;10(2):307–12.

15. Hutcheson KA, Barrow MP, Lisec A, Barringer DA, Gries K, Lewin JS. What is a clinically relevant difference in MDADI scores between groups of head and neck cancer patients? Laryngoscope. 2015;

16. Bjordal K, de Graeff A, Fayers PM, Hammerlid E, van Pottelsberghe C, Curran D, Ahlner-Elmqvist M, Maher EJ, Meyza JW, Bredart A, et al. A 12 country field study of the EORTC QLQ-C30 (version 3.0) and the head and neck cancer specific module (EORTC QLQ-H&N35) in head and neck patients. Eur J Cancer. 2000;36(14):1796–807.

17. Chalder T, Berelowitz G, Pawlikowska T, Watts L, Wessely S, Wright D, Wallace EP. Development of a fatigue scale. J Psychosom Res. 1993;37(2):147–53.

18. Mundt JC, Marks IM, Shear MK, Greist JM. The work and social adjustment scale: a simple measure of impairment in functioning. Br J Psychiatry. 2002;180(5):461–4.

19. Zigmond AS, Snaith RP. The hospital anxiety and depression scale. Acta Psychiatr Scand. 1983;67(6):361–70.

20. List MA, Mumby P, Haraf D, Siston A, Mick R, MacCracken E, Vokes E. Performance and quality of life outcome in patients completing concomitant chemoradiotherapy protocols for head and neck cancer. Qual Life Res. 1997;6(3):274–84.

21. Mittal BB, Pauloski BR, Haraf DJ, Pelzer HJ, Argiris A, Vokes EE, Rademaker A, Logemann JA. Swallowing dysfunction - preventative and rehabilitation strategies in patients with head-and-neck cancers treated with surgery, radiotherapy, and chemotherapy: a critical review. International Journal of Radiation Oncology Biology Physics. 2003;57(5):1219–30.

22. Villa C, Meregaglia M, Rognogni C, Pistillo P, Orlandi E, Iacovelli A, Granata R, Alfieri S, Bergamini C, Resteghini C, et al. Health and economic outcomes of two different follow up strategies in effectively cured advanced head and neck cancer patients. Annals of Oncology. 2016;27(suppl_4):iv87.

23. Richardson AE, Morton R, Broadbent E. Psychological support needs of patients with head and neck cancer and their caregivers: a qualitative study. Psychol Health. 2015;30(11):1288–305.

24. Roe JWG, Drinnan MJ, Carding PN, Harrington KJ, Nutting CM. Patient-reported outcomes following parotid-sparing intensity-modulated radiotherapy for head and neck cancer. How important is dysphagia? Oral Oncol. 2014;50(12):1182–7.

25. Mortensen HR, Jensen K, Aksglæde K, Lambertsen K, Eriksen E, Grau C. Prophylactic swallowing exercises in head and neck cancer radiotherapy. Dysphagia. 2015;

18

Anti-EGFR targeted therapy delivered before versus during radiotherapy in locoregionally advanced nasopharyngeal carcinoma: a big-data, intelligence platform-based analysis

Hao Peng[1†], Ling-Long Tang[1†], Xu Liu[1], Lei Chen[1], Wen-Fei Li[1], Yan-Ping Mao[1], Yuan Zhang[1], Li-Zhi Liu[2], Li Tian[2], Ying Guo[3], Ying Sun[1] and Jun Ma[1*]

Abstract

Background: Little is known about the prognostic difference of anti-EGFR therapy, cetuximab (CTX) or nimotuzumab (NTZ), concurrently with induction chemotherapy (IC, investigational arm) or RT (control arm) for patients with locoregionally advanced nasopharyngeal carcinoma (LA-NPC). We conducted this retrospective study to address this.

Methods: We identified 296 patients with newly diagnosed LA-NPC at Sun Yat-Sen University Cancer Center between January 2012 and May 2015. Patients were treated by IC with CCRT or RT and CTX/NTZ was delivered during IC or radiotherapy. Survival outcomes and toxicities between different arms were compared.

Results: In total, there were 149 patients in the investigational arm and 147 in control arm. The 3-year disease-free survival, overall survival, distant metastasis-free survival and locoregional relapse-free survival rates for investigational arm vs. control arm were 84.3% vs. 74.3% ($P = 0.027$), 94.0% vs. 92.1% ($P = 0.673$), 88.0% vs. 81.8% ($P = 0.147$) and 93.3% vs. 88.0% ($P = 0.093$). Multivariate analysis revealed patients in the control arm achieved significantly worse disease-free survival (HR, 1.497; 95% CI, 1.016–2.206; $P = 0.026$) compared with those in the investigational arm; however, no significant difference was identified for other endpoints. Patients in the investigational arm experienced more grade 3–4 skin reaction (15.4% vs. 2.0%, $P < 0.001$) and mucositis (10.1% vs. 3.4%, $P = 0.022$) during induction phase, but less skin reaction (5.4% vs. 25.9%, $P < 0.001$) and mucositis (24.8% vs. 36.7%, $P = 0.026$) during RT.

Conclusions: Our findings suggested that CTX/NTZ concurrently with IC may be a more effective and promising strategy for patients with LA-NPC receiving intensity-modulated radiotherapy.

Keywords: Nasopharyngeal carcinoma, Induction chemotherapy, Cetuximab, Nimotuzumab, Intensity-modulated radiotherapy, Prognosis

* Correspondence: majun2@mail.sysu.edu.cn
†Equal contributors
[1]Department of Radiation Oncology, Sun Yat-sen University Cancer Center, State Key Laboratory of Oncology in Southern China, Collaborative Innovation Center for Cancer Medicine, 651 Dongfeng Road East, Guangzhou 510060, People's Republic of China
Full list of author information is available at the end of the article

Background

Nasopharyngeal carcinoma (NPC) is a special type of head and neck malignancy for its extremely unbalanced geographic distribution and treatment modality. There are 86, 700 new cases reported worldwide in 2012 with the highest incidence in South China [1]. Unlike other head and neck cancers, radiotherapy (RT) is the primary and only cure for non-disseminated disease as a result of the anatomic constrain and sensitivity to radiation. Control of early stage disease with RT alone or chemo-radiation is usually excellent; however, management of locoregionally advanced NPC (LA-NPC) still remain unsatisfactory, with a 5-year overall survival (OS) of 67–77% [2]. Unfortunately, more than 70% of newly cases were locoregionally advanced disease at initial diagnosis [3]. Currently, concurrent chemo-radiation (CCRT) is the main standard care for LA-NPC. Although local and regional control has improved greatly, distant metastasis rates after treatment remain high and is the main source of treatment failure [4]. Therefore, identification of novel and effective therapeutic strategies is urgent and crucial for clinicians.

Epidermal growth factor receptor (EGFR), a transmembrane protein highly expressed in most human epithelial malignancies [5], is a promising therapeutic target in oncology for its correlation with aggressive phenotype, treatment resistance and poor prognosis [6, 7]. EGFR is also highly expressed in NPC [8] and numerous studies have evaluated the efficacy of anti-EGFR targeted therapy [9–15]. Cetuximab (CTX) or nimotuzumab (NTZ) (anti-EGFR monoclonal antibodies) concurrently with RT could achieved comparable outcomes compared with standard cisplatin-RT [12, 14]. When delivered during CCRT, different results were produced. You et al. and Xia et al. revealed CTX/NTZ additional to CCRT was more effective than CCRT alone [11, 13] while Li et al. did not identified any difference [10]. Regardless of the controversial efficacy, CTX/NTZ significantly increased acute mucositis and acneiform rash during RT [10, 12], resulting in poor quality of life or even disruption of RT. It seems that anti-EGFR therapy concurrent with RT may not be the best choice.

Induction chemotherapy (IC), given before RT, has been proven a promising treatment in LA-NPC for its satisfactory compliance and efficacy in reducing distant metastasis [16–19]. Possibly, CTX/NTZ in combination with IC may further reduce distant metastasis and improve survival outcomes. Notably, all abovementioned studies focus on the concurrent phase and no relative study to date has been carried out to assess the value of anti-EGFR therapy concurrently with IC. Given this concern, we initiated this retrospective study to evaluate the efficacy and toxicity difference of CTX/NTZ concurrently with IC or RT for LA-NPC.

Methods

Study patient

We identified 14,684 patients with newly diagnosed NPC on the big-data, intelligence database platform (YiduCloud Technology Ltd., Beijing, China) at Sun Yat-sen University Cancer center between January 2012 and May 2015. Inclusion criteria for this study were as follow: (i) stage III-IVB disease; (ii) age ≥ 18 years; (iii) karnofsky performance score (KPS) ≥ 70; (iv) did not have prior malignancies; (v) receiving IC followed by CCRT or RT alone; (vi) concurrent chemotherapy, if have, should be single-agent cisplatin; (vii) receiving intensity-modulated radiotherapy (IMRT).

Pre-treatment staging work-up

Conventional staging workup in our center included physical examination of head and neck, direct nasopharyngoscopy, chest radiography or computed tomography (CT), magnetic resonance imaging (MRI) of head and neck, abdominal sonography, whole-body bone scan and blood profile. Positron emission tomography (PET)-CT would also be recommended for patients with advanced N (N2–3) category. Magnetic resonance (MR) or CT scans of patients were reviewed separately by two radiologists employed at our center with more than 10-year experience, and any discrepancy was resolved by consensus. Tumor stage was grouped according to the 7th edition of the International Union against Cancer/American Joint Committee on Cancer (UICC/AJCC) system [20].

Treatment

All patients received radical IMRT at our center using the simultaneous integrated boost (SIB) technique as previously described. [18, 21] Briefly, prescribed radiation dose were 66–70 Gy at 2.12–2.27 Gy/fraction to the planning target volume (PTV) of nasopharyngeal gross tumor volume (GTV), 64–70 Gy to the PTV of GTV of metastatic lymph nodes, 60–63 Gy to the PTV of high-risk clinical target volume, and 50–56 Gy to the PTV of low-risk clinical target volume.

IC consisted of docetaxel (75 mg/m^2 d1) with cisplatin (75 mg/m^2 d1) (TP), fluorouracil (1000 mg/m^2 d1-d5) with cisplatin (80 mg/m^2 d1) (PF), or docetaxel (60 mg/m^2 d1) plus cisplatin (60 mg/m^2 d1) with fluorouracil (600–750 mg/m^2 d1-d5) (TPF) every three weeks for 2–4 cycles. Concurrent chemotherapy was tri-weekly cisplatin (80–100 mg/m^2) or weekly cisplatin (30–40 mg/m^2).

CTX was delivered at a dose of 400 mg/m^2 and NTZ was administered at a dose of 200 mg concurrently with IC (investigation arm) every three weeks. For patients receiving anti-EGFR therapy during RT (control arm), NTZ was administered at a dose of 200 mg weekly, and CTX was delivered at an initial dose of 400 mg/m^2 followed by 250 mg/m^2 weekly [13, 14]. Detailed information on treatment was presented in Additional file 1: Method S1.

Clinical endpoints and statistical analysis

The first endpoint is disease-free survival (DFS) defined as the time from diagnosis to disease progression or death from any cause. Other endpoints included OS (time from diagnosis to death from any cause), distant metastasis-free survival (DMFS, time from diagnosis to first distant metastasis) and locoregional relapse-free survival (LRRFS, time from diagnosis to local or regional recurrence or both). Tumor response to IC was evaluated based on Response Evaluation Criteria in Solid Tumors [22]. Acute toxicities during IC were graded according to the Common Terminology Criteria for Adverse Events (version 3.0).

The Chi-square test were adopted to compare categorical variables and Mann-Whitney test for continuous variables. Survival outcomes were calculated using Kaplan-Meier method and compared by log-rank test. Multivariate cox proportional hazards model was used to estimate hazard ratios (HRs), 95% confidence intervals (CIs) and independent prognostic factors. All tests were two-sided; $P < 0.05$ was considered significant. Stata Statistical Package 12 (StataCorp LP, College Station, TX, USA) was used for all analyses.

Results

Patient baseline characteristics

Flow chart of patient inclusion was presented in Fig. 1. In total, we identified 2999 patients and an eventual 296 patients were eligible for this study with 149 in the investigation arm and 147 in control arm. Baseline characteristics were summarized in Table 1. The median age for the whole cohort is 42 years (range, 18–73 years), and male-to-female ratio is 3.9:1. Host, tumor and treatment related factors were well balanced between the investigational arm and control arm. Moreover, patients in these two groups had similar pre-treatment imaging stage workups (Additional file 2: Table S1).

Among the investigational arm, 56 (37.6%) received CTX and the remaining 93 (62.4%) patients received NTZ. Within the control arm, 25 (17.0%) patients received CTX and 122 (83.0%) received NTZ. Obviously, more patients received NTZ during RT than that during IC ($P < 0.001$). Detailed information on dose and cycle of CTX/NTZ in each arm was shown in Additional file 3: Table S2. Undoubtedly, patients in the control arm received more cycles of CTX/NTZ. No dose reduction occurred in the two arms.

Short-term efficacy after IC

Sixteen patients with N0 category were not available for regional response evaluation, with 7 (4.7%) in the investigational arm and 9 (6.1%) in the control arm. After the completion of IC, 17 (11.4%), 121 (81.2%) and 11 (7.4%) in the investigational arm, and 13 (8.8%), 118 (80.3%)

and 16 (10.9%) in the control arm achieved complete response (CR), partial response (PR) and stable disease (SD), respectively ($P = 0.476$). No patient had progression disease (PD) in both arms. Additional file 4: Table S3 detailed the information on tumor response.

Long-term outcome analysis

Up to the last visit (September 30, 2017), the median follow-up duration is 42.0 months (range 1.27–64.8). Among the whole cohort, the overall rates of locoregional and distant failures were 11.1% (33/296) and 15.9% (47/296), respectively. In detail, 26 (17.4%) in the investigational arm and 42 (28.6%) in control arm experienced treatment failure ($P = 0.023$). Additionally, 14 (9.4%) and 16 (10.9%) in the investigational and control arms died ($P = 0.671$). Three-year DFS, OS, DMFS and LRRFS rates for the whole cohort were 79.3%, 93.1%, 84.9% and 90. 6%, respectively.

The 3-year DFS, OS, DMFS and LRRFS rates for investigational arm vs. control arm were 84.3% vs. 74.3% ($P = 0.027$), 94.0% vs. 92.1% ($P = 0.673$), 88.0% vs. 81.8% ($P = 0.147$) and 93.3% vs. 88.0% ($P = 0.093$, Fig. 2). After adjusting for various prognostic factors, patients in the control arm achieved significantly worse DFS (HR, 1.497; 95% CI, 1.016–2.206; $P = 0.026$) compared with those in the investigational arm; however, no significant difference was identified between the two arms in terms of OS (HR, 0.994; 95% CI, 0.466–2.122; $P = 0.988$), DMFS (HR, 1.409; 95% CI, 0.779–2.549; $P = 0.251$) and LRRFS (HR, 1.805; 95% CI, 0.883–3.686; $P = 0.105$; Table 2).

Grade 3–4 toxicities

Acute toxicity profiles during IC and RT were evaluated between the two groups and results were presented in Table 3. Generally, grade 3–4 toxic events were comparable between the investigational and control arms (58.4% vs. 58.5%, $P = 0.984$). However, patients in the investigational arm experienced more grade 3–4 skin reaction (15.4% vs. 2.0%, $P < 0.001$) and mucositis (10.1% vs. 3.4%, $P = 0.022$) during induction phase, but less skin reaction (5.4% vs. 25.9%, $P < 0.001$) and mucositis (24.8% vs. 36. 7%, $P = 0.026$) during RT compared with patients in the control arm. Haematological and gastrointestinal adverse events were similar between the two groups (all rates, $P > 0.005$).

Discussion

Managing advanced disease has always been a tough challenge not only in NPC management but also in many other cancers since prognosis of this subgroup is usually poor. Therefore, identification and establishment of novel and effective treatment is urgent and necessary. As far as we know, our study is the first one to compare the efficacy and safety of anti-EGFR therapy (CTX or

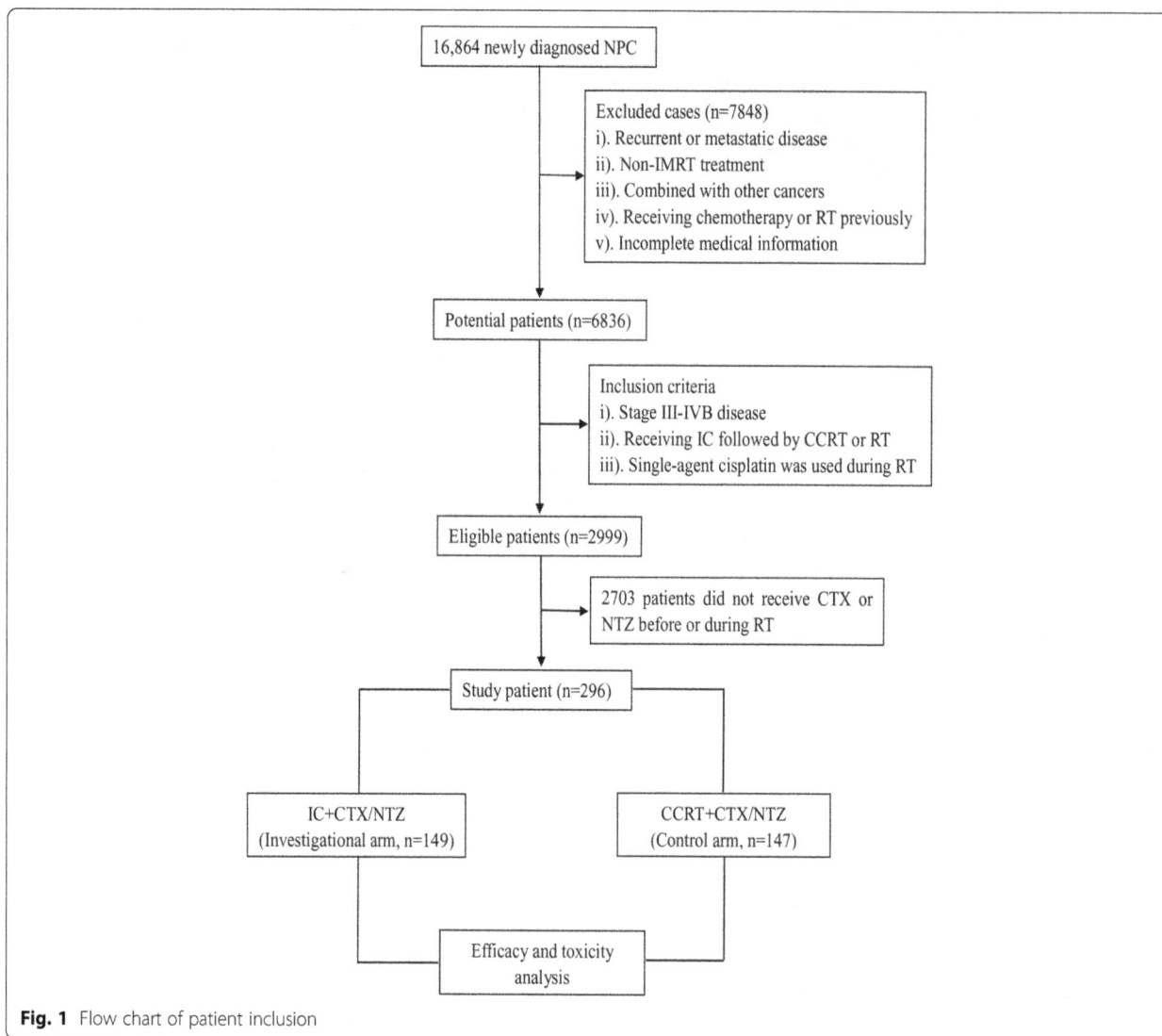

Fig. 1 Flow chart of patient inclusion

NTZ) concurrently with IC or RT in LA-NPC treated by IMRT. We found that CTX/NTZ delivered during IC could produce significantly better DFS than administered during RT while no significant difference was achieved with regard to OS, DMFS and LRRFS.

With the wide application of IMRT in NPC, local and regional control has improved greatly and distant metastasis has become the main failure pattern [4, 23]. Although CCRT is effective, it may be not powerful enough to reduce distant metastasis for LA-NPC [24]. Additional cycles of chemotherapy like IC to CCRT is warranted. Although IC followed by CCRT has achieved excellent efficacy [16, 17, 19], further improvement of prognosis is still needed. Therefore, novel and effective treatment strategies should be identified.

EGFR on tumor cells has been established as a factor predicting treatment resistance and poor prognosis [6, 7], making anti-EGFR a potential and promising treatment

strategy. Antitumor efficacy of CTX in combination with conventional chemotherapy has been proven in various EGFR-expressing malignancies like colorectal cancer, head and neck cancers and recurrent NPC [25–27]. In recurrent or metastatic head and neck squamous cell carcinoma (HNSCC), CTX combined with fluorouracil-cisplatin chemotherapy achieved significantly better DFS and OS compared with fluorouracil-cisplatin alone when given as the first-line therapy [28]. It seems that CTX could overcome resistance to previously administered chemotherapy and thereby improved survival outcomes [26]. You et al. [13] and Li et al. [10] enhanced the treatment intensity during concurrent phase by adding CTX/NTZ to standard concomitant cisplatin. However, the efficacy may be unsatisfactory and adverse events significantly increased [10, 12–14]. It's likely that concurrent administration of anti-EGFR therapy with cisplatin is a feasible strategy but not the best. These evidence reminded us that

Anti-EGFR targeted therapy delivered before versus during radiotherapy in locoregionally advanced...

177

Table 1 Baseline characteristics of the 296 patients with stage III-IVB nasopharyngeal carcinoma

Characteristics	Investigational arm (N = 149, %)	Control arm (N = 147, %)	P-value[a]
Gender			0.419
Male	116 (77.9)	120 (81.6)	
Female	33 (22.1)	27 (18.4)	
Age (years)			0.544
Median (IQR)	42 (36–51)	43 (36–52)	
Smoking			0.491
Yes	57 (38.3)	62 (42.2)	
No	92 (61.7)	85 (57.8)	
Drinking			0.095
Yes	30 (20.1)	19 (12.9)	
No	119 (79.9)	128 (87.1)	
Family history of cancer			0.668
Yes	47 (31.5)	43 (29.3)	
No	102 (68.5)	104 (70.7)	
LDH (U/L)			0.336
Median (IQR)	175 (154–216)	184 (161–215)	
Pre-DNA[b]			0.957
Median (IQR)	6880 (106–77,950)	7445 (494–52,050)	
T category[c]			0.112
T1	6 (4.0)	1 (0.7)	
T2	7 (4.7)	14 (9.5)	
T3	81 (54.4)	77 (52.4)	
T4	55 (36.9)	55 (37.4)	
N category[c]			0.873
N0	7 (4.7)	9 (6.1)	
N1	49 (32.9)	48 (32.7)	
N2	61 (40.9)	63 (42.9)	
N3	32 (21.5)	27 (18.3)	
Overall stage[c]			0.819
III	71 (47.7)	72 (49.0)	
IVA-B	78 (52.3)	75 (51.0)	
TPF regimen (cycles)			0.484
Two	15 (30.0)	14 (41.6)	
Three	33 (66.0)	18 (50.3)	
Four	2 (4.0)	2 (8.1)	
PF regimen (cycles)			0.495
Two	42 (93.3)	51 (96.3)	
Three	3 (6.7)	6 (2.9)	
Four	0 (0)	0 (0)	
TP regimen (cycles)			0.31
Two	43 (79.6)	45 (59.9)	
Three	7 (13.0)	10 (34.0)	

Table 1 Baseline characteristics of the 296 patients with stage III-IVB nasopharyngeal carcinoma (Continued)

Characteristics	Investigational arm (N = 149, %)	Control arm (N = 147, %)	P-value[a]
Four	4 (7.4)	1 (6.1)	
Concurrent chemotherapy			0.964
Yes	130 (87.2)	128 (87.1)	
No	19 (12.8)	19 (12.9)	

IC induction chemotherapy, *IQR* interquartile, *LDH* lactate dehydrogenase; *Pre-DNA* pre-treatment Epstein-Barr virus DNA, *TPF* docetaxel plus cisplatin with fluorouracil, *PF* cisplatin with fluorouracil, *TP* docetaxel with cisplatin
[a]P-values were calculated using Chi-square test for categorical variables and Mann-Whitney test for continuous variables
[b]Three patients in the control arm did not have this data
[c]According to the 7th edition of the International Union against Cancer/ American Joint Committee on Cancer (UICC/AJCC) system

CTX/NTZ in combination with IC may be a preferable choice. In our present study, we confirmed this view as patients in the investigational arm achieved significantly better DFS. Our findings provided a new insight in managing LA-NPC by enhancing the treatment intensity during IC.

Reasons contributing to the significantly difference of DFS were complicated. First, treatment intensity during IC was improved by adding CTX/NTZ which could help to further eradicate micro-metastasis lesions prior to RT and thereby reduce treatment failure events. Second, patients receiving CTX/NTZ during RT experienced more severe toxicities than those not. Consequently, these patients had poor quality of life during RT which could adversely affect prognosis [29, 30]. Furthermore, some patients even suffered RT interruption due to severe skin reaction or mucositis. Undoubtedly, the prolonged treatment time had a negative impact on prognosis [31, 32].

Notably, univariate and multivariate analysis only identified the significant difference between the two arms for DFS. As indicated by the survival curves, patients in the investigational arm also achieved better DMFS and LRRFS compared with patients in the control arm, although the difference was not significant. The main reason should be attributed to the small sample size which was not statistically powerful enough to identify the difference. Possibly, the improved DFS should originate from DMFS and LRRFS together. Due to the insufficient follow-up duration, no significant difference was achieved on OS although more patients in the control arm experienced treatment failure. Therefore, future studies with larger sample and longer follow-up duration are warranted to validate our results. Moreover, some other factors like program death ligand 1 (PD-L1) on tumor cells, human papillomavirus (HPV) status and lifetime cigarette smoking (pack-years) may also play important roles in prognosis and have an effect on the insignificant OS. However, these factors were not routinely evaluated in our center. Further studies were needed to evaluate these factors.

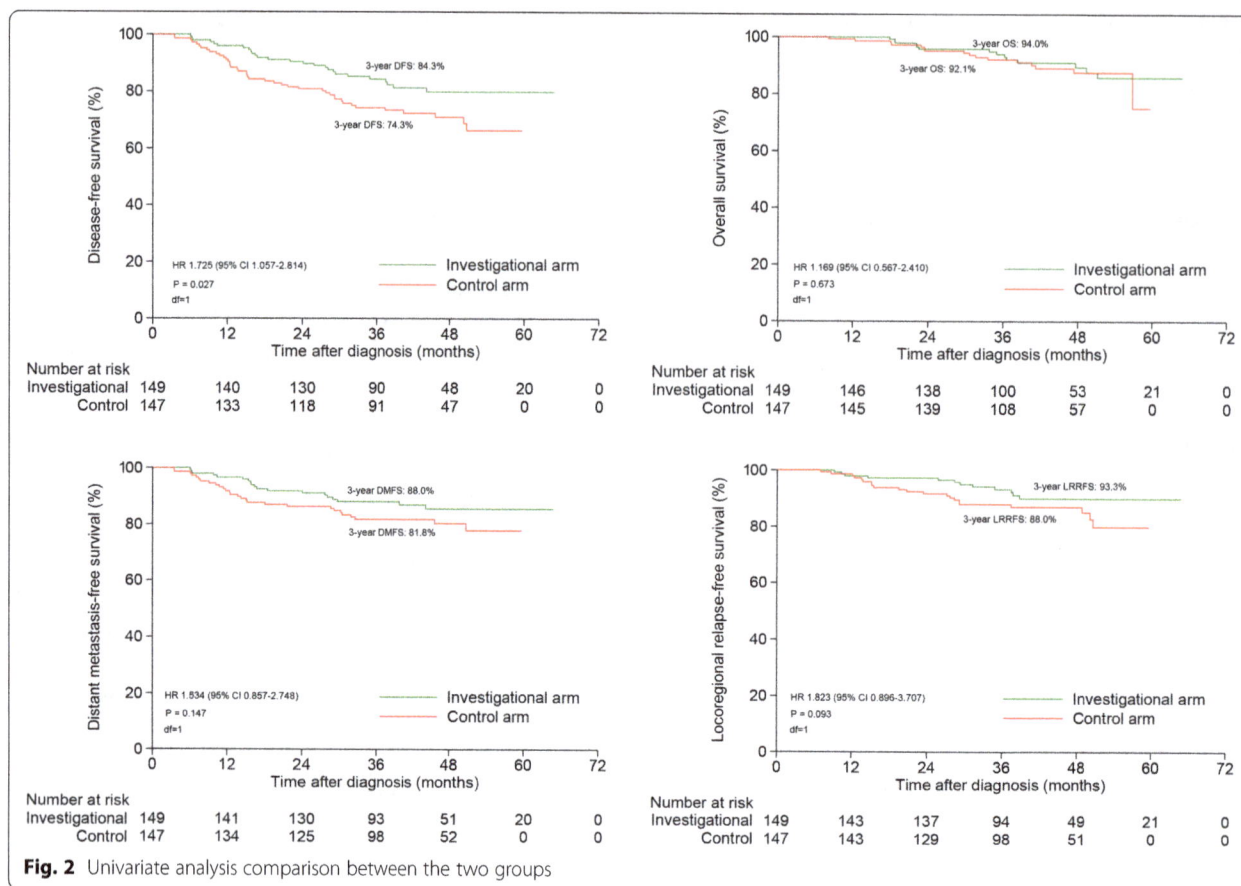

Fig. 2 Univariate analysis comparison between the two groups

Table 2 Multivariate regression analysis for prognostic factors

Variable	HR	95% CI	P value[a]
Disease-free survival			
N category (N2–3 vs. N0–1)	2.512	1.388–4.548	0.002
Overall stage (IV vs. III)	1.757	1.051–2.939	0.032
Treatment group (Control vs. investigational)	1.497	1.016–2.206	0.026
Overall survival			
Overall stage (IV vs. III)	4.995	1.907–13.083	0.001
Treatment group (Control vs. investigational)	0.994	0.466–2.122	0.988
Distant metastasis-free survival			
N category (N2–3 vs. N0–1)	2.791	1.344–5.793	0.006
Treatment group (Control vs. investigational)	1.409	0.779–2.549	0.251
Locoregional relapse-free survival			
IC regimen (TPF vs. PF)	0.204	0.059–0.707	0.012
IC regimen (TPF vs. TP)	0.823	0.398–1.701	0.598
Treatment group (Control vs. investigational)	1.805	0.883–3.686	0.105

HR hazard ratio, *CI* confidence interval, *IC* induction chemotherapy, *TPF* docetaxel plus cisplatin with fluorouracil, *PF* cisplatin with fluorouracil, *TP* docetaxel with cisplatin, *LDH* lactate dehydrogenase

[a]Multivariate P-values were calculated by Cox proportional hazard regression model with backward elimination for the following prognostic factors: gender (female vs. male), age (> 42y vs. ≤ 42y), smoking (yes vs. no), drinking (yes vs. no), family history of cancer (yes vs. no), LDH (> 245 vs. ≤ 245 U/L), IC regimen (TPF vs. PF, TPF vs. TP), concurrent chemotherapy (yes vs. no), T category (T3–4 vs. T1–2), N category (N2–3 vs. N0–1), Overall stage (IV vs. III) and treatment group (control vs. investigational)

Table 3 Grade 3–4 acute toxicity profiles during induction chemotherapy and radiotherapy

Grade 3–4 toxicity	Investigational arm (N = 149, %)	Control arm (N = 147, %)	P value[a]
Any	87 (58.4%)	86 (58.5%)	0.984
Induction phase			
Leucopenia	36 (24.2)	27 (18.4)	0.223
Neutropenia	61 (40.9)	45 (30.6)	0.064
Anaemia	2 (1.3)	2 (1.4)	0.989
Thrombocytopenia	5 (3.4)	1 (0.7)	0.102
Liver function	3 (2.0)	2 (1.4)	0.663
Renal function	0 (0)	0 (0)	1.000
Skin reaction	23 (15.4)	3 (2.0)	< 0.001
Mucositis	15 (10.1)	5 (3.4)	0.022
Nausea	3 (2.0)	2 (1.4)	0.663
Vomiting	8 (5.4)	12 (8.2)	0.338
Diarrhoea	3 (2.0)	1 (0.7)	0.321
Concurrent phase			
Leucopenia	31 (20.8)	40 (27.2)	0.197
Neutropenia	19 (12.8)	24 (16.3)	0.383
Anaemia	11 (7.4)	15 (10.2)	0.391
Thrombocytopenia	13 (8.7)	8 (5.4)	0.271
Liver function	3 (2.0)	5 (3.4)	0.462
Renal function	0 (0)	2 (1.4)	0.246
Skin reaction	8 (5.4)	38 (25.9)	< 0.001
Mucositis	37 (24.8)	54 (36.7)	0.026
Nausea	14 (9.4)	18 (12.2)	0.430
Vomiting	20 (13.4)	22 (15.0)	0.704
Diarrhoea	2 (1.3)	5 (3.4)	0.244

[a]P-values were calculated by Chi-square test or Fisher exact test

Generally, severe toxicities during RT in our study were similar as the findings in previous studies [10, 12–14]. Overall grade 3–4 toxic events were comparable between the two arms; however, anti-EGFR therapy related toxicities like skin reaction and mucositis significantly varied between the investigational and control arms during IC and RT. In detail, patients in the investigational arm experienced more grade 3–4 skin reaction and mucositis during IC but less during RT. Undoubtedly, CTX/NTZ could aggravate radiation-induced skin and oral mucositis. Another reason for the difference may be that the total dose used in induction phase is less than that used in concurrent phase. As both arms had similar chemotherapy intensity, severe heamatological and gastrointestinal events were parallel.

In our study, patients in the investigational arm had two main advantages compared with those in control arm. First, patients experienced significantly less anti-EGFR therapy related severe toxicities. Therefore, patients had better quality of life during treatment. Second, cycles of CTX/NTZ used during induction phase were usually less than that in concurrent phase. Hence, cost of anti-EGFR therapy is also less. However, limitations of this study should also be acknowledged. Our study is retrospective and the sample size may be small, meaning that potential bias existed and the power of identify difference may be insufficient. Moreover, the follow-up duration may be insufficient. Consequently, we set DFS as the first endpoint to address this. Furthermore, the cycles of IC were not uniform. In light of previous evidence, we recruited patients receiving at least two cycles because two cycles could produce the similar survival outcomes as three or more cycles [21]. Importantly, we balanced this factor between the two groups. The median age of included patients is younger than that in other reports, which should be attributed to the small sample size.

Conclusion

In summary, CTX/NTZ concurrently with IC could achieved better survival outcomes and less severe toxicities compared with CTX/NTZ concurrently with RT in LA-NPC treated by IMRT. Our study provided a new insight into managing LA-NPC for clinicians. However, findings of present study need to be validated in prospective studies.

Abbreviations

CCRT: concurrent chemo-radiation; CI: confidence interval; CT: computed tomography; CTX: Cetuximab; DFS: disease-free survival; DMFS: distant metastasis-free survival; EGFR: Epidermal growth factor receptor; GTV: gross tumor volume; HNSCC: head and neck squamous cell carcinoma; HR: hazard ratio; IC: Induction chemotherapy; IMRT: receiving intensity-modulated radiotherapy; KPS: karnofsky performance score; LA-NPC: locoregionally advanced nasopharyngeal carcinoma; LRRFS: locoregional relapse-free survival; MRI: magnetic resonance imaging; NPC: Nasopharyngeal carcinoma; NTZ: nimotuzumab; OS: overall survival; PET: positron emission tomography; PF: fluorouracil with cisplatin; PTV: planning target volume; RT: radiotherapy; SIB: simultaneous integrated boost; TP: docetaxel with cisplatin; TPF: docetaxel plus cisplatin with fluorouracil; UICC/AJCC: International Union against Cancer/American Joint Committee on Cancer

Acknowledgements

We sincerely thanked Dr. Wei Liang and Dr. Lei Shi (YiduCloud Technology Ltd., Beijing, China) for kindly providing technical support in searching data on the big-data intelligence platform.

Funding

This work was supported by grants from the National Science & Technology Pillar Program during the Twelfth Five-year Plan Period (2014BAI09B10), the Natural Science Foundation of Guangdong Province (2017A030312003), the National Natural Science Foundation of China (81572658), the Program of Introducing Talents of Discipline to Universities (B14035), and the Innovation Team Development Plan of the Ministry of Education (No. IRT_17R110).

Authors' contributions

HP, LLT, and JM contributed to study design and conception. HP, LZL, LT, YZ, XL and YPM contributed to data acquisition. HP, LC, JM, and YG analyzed and interpreted the data. HP, WFL, and YZ contributed to manuscript revision. YPM and YS contributed to quality control and review of the data and manuscript. All authors have read and approved the final version of the submitted manuscript.

Competing interests

The authors declare that they have no competing interests.

Author details

[1]Department of Radiation Oncology, Sun Yat-sen University Cancer Center, State Key Laboratory of Oncology in Southern China, Collaborative Innovation Center for Cancer Medicine, 651 Dongfeng Road East, Guangzhou 510060, People's Republic of China. [2]Imaging Diagnosis and Interventional Center, Sun Yat-sen University Cancer Center, State Key Laboratory of Oncology in Southern China, Collaborative Innovation Center for Cancer Medicine, Guangzhou, People's Republic of China. [3]Department of Clinical Trials Center, Sun Yat-sen University Cancer Center, State Key Laboratory of Oncology in Southern China, Collaborative Innovation Center for Cancer Medicine, Guangzhou, People's Republic of China.

References

1. Torre LA, Bray F, Siegel RL, Ferlay J, Lortet-Tieulent J, Jemal A. Global cancer statistics, 2012. CA Cancer J Clin. 2015;65:87–108.

2. Yi JL, Gao L, Huang XD, et al. Nasopharyngeal carcinoma treated by radical radiotherapy alone: ten-year experience of a single institution. Int J Radiat Oncol Biol Phys. 2006;65:161–8.

3. Mao YP, Xie FY, Liu LZ, et al. Re-evaluation of 6th edition of AJCC staging system for nasopharyngeal carcinoma and proposed improvement based on magnetic resonance imaging. Int J Radiat Oncol Biol Phys. 2009;73:1326–34.

4. Lai SZ, Li WF, Chen L, et al. How does intensity-modulated radiotherapy versus conventional two-dimensional radiotherapy influence the treatment results in nasopharyngeal carcinoma patients? Int J Radiat Oncol Biol Phys. 2011;80:661–8.

5. Zhang H, Berezov A, Wang Q, et al. ErbB receptors: from oncogenes to targeted cancer therapies. J Clin Invest. 2007;117:2051–8.

6. Ciardiello F, Tortora GA. Novel approach in the treatment of cancer: targeting the epidermal growth factor receptor. Clin Cancer Res. 2001;7:2958–70.

7. Mendelsohn J. Targeting the epidermal growth factor receptor for cancer therapy. J Clin Oncol. 2002;20(18 Suppl):1S–13S.

8. Ma BB, Poon TC, To KF, et al. Prognostic significance of tumor angiogenesis, Ki 67, p53 oncoprotein, epidermal growth factor receptor and HER2 receptor protein expression in undifferentiated nasopharyngeal carcinoma–a prospective study. Head Neck. 2003;25:864–72.

9. He X, Xu J, Guo W, et al. Cetuximab in combination with chemoradiation after induction chemotherapy of locoregionally advanced nasopharyngeal carcinoma: preliminary results. Future Oncol. 2013;9:1459–67.

10. Li Y, Chen QY, Tang LQ, et al. Concurrent chemoradiotherapy with or without cetuximab for stage II to IVb nasopharyngeal carcinoma: a case-control study. BMC Cancer. 2017;17:567.

11. Xia WX, Liang H, Lv X, et al. Combining cetuximab with chemoradiotherapy in patients with locally advanced nasopharyngeal carcinoma: a propensity score analysis. Oral Oncol. 2017;67:167–74.

12. Xu T, Liu Y, Dou S, Li F, Guan X, Zhu G. Weekly cetuximab concurrent with IMRT aggravated radiation-induced oral mucositis in locally advanced nasopharyngeal carcinoma: results of a randomized phase II study. Oral Oncol. 2015;51:875–9.

13. You R, Hua YJ, Liu YP, et al. Concurrent Chemoradiotherapy with or without anti-EGFR-targeted treatment for stage II-IVb nasopharyngeal carcinoma: retrospective analysis with a large cohort and long follow-up. Theranostics. 2017;7:2314–24.

14. You R, Sun R, Hua YJ, et al. Cetuximab or nimotuzumab plus intensity-modulated radiotherapy versus cisplatin plus intensity-modulated radiotherapy for stage II-IVb nasopharyngeal carcinoma. Int J Cancer. 2017;141:1265–76.

15. Huang JF, Zhang FZ, Zou QZ, et al. Induction chemotherapy followed by concurrent chemoradiation and nimotuzumab for locoregionally advanced nasopharyngeal carcinoma: preliminary results from a phase II clinical trial. Oncotarget. 2017;8:2457–65.

16. Cao SM, Yang Q, Guo L, et al. Neoadjuvant chemotherapy followed by concurrent chemoradiotherapy versus concurrent chemoradiotherapy alone in locoregionally advanced nasopharyngeal carcinoma: a phase III multicentre randomised controlled trial. Eur J Cancer. 2017;75:14–23.

17. Hui EP, Ma BB, Leung SF, et al. Randomized phase II trial of concurrent cisplatin-radiotherapy with or without neoadjuvant docetaxel and cisplatin in advanced nasopharyngeal carcinoma. J Clin Oncol. 2009;27:242–9.

18. Peng H, Chen L, Zhang J, et al. Induction chemotherapy improved long-term outcomes of patients with Locoregionally advanced nasopharyngeal carcinoma: a propensity matched analysis of 5-year survival outcomes in the era of intensity-modulated radiotherapy. J Cancer. 2017;8:371–7.

19. Sun Y, Li WF, Chen NY, et al. Induction chemotherapy plus concurrent chemoradiotherapy versus concurrent chemoradiotherapy alone in locoregionally advanced nasopharyngeal carcinoma: a phase 3, multicentre, randomised controlled trial. Lancet Oncol. 2016;17:1509–20.

20. Edge SB, Compton CC. The American joint committee on Cancer: the 7th edition of the AJCC cancer staging manual and the future of TNM. Ann Surg Oncol. 2010;17:1471–4.

21. Peng H, Chen L, Li WF, et al. Optimize the cycle of neoadjuvant chemotherapy for locoregionally advanced nasopharyngeal carcinoma treated with intensity-modulated radiotherapy: a propensity score matching analysis. Oral Oncol. 2016;62:78–84.

22. Therasse P, Arbuck SG, Eisenhauer EA, et al. New guidelines to evaluate the response to treatment in solid tumors. European Organization for Research and Treatment of Cancer, National Cancer Institute of the United States, National Cancer Institute of Canada. J Natl Cancer Inst. 2000;92:205–16.

23. Sun X, Su S, Chen C, et al. Long-term outcomes of intensity-modulated radiotherapy for 868 patients with nasopharyngeal carcinoma: an analysis of survival and treatment toxicities. Radiother Oncol. 2014;110:398–403.

24. Lin JC, Liang WM, Jan JS, Jiang RS, Lin AC. Another way to estimate outcome of advanced nasopharyngeal carcinoma–is concurrent chemoradiotherapy adequate? Int J Radiat Oncol Biol Phys. 2004;60:156–64.

25. Chan AT, Hsu MM, Goh BC, et al. Multicenter, phase II study of cetuximab in combination with carboplatin in patients with recurrent or metastatic nasopharyngeal carcinoma. J Clin Oncol. 2005;23:3568–76.

26. Cunningham D, Humblet Y, Siena S, et al. Cetuximab monotherapy and cetuximab plus irinotecan in irinotecan-refractory metastatic colorectal cancer. N Engl J Med. 2004;351:337–45.

27. Pfister DG, Su YB, Kraus DH, et al. Concurrent cetuximab, cisplatin, and concomitant boost radiotherapy for locoregionally advanced, squamous cell head and neck cancer: a pilot phase II study of a new combined-modality paradigm. J Clin Oncol. 2006;24:1072–8.

28. Vermorken JB, Mesia R, Rivera F, et al. Platinum-based chemotherapy plus cetuximab in head and neck cancer. N Engl J Med. 2008;359:1116–27.

29. Fang FM, Chiu HC, Kuo WR, et al. Health-related quality of life for nasopharyngeal carcinoma patients with cancer-free survival after treatment. Int J Radiat Oncol Biol Phys. 2002;53:959–68.

30. Fang FM, Tsai WL, Chien CY, et al. Pretreatment quality of life as a predictor of distant metastasis and survival for patients with nasopharyngeal carcinoma. J Clin Oncol. 2010;28:4384–9.

31. Kwong DL, Sham JS, Chua DT, Choy DT, Au GK, Wu PM. The effect of interruptions and prolonged treatment time in radiotherapy for nasopharyngeal carcinoma. Int J Radiat Oncol Biol Phys. 1997;39:703–10.

32. Li PJ, Jin T, Luo DH, et al. Effect of prolonged radiotherapy treatment time on survival outcomes after intensity-modulated radiation therapy in nasopharyngeal carcinoma. PLoS One. 2015;10:e0141332.

19

Gene-expression signature regulated by the KEAP1-NRF2-CUL3 axis is associated with a poor prognosis in head and neck squamous cell cancer

Akhileshwar Namani[1†], Md. Matiur Rahaman[2†], Ming Chen[2*] and Xiuwen Tang[1*] (ORCID)

Abstract

Background: NRF2 is the key regulator of oxidative stress in normal cells and aberrant expression of the NRF2 pathway due to genetic alterations in the KEAP1 (Kelch-like ECH-associated protein 1)-NRF2 (nuclear factor erythroid 2 like 2)-CUL3 (cullin 3) axis leads to tumorigenesis and drug resistance in many cancers including head and neck squamous cell cancer (HNSCC). The main goal of this study was to identify specific genes regulated by the KEAP1-NRF2-CUL3 axis in HNSCC patients, to assess the prognostic value of this gene signature in different cohorts, and to reveal potential biomarkers.

Methods: RNA-Seq V2 level 3 data from 279 tumor samples along with 37 adjacent normal samples from patients enrolled in the The Cancer Genome Atlas (TCGA)-HNSCC study were used to identify upregulated genes using two methods (altered KEAP1-NRF2-CUL3 versus normal, and altered KEAP1-NRF2-CUL3 versus wild-type). We then used a new approach to identify the combined gene signature by integrating both datasets and subsequently tested this signature in 4 independent HNSCC datasets to assess its prognostic value. In addition, functional annotation using the DAVID v6.8 database and protein-protein interaction (PPI) analysis using the STRING v10 database were performed on the signature.

Results: A signature composed of a subset of 17 genes regulated by the KEAP1-NRF2-CUL3 axis was identified by overlapping both the upregulated genes of altered versus normal (251 genes) and altered versus wild-type (25 genes) datasets. We showed that increased expression was significantly associated with poor survival in 4 independent HNSCC datasets, including the TCGA-HNSCC dataset. Furthermore, Gene Ontology, Kyoto Encyclopedia of Genes and Genomes, and PPI analysis revealed that most of the genes in this signature are associated with drug metabolism and glutathione metabolic pathways.

Conclusions: Altogether, our study emphasizes the discovery of a gene signature regulated by the KEAP1-NRF2-CUL3 axis which is strongly associated with tumorigenesis and drug resistance in HNSCC. This 17-gene signature provides potential biomarkers and therapeutic targets for HNSCC cases in which the NRF2 pathway is activated.

Keywords: Head and neck squamous cell cancer, KEAP1-NRF2-CUL3 mutations, Overall survival, Gene-expression signature

* Correspondence: mchen@zju.edu.cn; xiuwentang@zju.edu.cn
†Equal contributors
2Department of Bioinformatics, College of Life Sciences, Zhejiang University, Hangzhou 310058, People's Republic of China
1Department of Biochemistry, University School of Medicine, Hangzhou 310058, People's Republic of China

Background

Head and neck squamous cell cancer (HNSCC) is the sixth most prevalent form of cancer. It has a high incidence worldwide, and 90% of cases are histologically identified as squamous cell carcinomas [1, 2]. HNSCC is a broad category of cancers that predominantly arise in the oral cavity, oropharynx, hypopharynx, larynx, soft tissues of the neck, salivary glands, skin, and mucosal membranes [3, 4]. The most common causes are the consumption of tobacco and alcohol, and human papillomavirus infection [5].

NRF2 is the master transcription factor that regulates the genes involved in antioxidant and detoxification pathways. Under normal conditions, Kelch like-ECH-associated protein 1 (KEAP1) negatively regulates the NRF2 expression by cullin-3 (CUL3)-mediated ubiquitination and proteasomal degradation [6]. Under oxidative stress, NRF2 is liberated from the tight control of the KEAP1/CUL3 complex, is relocated to the nucleus where it forms heterodimers with small Maf proteins, and transactivates its downstream genes through binding with antioxidant responsive elements (AREs) [7]. Genetic alterations such as mutations (gain of function mutations of NRF2 and loss of function mutations in KEAP1 and CUL3), and copy-number changes (amplification of NRF2 and deletion of KEAP1 and CUL3) leads to oncogenesis and drug- and radio-resistance in different types of cancers including HNSCC [8, 9]. Due to the dysregulated NRF2 activity in different cancers, it is emerging as a promising therapeutic target in drug discovery [10, 11].

Stacy et al. [12] first reported the increased expression of NRF2 in HNSCC patients and suggested that NRF2 might be a biomarker. Another report from Huang et al. [13] found the increased expression of KEAP1 and NRF2 in oral squamous cell carcinoma. However, in their report, overall survival analysis of patients with increased expression of KEAP1 and NRF2 did not reveal significant differences. Recently, The Cancer Genome Atlas (TCGA) has provided a wealth of information about KEAP1-NRF2-CUL3 changes in HNSCC patients [14]. Therefore, examining the molecular mechanisms involved in these alterations by using publicly available data may contribute to the development and design of therapeutic targets for personalized/precision medicine in subsets of patients. Several emerging studies including our recent study on lung cancer have identified an NRF2-regulated gene signature and potential biomarkers for patient survival and NRF2 activity [15–18].

Given the importance of KEAP1-NRF2-CUL3 changes in HNSCC, it is important to identify the biomarkers that determine patient survival and NRF2 activity. A recent analysis on TCGA-HNSCC data revealed that patients with disruption of the KEAP1/CUL3/RBX1 E3-ubiquitin ligase complex have significantly poorer survival than non-disrupted counterparts [19]. However, their study specifically focused on the data from patients with a disrupted KEAP1/CUL3/RBX1 complex, but not the data from samples in which NRF2 was altered. In addition they utilized 302 patients data which contains provisional information in their study and overall survival analysis was limited to one cohort. In our study, we restricted the patients samples number ($n = 279$) which were reported in the TCGA publication [14] and excluded provisional data. Moreover, we analyzed the TCGA-HNSCC [14] RNA-Seq data and identified a 17-gene signature that was highly expressed in samples with altered KEAP1-NRF2-CUL3 compared with both normal and wild-type counterparts. Further, we showed that genomic changes in KEAP1-NRF2-CUL3 were key effectors of the overexpression of genes dependent on the NRF2 pathway. Furthermore, we identified known NRF2-regulated genes involved in drug and glutathione metabolism, along with 4 putative KEAP1-NRF2-CUL3-regulated genes. Finally, we found that higher expression of this gene signature was significantly associated with poorer survival in 4 HNSCC cohorts.

Methods

Samples and transcriptomic profile datasets

We obtained RNA-Seq gene expression version2 (RNA-SeqV2) level 3 data (Illumina Hiseq platform) from HNSCC patients along with adjacent normal tissues from the Broad GDAC Firehose website (http://gdac.broadinstitute.org/). We carried out the analysis of RNA-Seq data of 279 tumor samples and 37 adjacent normal samples listed in the TCGA network study [14]. All the alteration data for KEAP1-NRF2-CUL3 (KEAP1-mutation/deletion, NRF2-mutation/amplification, and CUL3-muatation/deletion) used in the present study was obtained from cBioportal [20, 21]. In addition to the TCGA-HNSCC RNA-Seq data, three independent HNSCC cohorts microarray data– Saintigny et al. (GSE26549) [22], Jung et al. (E-MTAB-1328) [23], and Cohen et al. (GSE10300) [24] – were also used for overall survival analysis. Our study meets the publication guidelines listed by the TCGA network.

RNA-Seq data analysis

The conventional method of differentially-expressed gene (DEG) analysis involves the comparison of tumor transcriptomic data with normal cell data. However, in recent studies, due to the availability of large sets of tumor samples and fewer adjacent normal datasets, researchers have performed DEG analysis of TCGA data by applying a new method in which the DEGs are identified by comparing altered or mutated tumor samples (including a particular gene/set of genes) with wild-type tumors (caused by factors other than alterations or mutations) [15, 25, 26].

Despite the fact that these two methods have been used separately for DEG analysis, in this study, we applied a combinatorial approach to obtain DEGs from HNSCC patients by using both conventional and new methods. We then integrated the resulting upregulated genes from both datasets to obtain overlapping genes. This approach led to the robust identification of more markedly upregulated genes specific to the samples with altered KEAP1-NRF2-CUL3 than in both normal and wild-type samples. Moreover, our method not only identified specific genes targeted by the KEAP1-NRF2-CUL3 axis but also minimized false-positive results.

We segregated the 279 HNSCC tumor samples into two groups: 54 altered KEAP1-NRF2-CUL3 samples (referred to below as 'altered') and 225 wild-type samples. Before performing transcriptomic data analysis, the TCGA barcodes of patient data were cross-checked to avoid technical errors. First, we carried out DEG analysis in the 54 altered versus 37 normal samples followed by 54 altered versus 225 wild-type samples using the R/Bioconductor package [27] – edgeR [28]. To crosscheck how our combinatorial approach effectively found specific genes targeted by the KEAP1-NRF2-CUL3 axis, we also subjected the 225 wild-type and 37 normal samples to DEG analysis. Briefly, the raw counts of RNA-SeqV2 level 3 data were filtered by removing the genes containing zero values. We then considered the genes with >100 counts per million in at least two samples for normalization using the trimmed mean of M-values method, followed by the estimation of dispersions using generalized linear models. Up- and down-regulated genes for altered versus normal and altered versus wild-type samples were identified separately by applying a Benjamini-Hochberg (BH) false-discovery rate (FDR) $p < 0.01$ with a log-fold change (logFC) > 1.5 and <−1.5. Finally, we used the overlapping upregulated genes obtained from both datasets using 'Venny 2.1' (http://bioinfogp.cnb.csic.es/tools/venny/index.html) for further analysis. Hierarchical clustering of overlapping upregulated genes was performed using the 'Heatmapper' web tool [29]. Box plots of the overlapping upregulated genes that represent the log (counts per million) expression values were generated using R-package 'ggplot2' [30]. The overall workflow of the study design is presented in Fig. 1.

Functional annotation and protein-protein interaction (PPI) network analysis

Functional annotation (Gene Ontology (GO) and Kyoto Encyclopedia of Genes and Genomes (KEGG) analysis) of overlapping upregulated genes was performed using the updated version of the Database for Annotation, Visualization and Integrated Discovery (DAVID) v6.8 web tool [31]. PPI network analysis was performed using the STRING v10 database [32].

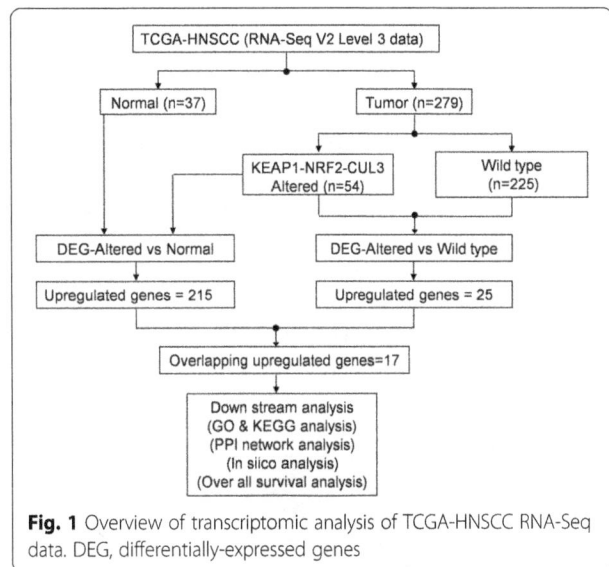

Fig. 1 Overview of transcriptomic analysis of TCGA-HNSCC RNA-Seq data. DEG, differentially-expressed genes

Identification of NRF2-binding sites by in silico analysis

To identify the NRF2 binding sites within the promoter regions of the putative KEAP1-NRF2-CUL3-regulated genes, we used the transcription factor-binding site finding tool LASAGNA-Search 2.0 [33] with cutoff p-values $\leq$ 0.001. The search was limited to the -5 kb upstream promoter region relative to the transcription start site.

Survival analysis

Cox proportional hazard regression was performed using the online survival analysis and biomarker validation tool SurvExpress [34]. We considered the data from a total of 502 patients in 4 independent HNSCC cohorts available in the SurvExpress database: the TCGA-HNSCC cohort ($n = 283$) with other three HNSCC cohorts – Saintigny et al. (GSE26549) ($n = 86$) [22], Jung et al. (E-MTAB-1328) ($n = 89$) [23], and Cohen et al. (GSE10300) ($n = 44$) [24] – for survival analysis. In the case of microarray-based survival data, we considered the average values for genes whose expression was associated with multiple probe sets such as duplicates or alternatives. SurvExpress separated the patient samples into two groups, high - and low-risk, based on average expression of the 17 genes signature values, and performed statistical analysis of survival probability of the two groups using the log-rank method. SurvExpress used the log-rank test to generate Kaplan-Meir plots based on the 'Survival' package of the R platform, which is integrated into its website. Log-rank test p-values < 0.05 were considered to be statistically significant.

Results

Overview of genetic alterations in the KEAP1-NRF2-CUL3axis

In HNSCC, changes in the KEAP1-NRF2-CUL3 axis occurred in ~20% of patients; of these, KEAP1 alterations accounted for 4.6%, NRF2 for 11.8%, and CUL3 for

5.7%. However, few samples overlapped (Fig. 2a). In order to better understand the KEAP1-NRF2-CUL3 mutational landscape in HNSCC, we used the cBioportal cancer genomics website [20, 21] to examine the types of mutation and their positions in the domain structure of proteins. All 13 KEAP1 and 18 NRF2 mutations were missense mutations, while 70% of the CUL3 mutations (7/10) were missense, 20% (2/10) were nonsense, and 10% (1/10) were splice mutations (Fig. 2b).

KEAP1 consists of 605 amino-acids with 3 domains in which 6 mutations were reported in the BTB (broad-complex, tramtrack, and bric-a-brac) domain, 1 in the IVR (intervening region), 1 in the C-terminal, 1 in the N-terminal region, and another 4 were in the Kelch domain, which is essential for the binding of NRF2. In the case of NRF2 structure, the majority of mutations (16) occurred in the crucial KEAP1-binding domain Neh2, and another 2 were found in each of the Neh7 and Neh3 domains. CUL3 contained 4 mutations in the N-terminal domain, 5 in the C-terminal domain, and 1 in the cullin repeat 3 domain (Fig. 2c). Overall, two samples contained both KEAP1 and NRF2 mutations, while one sample contained both NRF2 and CUL3 mutations. KEAP1 and CUL3 mutations were mutually exclusive.

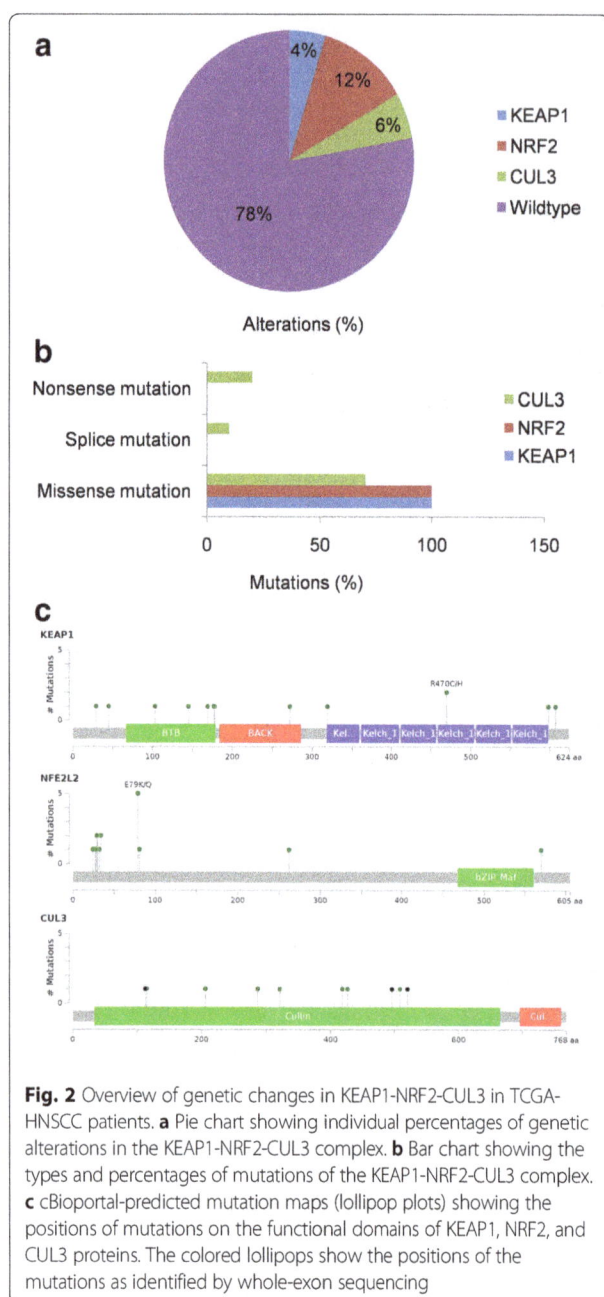

Fig. 2 Overview of genetic changes in KEAP1-NRF2-CUL3 in TCGA-HNSCC patients. **a** Pie chart showing individual percentages of genetic alterations in the KEAP1-NRF2-CUL3 complex. **b** Bar chart showing the types and percentages of mutations of the KEAP1-NRF2-CUL3 complex. **c** cBioportal-predicted mutation maps (lollipop plots) showing the positions of mutations on the functional domains of KEAP1, NRF2, and CUL3 proteins. The colored lollipops show the positions of the mutations as identified by whole-exon sequencing

Identification of genes regulated by the KEAP1-NRF2-CUL3 axis in HNSCC

In order to identify the genes regulated by the KEAP1-NRF2-CUL3 axis in HNSCC, we focused on the identification of differentially expressed genes by analyzing the RNA-Seq expression profiles in 54 altered versus 37 normal, and 54 altered versus 225 wild-type samples. A total of 215 upregulated genes and 9 downregulated genes were found in the altered versus normal analysis (Additional file 1: Table S1), and 25 upregulated genes and 13 downregulated genes in the altered versus wild-type analysis (Additional file 2: Table S2) with logFC >1.5 ($p < 0.01$ with BH-FDR adjustment). Since the ultimate effect of KEAP1-NRF2-CUL3 axis gene alterations leads to overexpression of NRF2 and its downstream genes, we focused on the upregulated genes for further analysis. By integrating both datasets using Venny web tool (http://bioinfogp.cnb.csic.es/tools/venny/index.html), we obtained 17 overlapping upregulated genes (Fig. 3a). We carried out literature survey to verify whether the downregulated genes obtained from both methods contains previously reported NRF2 regulated genes or not. Notably, we didn't observe any previously reported NRF2 target genes among all downregulated genes.

We also carried out DEG analysis in 225 wild-type versus 37 normal samples to assess the specificity of the 17 genes regulated by the KEAP1-NRF2-CUL3 axis. Strikingly, none of the 17 genes were found in the list of upregulated genes in the wild-type versus normal samples with logFC > 1.5 ($p < 0.01$ with BH-FDR adjustment; Additional file 3: Table S3). Thus, our analysis clearly showed that these 17 genes were significantly overexpressed in altered KEAP1-NRF2-CUL3 samples compared with their normal and wild-type counterparts (Fig. 3b, c). We then designated these 17 genes as the signature of gene expression regulated by the KEAP1-NRF2-CUL3 axis based on their specificity and higher expression (Table 1). Among these 17 genes, 13 – AKR1B10, AKR1C1, AKR1C2, AKR1C3, G6PD, GCLC, GCLM, GSTM3, OSGIN1, SRXN1, TXNRD1, SLC7A11 [11, 35, 36], and SPP1 [37]– are well-known NRF2-regulated genes, listed and reviewed in a wide variety of studies.

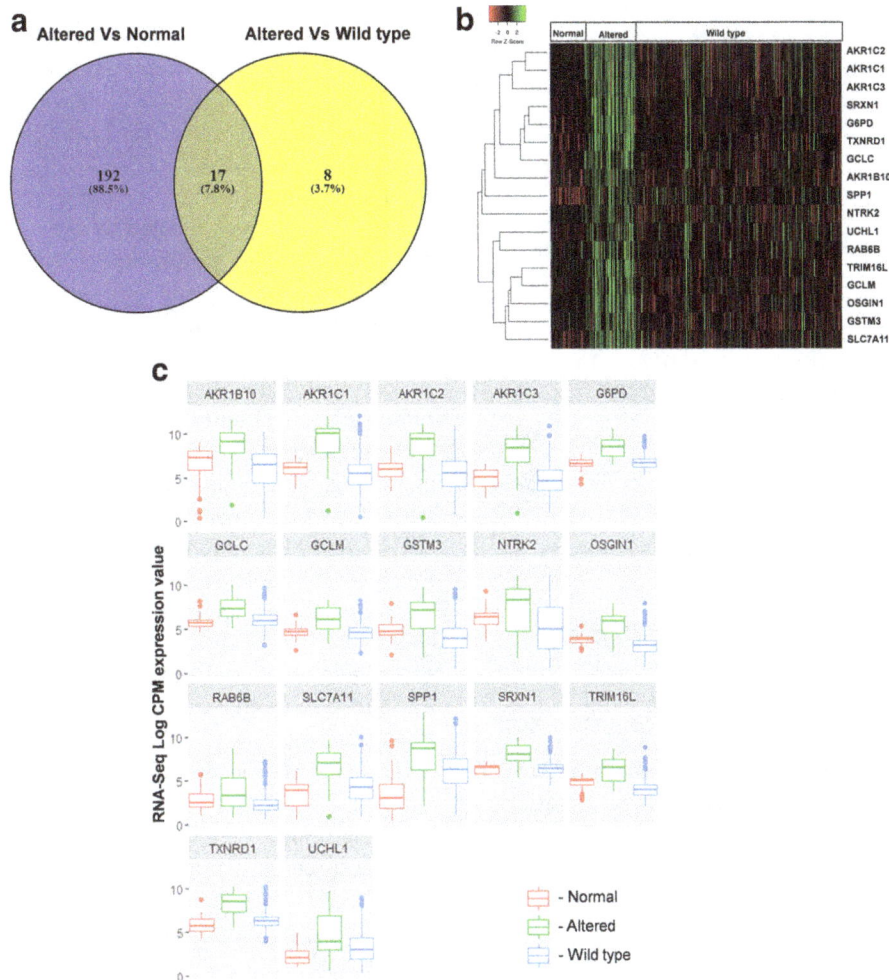

Fig. 3 Identification of expression signature of genes regulated by KEAP1-NRF2-CUL3 axis in TCGA-HNSCC. **a** Venn diagram of overlapping genes from both altered versus normal and altered versus wild-type upregulated gene analysis in HNSCC. **b** Hierarchical clustering of normal, altered, and wild-type cases showing the specific expression pattern of the 17-gene signature. Green, relatively high expression; red, relatively low expression. **c** Box plots of 17-gene signature illustrating significant differences of expression in normal, altered, and wild-type cases. X-axis, RNA-Seq V2 log CPM (counts per million) values

NRF2 binds with the ARE sequences of 3 putative genes identified in the 17-gene signature

Since the ultimate effect of KEAP1-NRF2-CUL3 gene alterations results in the overexpression of NRF2 and its target genes, it was not surprising that the majority of genes in our results were well-characterized NRF2-regulated genes. In addition, we found 4 putative KEAP1-NRF2-CUL3-regulated genes, NTRK2 (neurotrophic receptor tyrosine kinase 2), RAB6B, TRIM16L, and UCHL1 and investigated whether they were also regulated by NRF2. Interestingly, further in silico analysis using the 'LASAGNA-Search 2.0' [33] bioinformatics tool identified NRF2-ARE sequences within the -5 kb upstream promoter regions of the human RAB6B, UCHL1 and TRIM16L genes (Fig. 4a,b,c; Additional file 4: Table S4). However, we did not find an ARE sequence in the promoter region of the NTRK2 gene. Together, our results suggest that NRF2 directly binds with the promoter regions of 16 of the genes in the signature and triggers their overexpression; NTRK2 is the exception.

Functional annotation of the gene expression signature regulated by the KEAP1-NRF2-CUL3 axis

Functional annotation analysis from GO and KEGG pathway predictions using both DAVID and STRING v10 revealed that the 17 genes were significantly enriched ($p < 0.001$) in the biological processes daunorubicin metabolic process, doxorubicin metabolic process, oxidation-reduction process, cellular response to jasmonic acid stimulus, progesterone metabolic process, response to oxidative stress, and steroid metabolic process. In KEGG pathway analysis, we found significant enrichment ($p < 0.005$) in

Table 1 List of 17 upregulated KEAP1-NRF2-CUL3 axis genes identified in HNSCC

Gene symbol	Description
AKR1B10	Aldo-keto reductase family 1 member B10
AKR1C1	Aldo-keto reductase family 1 member C1
AKR1C2	Aldo-keto reductase family 1 member C2
AKR1C3	Aldo-keto reductase family 1 member C3
G6PD	Glucose-6-phosphate dehydrogenase
GCLC	Glutamate-cysteine ligase catalytic subunit
GCLM	Glutamate-cysteine ligase modifier subunit
GSTM3	Glutathione S-transferase mu 3
NTRK2	Neurotrophic receptor tyrosine kinase 2
OSGIN1	Oxidative stress induced growth inhibitor 1
RAB6B	RAB6B, member RAS oncogene family
SLC7A11	Solute carrier family 7 member 11
SPP1	Secreted phosphoprotein 1
SRXN1	Sulfiredoxin 1
TRIM16L	Tripartite motif containing 16-like
TXNRD1	Thioredoxin reductase 1
UCHL1	Ubiquitin C-terminal hydrolase L1

the three pathways glutathione metabolism, steroid hormone biosynthesis, and metabolism of xenobiotics by cytochrome P450 (Table 2).

The 17-gene signature is significantly associated with poor survival in TCGA-HNSCC patients

To evaluate the prognostic value of the 17-gene signature in patient survival, we first analyzed overall survival in the TCGA-HNSCC cohort available in the SurvExpress web tool. A total of 283 patient samples were divided into

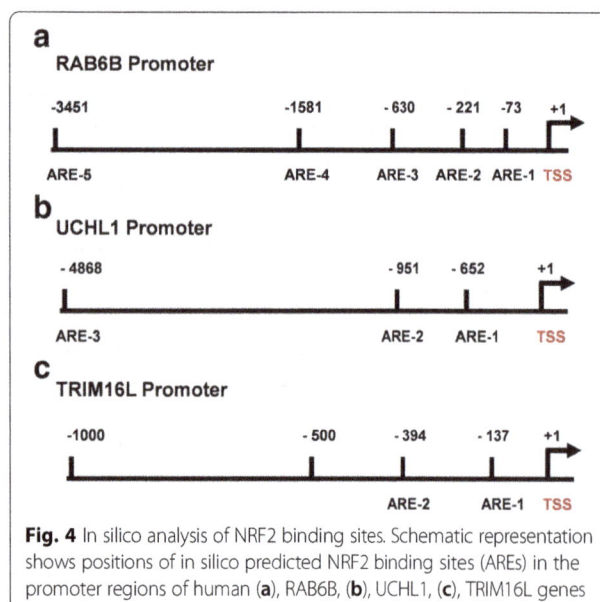

Fig. 4 In silico analysis of NRF2 binding sites. Schematic representation shows positions of in silico predicted NRF2 binding sites (AREs) in the promoter regions of human (**a**), RAB6B, (**b**), UCHL1, (**c**), TRIM16L genes

high-risk ($n = 141$) and low-risk groups ($n = 142$) based on their expression pattern (Fig. 5a). The survival probability estimates in the two risk groups were visualized as Kaplan-Meier plots. Strikingly, overall survival analysis revealed that the patients in the high-risk group had poorer survival (HR = 2.28; CI = 1.56–3.32; $p = 1.221e$-05) than the low-risk group (Fig. 5b). Thus, our analysis strongly suggests that genes regulated by the KEAP1-NRF2-CUL3 axis are powerful predictors of a poor prognosis in HNSCC patients. In addition, we also carried out the multivariate analysis with the limited variables present in Survexpress database. Consistent with the above results, patients with high-risk scores for clinical variables such as tumor grades G2 and G3, pathological stages T1 and T2, and pathological disease stages II and III were significantly associated with poor survival whereas the results were insignificant in other variables (Additional file 5: Table S5). Kaplan-Meier survival plots with log-rank test results for the significant clinical variables are shown in Additional file 6: Figure S1.

Association of 17-gene signature with disease-free survival (DFS), metastasis-free survival (MFS), and recurrence in HNSCC patients

After analyzing the prognostic value of the 17-gene signature in the TCGA cohort, we evaluated its prognostic value in another 3 HNSCC cohorts containing DFS, MFS, and recurrence data. Among these, Saintigny et al. (GSE26549) [22] contains DFS data, while Jung et al. (E-MTAB-1328) [23] contains MFS data. The third cohort, Cohen et al. (GSE10300) [24], contains recurrence data. Interestingly, our DFS analysis using the Saintigny et al. (GSE26549) [22] cohort showed that patients in the high-risk group with increased expression of the 17-gene signature had poorer survival (HR = 2.28; CI = 1.56–3.32; $p = 1.221e$-05) than the low-risk group (Fig. 6a). Likewise, we found a markedly shorter MFS (HR = 2.83, CI = 1.47–5.48; $p = 0.001$) in the high-risk group of the Jung et al. (E-MTAB-1328) [23] cohort (Fig. 6b). In the Cohen et al. (GSE10300) [24] cohort, we found lower recurrence-free survival (HR = 4.15; CI = 1.14–15.05; $p < 0.01$) in the high-risk group with the 17-gene signature than in the low-risk group (Fig. 6c). Thus, log-rank analysis revealed that the 17-gene signature was associated with a significantly increased risk of recurrence in HNSCC. The multivariate analysis results for the above cohorts were listed in Additional file 5: Table S5.

Discussion

The TCGA network provides valuable information about genetic changes in key genes involved in the oxidative-stress pathway, such as KEAP1, NRF2, and CUL3, in HNSCC patients. These particular data permit researchers to identify potential biomarkers, druggable

Table 2. GO and KEGG pathway analysis of 17 KEAP1-NRF2-CUL3 axis regulated genes in HNSCC

Term	p-value	Genes
GO_Biological Proceess (GO_BP)		
GO:0044597~daunorubicin metabolic process	3.22E-08	AKR1C3, AKR1C2, AKR1B10, AKR1C1
GO:0044598~doxorubicin metabolic process	3.22E-08	AKR1C3, AKR1C2, AKR1B10, AKR1C1
GO:0055114~oxidation-reduction process	3.29E-07	AKR1C3, AKR1C2, G6PD, AKR1B10, OSGIN1, TXNRD1, AKR1C1, SRXN1
GO:0071395~cellular response to jasmonic acid stimulus	4.46E-06	AKR1C3, AKR1C2, AKR1C1
GO:0042448~progesterone metabolic process	2.67E-05	AKR1C3, AKR1C2, AKR1C1
GO:0006979~response to oxidative stress	1.18E-04	GCLC, GCLM, SRXN1, SLC7A11
GO:0008202~steroid metabolic process	6.58E-04	AKR1C3, AKR1C2, AKR1B10
KEGG Pathway		
hsa00480:Glutathione metabolism	5.9956E-05	GSTM3, G6PD, GCLC, GCLM
hsa00140:Steroid hormone biosynthesis	0.00362777	AKR1C3, AKR1C2, AKR1C1
hsa00980:Metabolism of xenobiotics by cytochrome P450	0.00584594	AKR1C2, GSTM3, AKR1C1

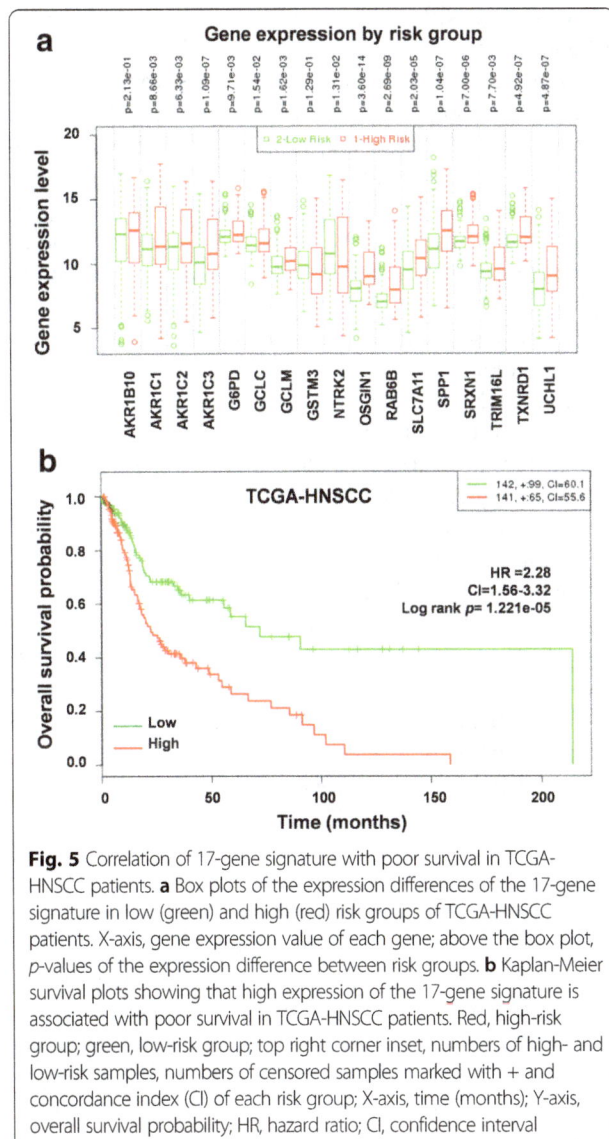

Fig. 5 Correlation of 17-gene signature with poor survival in TCGA-HNSCC patients. **a** Box plots of the expression differences of the 17-gene signature in low (green) and high (red) risk groups of TCGA-HNSCC patients. X-axis, gene expression value of each gene; above the box plot, p-values of the expression difference between risk groups. **b** Kaplan-Meier survival plots showing that high expression of the 17-gene signature is associated with poor survival in TCGA-HNSCC patients. Red, high-risk group; green, low-risk group; top right corner inset, numbers of high- and low-risk samples, numbers of censored samples marked with + and concordance index (CI) of each risk group; X-axis, time (months); Y-axis, overall survival probability; HR, hazard ratio; CI, confidence interval

mutations, and therapeutic targets for personalized medicine. In this study, using a new approach that consisted of two RNA-Seq DEG analysis methods, we identified a common set of 17 genes regulated by the KEAP1-NRF2-CUL3 axis that constitute an expression signature in TCGA-HNSCC patients. We further tested this signature in 4 independent clinical cohorts including the TCGA-HNSCC cohort. Kaplan-Meier survival plots generated for all 4 cohorts showed that higher expression of this gene signature is significantly correlated with poor survival outcomes.

The DFS data of Saintigny et al. (GSE26549) [22] suggested that patients with an increased 17-gene signature had poor benefit from chemotherapy because of aggressive expression of genes downstream of NRF2 that are involved in chemoresistance. Our GO and KEGG analysis of the 17-gene signature strongly supported the above conclusion. The top two enriched GO biological process terms were 'daunorubicin metabolic process' and 'doxorubicin metabolic process', clearly indicating that the genes involved in these processes, such as AKR (aldo-keto reductase) 1C3, AKR1C2, AKR1B10, and AKR1C1, are crucial drug-metabolizing enzymes whose overexpression is strongly associated with drug resistance in many cancers [38, 39] (Table 2). Aldo-keto reductases are well-characterized NRF2-regulated genes which contain consensus ARE sequences in their promoter regions for the binding and transactivation of NRF2 [39–41]. A recent lung cancer study emphasized that a panel of aldo-keto reductase family genes are markedly upregulated in patients harboring somatic alterations in the NRF2 pathway and considered to be biomarkers of NRF2 hyperactivation in lung cancer [17]. Consistent with their study, we showed that aldo-keto reductases were not only highly expressed in lung cancer but also in HNSCC patients with a dysregulated NRF2 pathway and could be used as biomarkers.

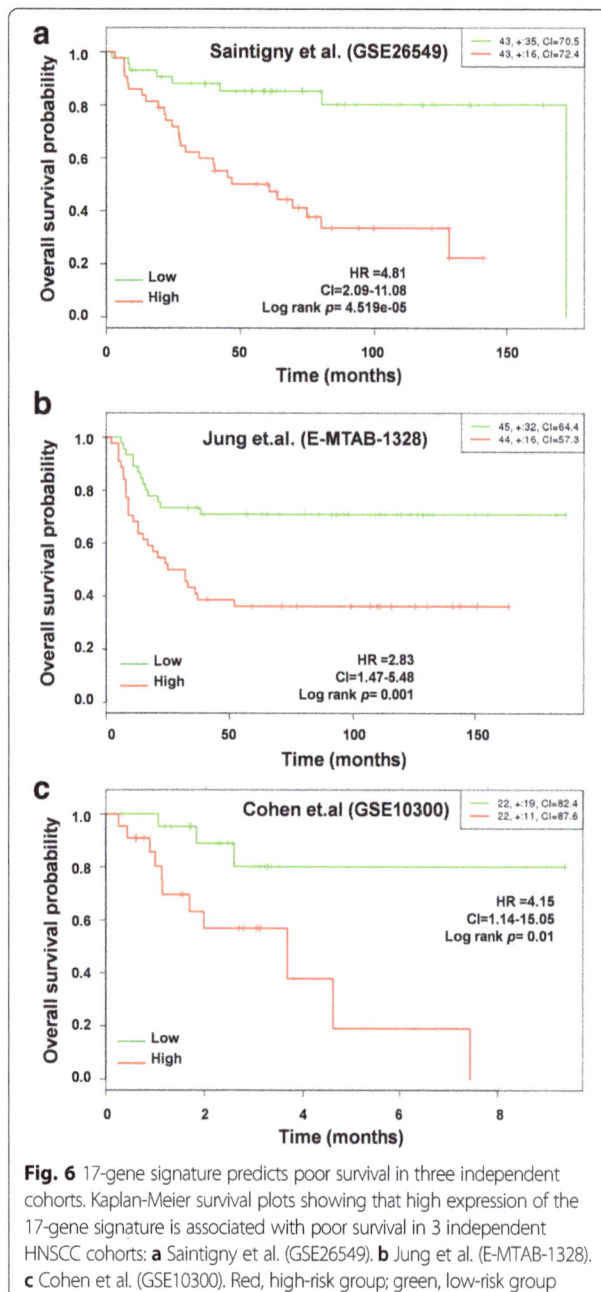

Fig. 6 17-gene signature predicts poor survival in three independent cohorts. Kaplan-Meier survival plots showing that high expression of the 17-gene signature is associated with poor survival in 3 independent HNSCC cohorts: **a** Saintigny et al. (GSE26549). **b** Jung et al. (E-MTAB-1328). **c** Cohen et al. (GSE10300). Red, high-risk group; green, low-risk group

More interestingly, the top hit in the KEGG pathway analysis of the 17-gene signature identified an important pathway involved in oxido-reductase activity known as 'glutathione metabolism'(Table 2). The genes listed in this pathway, such as GSTM3, G6PD, GCLC, and GCLM, play major roles in redox balance in normal cells. The redox imbalance in cancer cells because of the overexpression of these genes mainly leads to tumor growth and drug resistance [42]. Thus, our study revealed that NRF2 drives the expression of genes involved in glutathione metabolism, so the development of NRF2 inhibitors could be a means of altering tumor growth and drug resistance in HNSCC.

A very interesting recent study on the inhibition of NRF2, glutathione (GSH), and thioredoxin (Trx) in head and neck cancer (HNC) strongly supports our prediction that combined inhibition of the GSH, Trx, and NRF2 pathways could be an effective strategy to overcome therapeutic resistance in HNC [43].

In addition to the GO and KEGG analyses, we used the STRING v10 database to construct a PPI network of the 17-gene signature along with the KEAP1, NRF2, and CUL3 genes to reveal the complex associations between these genes. The enrichment results based on functional association between these genes revealed that the majority were closely associated with each other through a coordinated interactive network (Fig. 7). Thus, PPI network analysis suggested that the cross-talk of KEAP1, NRF2, and CUL3 with the 17-gene signature coordinately drives tumor progression and therapeutic resistance in HNSCC.

Apart from known NRF2-regulated genes, we found 4 putative KEAP1-NRF2-CUL3 axis-regulated genes: NTRK2, RAB6B, TRIM16L, and UCHL1. NTRK2, also known as tropomyosin receptor kinase B, is a neurotrophin-binding protein that phosphorylates members of the MAPK pathway. This receptor plays a major role in cell differentiation, specifically neuronal proliferation, differentiation, and survival, through its kinase signaling cascade [44]. Emerging evidence suggests that NTRK2 plays an important role in different cancers. For instance, it has been reported to be highly expressed in non-small cell lung cancer A549 cells [45] and is associated with a worse outcome in patients with Wilms' tumor [46].

Although NRF2-ARE sequences were not found in the NTRK2 promoter region, we looked into why NTRK2 was highly upregulated in altered samples. Surprisingly, a recent report revealed that NTRK2 inhibits KEAP1 expression in breast cancer cells and is involved in cancer proliferation, survival, and metastasis [47]. Thus, the overexpression of NTRK2 in altered samples clearly suggests that NTRK2 inhibits the expression of KEAP1, initiates the hyperactivation of genes downstream of NRF2, and is involved in HNSCC tumorigenesis. Another putative KEAP1-NRF2-CUL3 gene, UCHL1 (ubiquitin C-terminal hydrolase L1), has also been implicated in different types of human cancer such as breast [48, 49], melanoma [50], ovarian [51], colorectal [52], osteosarcoma [53], and gastric [54, 55] cancers, and multiple myeloma [56]. Most of the cancer studies on UCHL1 have revealed that overexpression and promoter methylation of UCHL1 are key reasons for UCHL1-mediated metastasis. Due to the adverse effect of overexpression of UCHL1, it is considered to be a biomarker and a therapeutic target in many cancers. The exact functions of the other two putative KEAP1-NRF2-CUL3axis-regulated genes, RAB6B and TRIM16L, are unknown in cancer cells and therefore are under investigation in our lab.

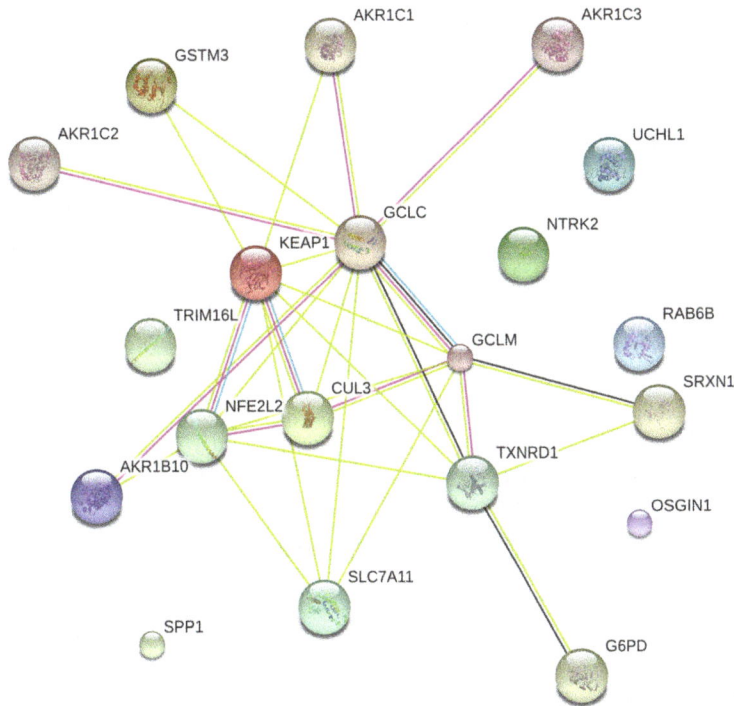

Fig. 7 Protein-protein interaction network analysis of the 17-gene signature predicting the functional correlation of the KEAP1-NRF2-CUL3 axis with genes involved in drug metabolism and glutathione metabolic pathways in HNSCC

Altogether, the above evidence suggests an oncogenic role of the 17-gene signature in many cancers.

Conclusions

In conclusion, we have identified a comprehensive gene signature of the KEAP1-NRF2-CUL3 axis, increased expression of which predicts poor survival in HNSCC. Moreover, the components of this 17-gene signature can be used as potential biomarkers to identify genetic alterations of the NRF2 pathway in HNSCC. Furthermore, the development of combined inhibitors for this 17-gene signature, along with NRF2, could pave the way for the development of personalized/precision medicine to suppress NRF2-mediated tumor growth and drug resistance.

Additional files

Additional file 1: Table S1. List of differentially expressed genes obtained from the RNA-Seq analysis of altered versus normal samples.

Additional file 2: Table S2. List of differentially expressed genes obtained from the RNA-Seq analysis of altered versus wild-type samples.

Additional file 3: Table S3. List of differentially expressed genes obtained from the RNA-Seq analysis of wild-type versus normal samples.

Additional file 4: Table S4. List of NRF2-AREs identified in the -5 kb promoter regions of RAB6B, UCHL1 and TRIM16L genes.

Additional file 5: Table S5. Multivariate analysis of 17-gene signature in 4 independent cohorts

Additional file 6: Figure S1. Kaplan-Meier plots showing the survival analysis of TCGA-HNSCC cohort clinical variables: tumor grades G2 (A) and G3 (B); pathologic T stagesT1 (C) and T2 (D); and pathologic disease stages II (E) and III (F).

Abbreviations

AKR1B10: Aldo-keto reductase family 1 member B10; AKR1C1: Aldo-keto reductase family 1 member C1; AKR1C2: Aldo-keto reductase family 1 member C2; AKR1C3: Aldo-keto reductase family 1 member C3; ARE: Antioxidant responsive element; BH: Benjamini-Hochberg; CUL3: Cullin-dependent E3 ligase; DAVID: Database for annotation visualization and integrated discovery; DEG: Differential Expression Genes; DFS: Disease free survival; edgeR: Empirical Analysis of Digital Gene Expression Data in R; FDR: False discovery rate; G6PD: Glucose-6-phosphate dehydrogenase; GCLC: Glutamate-cysteine ligase catalytic subunit; GCLM: Glutamate-cysteine ligase modifier subunit; GDAC: Genome Data Analysis Center; GO: Gene ontology; GSH: glutathione; GSTM3: Glutathione S-transferase mu 3; HNSCC: Head and Neck Squamous Cell Cancer; KEAP1: Kelch like-ECH-associated protein 1; KEGG: Kyoto Encyclopedia of Genes and Genomes; MFS: Metastasis-free survival; NRF2: Nuclear factor erythroid 2-related factor; NTRK2: Neurotrophic receptor tyrosine kinase 2; OSGIN1: Oxidative stress induced growth inhibitor 1; PPI: Protein-Protein interaction; RAB6B: RAB6B, member RAS oncogene family; RBX1: Ring-Box 1; RT-qPCR: Reverse transcription–quantitative polymerase chain reaction; SLC7A11: Solute carrier family 7 member 11; SPP1: Secreted phosphoprotein 1; SRXN1: Sulforedoxin 1; TCGA: The Cancer Genome Atlas; TRIM16L: Tripartite motif containing 16-like; TrkB: Tropomyosin receptor kinase B; Trx: Thioredoxin; TXNRD1: Thioredoxin reductase 1; UCHL1: Ubiquitin C-terminal hydrolase L1

Acknowledgements

The authors would like to thank the TCGA network for providing publicly available NGS data.

Funding

This work was supported by the National Natural Science Foundation of China to XT (31,170,743 and 81,172,230).

Authors' contributions

XT and AN conceived the project; AN, Md-MR, MC and XT analyzed the data and drafted the manuscript; MC had critically read the manuscript; XT edited and reviewed the manuscript. All authors read and approved the final manuscript.

Competing interests

The authors declare that they have no competing interests.

References

1. Mehanna H, Paleri V, West CM, Nutting C. Head and neck cancer–part 1: epidemiology, presentation, and prevention. BMJ. 2010;341:c4684.
2. Ferlay J, Soerjomataram I, Dikshit R, Eser S, Mathers C, Rebelo M, Parkin DM, Forman D, Bray F. Cancer incidence and mortality worldwide: sources, methods and major patterns in GLOBOCAN 2012. Int J Cancer. 2015;136(5):E359–86.
3. Pai SI, Westra WH. Molecular pathology of head and neck cancer: implications for diagnosis, prognosis, and treatment. Annu Rev Pathol. 2009;4:49–70.
4. Marron M, Boffetta P, Zhang ZF, Zaridze D, Wunsch-Filho V, Winn DM, Wei Q, Talamini R, Szeszenia-Dabrowska N, Sturgis EM, et al. Cessation of alcohol drinking, tobacco smoking and the reversal of head and neck cancer risk. Int J Epidemiol. 2010;39(1):182–96.
5. Leemans CR, Braakhuis BJ, Brakenhoff RH. The molecular biology of head and neck cancer. Nat Rev Cancer. 2011;11(1):9–22.
6. Namani A, Li Y, Wang XJ, Tang X. Modulation of NRF2 signaling pathway by nuclear receptors: implications for cancer. Biochim Biophys Acta. 2014; 1843(9):1875–85.
7. Ahmed SM, Luo L, Namani A, Wang XJ, Tang X. Nrf2 signaling pathway: pivotal roles in inflammation. Biochim Biophys Acta. 2017;1863(2):585–97.
8. Jaramillo MC, Zhang DD. The emerging role of the Nrf2-Keap1 signaling pathway in cancer. Genes Dev. 2013;27(20):2179–91.
9. Wang H, Liu K, Geng M, Gao P, Wu X, Hai Y, Li Y, Luo L, Hayes JD, Wang XJ, et al. RXRalpha inhibits the NRF2-ARE signaling pathway through a direct interaction with the Neh7 domain of NRF2. Cancer Res. 2013;73(10):3097–108.
10. Tang X, Wang H, Fan L, Wu X, Xin A, Ren H, Wang XJ. Luteolin inhibits Nrf2 leading to negative regulation of the Nrf2/ARE pathway and sensitization of human lung carcinoma A549 cells to therapeutic drugs. Free Radic Biol Med. 2011;50(11):1599–609.
11. Suzuki T, Motohashi H, Yamamoto M. Toward clinical application of the Keap1-Nrf2 pathway. Trends Pharmacol Sci. 2013;34(6):340–6.
12. Stacy DR, Ely K, Massion PP, Yarbrough WG, Hallahan DE, Sekhar KR, Freeman ML. Increased expression of nuclear factor E2 p45-related factor 2 (NRF2) in head and neck squamous cell carcinomas. Head Neck. 2006;28(9):813–8.
13. Huang CF, Zhang L, Ma SR, Zhao ZL, Wang WM, He KF, Zhao YF, Zhang WF, Liu B, Sun ZJ. Clinical significance of Keap1 and Nrf2 in oral squamous cell carcinoma. PLoS One. 2013;8(12):e83479.
14. The Cancer Genome Atlas Network (348 collaborators). Comprehensive genomic characterization of head and neck squamous cell carcinomas. Nature. 2015;517(7536):576–82.
15. Cescon DW, She D, Sakashita S, Zhu CQ, Pintilie M, Shepherd FA, Tsao MS. NRF2 pathway activation and adjuvant chemotherapy benefit in lung Squamous cell carcinoma. Clin Cancer Res. 2015;21(11):2499–505.
16. Qian Z, Zhou T, Gurguis CI, Xu X, Wen Q, Lv J, Fang F, Hecker L, Cress AE, Natarajan V, et al. Nuclear factor, erythroid 2-like 2-associated molecular signature predicts lung cancer survival. Sci Rep. 2015;5:16889.
17. MacLeod AK, Acosta-Jimenez L, Coates PJ, McMahon M, Carey FA, Honda T, Henderson CJ, Wolf CR. Aldo-keto reductases are biomarkers of NRF2 activity and are co-ordinately overexpressed in non-small cell lung cancer. Br J Cancer. 2016;115(12):1530–9.
18. Namani A, Cui QQ, Wu Y, Wang H, Wang XJ, Tang X. NRF2-regulated metabolic gene signature as a prognostic biomarker in non-small cell lung cancer. Oncotarget. 2017;8(41):69847 62.
19. Martinez VD, Vucic EA, Thu KL, Pikor LA, Lam S, Lam WL. Disruption of KEAP1/CUL3/RBX1 E3-ubiquitin ligase complex components by multiple genetic mechanisms: association with poor prognosis in head and neck cancer. Head Neck. 2015;37(5):727–34.
20. Cerami E, Gao J, Dogrusoz U, Gross BE, Sumer SO, Aksoy BA, Jacobsen A, Byrne CJ, Heuer ML, Larsson E, et al. The cBio cancer genomics portal: an open platform for exploring multidimensional cancer genomics data. Cancer Discovery. 2012;2(5):401–4.
21. Gao J, Aksoy BA, Dogrusoz U, Dresdner G, Gross B, Sumer SO, Sun Y, Jacobsen A, Sinha R, Larsson E, et al. Integrative analysis of complex cancer genomics and clinical profiles using the cBioPortal. Sci Signal. 2013;6(269):pl1.
22. Saintigny P, Zhang L, Fan YH, El-Naggar AK, Papadimitrakopoulou VA, Feng L, Lee JJ, Kim ES, Ki Hong W, Mao L. Gene expression profiling predicts the development of oral cancer. Cancer Prev Res (Phila). 2011;4(2):218–29.
23. Jung AC, Job S, Ledrappier S, Macabre C, Abecassis J, de Reynies A, Wasylyk B. A poor prognosis subtype of HNSCC is consistently observed across methylome, transcriptome, and miRNome analysis. Clin Cancer Res. 2013; 19(15):4174–84.
24. Cohen EE, Zhu H, Lingen MW, Martin LE, Kuo WL, Choi EA, Kocherginsky M, Parker JS, Chung CH, Rosner MR. A feed-forward loop involving protein kinase Calpha and microRNAs regulates tumor cell cycle. Cancer Res. 2009;69(1):65–74.
25. Goldstein LD, Lee J, Gnad F, Klijn C, Schaub A, Reeder J, Daemen A, Bakalarski CE, Holcomb T, Shames DS, et al. Recurrent loss of NFE2L2 exon 2 is a mechanism for Nrf2 pathway activation in human cancers. Cell Rep. 2016;16(10):2605–17.
26. Morris VK, Lucas FA, Overman MJ, Eng C, Morelli MP, Jiang ZQ, Luthra R, Meric-Bernstam F, Maru D, Scheet P et al: Clinicopathologic characteristics and gene expression analyses of non-KRAS 12/13, RAS-mutated metastatic colorectal cancer. Ann Oncol 2014, 25(10):2008-2014.
27. Gentleman RC, Carey VJ, Bates DM, Bolstad B, Dettling M, Dudoit S, Ellis B, Gautier L, Ge Y, Gentry J, et al. Bioconductor: open software development for computational biology and bioinformatics. Genome Biol. 2004;5(10):R80.
28. Robinson MD, McCarthy DJ, Smyth GK. edgeR: a bioconductor package for differential expression analysis of digital gene expression data. Bioinformatics. 2010;26(1):139–40.
29. Babicki S, Arndt D, Marcu A, Liang Y, Grant JR, Maciejewski A, Wishart DS. Heatmapper: web-enabled heat mapping for all. Nucleic Acids Res. 2016; 44(W1):W147–53.
30. Wickham H. ggplot2: elegant graphics for data analysis. New York: Springer-Verlag; 2009.
31. Huang d W, Sherman BT, Lempicki RA. Systematic and integrative analysis of large gene lists using DAVID bioinformatics resources. Nat Protoc. 2009; 4(1):44–57.
32. Szklarczyk D, Morris JH, Cook H, Kuhn M, Wyder S, Simonovic M, Santos A, Doncheva NT, Roth A, Bork P, et al. The STRING database in 2017: quality-controlled protein-protein association networks, made broadly accessible. Nucleic Acids Res. 2017;45(D1):D362–8.
33. Lee C, Huang CH. LASAGNA-search 2.0: integrated transcription factor binding site search and visualization in a browser. Bioinformatics. 2014; 30(13):1923–5.
34. Aguirre-Gamboa R, Gomez-Rueda H, Martinez-Ledesma E, Martinez-Torteya A, Chacolla-Huaringa R, Rodriguez-Barrientos A, Tamez-Pena JG, Trevino V. SurvExpress: an online biomarker validation tool and database for cancer gene expression data using survival analysis. PLoS One. 2013;8(9):e74250.
35. Chorley BN, Campbell MR, Wang X, Karaca M, Sambandan D, Bangura F, Xue P, Pi J, Kleeberger SR, Bell DA. Identification of novel NRF2-regulated genes by ChIP-Seq: influence on retinoid X receptor alpha. Nucleic Acids Res. 2012;40(15):7416–29.
36. Hayes JD, Dinkova-Kostova AT. The Nrf2 regulatory network provides an interface between redox and intermediary metabolism. Trends Biochem Sci. 2014;39(4):199–218.
37. Shibata T, Saito S, Kokubu A, Suzuki T, Yamamoto M, Hirohashi S. Global downstream pathway analysis reveals a dependence of oncogenic NF-E2-related factor 2 mutation on the mTOR growth signaling pathway. Cancer Res. 2010;70(22):9095–105.
38. Ma J, Luo DX, Huang C, Shen Y, Bu Y, Markwell S, Gao J, Liu J, Zu X, Cao Z, et al. AKR1B10 overexpression in breast cancer: association with tumor size, lymph node metastasis and patient survival and its potential as a novel serum marker. Int J Cancer. 2012;131(6):E862–71.

39. Jung KA, Choi BH, Nam CW, Song M, Kim ST, Lee JY, Kwak MK. Identification of aldo-keto reductases as NRF2-target marker genes in human cells. Toxicol Lett. 2013;218(1):39–49.

40. Lou H, Du S, Ji Q, Stolz A. Induction of AKR1C2 by phase II inducers: identification of a distal consensus antioxidant response element regulated by NRF2. Mol Pharmacol. 2006;69(5):1662–72.

41. Penning TM, Drury JE. Human aldo-keto reductases: function, gene regulation, and single nucleotide polymorphisms. Arch Biochem Biophys. 2007;464(2):241–50.

42. Trachootham D, Alexandre J, Huang P. Targeting cancer cells by ROS-mediated mechanisms: a radical therapeutic approach? Nat Rev Drug Discov. 2009;8(7):579–91.

43. Roh JL, Jang H, Kim EH, Shin D. Targeting of the glutathione, Thioredoxin, and Nrf2 antioxidant Systems in Head and Neck Cancer. Antioxid Redox Signal. 2017;27(2):106–14.

44. Minichiello L. TrkB signalling pathways in LTP and learning. Nat Rev Neurosci. 2009;10(12):850–60.

45. Zhang S, Guo D, Luo W, Zhang Q, Zhang Y, Li C, Lu Y, Cui Z, Qiu X. TrkB is highly expressed in NSCLC and mediates BDNF-induced the activation of Pyk2 signaling and the invasion of A549 cells. BMC Cancer. 2010;10:43.

46. Eggert A, Grotzer MA, Ikegaki N, Zhao H, Cnaan A, Brodeur GM, Evans AE. Expression of the neurotrophin receptor TrkB is associated with unfavorable outcome in Wilms' tumor. J Clin Oncol Off J Am Soc Clin Oncol. 2001;19(3):689–96.

47. Kim MS, Lee WS, Jin W. TrkB promotes breast cancer metastasis via suppression of Runx3 and Keap1 expression. Molecules Cells. 2016;39(3):258–65.

48. Schroder C, Milde-Langosch K, Gebauer F, Schmid K, Mueller V, Wirtz RM, Meyer-Schwesinger C, Schluter H, Sauter G, Schumacher U. Prognostic relevance of ubiquitin C-terminal hydrolase L1 (UCH-L1) mRNA and protein expression in breast cancer patients. J Cancer Res Clin Oncol. 2013;139(10):1745–55.

49. Jin Y, Zhang W, Xu J, Wang H, Zhang Z, Chu C, Liu X, Zou Q. UCH-L1 involved in regulating the degradation of EGFR and promoting malignant properties in drug-resistant breast cancer. Int J Clin Exp Pathol. 2015;8(10):12500–8.

50. Wulfanger J, Biehl K, Tetzner A, Wild P, Ikenberg K, Meyer S, Seliger B. Heterogeneous expression and functional relevance of the ubiquitin carboxyl-terminal hydrolase L1 in melanoma. Int J Cancer. 2013;133(11):2522–32.

51. Suong DN, Thao DT, Masamitsu Y, Thuoc TL. Ubiquitin carboxyl hydrolase L1 significance for human diseases. Protein Peptide Letters. 2014;21(7):624–30.

52. Heitzer E, Artl M, Filipits M, Resel M, Graf R, Weissenbacher B, Lax S, Gnant M, Wrba F, Greil R, et al. Differential survival trends of stage II colorectal cancer patients relate to promoter methylation status of PCDH10, SPARC, and UCHL1. Modern Pathol. 2014;27(6):906–15.

53. Zheng S, Qiao G, Min D, Zhang Z, Lin F, Yang Q, Feng T, Tang L, Sun Y, Zhao H, et al. Heterogeneous expression and biological function of ubiquitin carboxy-terminal hydrolase-L1 in osteosarcoma. Cancer Lett. 2015;359(1):36–46.

54. Wang G, Zhang W, Zhou B, Jin C, Wang Z, Yang Y, Chen Y, Feng X. The diagnosis value of promoter methylation of UCHL1 in the serum for progression of gastric cancer. Biomed Res Int. 2015;2015:741030.

55. YY G, Yang M, Zhao M, Luo Q, Yang L, Peng H, Wang J, Huang SK, Zheng ZX, Yuan XH, et al. The de-ubiquitinase UCHL1 promotes gastric cancer metastasis via the Akt and Erk1/2 pathways. Tumor Biol. 2015;36(11):8379–87.

56. Hussain S, Bedekovics T, Chesi M, Bergsagel PL, Galardy PJ. UCHL1 is a biomarker of aggressive multiple myeloma required for disease progression. Oncotarget. 2015;6(38):40704–18.

20

Lack of association between cigarette smoking and Epstein Barr virus reactivation in the nasopharynx in people with elevated EBV IgA antibody titres

Yufeng Chen[1,3,5†], Yifei Xu[1†], Weilin Zhao[1], Xue Xiao[1], Xiaoying Zhou[1], Longde Lin[2,3], Tingting Huang[1,2,5], Jian Liao[4], Yancheng Li[4], Xiaoyun Zeng[2,3], Guangwu Huang[1,2], Weimin Ye[5] and Zhe Zhang[1,2*]

Abstract

Background: Subjects with elevated Epstein-Barr virus (EBV) immunoglobulin A (IgA) titers have a higher risk of developing nasopharyngeal carcinoma (NPC), indicating that reactivation of EBV in the local mucosa might be important for NPC carcinogenesis. Cigarette smoking appears to be one of the environmental risk factors for NPC. However, it remains unclear whether smoking-induced nasopharyngeal carcinogenesis acts through reactivating EBV in the nasopharyngeal mucosa. Therefore, this study aims to investigate the association between cigarette smoking and nasopharyngeal EBV reactivation in a NPC high-risk population.

Methods: A NPC high-risk cohort study, established from a population-based NPC screening program of 22,816 subjects, consisted of 1045 subjects with elevated serum IgA antibodies against EBV viral capsid antigen (VCA/IgA). Among high-risk subjects, information on detailed cigarette smoking history was collected among 313 male subjects. The associations between cigarette smoking and EBV antibody levels, EBV DNA load of the nasopharynx were analyzed.

Results: No significant association was observed between either nasopharyngeal EBV DNA load or serum VCA/IgA titers and smoking status, age at smoking initiation, daily smoking intensity, smoking duration, cigarette type, or pack-years of smoking. Cigarette smoking characteristics in all subgroups did not correlate with nasopharyngeal EBV DNA positivity or EBV VCA/IgA seropositivity.

Conclusions: In a population at high risk of NPC, our study suggests that cigarette smoking is neither associated with nasopharyngeal EBV DNA load nor serum VCA/IgA antibody level. Smoking-associated NPC carcinogenesis may act through other mechanisms than reactivating nasopharyngeal EBV replication.

Keywords: Cigarette smoking, Epstein-Barr virus, Nasopharyngeal EBV load, Nasopharyngeal carcinoma, Nasopharyngeal EBV reactivation

* Correspondence: zhangzhe@gxmu.edu.cn
†Equal contributors
[1]Department of Otolaryngology-Head & Neck Surgery, First Affiliated Hospital of Guangxi Medical University, 6# Shuangyong Road, Nanning, Guangxi 530021, China
[2]Ministry of Education, Key Laboratory of High-Incidence-Tumor Prevention & Treatment (Guangxi Medical University), Nanning, Guangxi, China
Full list of author information is available at the end of the article

Background

Epstein-Barr virus (EBV) infection is a major etiologic factor for nasopharyngeal carcinoma (NPC), and EBV is detected in tumor cells of virtually all NPC cases [1]. The probability of developing NPC is 6.7–41.9 times higher for subjects seropositive for immunoglobulin A antibodies against viral capsid antigen (VCA/IgA) than those with undetectable antibodies [2].

Amongst potential non-viral causes of NPC, cigarette smoking has been intensively studied. Some early studies failed to show a link between tobacco smoking and NPC risk [3–7], while recent evidence supported a positive association between cigarette smoking and NPC risk [8–11]. Our recent population-based case-control study with a large sample size in southern China, observed that active smoking in males significantly increased the NPC risk, particularly among those heavy smokers. Moreover, exposure to passive smoking during childhood and from a spouse during adulthood was independently associated with an increased NPC risk [12]. In Taiwan, a large-scale 20-year follow-up cohort study reported that the NPC risk was closely associated with long and heavy cigarette smoking and the association persisted even when EBV seromarkers were included in the multivariate analysis [13]. In addition, cigarette smoking is an independent prognostic factor for poor NPC survival [14, 15], and is associated with a higher NPC mortality [16]. Besides epidemiological study, in vitro experiment showed that cigarette extracts could induce EBV reactivation in NPC cells [8], suggesting that cigarette smoking plays an important role in NPC carcinogenesis.

The high EBV titers in high risk NPC populations in endemic region indicate the reactivation of EBV in vivo. To date, the cell origin of reactivated EBV particles has not been addressed. Previously, we found that nasopharyngeal EBV load is correlated with serological EBV titers in high risk NPC population [17]. These clues lead us to hypothesize that cigarette smoking might be directly responsible for the reactivation of nasopharyngeal EBV and cause peripheral EBV IgA seropositivity. Thus, we investigated the association of cigarette smoking with nasopharyngeal EBV reactivation in a population based NPC high-risk cohort study.

Methods

Study population

The establishment of the study cohort has been described previously [17]. In brief, this study was based on a prospective NPC screening program conducted in three towns (Libu, Shatou and Shiqiao) of Cangwu County, southern China, between 2006 and 2013. Briefly, local residents ages 30–59 were enrolled in the screening program. A serum sample was taken from each subject for detection of EBV VCA/IgA antibody by immunoenzymatic assay, and each subject was offered an otorhinolaryngologic and neck lymphatic examination. A total of 22,186 individuals volunteered to take part in the initial screening program, and the participation rate was 56.2%. In total, 1045 healthy subjects seropositive with EBV VCA/IgA (VCA/IgA ≥1:5) identified from the 22,186 participants were defined as NPC high-risk population and followed up for NPC occurrence. During the follow-up period of 2010–2013, 8 individuals were diagnosed as NPC cases (5 in 2010, 3 in 2011). According to the American Joint Committee on Cancer (AJCC) TNM Staging System (7th ed., 2010), 7 of the 8 cases were early-stage NPCs (2 cases of stageI, 5 cases of stage II, and 1 case of stage III).

In 2010, a follow-up serological retest and endoscopy examination were performed in the 1045 subjects. Of them, 822 (78.4%) subjects agreed to both provide a nasopharyngeal swab and to complete a questionnaire about smoking and other lifestyle factors. Because fewer than 3% (15/509) of the participating females had ever smoked, only the 313 males were included in the analysis.

Ethics statement

Our study group has strictly abided by the principles of Helsinki Declaration and International Ethical Guidelines for Biomedical Research Involving Human Subjects developed by the Council for International Organizations of Medical Sciences (CIOMS). The NPC screening project involved in this study was started from 2006. From 2006 to 2008, staff in Cangwu Cancer Institute conducted screening program as a government-funded health promotion project, and no biological samples were preserved. Since 2010, we joined this project and conducted etiological studies after being approved by the Ethics Review Committee of First Affiliated Hospital of Guangxi Medical University in 2009. All the human materials, serological test results, and questionnaire data were collected during the follow-up stage in 2010. Written informed consents were obtained from all participants. Any published reports involved in the study would not reveal the participants' identification.

Cigarette smoking assessment

Questionnaire interviews were administered by trained local health workers. Individuals who had ever smoked at least one cigarette every 1–3 days for at least 6 months were defined as ever smokers, including current smokers and ex-smokers. Ex-smokers were defined as those who had quit smoking more than 1 year before the interview. Data on age at which the individual started and stopped smoking, daily cigarettes smoked, and type of cigarettes smoked (filtered, nonfiltered, or both) were collected.

EBV serology and DNA load measurement

Serum EBV VCA/IgA antibody levels were determined by immunoenzymatic assay as described previously [18]. Briefly, cell smears were prepared from B95–8 cultures, fixed in acetone and used in the indirect immunoenzymatic method with peroxidase-conjugated anti-human IgA antibody. Sera diluted to 1:5 were added to separate wells of slide. The slides were incubated at 37 °C for 30 min in a humid atmosphere, and washed 3 times with phosphate-buffered saline (PBS). Peroxidase-conjugated antihuman IgA antibody in appropriate dilution was added to the slides. The slides were incubated again for 30 min, washed 3 times with PBS, and flooded with di-aminobenzidine and H_2O_2 for 10 min. Positive and negative control sera were incubated in each experiment. A serum was considered positive if the cells in the well that contained the 1:5 dilution showed brown color characteristic of this test. The blood specimens from persons antibody-positive in the initial screening were tested in further dilutions. The highest dilution of serum still positive for IgA antibody to VCA was considered as the antibody titer of that serum.

Two real-time quantitative polymerase chain reaction (qPCR) systems were set up to detect EBV DNA load and the *β-globin* gene as described previously [19, 20]. The *β-globin* gene was used as a quality control for the nasopharyngeal swab sampling, DNA extraction and PCR reaction. A standard curve of the CT values obtained from plasmid DNA containing *BamHI-W* or *β-globin* fragment respectively was established in parallel. Each sample was tested in duplicate, and the mean of the two values was taken as the copy number of the sample. Samples were defined as negative if the CT values exceeded 40 cycles. In all experiments appropriate negative and positive controls were included during nucleic acid isolation and amplification. Swab DNA samples were renumbered before EBV DNA load detection to ensure a blind test. The copy numbers of EBV DNA or *β-globin* gene per swab (expressed in copies/swab) were calculated according to the following equation:

$$C = Q \times \frac{V_{DNA}}{V_{PCR}} \times \frac{1}{V_{EXT}}$$

C: target concentration in one swab (copies/swab).
Q: target quantity (copies) determined by PCR.
V_{DNA}: total volume of DNA obtained after extraction (50ul).
V_{PCR}: volume of DNA solution used for PCR (1ul).
V_{EXT}: volume of saline solution extracted (1 swab).

Statistical analysis

The SPSS statistical analysis software (Version 16.0, SPSS Inc., Chicago, IL) was used for all statistical analyses. Since the EBV DNA load and serum VCA/IgA antibody titers were non-normal distribution data, we conducted a log-transformed (log10-transformed) to obtain approximately normal distribution of the variables. To compare demographics, EBV DNA load and VCA/IgA antibody titers between different smoking subgroups, we used Chi-square test for categorical variables and one-way ANOVA for continuous variables. Linear trend tests for associations between smoking subgroups and EBV DNA load and serum VCA/IgA antibody titers were performed for ordinal variables. Multivariate unconditional logistic regression models were used to estimate odds ratios (ORs) and corresponding 95% confidence intervals (CIs) for associations between cigarette smoking and nasopharyngeal EBV DNA status or serum VCA/IgA status. All statistical tests were two-sided and a *P* value of < 0.05 was considered statistically significant.

Results

Study population characteristics

Demographic characteristics of the 313 males seropositive for VCA/IgA, stratified by smoking status, are shown in Table 1. Among them 75.4% (236/313) were current smokers, while former smokers and never smokers accounted for 12.8% (40/313) and 11.8% (37/313), with mean ages of 49.7, 49.5, and 47.3 years, respectively. Subjects with an ever smoking history were more likely to reside in Libu and Shatou than in Shiqiao, while the distribution of age and education level had no statistical difference among the three smoking groups (*P* > 0.05).

Associations between cigarette smoking and nasopharyngeal EBV DNA load, serum VCA/IgA titers

We found no significant associations between nasopharyngeal EBV DNA load and cigarette smoking characteristics, including smoking status, age at smoking initiation, number of cigarettes smoked per day, smoking duration, type of cigarettes and pack-years of smoking (*P* > 0.05, Table 2). Cigarette smoking also was not associated with serum VCA/IgA titers (*P* > 0.05 for all subgroups, Table 2).

As shown in Tables 3, 87% (272/313) of male high-risk individuals was positive for nasopharyngeal EBV DNA, and 13% (41/313) was EBV DNA negative. In the follow-up serological retest, 7% (23/313) subjects' VCA/IgA antibodies turned to be negative, and because of the small number of seronegative subjects we classified VCA/IgA negative and titer of 1:5 subjects into one group (30%, 95/313), thus the rest was another group with VCA/IgA ≥ 1:10 (70%, 218/313). Cigarette smoking variables in all aspects did not show any positive association either with

Table 1 Characteristics of male nasopharyngeal carcinoma high-risk population by smoking status, Cangwu county, China, 2006–2013

Characteristics	Smoking status						P Value[a]
	Never (N = 37)		Former (N = 40)		Current (N = 236)		
	No.	%	No.	%	No.	%	
Residential area							0.039
Libu	4	11.1	2	5.6	30	83.3	
Shatou	9	6.5	21	15.1	109	78.4	
Shiqiao	24	17.4	17	12.3	97	70.3	
Age							0.176
Mean(SD)	47.3(7.5)		49.5(9.3)		49.7(8.0)		0.323
30–39	4	10.0	6	15.0	30	75.0	
40–49	19	18.3	12	11.5	73	70.2	
50–59	14	8.3	22	13.1	133	78.7	
Education level							0.329
Primary school or below	16	10.1	20	12.6	123	77.4	
Secondary school	15	13.6	18	16.4	77	70.0	
High school or above	6	13.6	2	4.5	36	81.8	

[a]P value for the comparison of means of age was determined by a one-way ANOVA, other P values were determined by a chi-square test. Abbreviation: SD, standard deviation

nasopharyngeal EBV DNA status or serum VCA/IgA status (Table 3).

Discussion

Epidemiologic studies have demonstrated cigarette smoking is associated with excess NPC risk. In vitro experiments also found that cigarette extracts promote EBV replication in B cells and NPC cells [8]. Therefore, it has been proposed that cigarette smoking may play a role in NPC development and induction of EBV reactivation. However, whether cigarette smoking directly induces EBV replication in the nasopharynx and causes EBV IgA seropositivity is unknown. In this population-based study, we found no evidence of a positive association between cigarette smoking and the EBV DNA load in the nasopharynx or with serum EBV VCA/IgA antibody titers. Our results suggest that cigarette smoking does not directly affect EBV reactivation in the nasopharynx. Thus, cigarette-smoking-associated NPC carcinogenesis might act through other mechanisms.

Except IgA antibodies of mucosa origin, smoking also induces IgG antibodies against EBV replication. For instance, cigarette smoking has been associated with titers of VCA/IgG [21], which is in turn associated with an increased risk of EBV-positive Hodgkin lymphoma [22]. These findings, combined with ours, indicate that rather than being specific to the nasopharyngeal mucosa, smoking-induced activation of EBV might be a systemic effect.

On the other hand, serologic responses to EBV, as determined by antibody levels in circulation, were used as a proxy for evaluation of the degree of EBV exposure in previous studies. Elevated serum levels of antibodies against EBV viral capsid antigen and EBV DNase may reflect the reactivation of EBV in human body [13]. The antibody production has underlying host exogenous determinants such as genetic susceptibility or the subtype of EBV [23]. What is more, other etiologic factors may also be involved as confounders. Cigarette smoking is associated with lower socioeconomic status in many populations. In addition, socioeconomic and race/ethnic differences were demonstrated in the seroprevalence of EBV [24]. Thus, in EBV related diseases, EBV antibody seropositivity, host genetic background and the habit of smoking might not act independently. Instead, they might have combined or synergistic effects on the etiology. The complicated synergistic effects result in conflicting conclusions as regard to the association between smoking, EBV seropositivity and cancer risks.

Compared to the lower aero-digestive tracts, the nasopharynx is a site which is more directly exposed to cigarette smoking. However, the magnitude of excess risks associated with smoking in cancer of the nasopharynx (OR less than 2) [8–10, 12, 25] is much lower than that for cancers of the lung and larynx (OR~ 20) [26], indicating that the nasopharyngeal epithelium might not be sensitive target cells of carcinogens from tobacco smoking. Furthermore, previous studies did not find any significant interaction between anti-EBV seromarkers and cigarette smoking for NPC development [13, 27]. These observations are plausibly consistent with our current results, indicating that the induction of NPC

Table 2 Relationship between smoking and nasopharyngeal EBV load, EBV VCA/IgA antibody

Smoking characteristics	No.	EBV DNA copies, $\log_{10}$ (Mean ± SD)	P value[a]	VCA/IgA titer, $\log_{10}$ (Mean ± SD)	P value[a]
Smoking status					
Never smoker	37	2.87 ± 1.60	0.384	1.05 ± 0.21	0.228
Former smoker	40	3.36 ± 1.55		1.00 ± 0.21	
Current smoker	236	3.19 ± 1.58		1.07 ± 0.23	
P_{trend}			0.251		0.551
Age at smoking initiation (years)					
< 20	127	3.05 ± 1.68	0.123	1.07 ± 0.22	0.924
20–29	123	3.29 ± 1.53		1.06 ± 0.24	
≥30	26	3.71 ± 1.10		1.04 ± 0.24	
P_{trend}			0.025		0.911
Smoking intensity (cigarettes/day)					
≤10	51	3.27 ± 1.47	0.604	1.06 ± 0.23	0.282
11–30	159	3.19 ± 1.62		1.07 ± 0.23	
> 30	31	3.33 ± 1.49		1.00 ± 0.20	
P_{trend}			0.273		0.327
Smoking duration (years)					
≤15	24	3.23 ± 1.54	0.551	0.99 ± 0.24	0.350
16–30	123	3.14 ± 1.59		1.06 ± 0.22	
> 30	129	3.29 ± 1.58		1.08 ± 0.23	
P_{trend}			0.224		0.240
Type of cigarettes smoked					
Filtered cigarettes	174	3.23 ± 1.56	0.635	1.07 ± 0.23	0.895
Non-filtered cigarettes	34	3.26 ± 1.35		1.08 ± 0.24	
Both type	68	3.15 ± 1.72		1.05 ± 0.22	
P_{trend}			0.392		0.926
Cumulative smoking (pack-years[b])					
< 20	95	3.16 ± 1.53	0.202	1.03 ± 0.23	0.252
20–39	136	3.37 ± 1.59		1.09 ± 0.24	
≥40	45	2.91 ± 1.58		1.04 ± 0.19	
P_{trend}			0.768		0.846

[a]Comparisons were performed using one-way ANOVA; [b] pack-years = (number of cigarettes smoked per day/20) × number of years smoked. Abbreviation: EBV, Epstein-Barr virus; VCA/IgA, IgA antibodies against viral capsid antigen; SD, standard deviation

carcinogenesis might not be a synergistic effect of carcinogens from tobacco smoking and EBV reactivation.

Some other factors might be involved in the reactivation of nasopharyngeal EBV. The nasopharyngeal cavity is an ideal ecological niche with suitable conditions for colonization of micro-organisms which normally inhabit the nasopharynx. Some bacteria can produce short chain fatty acids such as butyric acid, which is known as an inducer of EBV replication, suggesting that microflora could be a risk factor in the development of NPC by effecting on the lytic cycle of EBV. Interestingly, one study shows that microbial communities in the upper respiratory tract can be distorted by cigarette smoking [28], thus it may be one of the potential mechanisms for

cigarette-smoking-related NPC carcinogenesis, as observed by other studies [29, 30].

The advantage of this study is that it is the first population based study to investigate the association between cigarette smoking and EBV reactivation, by assessing nasopharyngeal EBV DNA load or serum VCA-IgA antibody level in an EBV seropositive high-risk population. However, there are also limitations. First, our major concern is the self-reported nature of smoking information, which might be misclassified by recall bias. Second, the influence of passive smoking on EBV load and VCA/IgA titers was not assessed as we did not collect such information. Finally, although the 1045 high-risk subjects were enrolled from a large sample size of 22,186, the

Table 3 The association between cigarette smoking and nasopharyngeal EBV DNA positivity, serum VCA/IgA antibody status

Variable	Nasopharyngeal EBV DNA				VCA/IgA titer			
	Negative	Positive	OR[a] (95% CI)	OR[b] (95% CI)	Negative or 1:5	≥ 1:10	OR[a] (95% CI)	OR[c] (95% CI)
Smoking status								
Never smoker[d]	6	31	1.00 (reference)	1.00 (reference)	11	26	1.00 (reference)	1.00 (reference)
Former smoker	4	36	1.28 (0.49–3.32)	1.34 (0.51–3.54)	12	28	0.96 (0.45–2.06)	0.72 (0.32–1.58)
Current smoker	31	205	1.74 (0.45–6.74)	1.73 (0.43–6.69)	72	164	0.99 (0.37–2.62)	0.76 (0.27–2.09)
Age at smoking initiation (years)								
< 20	20	107	1.04 (0.38–2.80)	1.06 (0.38–2.95)	41	86	0.89 (0.40–1.97)	0.64 (0.28–1.49)
≥20	15	134	1.73 (0.62–4.82)	1.79 (0.63–5.07)	43	106	1.04 (0.47–2.30)	0.79 (0.35–1.81)
Smoking intensity (cigarettes/day)								
≤10	6	45	1.60 (0.46–5.58)	1.75 (0.50–6.21)	20	31	0.61 (0.24–1.56)	0.54 (0.21–1.39)
11–30	27	167	1.19 (0.44–3.21)	1.20 (0.44–3.24)	51	143	1.01 (0.45–2.25)	0.92 (0.41–2.08)
> 30	2	29	2.91(0.53–15.80)	3.08 (0.56–16.85)	13	18	0.51 (0.18–1.43)	0.45 (0.16–1.29)
Smoking duration (years)								
≤15	3	21	1.36 (0.31–6.03)	2.12(0.42–10.80)	9	15	0.71 (0.24–2.09)	0.80 (0.24–2.68)
16–30	17	106	1.21 (0.44–3.32)	1.37 (0.49–3.84)	42	81	0.82 (0.37–1.81)	0.71 (0.31–1.64)
> 30	15	114	1.47 (0.53–4.11)	1.20 (0.36–3.93)	33	96	1.23 (0.55–2.76)	0.71 (0.28–1.79)
Type of cigarettes smoked								
filtered cigarettes	21	153	1.41 (0.53–3.78)	1.55 (0.57–4.23)	48	126	1.11 (0.51–2.42)	2.32 (0.94–5.75)
non-filtered cigarettes	3	31	2.00 (0.46–8.72)	1.52 (0.33–7.05)	9	25	1.18 (0.42–3.32)	2.30 (0.88–4.39)
both type	11	57	1.00 (0.38–2.97)	0.97 (0.31–3.01)	27	41	0.64 (0.27–1.51)	1.90 (0.72–4.81)
Cumulative smoking (pack-years)								
< 20	13	82	1.22 (0.43–3.50)	1.03 (0.30–2.58)	35	60	0.73 (0.32–1.65)	0.64 (0.27–1.50)
20–39	15	121	1.56 (0.56–4.35)	1.44 (0.49–4.27)	35	101	1.22 (0.55–2.73)	0.83 (0.36–1.95)
≥40	7	38	1.05 (0.32–3.45)	1.59 (0.59–4.29)	14	31	0.94 (0.36–2.41)	0.68 (0.25–1.86)

[a]The OR without adjustment; [b] OR adjusted for residential area, age, education level, VCA/IgA antibody titers; [c] OR adjusted for residential area, age, education level, nasopharyngeal EBV DNA load; [d] Never smokers were the reference group for all comparisons. Abbreviation: EBV, Epstein-Barr virus; VCA/IgA, IgA antibodies against viral capsid antigen; CI, confidence interval

number of study subjects (313 high-risk males) was relatively small.

Conclusions

We found null association between either nasopharyngeal EBV DNA load or serum VCA/IgA titers and cigarette smoking. Cigarette smoking-associated NPC carcinogenesis might not act through reactivating nasopharyngeal EBV replication, but by other mechanisms. Our study leads to a better understanding of the etiologic interactions between viral and environmental factors in the pathogenesis of NPC.

Abbreviations
EBV: Epstein-Barr virus; IgA: Immunoglobulin A; NPC: Nasopharyngeal carcinoma; VCA: Viral capsid antigen

Acknowledgements
We thank all of the participants for their long-term and dedicated contribution to the study. We also thank the staffs at the Cancer Institute of Cangwu County, for their efforts in data linkage and follow-up.

Funding
This study was supported by grants from the Natural Science Foundation of Guangxi Province (grant number: 2013GXNSFGA019002, recipient: ZZ), Natural Science Foundation of China, (grant number: 81272983, recipient: ZZ), Program for New Century Excellent Talents in University of the Ministry of Education of China (grant number: NCET-12-0654, recipient: ZZ). The funders had no role in study design, data collection and analysis, decision to publish, or preparation of the manuscript.

Authors' contributions
Conceived and designed the study: ZZ and WMY. Performed the experiments: YFC and WLZ. Contributed reagents/materials: LDL, XY Zeng and GWH. Statistically analyzed and drafted the manuscript: YFC, YFX and TTH. Literature reviewed and revised the manuscript: XX and XY Zhou. Clinical data collection and follow-up: JL and YCL. All authors read and approved the final manuscript.

Competing interests
The authors declare that they have no competing interests.

Author details

[1]Department of Otolaryngology-Head & Neck Surgery, First Affiliated Hospital of Guangxi Medical University, 6# Shuangyong Road, Nanning, Guangxi 530021, China. [2]Ministry of Education, Key Laboratory of High-Incidence-Tumor Prevention & Treatment (Guangxi Medical University), Nanning, Guangxi, China. [3]Department of Epidemiology, School of Public Health, Guangxi Medical University, Nanning, Guangxi, China. [4]Cancer Institute of Cangwu County, Wuzhou, Guangxi, China. [5]Department of Medical Epidemiology and Biostatistics, Karolinska Institutet, Stockholm, Sweden.

References

1. Wu HC, Lin YJ, Lee JJ, Liu YJ, Liang ST, Peng Y, Chiu YW, Wu CW, Lin CT. Functional analysis of EBV in nasopharyngeal carcinoma cells. Lab Investig. 2003;83(6):797–812.
2. Cao SM, Liu Z, Jia WH, Huang QH, Liu Q, Guo X, Huang TB, Ye W, Hong MH. Fluctuations of epstein-barr virus serological antibodies and risk for nasopharyngeal carcinoma: a prospective screening study with a 20-year follow-up. PLoS One. 2011;6(4):e19100.
3. Sriamporn S, Vatanasapt V, Pisani P, Yongchaiyudha S, Environmental RV. Risk factors for nasopharyngeal carcinoma: a case-control study in northeastern Thailand. Cancer Epidemiol Biomark Prev. 1992;1(5):345–8.
4. Friborg JT, Yuan JM, Wang R, Koh WP, Lee HP, Yu MC. A prospective study of tobacco and alcohol use as risk factors for pharyngeal carcinomas in Singapore Chinese. Cancer. 2007;109(6):1183–91.
5. Feng BJ, Khyatti M, Ben-Ayoub W, Dahmoul S, Ayad M, Maachi F, et al. Cannabis, tobacco and domestic fumes intake are associated with nasopharyngeal carcinoma in North Africa. Br J Cancer. 2009;101(7):1207–12.
6. Guo X, Johnson RC, Deng H, Liao J, Guan L, Nelson GW, et al. Evaluation of nonviral risk factors for nasopharyngeal carcinoma in a high-risk population of southern China. Int J Cancer. 2009;124(12):2942–7.
7. Jia WH, Qin HD. Non-viral environmental risk factors for nasopharyngeal carcinoma: a systematic review. Semin Cancer Biol. 2012;22(2):117–26.
8. Xu FH, Xiong D, Xu YF, Cao SM, Xue WQ, Qin HD, et al. An epidemiological and molecular study of the relationship between smoking, risk of nasopharyngeal carcinoma, and Epstein-Barr virus activation. J Natl Cancer Inst. 2012;104(18):1396–410.
9. He YQ, Xue WQ, Shen GP, Tang LL, Zeng YX, Jia WH. Household inhalants exposure and nasopharyngeal carcinoma risk: a large-scale case-control study in Guangdong, China. BMC Cancer. 2015;15:1022.
10. Xie SH, Yu IT, Tse LA, Au JS, Lau JS. Tobacco smoking, family history, and the risk of nasopharyngeal carcinoma: a case-referent study in Hong Kong Chinese. Cancer Causes Control. 2015;26(6):913–21.
11. Yong SK, Ha TC, Yeo MC, Gaborieau V, McKay JD, Wee J. Associations. Of lifestyle and diet with the risk of nasopharyngeal carcinoma in Singapore: a case-control study. Chin J Cancer. 2017;36(1):3.
12. Chang ET, Liu Z, Hildesheim A, Liu Q, Cai Y, Zhang Z, et al. Active and passive smoking and risk of nasopharyngeal carcinoma: a population-based case-control study in southern China. Am J Epidemiol. 2017;185(12):1272-80.
13. Hsu WL, Chen JY, Chien YC, Liu MY, You SL, Hsu MM, Yang CS, Chen CJ. Independent effect of EBV and cigarette smoking on nasopharyngeal carcinoma: a 20-year follow-up study on 9,622 males without family history in Taiwan. Cancer Epidemiol Biomark Prev. 2009;18(4):1218–26.
14. Zeng Q, Shen LJ, Li S, Chen L, Guo X, Qian CN, Wu PH. The effects of hemoglobin levels and their interactions with cigarette smoking on survival in nasopharyngeal carcinoma patients. Cancer Med. 2016;5(5):816–26.
15. Lv JW, Chen YP, Zhou GQ, Tang LL, Mao YP, Li WF, et al. Cigarette smoking complements the prognostic value of baseline plasma Epstein-Barr virus deoxyribonucleic acid in patients with nasopharyngeal carcinoma undergoing intensity-modulated radiation therapy: a large-scale retrospective cohort study. Oncotarget. 2016;7(13):16806–17.
16. Lin JH, Jiang CQ, Ho SY, Zhang WS, Mai ZM. Xu L, lo CM, lam TH. Smoking and nasopharyngeal carcinoma mortality: a cohort study of 101,823 adults in Guangzhou, China. BMC Cancer. 2015;15:906.
17. Chen Y, Zhao W, Lin L, Xiao X, Zhou X, Ming H, et al. Nasopharyngeal Epstein-Barr virus load: an efficient supplementary method for population-based nasopharyngeal carcinoma screening. PLoS One. 2015;10(7):e0132669.
18. Yi Z, Yuxi L, Chunren L, Sanwen C, Jihneng W, Jisong Z, Huijong Z. Application of an immunoenzymatic method and an immunoautoradiographic method for a mass survey of nasopharyngeal carcinoma. Intervirology. 1980;13(3):162–8.
19. Lo YM, Tein MS, Lau TK, Haines CJ, Leung TN, Poon PM, et al. Quantitative analysis of fetal DNA in maternal plasma and serum: implications for noninvasive prenatal diagnosis. Am J Hum Genet. 1998;62(4):768–75.
20. Lo YM, Chan LY, Lo KW, Leung SF, Zhang J, Chan AT, et al. Quantitative analysis of cell-free Epstein-Barr virus DNA in plasma of patients with nasopharyngeal carcinoma. Cancer Res. 1999;59(6):1188–91.
21. Nielsen TR, Pedersen M, Rostgaard K, Frisch M, Hjalgrim H. Correlations between Epstein-Barr virus antibody levels and risk factors for multiple sclerosis in healthy individuals. Mult Scler. 2007;13(3):420–3.
22. Levin LI, Chang ET, Ambinder RF, Lennette ET, Rubertone MV, Mann RB, et al. Atypical prediagnosis Epstein-Barr virus serology restricted to EBV-positive Hodgkin lymphoma. Blood. 2012;120(18):3750–5.
23. Tang M, Lautenberger JA, Gao X, Sezgin E, Hendrickson SL, Troyer JL, et al. The principal genetic determinants for nasopharyngeal carcinoma in China involve the HLA class I antigen recognition groove. PLoS Genet. 2012;8(11): e1003103.
24. Dowd JB, Palermo T, Brite J, McDade TW, Aiello A. Seroprevalence of Epstein-Barr virus infection in U.S. children ages 6-19, 2003-2010. PLoS One. 2013;8(5):e64921.
25. Xue WQ, Qin HD, Ruan HL, Shugart YY, Jia WH. Quantitative association of tobacco smoking with the risk of nasopharyngeal carcinoma: a comprehensive meta-analysis of studies conducted between 1979 and 2011. Am J Epidemiol. 2013;178(3):325–38.
26. Jung KJ, Jeon C, Jee SH. The effect of smoking on lung cancer: ethnic differences and the smoking paradox. Epidemiol Health. 2016;38:e2016060.
27. Lin TM, Yang CS, Tu SM, Chen CJ, Kuo KC, Hirayama T. Interaction of factors associated with cancer of the nasopharynx. Cancer. 1979;44(4):1419–23.
28. Charlson ES, Chen J, Custers-Allen R, Bittinger K, Li H, Sinha R, Hwang J, Bushman FD, Collman RG. Disordered microbial communities in the upper respiratory tract of cigarette smokers. PLoS One. 2010;5(12):e15216.
29. Charriere M, Poirier S, Calmels S, De Montclos H, Dubreuil C, Poizat R, Hamdi Cherif M, de The G. Microflora of the nasopharynx in Caucasian and Maghrebian subjects with and without nasopharyngeal carcinoma. IARC Sci Publ. 1991;105:158–61.
30. Brook I, Gober AE. Recovery of potential pathogens and interfering bacteria in the nasopharynx of smokers and nonsmokers. Chest. 2005;127(6):2072–5.

21

Radiotherapy related skin toxicity (RAREST-01): Mepitel® film versus standard care in patients with locally advanced head-and-neck cancer

Carlos Narvaez[1], Claudia Doemer[1], Christian Idel[2], Cornelia Setter[3], Denise Olbrich[4], Zaza Ujmajuridze[5], Jesper Hansen Carl[5] and Dirk Rades[1*]

Abstract

Background: The aim of the present trial is to investigate a new option of skin protection in order to reduce the rate of grade ≥ 2 skin toxicity in patients receiving radiotherapy alone or radiochemotherapy for locally advanced squamous cell carcinoma of the head-and-neck (SCCHN).

Methods / Design: This is a randomized, active-controlled, parallel-group multi-center trial that compares the following treatments of radiation dermatitis in patients with head-and-neck cancer: Mepitel® Film (Arm A) vs. standard care (Arm B). The primary aim of this trial is to investigate the rate of patients experiencing grade ≥ 2 radiation dermatitis (according to Common Toxicity Criteria for Adverse Events (CTCAE) Version 4.03) until 50 Gy of radiotherapy. Evaluation until 50 Gy of radiotherapy has been selected as the primary endpoint, since up to 50 Gy, the irradiated volume includes the primary tumor and the bilateral cervical and supraclavicular lymph nodes, and, therefore, is similar in all patients. After 50 Gy, irradiated volumes are very individual, depending on location and size of the primary tumor, involvement of lymph nodes, and the treatment approach (definitive vs. adjuvant). In addition, the following endpoints will be evaluated: Time to grade 2 radiation dermatitis until 50 Gy of radiotherapy, rate of patients experiencing grade ≥ 2 radiation dermatitis during radio(chemo)therapy, rate of patients experiencing grade ≥ 3 skin toxicity during radio(chemo)therapy, adverse events, quality of life, and dermatitis-related pain. Administration of Mepitel® Film will be considered to be clinically relevant, if the rate of grade ≥ 2 radiation dermatitis can be reduced from 85% to 65%.

Discussion: If administration of Mepitel® Film instead of standard care will be able to significantly reduce the rate of grade ≥ 2 radiation dermatitis, it could become the new standard of skin care in patients irradiated for SCCHN.

Keywords: Head-and-neck cancer, Radio(chemo)therapy, Radiation dermatitis, Mepitel® film, Standard care

* Correspondence: Rades.Dirk@gmx.net
[1]Department of Radiation Oncology, University of Lübeck, Ratzeburger Allee 160, D-23562 Lübeck, Germany
Full list of author information is available at the end of the article

Background

Locally advanced squamous head-and-neck cancer is a serious malignant disease. In about 90% of head-and-neck cancers, the histology is squamous cell carcinoma (SCCHN). The vast majority of patients with locally advanced SCCHN receive radiotherapy, either as a part of a definitive treatment approach, or as an adjuvant treatment following surgery. If radiotherapy is administered as definitive treatment, it is usually combined with concurrent cisplatin-based chemotherapy [1]. In an adjuvant situation, chemotherapy will be added to radiotherapy in case of risk factors, namely microscopically or macroscopically incomplete resection or in case of extra-capsular spread of lymph nodes metastases.

Radiotherapy of locally advanced SCCHN may be associated with severe acute toxicities including skin reaction such as erythema or desquamation. Skin toxicity is enhanced if concurrent chemotherapy is administered. If the skin toxicity becomes severe (grade ≥ 3 according to the Common Toxicity Criteria for Adverse Events (CTCAE) Version 4.03), it may lead to a reduction of the planned chemotherapy dose and to interruptions of radiotherapy. Interruptions of radiotherapy have been reported to be associated with poorer treatment outcomes in patients with SCCHN [2, 3].

In order to successfully avoid grade ≥ 3 skin toxicity, it appears mandatory to avoid or at least postpone the development of grade 2 skin toxicity. In previous studies of patients receiving radiotherapy or radio(chemo)therapy for locally advanced head-and-neck cancer, rates of grade ≥ 2 skin toxicity ranging between 86% and 92% have been reported, although the standard procedures of skin care and protection had been applied [1, 4, 5]. These figures demonstrate that the results of standard care need to be improved.

A few years ago, the results of a systematic inpatient controlled clinical trial were published that had investigated the use of an absorbent, self-adhesive dressing (Mepilex® Lite) for skin protection in patients irradiated for breast cancer [6]. According to this study the dressings were able to significantly reduce the radiation-related skin erythema. Similar dressings (Mepilex® Border Sacrum and Mepilex® Heel dressings) have been demonstrated in a randomized trial to be effective also in the prevention of sacral and heel pressure ulcers in trauma and critically ill patients [7]. In another randomized trial a silver-containing soft silicone foam dressing (Mepilex® Ag dressing) was as effective in the treatment of partial-thickness thermal burns when compared to the standard care (silver sulfadiazine) [8]. In addition, the group of patients treated with the Mepilex® Ag dressing demonstrated decreased pain and lower costs associated with treatment. More recently, a new dressing (Mepitel® Film) has been developed, which is thinner, softer and more comfortable than previous dressings.

The rationale for the present study is to investigate a new option of skin protection in order to reduce the rate of grade ≥ 2 skin toxicity in patients receiving radiotherapy alone or radiochemotherapy for locally advanced SCCHN.

Methods / Design
Endpoints of the study

The primary aim of this randomized multi-center trial is to investigate the rate of patients experiencing grade ≥ 2 radiation dermatitis (CTCAE v4.03) until 50 Gy of radiotherapy. Evaluation until 50 Gy of radiotherapy has been selected as the primary endpoint, since up to 50 Gy, the irradiated volume includes the primary tumor and the bilateral cervical and supraclavicular lymph nodes, and, therefore, is similar in all patients. After 50 Gy, irradiated volumes are very individual, depending on location and size of the primary tumor, involvement of lymph nodes, and the treatment approach (definitive vs. adjuvant).

In addition, the following endpoints will be evaluated:

1. Time to grade 2 radiation dermatitis until 50 Gy of radiotherapy
2. Rate of patients experiencing grade ≥ 2 radiation dermatitis during radio(chemo)therapy
3. Rate of patients experiencing grade ≥ 3 skin toxicity during radio(chemo)therapy
4. Adverse Events
5. Quality of life: Evaluation prior to radiotherapy, at the end of radiotherapy weeks 3 + 5, and at 3 weeks following radiotherapy
6. Pain: Evaluation prior to radiotherapy, at the end of radiotherapy weeks 3 + 5, and at 1 and 3 weeks following radiotherapy

Study design

This is a randomized, active-controlled, parallel-group trial, which will compare the following treatments of radiation related skin toxicity in patients with head-and-neck cancer: Mepitel® Film (Arm A) vs. Standard Care (Arm B).

The recruitment of all 168 patients should be completed within 24 months. The follow-up period will be 3 weeks. Stratification will be done using the following factors:

1. Tumor site: oropharynx/oral cavity vs. hypopharynx/larynx
2. Treatment approach: radiochemotherapy vs. radiotherapy alone
3. Participating site

Inclusion criteria

1. Histologically proven locally advanced squamous cell carcinoma of the head-and-neck (SCCHN)

2. Conventionally fractionated (5 × 2 Gy per week) definitive or adjuvant radio(chemo)therapy
3. Age ≥ 18 years
4. Written informed consent
5. Capacity of the patient to contract

Exclusion criteria

1. N3 stage (lymph nodes > 6 cm)
2. Distant metastases (M1)
3. Pregnancy, Lactation
4. Treatment with EGFR-antibodies (either given or planned)
5. Expected non-compliance

Treatment

Radiotherapy

Radiotherapy is administered using conventional fractionation (5 × 2.0 Gy per week). The initial target volume includes the region of the primary tumor plus bilateral cervical and supraclavicular lymph nodes up to 50 Gy. Patients treated with adjuvant radiotherapy following complete resection of the primary tumor and the involved lymph nodes receive a radiation boost of 10 Gy (5 × 2.0 Gy per week) to the regions of the primary tumor and the involved lymph nodes. In case of a microscopically incomplete resection, the boost dose to the primary tumor region is 16 Gy. In case of extra-capsular spread (ECS) of lymph nodes, the lymph nodes showing ECS receive an additional boost of 6 Gy (i.e. a cumulative boost dose of 16 Gy). Patients receiving definitive radiotherapy, receive a boost of 10 Gy (5 × 2.0 Gy per week) to the primary tumor, the involved lymph nodes, and the lymph node levels adjacent to the involved lymph nodes. An additional boost of another 10 Gy (5 × 2.0 Gy per week) is administered to the primary tumor and the involved lymph nodes. Treatment should be performed as intensity-modulated radiotherapy (IMRT) or volumetric modulated arc therapy (VMAT) radiotherapy.

Chemotherapy

In patients who receive definitive radiotherapy, concomitant chemotherapy with cisplatin is administered. The cumulative cisplatin dose at the end of the fifth week of radiotherapy (50 Gy) should be 200 mg/m2. This cumulative dose may either be achieved with 20 mg/m2 given with radiotherapy fractions 1–5 and 21–25, 25 mg/m2 given with radiotherapy fractions 1–4 and 21–24, or weekly doses of 40/m2.

Skin care

Arm a (Mepitel® film) Starting on the first day of radiotherapy, Mepitel® Film will be applied. Skin care will be continued until the end of the study period or until a patient experiences grade ≥ 2 moist desquamation or grade ≥ 3 radiation dermatitis. In case of grade ≥ 2 moist desquamation or grade ≥ 3 radiation dermatitis, antiseptic agents will be used daily followed by administration of silicon or calcium alginate bandage until moist desquamation disappears and radiaton dermatitis improves to grade 2.

Arm B (standard care) Standard skin care will be applied starting on radiotherapy day 1 including fatty cream with 2–5% urea (fatty cream alone, if patients do not tolerate urea) and mometasone furoate cream. The treatment will be continued until the end of the study period or until a patient experiences grade ≥ 2 moist desquamation or grade ≥ 3 radiation dermatitis. In case of grade ≥ 2 moist desquamation or grade ≥ 3 radiation dermatitis, the same skin care regimen is used as in Arm A.

Assessments

The following parameters will be recorded at the start of the trial: Medical history, physical examination, complications from head-and-neck surgery, age, gender, performance status, site of primary tumor, tumor stage, histology, HPV-status, histologic grading, surgery of primary tumor, extent of resection, neck dissection, complications of surgery, chemotherapy planned, skin status of the head-and neck region, and quality of life.

The following parameters will be assessed continuously throughout the course of the trial:

1. Radiation dermatitis: Radiation dermatitis will be assessed by two independent observers (specially trained nurses, technicians, or physicians) prior to radio(chemo)therapy, daily during radio(chemo)therapy and up to three weeks following radio(chemotherapy) according to CTCAE v4.03. If the graduation of radiation dermatitis varies between the two observers, skin toxicity will be assessed by an additional observer. Observers are required to be very experienced in rating skin reactions and will additionally undergo a particular briefing prior to the start of this study.
2. Adverse Events: Adverse events, other than radiation dermatitis will be assessed on an ongoing basis according to CTCAE v4.03.
3. Quality of life: Quality of life will be assessed prior to radio(chemo)therapy, at the end of radiotherapy weeks 3 and 5, and at three weeks following radio(chemo)therapy using EORTC QLQ-C30 Version 3.0 and EORTC QLQ-H&N35.
4. Pain: Dermatitis-related pain is assessed with a visual analogue scale (self-assessment: from 0 = No pain; 1 = Mild pain to 10 = Very severe pain) prior to, daily during and up to three weeks following radio(chemotherapy). Pain scores will be correlated with grade of skin reactions.

Sample size calculation

The primary goal of this randomized trial is to demonstrate that Mepitel® Film is superior to Standard Care with respect to prevent grade 2 radiation dermatitis in patients receiving radio(chemo)therapy up to 50 Gy for locally advanced SCCHN. The null hypothesis of equal rates of grade ≥ 2 skin toxicity is tested against the two-sided alternative hypothesis of different rates. Based on this hypothesis system, the sample size required for this trial is calculated taking into account the following assumptions:

- A Chi-square Test will be applied
- The two-sided significance level is set to 5%
- In patients treated with radio(chemo)therapy for locally advanced SCCHN, previous studies have suggested rates of grade ≥ 2 skin toxicity of 86–92% if standard skin care was administered.
- Based on these data, a rate of grade ≥ 2 skin toxicity of 85% can be assumed in the reference group ("worst-case"), i.e. in patients receiving standard care for skin toxicity.
- Administration of Mepitel® Film will be considered to be clinically relevant, if the rate of grade ≥ 2 skin toxicity can be reduced to 65%.
- The power to yield statistical significance if the difference in rates is in fact 20 percentage points is set to 80%.

Based on these assumptions, 80 patients are required per study arm within the full analysis set. Taking into account that 5% of patients will not qualify for the set, a total of 168 patients should be randomized.

The rates of patients experiencing grade ≥ 2 radiation dermatitis in patients receiving radio(chemo)therapy up to 50 Gy will be statistically compared using the Cochran-Mantel-Haenszel Chi-square test on a two-sided significance level of 5%. This test is the natural non-parametric extension of the Chi-square test for testing the treatment effect, while adjusting for the effects of the stratification variables used for randomization. For further assessment of the robustness of the results, a logistic regression model for grade ≥ 2 radiation dermatitis will be applied including the parameters used for stratification. In addition, a model including also additional patient characteristics will be fitted. The confirmatory evaluation will be performed within the Full Analysis Set, the Per Protocol Set serves for further sensitivity analyses.

Discussion

Radiotherapy is the most frequently administered treatment modality in patients with locally advanced SCCHN. A considerable number of these patients receive concurrent chemotherapy, generally including cisplatin or carboplatin [1]. Many of these patients, particularly those receiving radio-chemotherapy, experience severe acute side effects including radiation dermatitis. Severe skin reactions may require an interruption of the radiotherapy series, which can lead to a worsening of the patients' prognoses. On multivariate analyses of a retrospective study of 153 patients irradiated for SCCHN, better overall survival was significantly associated with no interruptions of radiotherapy longer than one week (relative risk: 2.59, 95% confidence interval: 1.15–5.78, $p = 0.021$) [2]. So was local control (relative risk: 3.32, 95% confidence interval: 1.26–8.79, $p = 0.015$). In a SEER database analysis, patients irradiated for larynx cancer with an interruption of their radiotherapy had a 68% (95% confidence interval: 41% to 200%) increased risk of death than those patients without an interruption. Patients with head-and-neck cancers at other sites showed similar associations. However, due to the relatively small numbers of patients, the difference between patients who did and who did experience interruptions of radiotherapy did not reach significance [3]. To avoid such interruptions of radiotherapy due to radiation dermatitis, it is reasonable to avoid or at least significantly postpone grade 2 skin reactions. This appears a challenge for radiation oncologists, since in previous studies grade ≥ 2 radiation dermatitis occurred in 86% to 92% of patients, despite administration of standard skin care procedures from the first day of radiotherapy [1, 4, 5]. Therefore, skin care in patients irradiated for SCCHN needs to be improved, particularly to avoid interruptions of radiotherapy and a subsequent impairment of the patient's prognoses in terms of local control and overall survival [2, 3]. The use of an absorbent, self-adhesive dressing represents a promising approach. According to a systematic inpatient controlled clinical, such dressings can significantly decrease radiation-related erythema of the skin in breast cancer patients [6]. Promising results have also been reported for the prevention of sacral and heel pressure ulcers in trauma and critically ill patients and the treatment of partial-thickness thermal burns [7, 8]. More recently, a new dressing named Mepitel® Film was developed that is thinner and softer than previous dressings and, therefore, appears more comfortable for the patients than the previous dressings. The randomized RAREST-01 compares this new dressing to standard procedures of skin care in patients with locally advanced SCCHN receiving radiotherapy or radiochemotherapy. If Mepitel® Film can significantly reduce the rate of grade ≥ 2 radiation dermatitis in patients irradiated for locally advanced SCCHN it would have the potential to become the new standard of skin care in this group of patients.

Abbreviations
CTCAE: Common Terminology Criteria for Adverse Events; ECOG: Eastern Cooperative Oncology Group; ECS: Extra-capsular spread; EORTC: European Organisation for Research and Treatment of Cancer; IMRT: Intensity-modulated radiotherapy; QLQ: Quality of life questionnaire; SCCHN: Squamous cell carcinoma; VMAT: Volumetric modulated arc therapy

Acknowledgements
The study is part of the INTERREG-project InnoCan. The authors wish to thank all colleagues and project partners working within the InnoCan project for their excellent collaboration.

Funding
The study is part of the INTERREG-project InnoCan, which is funded by the European Union (reference: Innoc 11–1.0-15). The funding body has no role in the design of the study, in collection, analysis and interpretation of the data and in writing of the manuscript.

Authors' contributions
CN, CD, CI, CS, DO, ZU, JHC, and DR participated in the generation of the study protocol of the RAREST-01 trial. CN and DR drafted the manuscript, which has been reviewed by the other authors. The final version of the manuscript has been approved by the authors.

Competing interests
D.R. is an associate editor for BMC Cancer. Otherwise, the authors declare that they have no competing interest related to the study presented here.

Author details
[1]Department of Radiation Oncology, University of Lübeck, Ratzeburger Allee 160, D-23562 Lübeck, Germany. [2]Departments of Radiation Oncology and Oto-Rhino-Laryngology and Head and Neck Surgery, University of Lübeck, Lübeck, Germany. [3]Department of Radiation Oncology, Christian-Albrechts University Kiel, Kiel, Germany. [4]Centre for Clinical Trials Lübeck, Lübeck, Germany. [5]Department of Oncology, Zealand University Hospital, Naestved, Denmark.

References
1. Rades D, Kronemann S, Meyners T, Bohlen G, Tribius S, Kazic N, Schroeder U, Hakim SG, Schild SE, Dunst J. Comparison of four cisplatin-based radiochemotherapy regimens for nonmetastatic stage III/IV squamous cell carcinoma of the head and neck. Int J Radiat Oncol Biol Phys. 2011;80:1037–44.
2. Rades D, Stoehr M, Kazic N, Hakim SG, Walz A, Schild SE, Dunst J. Locally advanced stage IV squamous cell carcinoma of the head and neck: impact of pre-radiotherapy hemoglobin level and interruptions during radiotherapy. Int J Radiat Oncol Biol Phys. 2008;70:1108–14.
3. Fesinmeyer MD, Mehta V, Blough D, Tock L, Ramsey SD. Effect of radiotherapy interruptions on survival in medicare enrollees with local and regional head-and-neck cancer. Int J Radiat Oncol Biol Phys. 2010;78:675–81.
4. Rades D, Fehlauer F, Wroblesky J, Albers D, Schild SE, Schmidt R. Prognostic factors in head-and-neck cancer patients treated with surgery followed by intensity-modulated radiotherapy (IMRT), 3D-conformal radiotherapy, or conventional radiotherapy. Oral Oncol. 2007;43:535–43.
5. Rades D, Stoehr M, Meyners T, Bohlen G, Nadrowitz R, Dunst J, Schild SE, Wroblewski J, Albers D, Schmidt R, Alberti W, Tribius S. Evaluation of prognostic factors and two radiation techniques in patients treated with surgery followed by radio(chemo)therapy or definitive radio(chemo)therapy for locally advanced head-and-neck cancer. Strahlenther Onkol. 2008;184:198–205.
6. Diggelmann KV, Zytkovicz AE, Tuaine JM, Bennett NC, Kelly LE, Herst PM. Mepilex lite dressings for the management of radiation-induced erythema: a systematic inpatient controlled clinical trial. Br J Radiol. 2010;83:971–8.
7. Santamaria N, Gerdtz M, Sage S, McCann J, Freeman A, Vassiliou T, De Vincentis S, Ng AW, Manias E, Liu W, Knott J. A randomised controlled trial of the effectiveness of soft silicone multi-layered foam dressings in the prevention of sacral and heel pressure ulcers in trauma and critically ill patients: the border trial. Int Wound J. 2015;12:302–8.
8. Silverstein P, Heimbach D, Meites H, Latenser B, Mozingo D, Mullins F, Garner W, Turkowski J, Shupp J, Glat P, Purdue G. An open, parallel, randomized, comparative, multicenter study to evaluate the cost-effectiveness, performance, tolerance, and safety of a silver-containing soft silicone foam dressing (intervention) vs silver sulfadiazine cream. J Burn Care Res. 2011;32:617–26.

22

Preoperative serum immunoglobulin G and A antibodies to *Porphyromonas gingivalis* are potential serum biomarkers for the diagnosis and prognosis of esophageal squamous cell carcinoma

She-Gan Gao[1], Jun-Qiang Yang[1], Zhi-Kun Ma[1], Xiang Yuan[1], Chen Zhao[1], Guang-Chao Wang[2], Hua Wei[3], Xiao-Shan Feng[1*] and Yi-Jun Qi[1*]

Abstract

Background: The key-stone-pathogen, *Porphyromonas gingivalis* associates not only with periodontal diseases but with a variety of other chronic diseases such as cancer. We previously reported an association between the presence of *Porphyromonas gingivalis* in esophageal squamous cell carcinoma (ESCC) and its progression. We now report the diagnostic and prognostic potential of serum immunoglobulin G and A antibodies (IgG/A) against *Porphyromonas gingivalis* for ESCC.

Methods: An enzyme-linked immunosorbent assay (ELISA) was used to determine the serum levels of *Porphyromonas gingivalis* IgG and IgA in 96 cases with ESCC, 50 cases with esophagitis and 80 healthy controls.

Results: The median serum levels of IgG and IgA for *P. gingivalis* were significantly higher in ESCC patients than non-ESCC controls. *P. gingivalis* IgG and IgA in serum demonstrated sensitivities/specificities of 29.17%/96.90% and 52.10%/70.81%, respectively, and combination of IgG and IgA produced a sensitivity/specificity of 68.75%/68.46%. The diagnostic performance of serum *P. gingivalis* IgA for early ESCC was superior to that of IgG (54.54% vs. 20.45%). Furthermore, high serum levels of *P. gingivalis* IgG or IgA were associated with worse prognosis of ESCC patients, in particular for patients with stage 0-IIor negative lymphnode metastasis, and ESCC patients with high levels of both IgG and IgA had the worst prognosis. Multivariate analysis revealed that lymph node status, IgG and IgA were independent prognostic factors.

Conclusions: The IgG and IgA for *P. gingivalis* are potential serum biomarkers for ESCC and combination of IgG and IgA improves the diagnostic and prognostic performance. Furthermore, serum *P. gingivalis* IgG and IgA can detect early stage ESCC.

Keywords: Esophageal squamous cell carcinoma, *Porphyromonas gingivalis*, Antibody, Immunoglobulin G/A, Diagnosis, Prognosis

* Correspondence: samfeng137@hotmail.com; qiqiyijun@163.com
[1]Henan Key Laboratory of Cancer Epigenetics; Cancer Hospital, The First Affiliated Hospital, College of Clinical Medicine, Medical College of Henan University of Science and Technology, Luoyang, Henan 471003, People's Republic of China
Full list of author information is available at the end of the article

Background

Esophageal squamous cell carcinoma (ESCC) remains the predominant histological subtype of esophageal carcinoma and ranks as the fourth most common cancer in terms of both incidence and mortality in China [1, 2]. Although significant advances in diagnostic and therapeutic modalities have improved the prognosis of ESCC patients, the overall 5-year survival rate still ranges from 25% to 30%, mainly due to advanced stage at initial presentation [1, 3–7]. On the other hand, accurate staging and prognosis is difficult to assess at diagnosis, which hampers ESCC tailoring therapy, treatment efficiency and recurrence monitoring. It is, therefore, imperative to identify novel biomarkers for early detection, metastasis and recurrence to reduce ESCC-related morbidity and mortality.

A number of epidemiological and clinical studies have reported a positive association between the conditions of oral microbiome, periodontal disease or tooth loss and the progression of multiple cancers [8–25], and even gastric precancerous lesions [26, 27]. The oral microbiome inhabiting the oral cavity contains multiple species in a complex community that generally exist in a balanced immunoinflammatory state with the host [28]. Disruption of this equilibrium has deleterious effects on the mucosal lining, surrounding tissues and even distant organs and systems of human body through the combined effects of a dysbiotic microbial community and a dysregulated immune response [12, 13, 29]. *Porphyromonas gingivalis* has become regarded as a key-stone pathogen and is closely associated with periodontal diseases, a variety of presumably unrelated chronic diseases and multiple cancers [30, 31]. Although the self-reported tooth loss may have a microbial basis in the case of esophageal cancer [16, 17], there is no convincing evidence of direct and specific microbial etiologic agents until our recent findings, which revealed a higher frequency (61%) of *P. gingivalis* presence in ESCC [18].

As *P. gingivalis*is is an important periodontal pathogen in various types of periodontal disease, numerous studies have reported that antibody responses to *P. gingivalis* correlate with severity and progression of periodontitis, extent of attachment loss and treatment effects [32–36]. In a cohort study of NHANES III, not only the increasing severity of periodontitis but the higher serum IgG for *P. gingivalis* was associated with increased orodigestive cancer mortality [25]. In another European prospective cohort study, high levels of antibodies to *P. gingivalis* rendered a > 2-fold increased risk to pancreatic cancer [21]. In clinical settings, serum tumor biomarkers take priority over other measures for screening, diagnosis and clinical management of cancer. However, conventional serum markers for ESCC, such as squamous cell carcinoma antigen (SCCA), carcinoembryonic antigen (CEA), CYFRA21-1 and carbohydrate antigen (CA)19-9, lack sufficient sensitivity and specificity for the early detection and progression of ESCC [37–41].

On the grounds of our recent study establishing the association between the infection of *P. gingivalis* in esophageal epithelium and progression of ESCC, herein we investigate the serum levels of immunoglobulin G and A (IgG and IgA) for *P. gingivalis* and their clinical significance for the diagnosis and postoperative prognosis of ESCC.

Methods

Patients

The first cohort of 96 preoperative serum samples were recruited from ESCC patients, who underwent curative esophagectomy at the First Affiliated Hospital of Henan University of Science & Technology and Anyang people's hospital. None of ESCC patients received preoperative neoadjuvant chemoradiotherapy. The clinical stage of ESCC was classified in accordance with the seventh edition of AJCC and early stage was defined as AJCC stage 0 + I + IIA. Another cohort of 50 serum samples were collected from patients with esophagitis, who underwent gastroscopy. In addition, 80 healthy individuals without evidence of comorbid disease were recruited as healthy controls from the physical examination center of our hospital.

Enzyme-linked immunosorbent assay

P. gingivalis ATCC 33277, used as the antigen in our experiment, was cultured and prepared as previously described. For enzyme-linked immunosorbent assay (ELISA), 100 ul of reconstituted protein extracts of *P. gingivalis* (10 μg/ml) was used to coat microtiter plates followed by incubation with 1:200 diluted serum incubation, 1: 1000 biotin-conjugated anti-human IgG and IgA, and 1:400 avidin-conjugated peroxidase. Antibodies levels were expressed as ELISA units (EUs) with the use of a reference serum pool [42].

Statistical analysis

The statistical analyses were performed using SPSS 19.0 software package (SPSS, Chicago, IL, USA). Data are expressed as mean ± standard deviation (SD). Comparisons between groups were performed using t tests. The receiver operating characteristic (ROC) was used to determine the optimal cut-off value of IgG and IgA. The accuracy, sensitivity, specificity, false negative rate (FNR), false positive rate (FPR) and area under the ROC (AUC) were used to assess the classification efficiency. Overall survival (OS) was defined as the interval between the date of surgery and the date of death or the date of last follow-up. Follow-up data was available for 80 ESCC patients with a median follow-up interval of

10.5 months (3.0-42.6 months). Clinical stage and lymph node metastasis were available for 78 ESCC patients. Survival curves were plotted using the Kaplan-Meier method and differences between curves were tested by log-rank tests. The significance of prognostic factors on survival was studied by Cox regression model.

Results

Levels of serum IgG and IgA for *P. gingivalis* in ESCC

The details of ESCC characteristics are presented in Table 1. Figure 1 shows the frequency distributions of IgG and IgA for *P. gingivalis* across the three cohorts. As there were no significant differences between healthy controls and non-ESCC patients with esophagitis with regards to serum levels of *P. gingivalis* IgG or IgA, we combined these two cohorts as non-ESCC controls hereafter. The median serum levels of IgG and IgA for *P. gingivalis* were significantly higher in ESCC patients than in non-ESCC controls (150.69 EU vs. 109.13 EU, $P < 0.001$ for IgG; 33.16 EU vs. 19.14 EU, $P < 0.01$ for IgA). However, no significant correlation was found between serum levels of *P. gingivalis* IgG and IgA ($r^2 = 0.03$, $P > 0.05$, data not shown).

Seeking to determine the diagnostic potential of *P. gingivalis* IgG and IgA, ROC curves were plotted to distinguish 96 patients of ESCC from 130 non-ESCC controls. As shown in Fig. 2a, AUCs of IgG and IgA for *P. gingivalis* were 0.612 and 0.632, with optimal cut-off values of 189.17 EU and 21.25 EU, respectively. The specificity for IgG was higher (96.90%) than that of IgA

(70.81%) but not the sensitivity (29.17% vs. 52.10%, Fig. 2b). Combination of IgG and IgA, i.e. seropositivity for at least one subtype of IgG or IgA antibody, produced an AUC of 0.686 with a sensitivity of 68.75% and a specificity of 68.46%, respectively (Fig. 2a). Figure 2b shows the diagnostic performance of IgG, IgA, and combination of IgG and IgA in terms of accuracy, sensitivity, specificity, FNR and FPR.

Diagnostic value of IgG and IgA for *P. gingivalis* in early stage of ESCC.

There were 44 patients with early stage disease in our cohort of ESCC. The mean value of *P. gingivalis* IgA in early stage ESCC was lower (32.08 EU) than that of late stage ESCC (41.76 EU) without statistical significance ($P = 0.29$), whereas the mean IgG value was marginally higher in early stage ESCC (114.35 EU vs. 113.62 EU, $P = 0.058$). The sensitivity of *P. gingivalis* IgA for detection of early stage ESCC was 54.54% (24/44) with a specificity of 70.82%, and was far better than that of IgG (20.45%, (9/44)).

Associations between *P. gingivalis* IgG and IgA with clinicopathological features and overall survival of ESCC

The associations between clinicopathological features of ESCC and serum levels of IgG or IgA for *P. gingivalis* were determined by *t* test. No significant associations were observed between any clinicopathological features with IgG or IgA serum levels. Likewise, ROCs were plotted to predict the 3-year OS rate of ESCC. Figure 2c shows the time-dependent ROC

Table 1 Associations between serum IgG and IgA antibodies for *P. gingivalis* with clinicopathological features of ESCC

Variables		IgG Titer (EU)	P	IgA Titer (EU)	P
Age (n(%))	≤ 60(26(32.5%))	132.15 ± 62.13	0.46	31.54 ± 25.93	0.52
	> 60(54(67.5%))	121.07 ± 62.65		38.23 ± 49.45	
Gender (n(%))	Male(55(68.8%))	127.80 ± 62.18	0.51	37.52 ± 48.10	0.65
	Female(25(31.2%))	116.77 ± 63.30		32.84 ± 30.22	
Tobacco use (n(%))	No(43(%))	122.62 ± 58.81	0.75	34.52 ± 30.12	0.73
	Yes(37(%))	127.05 ± 66.87		37.84 ± 55.00	
Alcohol use (n(%))	No(74(%))	125.57 ± 63.66	0.65	61.30 ± 74.42	0.60
	Yes(6(%))	113.47 ± 44.82		54.28 ± 25.41	
Differentiation grade (n(%))	Well(17(21.2%))	166.72 ± 71.77	0.15	36.47 ± 36.07	0.83
	Moderately(47(58.8%))	105.27 ± 45.26		35.12 ± 49.55	
	Poorly(15(18.8))	140.28 ± 72.94		40.17 ± 29.95	
T stage (n(%))	T1 + T2(17(21.5%))	121.72 ± 48.57	0.80	27.17 ± 20.14	0.33
	T3 + T4(62(78.5%))	126.08 ± 66.19		38.89 ± 47.61	
Lymph node metastasis (n(%))	No(44(56.4%))	115.07 ± 57.03	0.19	42.94 ± 57.45	0.27
	Yes(34(43.6%))	134.05 ± 66.21		31.97 ± 28.31	
TNM stage (n(%))	I–II(51(63.8%))	130.18 ± 62.58	0.34	31.77 ± 27.59	0.21
	III–IV(28(36.2%))	115.95 ± 62.60		44.73 ± 62.51	

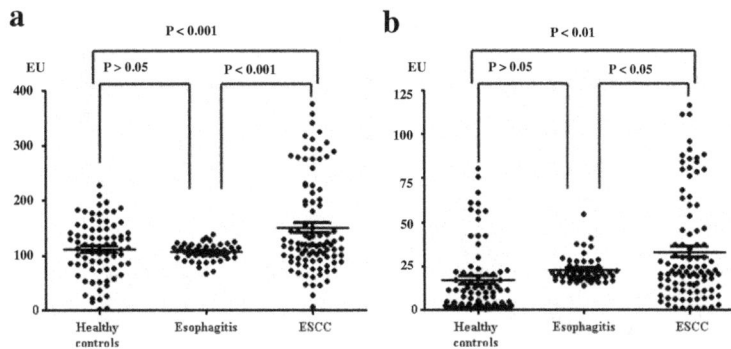

Fig. 1 Enzyme-linked immunosorbent assay (ELISA) of serum IgG and IgA antibodies to *P. gingivalis* in healthy controls (*n* = 80), patients with esophagitis (*n* = 50) and ESCC (*n* = 96). **a** Scatter plots of ELISA units (EUs) of *P. gingivalis* IgG antibody in serum of healthy controls, patients with esophagitis and ESCC. **b** Scatter plots of ELISA units (EUs) of *P. gingivalis* IgA antibody in serum of healthy controls, patients with esophagitis and ESCC

curves of *P. gingivalis* antibodies as predictors of ESCC-related 3-year survival rates and the AUCs were 0.595 and 0.719 with optimal cut-off values of 125.08 EU and 37.12 EU for IgG and IgA, respectively. The sensitivity of *P. gingivalis* IgA was higher than that of IgG (86.25% vs. 47.82%) but not the specificity (57.54% vs. 71.92%, Fig. 2d). Likewise, combination of IgG and IgA produced a maximal AUC (0.746), a maximal sensitivity (87.16%) but a modest

specificity (62.07%) in comparison with individual IgG or IgA (Fig. 2d).

Figure 3a shows the postoperative survival of 80 ESCC patients with a median survival time of 31.58 months, 61 surviving patients and 19 ESCC-related deaths at the last clinical follow-up (Fig. 3a). Using the optimal cut-off value of 138.23 EU, Kaplan-Meier survival analysis revealed that ESCC patients with higher serum level of *P. gingivalis* IgG had a significantly worse prognosis than

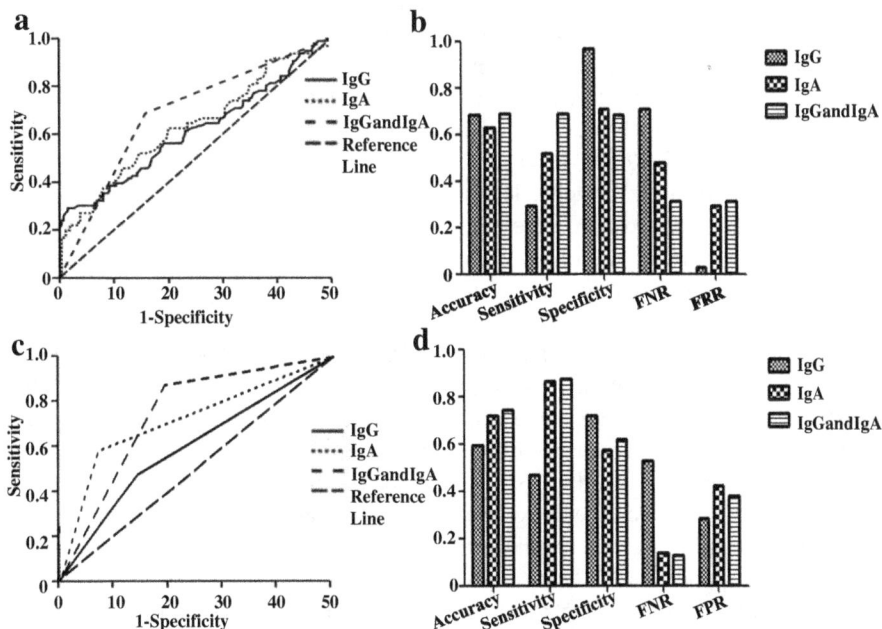

Fig. 2 Receiver operating characteristic (ROC) curves and clinical performances of *P. gingivalis* IgG and IgA. **a** ROC curves of IgG, IgA and combination of IgG and IgA for *P. gingivalis* as a diagnostic marker for discrimination of ESCC and non-ESCC controls. **b** Clinical performances of IgG, IgA and combination of IgG and IgA for *P. gingivalis* as a diagnostic marker for discrimination of ESCC and non-ESCC controls in terms of accuracy, sensitivity, specificity, false negative rate (FNR), false positive rate (FPR). **c** Time-dependent ROC curves of IgG, IgA and combination of IgG and IgA for *P. gingivalis* as predictors of ESCC-related 3-year survival rates. **d** Clinical performances of IgG, IgA and combination of IgG and IgA for *P. gingivalis* predictors of ESCC-related 3-year survival rates in terms of accuracy, sensitivity, specificity, false negative rate (FNR), false positive rate (FPR)

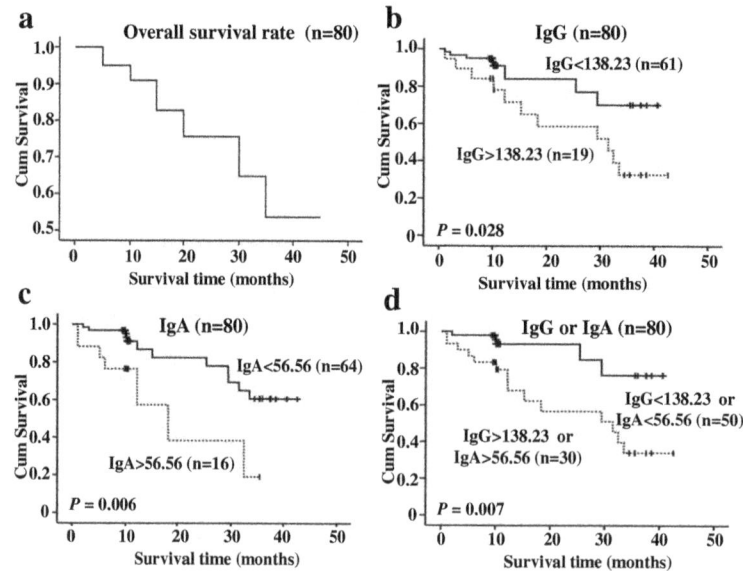

Fig. 3 Kaplan-Meier survival curves of ESCC patients. **a** The 3-year OS rate of 80 ESCC patients was 52.23%. **b** The 3-year OS rates in ESCC patients with IgG < 138.23 EU (*n* = 61) and IgG > 138.23 EU (*n* = 19) were 70.145% and 32.68%, respectively, with a significant difference (*P* = 0.028). **c** The 3-year OS rates in ESCC patients with IgA < 56.56 EU (*n* = 64) and IgG > 56.56 EU (*n* = 16) were 60.82% and 18.83%, respectively, with a significant difference (*P* = 0.006). **d** The 3-year OS rates in ESCC patients with IgG < 138.23 EU or IgA < 56.56 (*n* = 50) and IgG > 138.23 EU or IgA > 56.56 (*n* = 30) were 76.38% and 34.04%, respectively, with a significant difference (*P* = 0.007)

ESCC with lower serum level (log-rank test, x^2 = 4.852, *P* = 0.028, median OS of 26.25 (*n* = 19) months vs. 33.68 months (*n* = 61), Fig. 3b). The prognostic effect of *P. gingivalis* IgA resembled that of IgG (log-rank test, x^2 = 6.800, *P* = 0.006, median OS of 19.59 months (*n* = 16) vs. 34.15 months (*n* = 64), Fig. 3c). In 50 ESCC patients with lower IgG or IgA serum level, the median OS was 36.12 months compared with 25.89 months of their counterparts (log-rank test, x^2 = 7.208, *P* = 0.007, Fig. 3d). Furthermore, 5 ESCC patients with higher levels of both IgG and IgA had the worst prognosis and the median OS for these 5 patients was 16.62 months versus 32.93 months of the other 75 patients (log-rank test, x^2 = 8316, *P* = 0.004, Data now shown).

The prognostic values of histopathological features were also evaluated by Kaplan-Meier method and log-rank test. With regards to clinical TNM stage, stage I–II ESCC patients (stage I–II, 63.75%, *n* = 51) survived longer than stage III–IV ESCC cases (Stage III–IV, 36.25%, *n* = 27, Additional file 1: Figure S1A). For the subgroup ESCC patients with early clinical stage, a significant benefit in OS was observed in patients with low serum level of *P. gingivalis* IgA but non-significant for IgG than in patients with high level (log-rank test, x^2 = 9.141, *P* = 0.003, Additional file 1: Figure S1B & D), and neither IgG nor IgA was associated with OS of late stage ESCC (Additional file 1: Figure S1C &E). In addition, lymph node metastasis was significantly associated with shorter OS ((log-rank test, x^2 = 5.61, *P* = 0.018,

Additional file 2: Figure S2A). In ESCC patients with negative lymph node metastasis, those with high levels of *P. gingivalis* IgG or IgA had worse OS than patients with low IgG or IgA serum level (log-rank test, x2 = 6.097/6.097, *P* = 0.014/0.011, Additional file 2: Figure S2B & D), whereas no significant differences were observed between *P. gingivalis* IgG or IgA and OS in positive lymph node metastasis (Additional file 2: Figure S2C & E).

To identify independent prognostic factors for ESCC patients, clinicopathological factors were assessed by univariate and multivariate Cox regression models. Univariate Cox proportional hazard regression analysis revealed that N-stage (Hazard ratio = 3.169, 95% CI = 1.175 – 8.545, *P* = 0.023), IgG (Hazard ratio = 3.039, 95% CI = 1.148 – 8.041, *P* = 0.025) and IgA (Hazard ratio = 3.588, 95% CI = 1.368 – 9.409, *P* = 0.009) were significant prognostic predictors for OS of ESCC patients (Table 2). When N-stage, IgG and IgA were analysed by multivariate analysis using Cox's proportional hazards model, N-stage (Hazard ratio = 12.292, 95% CI = 1.399 – 108.003, *P* = 0.024), IgG (Hazard ratio = 4.910, 95% CI = 1.473– 16.364, *P* = 0.010) and IgA (Hazard ratio = 4.686, 95% CI = 1.492 – 14.722, *P* = 0.008) were independent prognostic factors of ESCC (Table 2).

Discussion

Early diagnosis remains one of the key determinants to improve the long-term survival of patients with ESCC. The majority of patients with ESCC present at

Table 2 Univariate and multivariate Cox regression analyses of the prognostic variables in ESCC patients

Variables	Subsets	Univariate analysis (n = 79)			Multivariate analysis (n = 79)		
		Hazard ratio	95% CI	P	Hazard ratio	95% CI	P
Age	≤ 60 vs. >60	1.779	0.628–5.042	0.278	–	–	–
Gender	Male vs. Female	0.601	0.212–1.703	0.338	–	–	–
T-stage	T1 + T2 vs. T3 + T4	0.875	0.252–3.037	0.834	–	–	–
N-stage	No vs. Yes	3.169	1.175–8.545	0.023	12.292	1.399–108.003	0.024
Histological grade	G1 vs. G2–G3	2.470	0.920–6.631	0.073	–	–	–
Clinical stage	I–II vs. III–IV	0.407	0.150–1.104	0.077	–	–	–
IgG (EU)	≤ 2760 vs. >2760	3.039	1.148–8.041	0.025	4.910	1.473–16.364	0.010
IgA (EU)	≤ 1130 vs. >1130	3.588	1.368–9.409	0.009	4.686	1.492–14.722	0.008

an advanced stage and have limited treatment options, resulting in dismal prognosis [1, 3–7]. Although gastroscopy with biopsy offers an efficient method for diagnosis of patients with ESCC, poor compliance of gastroscopy in asymptomatic patients precludes early detection. Compared with gastroscopy, blood testing is less invasive and cost-effective. Therefore, serum biomarkers have the priority over other measures for clinical application to detect ESCC at an early stage [43].

First and foremost, the present study demonstrates that serum antibody levels against *P. gingivalis* have the potential for diagnosis of ESCC. Although inflammation plays a key role in esophageal carcinogenesis, our results revealed that morphological esophagitis harboring inflammatory cells without transformed cells in esophageal mucosa failed to show increased IgG and IgA antibody response to *P. gingivalis*. This finding indicates that *P. gingivalis* may not be involved in the process of esophagitis, but do not rule out the possibility that *P. gingivalis* or host responses against *P. gingivalis* contribute to the development and progression of ESCC. In sharp contrast, titers of IgG and IgA against *P. gingivalis* in serum of patients with ESCC increased remarkably compared to patients with esophagitis and healthy controls, which provides direct evidence that *P. gingivalis* is implicated in the pathogenesis of ESCC. Using an optimal diagnostic cut off value of 425 EU, individual IgA had the highest sensitivity (52.1%) for discrimination of ESCC from non-ESCC controls compared with conventional serum markers for ESCC, such as SCCA, CYFRA21-1, CEA, CA19-9 [37–41], whereas the specificity was low (70.8%). However, ELISA results of SCCA1, SCCA2, CYFRA21-1 and CEA did not show diagnostic value in our cohort (data not shown). Growing evidence indicates that combination of several individual biomarkers is superior to any single biomarker [44]. Combination of IgG and IgA for *P. gingivalis* had an increased AUC (0.671) compared with an individual IgG or IgA.

For detection of early stage ESCC, conventional serum biomarkers of ESCC have little diagnostic benefit. For instance, the positive frequencies of both CYFRA21-1 and SCCA in patients with early stage ESCC (stage 0-II) varied from 4.7% to 24% [37, 40]. In contrast, the diagnostic performance of serum *P. gingivalis* IgA for early ESCC was superior as evidenced by a sensitivity of 54.54% in our study. Although the specificity of single IgA was not sufficient, combination of IgG and IgA produced a specificity of 91.5%.

Mounting clinical evidence indicates a positive association between *P. gingivalis* or periodontal disease and an increased risk for a variety of cancers and even poor prognosis [11, 12, 18, 21, 25]. In normal distal esophagus, bacterial colonization was not uncommon [45]. Furthermore, the global esophageal microbiome in both esophagitis and Barrett's esophagus altered from typeI bacteria in normal esophageal mucosa to typeII bacteria, many of which are Gram-negative anaerobes/microaerophiles and putative pathogens of periodontal disease [46]. Our previous study demonstrated that *P. gingivalis* infection in ESCC was prevalent (61%) and negatively correlated with OS of ESCC [18]. In the present study, we looked into the prognostic potential of human immune response to *P. gingivalis* in terms of IgG and IgA. In line with the presence of *P. gingivalis* in ESCC, higher serum levels of *P. gingivalis* IgG and IgA were associated with worse prognosis of patients with ESCC. In particular for early stage ESCC, i.e. ESCC with stage 0-II or negative lymphnode metastasis, patients with high level of *P. gingivalis* IgG or IgA had a significantly lower OS relative to ESCC patients with low level, and patients with high level of both IgG and IgA had the worst prognosis. Multivariate analysis identified lymph node status, IgG and IgA as independent prognostic factors. Therefore, IgG and IgA were combined and we found that the combination produced higher predictive accuracy than an individual IgG or IgA.

Conclusions

To our knowledge, we are the first to report that the human immune response against *P. gingivalis* is implicated in the malignant progression of ESCC. IgG and IgA for *P. gingivalis* are potential serum biomarkers for ESCC and combination of IgG and IgA improves the diagnostic and prognostic performance. Furthermore, serum IgG and IgA for *P. gingivalis* could differentiate early stage ESCC patients. Further investigations are warranted to compare or combine with current serum biomarkers for ESCC, to identify the optimal panel for clinical application.

Additional files

Additional file 1: Figure S1. Kaplan-Meier survival curves of ESCC patients with regards to clinical stage. A The 3-year OS rates in ESCC patients with TNM I-II ($n = 51$) and patients with TNM III-IV ($n = 27$) were 59.95% and 33.26%, respectively ($P = 0.069$). B The 3-year OS rates in ESCC patients with IgG < 138.23 EU ($n = 59$) and IgG > 138.23 EU ($n = 19$) were 77.59% and 37.65%, respectively, in early clinical stage ($P = 0.055$). B The 3-year OS rates in ESCC patients with IgG < 138.23 EU ($n = 59$) and IgG > 138.23 EU ($n = 19$) were 44.63% and 20.89%, respectively, in late clinical stage ($P = 0.055$). D The 3-year OS rates in ESCC patients with IgA < 56.56 EU ($n = 62$) and IgA > 56.56 EU ($n = 16$) were 68.95% and 23.34%, respectively, in early clinical stage ($P = 0.003$). D The 3-year OS rates in ESCC patients with IgA < 56.56 EU ($n = 62$) and IgA > 56.56 EU ($n = 16$) were 41.45% and 0, respectively, in late clinical stage ($P = 0.48$).

Additional file 2: Figure S2. Kaplan-Meier survival curves of ESCC patients with regards to lymph node stage. A The 3-year OS rates in ESCC patients without lymph node metastasis ($n = 44$) and patients with lymph node metastasis ($n = 34$) were 63.87% and 27.85%, respectively ($P = 0.018$). B The 3-year OS rates in ESCC patients with IgG < 138.23 EU ($n = 59$) and IgG > 138.23 EU ($n = 19$) were 87.19% and 37.64%, respectively, in negative lymph node metastasis ($P = 0.014$). C The 3-year OS rates in ESCC patients with IgG < 138.23 EU ($n = 59$) and IgG > 138.23 EU ($n = 19$) were 29.43% and 20.80%, respectively, in lymph node metastasis ($P = 0.293$). D The 3-year OS rates in ESCC patients with IgA < 56.56 EU ($n = 62$) and IgA > 56.56 EU ($n = 16$) were 72.91% and 25.96%, respectively, in negative lymph node metastasis ($P = 0.011$). E The 3-year OS rates in ESCC patients with IgA < 56.56 EU ($n = 62$) and IgA > 56.56 EU ($n = 16$) were 34.52% and 0, respectively, in lymph node metastasis ($P = 0.092$).

Abbreviations

AUC: Area under the ROC curve; ESCC: Esophageal squamous cell carcinoma; IgG/A: Immunoglobulin G/A; ROC: Receiving operating characteristic

Acknowledgements

We thank Dr. Huizhi Wang and Dr. David A. Scott from Department of Oral Immunology and Infectious Diseases, University of Louisville School of Dentistry, for providing *P. gingivalis* protein extract for ELISA assay.

Funding

This study was supported by the National Natural Science Foundation of China (81,472,234, U1604191), Science and Technology Innovation Team Program for Universities of Henan (15IRTSTHN024), Science and Technology Major Project of Henan (161100311200). The funding body had no role in the design of the study, collection, analysis, and interpretation of data or in writing the manuscript.

Authors' contributions

SGG and XSF conceived and designed the study. YJQ drafted the manuscript. ZKM and XY collected the blood samples and performed ELISA assays. HW collected part of blood samples and JQY collected the follow-up data of ESCC patients. JQY, CZ and GCW were responsible for statistical analyses. All authors read and approved the final manuscript.

Competing interests

The authors declare that they have no competing interests.

Author details

[1]Henan Key Laboratory of Cancer Epigenetics; Cancer Hospital, The First Affiliated Hospital, College of Clinical Medicine, Medical College of Henan University of Science and Technology, Luoyang, Henan 471003, People's Republic of China. [2]Department of Oral Mucosal Diseases, Shanghai Ninth People's Hospital, Shanghai Jiao Tong University School of Medicine, Shanghai 200011, People's Republic of China. [3]Huaihe Hospital, Henan University, Kaifeng, Henan 475004, People's Republic of China.

References

1. Jemal A, Bray F, Center MM, Ferlay J, Ward E, Forman D. Global cancer statistics. CA Cancer J Clin. 2011;61(2):69–90.
2. Lin Y, Totsuka Y, He Y, Kikuchi S, Qiao Y, Ueda J, Wei W, Inoue M, Tanaka H. Epidemiology of esophageal cancer in Japan and China. J Epidemiol. 2013; 23(4):233–42.
3. Enzinger PC, Mayer RJ. Esophageal cancer. N Engl J Med. 2003;349(23):2241–52.
4. Pennathur A, Gibson MK, Jobe BA, Luketich JD. Oesophageal carcinoma. Lancet. 2013;381(9864):400–12.
5. Shimada H, Nabeya Y, Okazumi S, Matsubara H, Shiratori T, Gunji Y, Kobayashi S, Hayashi H, Ochiai T. Prediction of survival with squamous cell carcinoma antigen in patients with resectable esophageal squamous cell carcinoma. Surgery. 2003;133(5):486–94.
6. Tang KH, Dai YD, Tong M, Chan YP, Kwan PS, Fu L, Qin YR, Tsao SW, Lung HL, Lung ML, et al. A CD90(+) tumor-initiating cell population with an aggressive signature and metastatic capacity in esophageal cancer. Cancer Res. 2013;73(7):2322–32.
7. Falk GW. Risk factors for esophageal cancer development. Surg Oncol Clin N Am. 2009;18(3):469–85.
8. Nagy KN, Sonkodi I, Szoke I, Nagy E, Newman HN. The microflora associated with human oral carcinomas. Oral Oncol. 1998;34(4):304–8.
9. Mager DL, Haffajee AD, Devlin PM, Norris CM, Posner MR, Goodson JM. The salivary microbiota as a diagnostic indicator of oral cancer: a descriptive, non-randomized study of cancer-free and oral squamous cell carcinoma subjects. J Transl Med. 2005;3:27.
10. Katz J, Onate MD, Pauley KM, Bhattacharyya I, Cha S. Presence of Porphyromonas gingivalis in gingival squamous cell carcinoma. Int J Oral Sci. 2011;3(4):209–15.
11. Whitmore SE, Lamont RJ. Oral bacteria and cancer. PLoS Pathog. 2014;10(3): e1003933.
12. Hooper SJ, Wilson MJ, Crean SJ. Exploring the link between microorganisms and oral cancer: a systematic review of the literature. Head Neck. 2009;31(9): 1228–39.
13. Ahn J, Chen CY, Hayes RB. Oral microbiome and oral and gastrointestinal cancer risk. Cancer Causes Control. 2012;23(3):399–404.

14. Groeger S, Domann E, Gonzales JR, Chakraborty T, Meyle J. B7-H1 and B7-DC receptors of oral squamous carcinoma cells are upregulated by Porphyromonas gingivalis. Immunobiology. 2011;216(12):1302–10.

15. Tezal M, Sullivan MA, Hyland A, Marshall JR, Stoler D, Reid ME, Loree TR, Rigual NR, Merzianu M, Hauck L, et al. Chronic periodontitis and the incidence of head and neck squamous cell carcinoma. Cancer Epidemiol Biomark Prev. 2009;18(9):2406–12.

16. Hiraki A, Matsuo K, Suzuki T, Kawase T, Tajima K. Teeth loss and risk of cancer at 14 common sites in Japanese. Cancer Epidemiol Biomark Prev. 2008;17(5):1222–7.

17. Abnet CC, Qiao YL, Mark SD, Dong ZW, Taylor PR, Dawsey SM. Prospective study of tooth loss and incident esophageal and gastric cancers in China. Cancer Causes Control. 2001;12(9):847–54.

18. Gao S, Li S, Ma Z, Liang S, Shan T, Zhang M, Zhu X, Zhang P, Liu G, Zhou F, et al. Presence of Porphyromonas gingivalis in esophagus and its association with the clinicopathological characteristics and survival in patients with esophageal cancer. Infect Agent Cancer. 2016;11:3.

19. Abnet CC, Kamangar F, Dawsey SM, Stolzenberg-Solomon RZ, Albanes D, Pietinen P, Virtamo J, Taylor PR. Tooth loss is associated with increased risk of gastric non-cardia adenocarcinoma in a cohort of Finnish smokers. Scand J Gastroenterol. 2005;40(6):681–7.

20. Watabe K, Nishi M, Miyake H, Hirata K. Lifestyle and gastric cancer: a case-control study. Oncol Rep. 1998;5(5):1191–4.

21. Michaud DS, Izard J, Wilhelm-Benartzi CS, You DH, Grote VA, Tjonneland A, Dahm CC, Overvad K, Jenab M, Fedirko V, et al. Plasma antibodies to oral bacteria and risk of pancreatic cancer in a large European prospective cohort study. Gut. 2013;62(12):1764–70.

22. Michaud DS. Role of bacterial infections in pancreatic cancer. Carcinogenesis. 2013;34(10):2193–7.

23. Stolzenberg-Solomon RZ, Dodd KW, Blaser MJ, Virtamo J, Taylor PR, Albanes D. Tooth loss, pancreatic cancer, and helicobacter pylori. Am J Clin Nutr. 2003;78(1):176–81.

24. Michaud DS, Joshipura K, Giovannucci E, Fuchs CS. A prospective study of periodontal disease and pancreatic cancer in US male health professionals. J Natl Cancer Inst. 2007;99(2):171–5.

25. Ahn J, Segers S, Hayes RB. Periodontal disease, Porphyromonas gingivalis serum antibody levels and orodigestive cancer mortality. Carcinogenesis. 2012;33(5):1055–8.

26. Salazar CR, Sun J, Li Y, Francois F, Corby P, Perez-Perez G, Dasanayake A, Pei Z, Chen Y. Association between selected oral pathogens and gastric precancerous lesions. PLoS One. 2013;8(1):e51604.

27. Salazar CR, Francois F, Li Y, Corby P, Hays R, Leung C, Bedi S, Segers S, Queiroz E, Sun J, et al. Association between oral health and gastric precancerous lesions. Carcinogenesis. 2012;33(2):399–403.

28. Hajishengallis G, Lamont RJ. Beyond the red complex and into more complexity: the polymicrobial synergy and dysbiosis (PSD) model of periodontal disease etiology. Mol Oral Microbiol. 2012;27(6):409–19.

29. Jenkinson HF. Beyond the oral microbiome. Environ Microbiol. 2011;13(12):3077–87.

30. Meyer MS, Joshipura K, Giovannucci E, Michaud DS. A review of the relationship between tooth loss, periodontal disease, and cancer. Cancer Causes Control. 2008;19(9):895–907.

31. Atanasova KR, Yilmaz O. Looking in the Porphyromonas gingivalis cabinet of curiosities: the microbium, the host and cancer association. Mol Oral Microbiol. 2014;29(2):55–66.

32. Tribble GD, Kerr JE, Wang BY. Genetic diversity in the oral pathogen Porphyromonas gingivalis: molecular mechanisms and biological consequences. Future Microbiol. 2013;8(5):607–20.

33. Naito Y, Okuda K, Takazoe I. Detection of specific antibody in adult human periodontitis sera to surface antigens of Bacteroides Gingivalis. Infect Immun. 1987;55(3):832–4.

34. Ebersole JL, Taubman MA, Smith DJ, SocranskySS. Humoral immune responses and diagnosis of human periodontal disease. J Periodontal Res. 1982;17(5):478–80.

35. Vincent JW, Falkler WA Jr, Cornett WC, Suzuki JB. Effect of periodontal therapy on specific antibody responses to suspected periodontopathogens. J Clin Periodontol. 1987;14(7):412–7.

36. Mooney J, Adonogianaki E, Riggio MP, Takahashi K, Haerian A, Kinane DF. Initial serum antibody titer to Porphyromonas gingivalis influences development of antibody avidity and success of therapy for chronic periodontitis. Infect Immun. 1995;63(9):3411–6.

37. Kosugi S, Nishimaki T, Kanda T, Nakagawa S, Ohashi M, Hatakeyama K. Clinical significance of serum carcinoembryonic antigen, carbohydrate antigen 19-9, and squamous cell carcinoma antigen levels in esophageal cancer patients. World J Surg. 2004;28(7):680–5.

38. Shimada H, Nabeya Y, Tagawa M, Okazumi S, Matsubara H, Kadomatsu K, Muramatsu T, Ikematsu S, Sakuma S, Ochiai T. Preoperative serum midkine concentration is a prognostic marker for esophageal squamous cell carcinoma. Cancer Sci. 2003;94(7):628–32.

39. Mealy K, Feely J, Reid I, McSweeney J, Walsh T, Hennessy TP. Tumour marker detection in oesophageal carcinoma. Eur J Surg Oncol. 1996;22(5):505–7.

40. Shimada H, Nabeya Y, Okazumi S, Matsubara H, Miyazawa Y, Shiratori T, Hayashi H, Gunji Y, Ochiai T. Prognostic significance of CYFRA 21-1 in patients with esophageal squamous cell carcinoma. J Am Coll Surg. 2003;196(4):573–8.

41. Zheng X, Xing S, Liu XM, Liu W, Liu D, Chi PD, Chen H, Dai SQ, Zhong Q, Zeng MS, et al. Establishment of using serum YKL-40 and SCCA in combination for the diagnosis of patients with esophageal squamous cell carcinoma. BMC Cancer. 2014;14:490.

42. Ogawa T, Kusumoto Y, Hamada S, McGhee JR, Kiyono H. Bacteroides Gingivalis-specific serum IgG and IgA subclass antibodies in periodontal diseases. Clin Exp Immunol. 1990;82(2):318–25.

43. Hsu FM, Cheng JC, Chang YL, Lee JM, Koong AC, Chuang EY. Circulating mRNA profiling in esophageal Squamous cell carcinoma identifies FAM84B as a biomarker in predicting pathological response to Neoadjuvant Chemoradiation. Sci Rep. 2015;5:10291.

44. Xu YW, Peng YH, Chen B, Wu ZY, Wu JY, Shen JH, Zheng CP, Wang SH, Guo HP, Li EM, et al. Autoantibodies as potential biomarkers for the early detection of esophageal squamous cell carcinoma. Am J Gastroenterol. 2014;109(1):36–45.

45. Pei Z, Bini EJ, Yang L, Zhou M, Francois F, Blaser MJ. Bacterial biota in the human distal esophagus. Proc Natl Acad Sci U S A. 2004;101(12):4250–5.

46. Yang L, Lu X, Nossa CW, Francois F, Peek RM, Pei Z. Inflammation and intestinal metaplasia of the distal esophagus are associated with alterations in the microbiome. Gastroenterology. 2009;137(2):588–97.

Improving quality of life through the routine use of the patient concerns inventory for head and neck cancer patients: a cluster preference randomized controlled trial

Simon N. Rogers[1,2,10*] ⓘ, Derek Lowe[1,2], Cher Lowies[3], Seow Tien Yeo[4], Christine Allmark[5], Dominic Mcavery[1], Gerald M. Humphris[6], Robert Flavel[7], Cherith Semple[8], Steven J. Thomas[9] and Anastasios Kanatas[5]

Abstract

Background: The consequences of treatment for Head and Neck cancer (HNC) patients has profound detrimental impacts such as impaired QOL, emotional distress, delayed recovery and frequent use of healthcare. The aim of this trial is to determine if the routine use of the Patients Concerns Inventory (PCI) package in review clinics during the first year following treatment can improve overall quality of life, reduce the social-emotional impact of cancer and reduce levels of distress. Furthermore, we aim to describe the economic costs and benefits of using the PCI.

Methods: This will be a cluster preference randomised control trial with consultants either 'using' or 'not using' the PCI package at clinic. It will involve two centres Leeds and Liverpool. 416 eligible patients from at least 10 consultant clusters are required to show a clinically meaningful difference in the primary outcome. The primary outcome is the percentage of participants with less than good overall quality of life at the final one-year clinic as measured by the University of Washington QOL questionnaire version 4 (UWQOLv4). Secondary outcomes at one-year are the mean social-emotional subscale (UWQOLv4) score, Distress Thermometer (DT) score ≥ 4, and key health economic measures (QALY-EQ-5D-5 L; CSRI).

Discussion: This trial will provide knowledge on the effectiveness of a consultation intervention package based around the PCI used at routine follow-up clinics following treatment of head and neck cancer with curative intent. If this intervention is (cost) effective for patients, the next step will be to promote wider use of this approach as standard care in clinical practice.

Keywords: Head and neck Cancer, Patient concerns inventory, Quality of life, Patient reported outcomes, Intervention

* Correspondence: simonn.rogers@aintree.nhs.uk
[1]Regional Maxillofacial Unit, University Hospital Aintree, Liverpool, UK
[2]Edge Hill University, Liverpool and Evidence-Based Practice Research Centre (EPRC), Faculty of Health and Social Care, Road, L39 4QP, Ormskirk, St Helens, UK
Full list of author information is available at the end of the article

Background

The incidence of Head and neck cancer (HNC) is increasing, the three main sites being oral cavity (mouth), oropharynx (throat) and larynx (voice box) with about 11,000 new cancers in the UK each year http://www.cancerresearchuk.org/about-cancer/mouth-cancer. Treatments such as surgery and chemo-radiotherapy have a detrimental effect on basic functions including speech, swallowing and appearance. These in turn can have a profound negative influence on emotional well-being and social integration http://www.handle-on-qol.com/About.aspx. Patients often do not raise issues of concern in their follow-up consultations and it can be a challenge for clinicians to facilitate this in a busy clinic [1]. Questionnaire prompt lists (QPL) are a means to allow patients to raise their agenda and help focus consultations [2–5]. The Patient Concerns Inventory (PCI-HN) is an item prompt list specific to head and neck cancer [6] http://www.headandneckcancer.co.uk/professionals/patient-concerns-inventory, and differs from many QPLs, which are more general cancer tools [7]. The PCI-HN was designed for routine clinic consultations within the context of NHS financial constraints. It is freely available http://www.patient-concerns-inventory.co.uk and is in the early phases of development for other cancers and chronic conditions. The PCI consists of 56 clinical items, which patients select from before their appointment, to help guide the outpatient consultation through the symptoms and problems that they may experience following their treatment for HNC. It helps to focus the consultation, aid doctor-patient communication, and can assist in signposting patients to other professional for advice and support.

The PCI supports several national initiatives and is set in the context of the national debate about how to bring about more person-centred care [8, 9] and the National Cancer Survivorship Initiative http://www.ncin.org.uk/cancer_type_and_topic_specific_work/topic_specific_work/survivorship which 'aims to ensure that those living with and beyond cancer get the care and support they need to lead as healthy and active a life as possible, for as long as possible'. In a survey of the British Association of Head and Neck Oncology Nurses (BAHNON), the PCI at that time, was the preferred assessment and the majority (60%) felt, as a head and neck specific tool, it was 'most appropriate' [10].

Oncology review clinics are busy and barriers such as time constraints, a medical focus of the consultation, and lack of level 1 evidence of patient benefit from the use of the PCI, prevents its wider implementation. Although pilot work has shown that patients completing the PCI would like to continue to use it in clinic and that it is feasible, [11, 12] clinicians tend to focus on traditional medical aspects. There is evidence that consultations can be improved through clinicians developing skills in detecting and responding to patient distress, thereby improving their patients' emotional functioning

and reducing psychological distress [13, 14]. Preliminary findings around the PCI suggest that its use in clinic allows emotional issues to be discussed more openly - notably fears of recurrence, anxiety and depression [15, 16]. Hence the PCI could help clinician communication with patients in these important areas and consequently impact on how consultations are constructed.

The PCI provides a process by which the patient has repeated opportunities to raise issues they feel are important and that they want to discuss. It can be argued that the routine repeated use of the PCI in follow-up clinics will benefit patients wanting support to speak more openly about problems or concerns e.g. psychosocial causes of symptoms; need for psychosocial help; to seek explanation and reassurance for more physical explanations about their cancer and about the side-effects of treatment. It is postulated that this will have a positive impact on quality of life and emotional distress and be demonstrable by one year following HNC treatment [17]. Thus far, the majority of evidence related to the PCI-HN has been derived from one clinic setting. By conducting a randomised controlled trial (RCT) across multiple consultants, it will be possible to rigorously evaluate if the repeated inclusion of the PCI-HN in routine post-treatment consultations does make a significant and clinically meaningfully difference in patient reported quality of life and distress.

Methods/design

This is a preference cluster randomised control trial with consultants either 'using or 'not using' the PCI at clinic. 416 HNC eligible patients from at least 10 consultant clusters are required to show a clinically meaningful difference in the primary outcome, that is having less than good overall QOL at the final one-year clinic as measured by the relevant question on the UWQOL-v4 [18].

Before treatment, eligible patients will be asked to consent to participation in the 'research cohort'. Patients agree to their clinical data being used (Table 1) and to completing research questionnaires before each post-treatment consultation, some of which might be used in their consultation. Completion of all pre-consultation questionnaires including the PCI items will be by computer (desktop, tablet, IPAD). Quality Assurance is by initial training and later booster sessions for consultants and a post consultation survey of those in the PCI arm. Also, in the first six months of the study a random selection of clinic consultations will be taped in order to check how consultants do or do not use the PCI package.

A Steering Group is guiding the research and a joint-site Management group will manage it. Each site will have regular Project Team meetings to review progress. Day to day management issues will be addressed with each unit Lead Researcher. A data manager (based at Aintree R&D) will have overall responsibility for ensuring data quality

Table 1 Schedule for collecting clinical and demographic details

Timepoint		Trial Period	
	Enrolment	Baseline clinic	Follow up clinics
Gender	X		
DOB	X		
IMD 2015	X		
Smoking and Drinking Details		X	X[a]
Living Situation		X	
Employment		X	
Income		X	
Primary Diagnosis (ICD code)	X		
Tumour Site	X		
Treatment Plan	X		
Ethnicity	X		
TNM Stage	X		
Cancer Staging	X		
Histology (SNOMED)	X		
HPV Status	X		
Co-Morbidity	X		
ACE 27	X		

[a]Completion at patient 6 and 12 month study visit

and integrity. The study will last three years comprising of set-up and piloting, 12 months of recruitment, 15 months of follow-up and analysis, and then write-up and initial dissemination.

In analysis, the two patient groups will be compared after adjusting for relevant case-mix and for effects of patients being within consultant clusters. A summary flowchart of the key features of this trial is shown as Fig. 1.

Purpose of the study and hypotheses

The main purpose of this three-year research project is to investigate whether incorporating the PCI into routine head and neck cancer (HNC) follow-up consultations improves the overall QOL of patients. The Null hypothesis is that there is no difference between trial groups in the percentage of patients with less than good overall QOL at one year following the first baseline routine clinic post-treatment.

Participant eligibility

Eligible patients will have a first occurrence of HNC, and be treated curatively (all sites, stage of disease, treatments). To ensure participation of patients with little or no written or spoken English, translation services will be provided as necessary.

Patients treated with palliative intent and patients with a history of previous HNC or recurrence will be excluded from the study. Although the PCI could benefit these patients the primary endpoint of this study is QOL at one year. For reasons of engagement and ethics, patients with a history of cognitive impairment, psychoses or dementia are excluded, as discussed and identified at the staging/treatment decision-making Multi-Professional Team meeting (MDT). Patients who initially are included and treated curatively but who later start receiving treatment with palliative intent will no longer be asked to continue their participation in the research.

Method of randomisation

Problems of consultant contamination (from switching back and forth from using to not using the PCI package as would be required with conventional randomisation) indicate this should be a cluster RCT, in that consultants are randomised to 'using' or 'not using' the PCI at all their trial clinics. The steering group approved a randomisation process incorporating consultant preference; a method reported previously [19]. The aim is to limit the chance occurrence of PCI-sceptic consultants dominating the PCI group and PCI-enthusiastic consultants the non-PCI group. Those with a strong preference are offered their preferred group and those with no preference are randomised. The allocation process was overseen by the medical statistician involved, before any patient recruitment occurred. At Leeds, three of six consultants preferred to be in the PCI group, while the other three consultants had no preference as to group and were all allocated to the non-PCI control group. At Liverpool, three of eight consultants preferred to be in the non-PCI control group. One of the other five consultants was randomly allocated to the non-PCI control group, leaving four to be in the PCI group. Thus, at the two sites, seven consultants were in each arm of the trial.

Study intervention

Patient completion of the PCI and its inclusion into the regular review clinic consultation within a summary paper output is the 'intervention' and is compared to standard out-patient follow-up. The pre-consultation questionnaires and PCI will be used from the first post-treatment clinic (baseline) onwards for one year. The trial will only apply for routine out-patient follow-ups. Completion of all pre-consultation questionnaires and the PCI is by computer (desktop, tablet, IPAD). Assistance (from trained volunteers) will be available to patients as required. Patients of intervention consultants complete the PCI throughout the trial while patients of control consultants do not complete the PCI at all. All study patients will see their consultant surgeon at 6–8 weekly intervals for planned out-patient review. This might be as joint consultation with the oncologist depending on the configuration of the clinic.

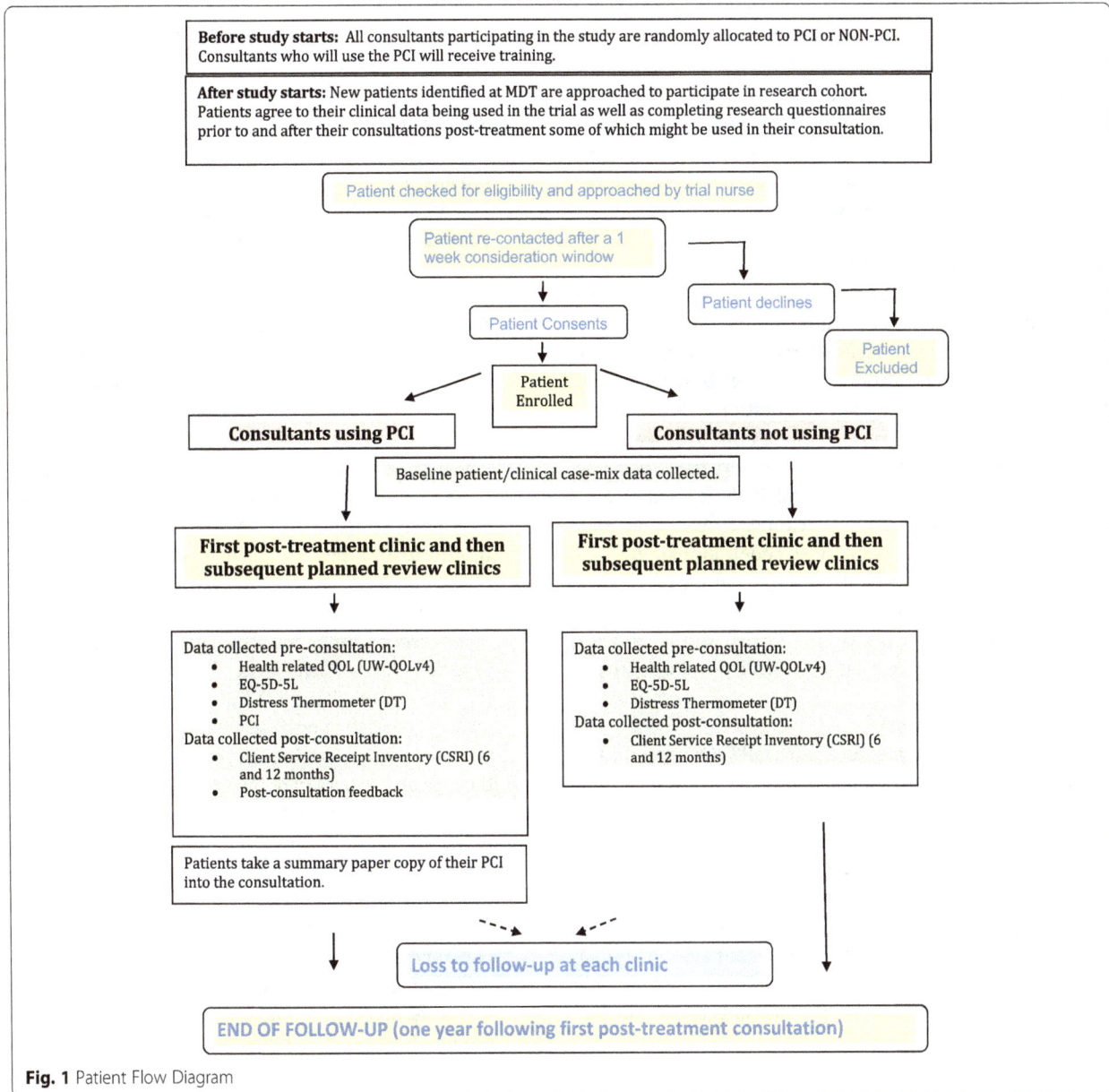

Fig. 1 Patient Flow Diagram

While waiting for each consultation the Intervention group patients complete the following:

- Health related QOL (UW-QOLv4)
- EQ-5D-5 L
- Distress Thermometer (DT)
- PCI

Intervention patients then take a summary paper output of their data into the clinic consultation (Fig. 2). Post-consultation they will be asked to complete:

- Post-Consultation Patient Feedback about the use of the PCI.

- Client Service Receipt Inventory (CSRI) at 6 and 12 months.

The post consultation data collection will involve self-completion in clinic but either research assisted completion or telephone completion is possible if the patient prefers.

Control patients will complete exactly the same information as intervention patients apart from the PCI and the post consultation feedback on the PCI. They do not take any summary output with them into the consultation. The summary output is a product of the raw inputted data from the patient being run through a software programme that indicates (1) all the items selected from the PCI that the patient wants to discuss (2) those domains from the UWQOL questionnaire for which the patient responses suggest a significant problem or dysfunction (using software algorithms derived from earlier work with the UWQOL [20], (3) the patient's overall QOL and (4) the Distress Thermometer score. The presence of this summary output during the consultation is the difference in reality between the intervention and control groups as far as the interaction between consultant and patient is concerned.

Data collection and outcome measures

Unit Clinical Trials Nurses who recruit eligible patients will keep recruitment and clinic attendance logs. The dedicated funded Unit researchers will collect baseline clinical/demographic data either via a baseline clinic questionnaire, with demographic questions chosen as far as possible to match those included in the head and neck 5000 project [21], or by extraction from baseline clinical records. Baseline data will include cancer site, disease severity, HPV status, treatment details, gender, age, deprivation [IMD from post code], smoking, alcohol, and ACE-27 comorbidity. All clinical outcome data will be collected automatically via IPAD at each consultation. A data manager (based at Aintree) will have overall responsibility for ensuring data quality and integrity.

Primary outcome measure

The primary outcome measure is overall QOL, specifically the percentage with less than good overall QOL at the final one-year clinic as measured by the single UWQOL-v4 question [18]. The anticipated result in the control group is 30%. The UW-QOLv4 is a commonly used HNC specific HRQOL questionnaire [22, 23] and has been used with HNC patients at the Aintree Regional Head and Neck Unit since 1995. Over 1000 patients have completed over 5000 UW-QOL questionnaires giving the research team considerable experience in analysing and reporting this QOL measure.

Secondary outcome measures

1. Mean social-emotional subscale score of UW-QOL
   The Aintree Research team was involved in developing the UW-QOL subscales, and the social-emotional subscale [20] is the mean of 6 domain scores (each 0–100) - anxiety, mood, pain, activity, recreation and shoulder function. The anticipated result in the control group is a mean score of 75.

2. Distress Thermometer (DT) score of 4 or more (range 0 to 10). The anticipated result in the control group is 34%. The Distress Thermometer (DT) is a single item self-report measure and has been used to screen for distress in various cancers [24–27]. A score of four and above denotes

significant distress as this correlates with optimal sensitivity and specificity to the Hospital Anxiety Depression Scale [25, 28].

Cost-effectiveness

1. Quality-adjusted life year (QALY).
   Quality-adjusted life year (QALY) is used as a summary measure of health benefit for economic evaluation, using the EQ-5D-5 L health index to adjust for patient QOL [29, 30]. QALY is used as a common unit to allow comparisons across different interventions or disease areas [31]. EQ-5D-5 L is a validated generic, health-related, preference-based measure comprising mobility, self-care, usual activities, pain and discomfort, anxiety and depression. These are complemented by a visual analogue scale (VAS) [32], on which patients are asked to indicate their current health from 0 (worst imaginable health) to 100 (best imaginable health) [33].

2. Health service use and costs
   Health service use by participating patients will be collected using a Client Service Receipt Inventory (CSRI). CSRI is a form that is usually administered in an interview setting or by self-completion via postal surveys or at clinics – asking them to recall retrospectively the type and frequency of their contacts with primary and secondary care NHS services. A CSRI form adapted to the study was developed using existing CSRIs, available from the DIRUM open access database http://www.dirum.org, as a reference and guidance with input from study researchers. For this trial, services such as physiotherapist, occupational therapist, social worker and others are included. To translate the service use into costs, unit costs from published sources will be applied to the patients' self-reported service use data and the mean total cost of care per patient over 12 months will be calculated in each group. CSRI is the most common means of collecting service use data, usually with a short recall period of up to 6 months [34, 35], in health economics studies that require data across a range of health care settings. CSRIs were developed first in the field of mental health economics [36], and a review of their use is published by Ridyard and Hughes [37].

6. Cost of the PCI intervention
   Resources and materials use for the delivery of the PCI intervention will be recorded and costed and the total cost of the PCI intervention will be calculated.

Sample size calculation

We have used nearly 20 years of accumulated experience with the UW-QOL to estimate a sample size that is

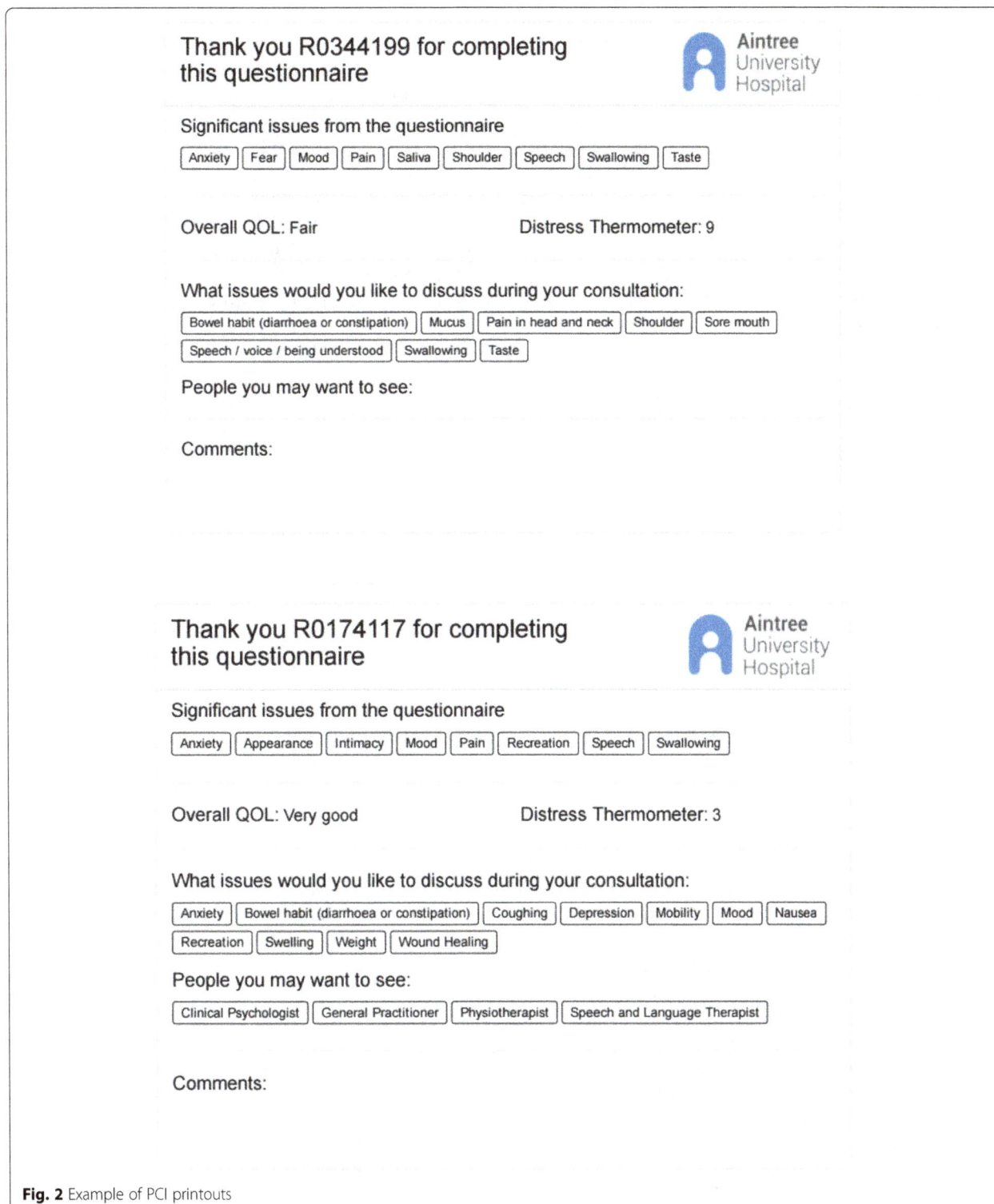

Fig. 2 Example of PCI printouts

pragmatic enough for a trial to be doable, yet able to detect meaningful differences if they exist. In regard to all UWQOL records collected the percentages of patients reporting less than good overall quality of life were relatively similar over different time periods from diagnosis and the expectation for the trial control group was taken as 30% after about 12 months. Cluster randomized trials require larger sample sizes than the individually randomised design because observations on individuals in the same cluster tend to be correlated, thereby reducing the effective sample size. The degree of correlation within consultant clusters, as estimated by the intra-class correlation (ICC) was estimated as barely above zero (6.7e-05) for consultants at Aintree. Assuming a likely control group outcome of 30%, an ICC value of 0.01 for the trial and not wishing to miss a halving in outcome rate, then a total of 312 patients from at least 10 consultants were required. After factoring a likely loss of 15% through patient mortality during the follow-up period and a possible maximum loss of 10% from initial non-consent, this then implied a total of 416 eligible patients needing to be approached for participation to the research. This number would also detect a moderate-sized clinical difference of 10 units (75 Vs. 85) in the mean composite social-emotional subscale score, for which an ICC estimate of 0.025 was obtained for consultants within Aintree. Data from an MD project with 325 HNC patients at Aintree gave an estimated 34% with a Distress Thermometer score ≥ 4, and the trial numbers would be sufficient to detect a halving in this outcome.

Statistical analysis

As inference will target the individual patient level, analyses will need to adjust for potential clustering in the data. We will report results for each group (PCI, non-PCI) and the estimated effect size from the use of PCI and its precision (95% confidence interval). For the primary outcome, we will report the intra-cluster correlation coefficient to assess the amount of clustering. In reporting results, we will follow the CONSORT statement extension applicable to cluster RCTs. We will use random effects (multi-level) logistic regression methods and will estimate the effect of PCI after making adjustment for relevant case-mix and for clustering effects of patients being within consultant clusters. Only baseline patient factors will be considered as case-mix adjusters and these include age, gender, treatment, overall clinical stage, tumour site and baseline clinic assessment of whether overall UWQOL was less than good (Y/N). A P value ≤ 0.05 is considered statistically significant. Secondary clinical outcomes will be analysed as per protocol.

We will fully cost the delivery of the PCI intervention and associated costs such as training and other materials used. We will use published national average NHS reference consultant costs, accounting for overheads. From an NHS perspective, we will undertake a primary cost-effectiveness analysis of the PCI approach, using the change in % of patients with 'less than good' overall QOL between baseline and one-year as the outcome effect, and a subsequent cost-utility analysis using QALY as the outcome effect measured using the EQ-5D-5 L questionnaire. Costs of service use and QALY data will be derived from the CSRI and EQ-5D-5 L questionnaires collected at baseline, 3, 6, 9 and 12 months. The area under the curve method will be used to calculate QALYs, weighting survival by QOL

weights obtained from the EQ-5D-5 L. We will compare our findings with unofficial NICE thresholds (ceilings) of £20,000 to £30,000 per QALY. Discounting is unnecessary given the time period. We will account for patient clustering, producing cost-effectiveness planes and acceptability curves (CEACs) to convey to policy makers the probability that PCI approach is cost-effective at different payer thresholds. We will undertake 5000 bootstrapped replications to generate confidence intervals around point estimates. The CSRI also allows us to account for the impact on healthcare service use from intervention participation, important when further rolling out the PCI approach.

Quality assurance (QA)

Quality Assurance will be ensured by initial training and booster sessions for consultants, together with post consultation patient feedback and audio taping of a number of consultations.

Training

There will be a short training programme for staff using the PCI before any patient recruitment. A brief manual/instruction booklet is used to talk through how the PCI should be used in consultations. There will also be two refresher sessions at 4 and 8 months into the trial recruitment phase.

Patients completing the PCI will be asked to complete a post-consultation feedback on paper identified by unique study number and date of clinic; they will be asked to leave this in clinic with the research team; telephone completion of this will also be available. The question is: Did the doctor make reference to the PCI prompt list during the consultation? Response options are 'Not at all', 'A little', 'Somewhat', 'A great deal'.

Any 'Not at all' response will be followed through with the relevant consultant with a view to resolving the issue for future clinics conducted.

Fidelity

In the first months of the study a random selection of clinic consultations will be taped. The additional burden of taping is an argument for focusing on the set-up period in order to check how consultants do or do not use the PCI. The tapes will allow a check on if and how the PCI print out is being used and it will allow for a check for contamination in the non-PCI group. It would be expected that between 3 and 6 months into the study, two clinics from each consultant would be taped.

Management and governance

The trial will be guided by the Steering Group, meeting during the set-up and six-monthly thereafter to ensure progress towards reaching the study's purpose and to give oversight regarding research governance. Its' membership includes an independent chairman, at least two other independent members, the two Unit Lead Investigators, Trial Coordinator (Full Time), Research Practitioner (Part-Time), Medical Statistician, Health Economist, IT/data management representation and a patient representative from each Unit.

There will be joint-Unit management group meetings every three months, membership comprising the two Unit Lead Investigators, dedicated funded researchers, IT/data management representation and a patient representative from each Unit. Statistical and Economic representation as required. Within Unit, there will be monthly Project Team meetings, membership comprising Unit Lead investigator, dedicated funded researchers, Clinical Trials Nurse(s), and patient representative. Day to day management issues will be addressed by Unit Researchers and escalate to the Unit Lead Investigator.

Discussion

There is growing evidence that enhanced symptom monitoring during routine cancer care using patient-reported outcomes benefits patients in respect to HRQOL and survival [38]. The premise of this trial is that the PCI can be integrated into routine clinical consultations with minimal cost implication as the doctor-patient interaction will be more time efficient and facilitate appropriate and targeted multi-professional referrals. The item prompt list approach of the PCI should have direct benefit for the participants. A key issue limiting successful implementation of patient reported outcomes in clinical practice is clinicians' lack of knowledge on how to effectively utilise PROs data in their clinical encounters [39]. Hence, for this trial there is an educational component and training around the use of the PCI. Also, the patient feedback and analysis of taped consultations will help underpin the evidence related to use of the PCI in the consultation. From this material, it would be possible in the future to develop a more robust training package, informed from the lessons learnt from this trial. In addition, the need for clear system guidelines built into how to most effectively use the PCI for the clinician, the patient and other members of the multi-professional team is recognised [40]. The findings from this trial will inform the development of a PCI manual both for patients and professionals.

The collection of the data in both arms of the trial by touch screen computer-assisted technology (IPAD) has distinct advantages in terms of data capture. With advances in digital health it could be expected that this approach would become regularly employed. Touch screen health-related QOL data collection can be used for scientific documentation as well as in clinical settings [41]. For the purpose of the trial the computer system has been transferred from Aintree to the other sites. This has not been as straightforward as expected. This has caused delays in the use of the IPADs in the other clinics. After completion of this trial, in order to support wider adoption of the PCI approach to patient care, progress is being made in respect to a cloud based platform which should be more readily accessible and easier to use than the current system.

The use of the PCI is a form of intervention in clinic by the consultant. There are other intervention trials that focus to improve function and wellbeing in patients with head and neck cancer. Hansson and colleagues [42] compare a person-centred care intervention in terms of health-related quality of life, disease-specific symptoms or problems, with traditional care as a control group for patients with head and neck cancer. Another trial by van der Hout and co-workers [43] is testing the efficacy, cost-utility and reach of an eHealth self-management application 'Oncokompas' to obtain optimal supportive care. Both trials explore different tools in a different context to the PCI in this trial. There are many different ways to help enable patients to recover from head and neck cancer, and the possibility of having several evidence based interventions can only help to improve patient's outcomes and allow centres to select the most appropriate intervention with their healthcare environment. This study has QOL as the primary outcome. This reflects the importance QOL has in terms of outcome following HNC. Also, given the inherent difficulties in QOL evaluation, such as adaptation, response shift, limitations in questionnaire wording, scaling and scoring, it demonstrates the potential power of the PCI to impact positively in patient care. A positive finding from this research will not only serve to promote wider use of the PCI in HNC, but also accelerate the development, piloting and introduction of the PCI in other cancers and chronic conditions. Level 1 evidence as to the benefits of the PCI in HNC care will help drive up standards of care. This research will add substantially to the evidence supporting the use of question prompt lists in NHS practice.

Abbreviations

ACE-27: Adult Co-Morbidity Evaluation 27; AUH: Aintree University Hospital; BAHNON: British Association of Head and Neck Oncology Nurses; CEAC: cost-effectiveness planes and acceptability curves; CHEME: Centre for Health Economics and Medicines Evaluation; CoHaBS: College of Health and Behavioural Sciences; CONSORT: Consolidated standards of reporting trials; CSRI: Client Service Receipt Inventory (CSRI); DIRUM: Database of Instruments for Resource Use Measurement; DT: Distress Thermometer; EHU: Edge Hill University; EPRC: Evidence based Practice Research Centre; EQ-5D-5 L: EuroQol 5 dimension questionnaire; HNC: Head and Neck Cancer; HPV: Herpes Papilloma Virus; HRQOL: Health Related Quality of Life; ICC: Intra-Class Correlation; IMD: Index of Multiple Deprivation; MDT: Multi-Professional Team; NICE: National Institute for Health and Care Excellence; PCI: Patients Concerns Inventory; PCI HN: Patient Concerns Inventory-Head Neck; PROs: Patient Reported Outcomes; QA: Quality Assurance; QALY: Quality-Adjusted Life Year; QOL: Quality of Life; QPL: Questionnaire prompt lists; R&D: Research and Development; RCT: Randomised Controlled Trial; UWQOL: University of Washington QOL questionnaire; UWQOLv4: University of Washington QOL questionnaire version 4; VAS: Visual Analogue Scale

Acknowledgements

The authors recognise the collaboration between the Research and Development Department at AUH and Edge Hill University with respect the intellectual property related to the PCI. The authors would like to thank Christopher Hughes; Head of Research Support for his help is submitting the grant application.

This paper presents independent research funded by the National Institute for Health Research (NIHR) under its Research for Patient Benefit (RfPB) Programme (Grant Reference Number PB-PG-0215-36047). The views expressed are those of the authors and not necessarily those of the NHS, the NIHR or the Department of Health.

Funding

This trial is funded by the RfPB on behalf of the NIHR (PB-PG-0215-36047).

Authors' contributions

SNR, DL, STY, CA, DM, GMH, RF, CS, AK are responsible for the research question, design of the trial and contributed to the writing of the study protocol. DL is the trial statistician. SNR is the Principle Investigator and corresponding author. CL is the trial manager. CA, DM and RF are patient representatives. All authors sit on the trials Steering group. SNR is responsible for the manuscript. All authors have read and approved the final manuscript.

Competing interests

The authors declare that they have no competing interests.

Author details

[1]Regional Maxillofacial Unit, University Hospital Aintree, Liverpool, UK. [2]Edge Hill University, Liverpool and Evidence-Based Practice Research Centre (EPRC), Faculty of Health and Social Care, Road, L39 4QP, Ormskirk, St Helens, UK. [3]Head and Neck Clinical Trials, University Hospital Aintree, Clinical Sciences Building, Liverpool, UK. [4]Centre for Health Economics and Medicines Evaluation (CHEME), School of Healthcare Sciences, College of Health and Behavioural Sciences (CoHaBS), Bangor University, Ardudwy Building, Normal Site, Bangor, UK. [5]Leeds Teaching Hospitals and St James Institute of Oncology, Leeds Dental Institute and Leeds General Infirmary, Leeds, UK. [6]School of Medicine, Medical & Biological Sciences, North Haugh, St Andrews, UK. [7]Southway, Guildford, Surrey, UK. [8]Macmillan Health and Wellbeing Service, Ulster Hospital, Upper Newtownards Road, Dundonald, Belfast, UK. [9]Oral and Maxillofacial Surgery Department, University, Bristol, Lower Maudlin Street, Bristol, UK. [10]Consultant Regional Maxillofacial Unit, University Hospital Aintree, L9 1AE, Liverpool, UK.

References

1. Rogers SN, Clifford N, Lowe D. Patient and carer unmet needs: a survey of the British Association of Head and Neck Oncology Nurses. Br J Oral Maxillofac Surg. 2011;49(5):343–8.
2. Yeh JC, Cheng MJ, Chung CH, Smith TJ. Using a question prompt list as a communication aid in advanced cancer care. J Oncol Pract. 2014;10(3):e137–41.
3. Brown RF, Bylund CL, Li Y, Edgerson S, Butow P. Testing the utility of a cancer clinical trial specific question prompt list (QPL-CT) during oncology consultations. Patient Educ Couns. 2012;88(2):311–7.
4. Dimoska A, Butow PN, Lynch J, Hovey E, Agar M, Beale P, Tattersall MH. Implementing patient question-prompt lists into routine cancer care. Patient Educ Couns. 2012;86(2):252–8.
5. Brown RF, Butow PN, Dunn SM, Tattersall MH. Promoting patient participation and shortening cancer consultations: a randomised trial. Br J Cancer. 2001;85(9):1273–9.

6. Rogers SN, El-Sheikha J, Lowe D. The development of a patients concerns inventory (PCI) to help reveal patients concerns in the head and neck clinic. Oral Oncol. 2009;45(7):555–61.
7. Miller N, Rogers SNA. Review of question prompt lists used in the oncology setting with comparison to the patient concerns inventory. Eur J Cancer Care (Engl). 2016 Mar 14; https://doi.org/10.1111/ecc.12489. [Epub ahead of print].
8. Transforming Patients Experience. https://www.kingsfund.org.uk/events/transforming-patient-experience-2015
9. Ideas into action: person-centre care in Practice. The Health Foundation 2014 https://www.health.org.uk/publication/ideas-action-person-centred-care-practice.
10. Wells M, Semple CJ, Lane C. A national survey of healthcare professionals' views on models of follow-up, holistic needs assessment and survivorship care for patients with head and neck cancer. Eur J Cancer Care (Engl). 2015; 24(6):873–83.
11. Rogers SN, Lowe D. An evaluation of the head and neck Cancer patient concerns inventory across the Merseyside and Cheshire network. Br J Oral Maxillofac Surg. 2014 Sep;52(7):615–23.
12. Ghazali N, Roe B, Lowe D, Rogers SN. Patients concerns inventory highlights perceived needs and concerns in head and neck cancer survivors and its impact on health-related quality of life. Br J Oral Maxillofac Surg. 2015;53(4):371–9.
13. Girgis A, Cockburn J, Butow P, Bowman D, Schofield P, Stojanovski E, D'Este C, Tattersall MH, Doran C, Turner J. Improving patient emotional functioning and psychological morbidity: evaluation of a consultation skills training program for oncologists. Patient Educ Couns. 2009;77(3):456–62.
14. Zhou Y, Humphris G, Ghazali N, Friderichs S, Grosset D, Rogers SN. How head and neck consultants manage patients' emotional distress during cancer follow-up consultations: a multilevel study. Eur Arch Otorhinolaryngol. 2015;272(9):2473–81.
15. Ghazali N, Cadwallader E, Lowe D, Humphris G, Ozakinci G, Rogers SN. Fear of recurrence among head and neck cancer survivors: longitudinal trends. Psychooncology. 2013;22(4):807–13.
16. Kanatas A, Humphris G, Lowe D, Rogers SN. Further analysis of the emotional consequences of head and neck cancer as reflected by the Patients' concerns inventory. Br J Oral Maxillofac Surg. 2015;53(8):711–8.
17. Ghazali N, Roe B, Lowe D, Tandon S, Jones T, Brown J, Shaw R, Risk J, Rogers SN. Screening for distress using the distress thermometer and the University of Washington Quality of life in post-treatment head and neck cancer survivors. Eur Arch Otorhinolaryngol. 2017;274(5):2253–60.
18. Rogers SN, Gwane S, Lowe D, Humphris G, Yueh B, Weymuller EA. The addition of mood and anxiety domains to the University of Washington Quality of life scale. Head Neck. 2002;24(6):521–9.
19. Verhaeghe N, Clays E, Vereecken C, De Maeseneer J, Maes L, Van Heeringen C, De Bacquer D, Annemans L. Health promotion in individuals with mental disorders: a cluster preference randomized controlled trial. BMC Public Health. 2013;13:657. https://doi.org/10.1186/1471-2458-13-657.
20. Rogers SN, Lowe D, Yueh B, Weymuller EA. The physical function and social-emotional function subscales of the University of Washington Quality of life questionnaire (UW-QOL). Arch Otolaryngol Head Neck Surg. 2010;136(4):352–7.
21. Ness AR, Waylen A, Hurley K, Jeffreys M, Penfold C, Pring M, Leary S, Allmark C, Toms S, Ring S, Peters TJ, Hollingworth W, Worthington H, Nutting C, Fisher S, Rogers SN, Thomas SJ. Head and neck 5000 study team. Establishing a large prospective clinical cohort in people with head and neck cancer as a biomedical resource: head and neck 5000. BMC Cancer. 2014;14:973. https://doi.org/10.1186/1471-2407-14-973.
22. Kanatas AN, Mehanna H, Lowe D, Rogers SN. A second national survey of health-related quality of life questionnaires in head and neck oncology. Ann R Coll Surg Engl. 2009 Jul;91(5):420–5.
23. Laraway DC, Rogers SN. A structured review of journal articles reporting outcomes using the University of Washington Quality of life scale. Br J Oral Maxillofac Surg. 2012 Mar;50(2):122–31.
24. Roth AJ, Kornblith AB, Batel-Copel L, Peabody E, Scher HI, Holland JC. Rapid screening for psychologic distress in men with prostate carcinoma: a pilot study. Cancer. 1998;82(10):1904–8.
25. Jacobsen PB, Donovan KA, Trask PC, Fleishman SB, Zabora J, Baker F, Holland JC. Screening for psychologic distress in ambulatory cancer patients. Cancer. 2005;103(7):1494–502.
26. Keir ST, Calhoun-Eagan RD, Swartz JJ, Saleh OA, Friedman HS. Screening for distress in patients with brain cancer using the NCCN's rapid screening measure. Psychooncology. 2008 Jun;17(6):621–5.

Improving quality of life through the routine use of the patient concerns inventory for head and neck cancer...

221

27. Hegel MT, Collins ED, Kearing S, Gillock KL, Moore CP, Ahles TA. Sensitivity and specificity of the distress thermometer for depression in newly diagnosed breast cancer patients. Psychooncology. 2008 Jun;17(6):556–60.

28. Shim EJ, Shin YW, Jeon HJ, Hahm BJ. Distress and its correlates in Korean cancer patients: pilot use of the distress thermometer and the problem list. Psychooncology. 2008 Jun;17(6):548–55.

29. Drummond MF, Sculpher MJ, Torrance GW, O'Brien BJ, Stoddart GL. Methods for the economic evaluation of health care programmes. 3rd ed. Oxford: Oxford University Press; 2005.

30. Morris S, Devlin N, Parkin D. Economic analysis in health care. Chichester: John Wiley & Sons Ltd, 2007.

31. National Institute for Health and Clinical Excellence. (NICE). Process and methods guides: guide to the methods of technology. Appraisal. 2013; https://www.nice.org.uk/process/pmg9/chapter/foreword.

32. Dolan P, Gudex C, Kind P, Williams A. A social tariff for EuroQoL: Results from a UK general population survey, Discussion paper No. 138. York: Centre for Health Economics, University of York; 1995.

33. EuroQoL. EQ-5D User Guide version. 2015;5:0. https://euroqol.org/eq-5d-instruments/eq-5d-5l-about/.

34. Jobe JB, White AA, Kelley CL, Mingay DJ, Sanchez MJ, Loftus EF. Recall strategies and memory for health care visits. Milbank Mem Fund Q. 1990; 68(2):171–89.

35. Chisholm D, Knapp MRJ, Knudsen HC, Amaddeo F, Gaite L, Van Wijngaarden B. Client socio-demographic and service receipt inventory - European version : development of an instrument for international research: EPSILON study 5. European Psychiatric Services: Inputs Linked to Outcome Domains and Needs Br J Psychiatry Suppl. 2000;39:s28–33.

36. Knapp M, Beecham J. Costing mental health services. Psychol Med. 1990; 20(4):893–908. Review

37. Ridyard CH, Hughes DA. Methods for the collection of resource use data within clinical trials: a systematic review of trials funded by the UK health technology assessment programme. Value Health. 2010;13(8):867–72.

38. Basch E, Deal AM, Kris MG, Scher HI, Hudis CA, Sabbatini P, Rogak L, Bennett AV, Dueck AC, Atkinson TM, Chou JF, Dulko D, Sit L, Barz A, Novotny P, Fruscione M, Sloan JA, Schrag D. Symptom monitoring with patient-reported outcomes during routine Cancer treatment: a randomized controlled trial. J Clin Oncol. 2016;34(6):557–65.

39. Santana MJ, Haverman L, Absolom K, Takeuchi E, Feeny D, Grootenhuis M, Velikova G. Training clinicians in how to use patient-reported outcome measures in routine clinical practice. Qual Life Res. 2015;24(7):1707–18.

40. Kotronoulas G, Kearney N, Maguire R, Harrow A, Di Domenico D, Croy S, MacGillivray S. What is the value of the routine use of patient-reported outcome measures toward improvement of patient outcomes, processes of care, and health service outcomes in cancer care? A systematic review of controlled trials. J Clin Oncol. 2014;32(14):1480–501.

41. de Bree R, Verdonck-de Leeuw IM, Keizer AL, Houffelaar A, Leemans CR. Touch screen computer-assisted health-related quality of life and distress data collection in head and neck cancer patients. Clin Otolaryngol. 2008; 33(2):138–42.

42. Hansson E, Carlström E, Olsson LE, Nyman J, Koinberg I. Can a person-centred-care intervention improve health-related quality of life in patients with head and neck cancer? A randomized, controlled study. BMC Nurs. 2017;16:9. https://doi.org/10.1186/s12912-017-0206-6. eCollection 2017.

43. van der Hout A, van Uden-Kraan CF, Witte BI, VMH C, Jansen F, Leemans CR, Cuijpers P, van de Poll-Franse LV, Verdonck-de Leeuw IM. Efficacy, cost-utility and reach of an eHealth self-management application 'Oncokompas' that helps cancer survivors to obtain optimal supportive care: study protocol for a randomised controlled trial. Trials. 2017;18(1):228. https://doi.org/10.1186/s13063-017-1952-1.

Permissions

All chapters in this book were first published in CANCER, by BioMed Central; hereby published with permission under the Creative Commons Attribution License or equivalent. Every chapter published in this book has been scrutinized by our experts. Their significance has been extensively debated. The topics covered herein carry significant findings which will fuel the growth of the discipline. They may even be implemented as practical applications or may be referred to as a beginning point for another development.

The contributors of this book come from diverse backgrounds, making this book a truly international effort. This book will bring forth new frontiers with its revolutionizing research information and detailed analysis of the nascent developments around the world.

We would like to thank all the contributing authors for lending their expertise to make the book truly unique. They have played a crucial role in the development of this book. Without their invaluable contributions this book wouldn't have been possible. They have made vital efforts to compile up to date information on the varied aspects of this subject to make this book a valuable addition to the collection of many professionals and students.

This book was conceptualized with the vision of imparting up-to-date information and advanced data in this field. To ensure the same, a matchless editorial board was set up. Every individual on the board went through rigorous rounds of assessment to prove their worth. After which they invested a large part of their time researching and compiling the most relevant data for our readers.

The editorial board has been involved in producing this book since its inception. They have spent rigorous hours researching and exploring the diverse topics which have resulted in the successful publishing of this book. They have passed on their knowledge of decades through this book. To expedite this challenging task, the publisher supported the team at every step. A small team of assistant editors was also appointed to further simplify the editing procedure and attain best results for the readers.

Apart from the editorial board, the designing team has also invested a significant amount of their time in understanding the subject and creating the most relevant covers. They scrutinized every image to scout for the most suitable representation of the subject and create an appropriate cover for the book.

The publishing team has been an ardent support to the editorial, designing and production team. Their endless efforts to recruit the best for this project, has resulted in the accomplishment of this book. They are a veteran in the field of academics and their pool of knowledge is as vast as their experience in printing. Their expertise and guidance has proved useful at every step. Their uncompromising quality standards have made this book an exceptional effort. Their encouragement from time to time has been an inspiration for everyone.

The publisher and the editorial board hope that this book will prove to be a valuable piece of knowledge for researchers, students, practitioners and scholars across the globe.

List of Contributors

Roganie Govender
University College London, Health Behaviour Research Centre and University College London Hospital, Head and Neck Cancer Centre, Ground Floor Central, 250 Euston Road, London NW1 2PQ, UK

Christina H. Smith
Division of Psychology and Language Sciences University College London, London, UK

Stuart A. Taylor
Centre for Medical Imaging, University College London, London, UK

Helen Barratt
Department of Applied Health Research, University College London, London, UK

Benjamin Gardner
Department of Psychology, Institute of Psychiatry, Psychology and Neuroscience (IoPPN), Kings College London, London, UK and UCL Department of Epidemiology and Public Health, University College London, London, UK

Shiang-Fu Huang
Department of Otolaryngology, Head and Neck Surgery, Chang Gung Memorial Hospital, No. 5 Fu-Shin Street, Kwei-Shan, Taoyuan, Taiwan
Department of Public Health, Chang Gung University, Tao-Yuan, Taiwan
Taipei CGMH Head and Neck Oncology Group, Tao-Yuan, Taiwan

Chun-Ta Liao
Department of Otolaryngology, Head and Neck Surgery, Chang Gung Memorial Hospital, No. 5 Fu-Shin Street, Kwei-Shan, Taoyuan, Taiwan
Taipei CGMH Head and Neck Oncology Group, Tao-Yuan, Taiwan

Huei-Tzu Chien
Department of Public Health, Chang Gung University, Tao-Yuan, Taiwan
Department of Nutrition and Health Sciences, Chang Gung University of Science and Technology, Tao-Yuan, Taiwan

Sou-De Cheng
Department of Anatomy, Chang Gung University, Tao-Yuan, Taiwan

Wen-Yu Chuang
Department of Pathology, Chang Gung Memorial Hospital, Tao-Yuan, Taiwan

Hung-Ming Wang
Taipei CGMH Head and Neck Oncology Group, Tao-Yuan, Taiwan
Division of Hematology/Oncology, Department of Internal Medicine, Chang Gung Memorial Hospital, Tao-Yuan, Taiwan

Juan Fang, Xiaoxu Li, Da Ma, Xiangqi Liu, Yichen Chen, Yun Wang, Juan Xia, Bin Cheng and Zhi Wang
Guangdong Provincial Key Laboratory of Stomatology, Guanghua School of Stomatology, Sun Yat-Sen University, No. 56, Lingyuanwest Road, Guangzhou, Guangdong 510055, China

Vivian Wai Yan Lui
School of Biomedical Sciences, Faculty of Medicine, The Chinese University of Hong Kong, Hong Kong, SAR, China

Hye Sook Chon, Sachin M. Apte, Mian M. Shahzad and Robert M. Wenham
Department of Gynecologic Oncology, H. Lee Moffitt Cancer Center and Research Institute, 12902 Magnolia Drive, Tampa, FL 33647, USA

Sokbom Kang
Division of Gynecologic Cancer Research, Center for Uterine Cancer, National Cancer Center, Ilsan-gu Madu-dong, Goyang 410-768, Korea

Jae K. Lee
Department of Biostatistics and Bioinformatics, H. Lee Moffitt Cancer Center and Research Institute, 12902 Magnolia Drive, Tampa, FL 33647 USA

Irene Williams-Elson
Clinical Trials Office, Phase 1 Clinical trials, H. Lee Moffitt Cancer Center and Research Institute, 12902 Magnolia Drive, Tampa, FL 33647, USA

Kaoru Midorikawa, Yusuke Hiraku, Shinji Oikawa and Mariko Murata
Department of Environmental and Molecular Medicine, Mie University Graduate School of Medicine, 2-174, Edobashi, Tsu, Mie 514-8507, Japan

Kazuhiko Takeuchi
Department of Otorhinolaryngology, Head and Neck Surgery, Mie University Graduate School of Medicine, Tsu, Mie, Japan

Weilin Zhao
Department of Environmental and Molecular Medicine, Mie University Graduate School of Medicine, 2-174, Edobashi, Tsu, Mie 514-8507, Japan
Department of Otorhinolaryngology, Head and Neck Surgery, Mie University Graduate School of Medicine, Tsu, Mie, Japan
Department of Otolaryngology Head and Neck Surgery, First Affiliated Hospital of Guangxi Medical University, Nanning, China

Guangwu Huang and Zhe Zhang
Department of Otolaryngology Head and Neck Surgery, First Affiliated Hospital of Guangxi Medical University, Nanning, China

Yingxi Mo
Department of Environmental and Molecular Medicine, Mie University Graduate School of Medicine, 2-174, Edobashi, Tsu, Mie 514-8507, Japan
3Department of Otolaryngology Head and Neck Surgery, First Affiliated Hospital of Guangxi Medical University, Nanning, China
Department of Research, Affiliated Tumor Hospital of Guangxi Medical University, Nanning, Guangxi, China

Shumin Wang
Department of Environmental and Molecular Medicine, Mie University Graduate School of Medicine, 2-174, Edobashi, Tsu, Mie 514-8507, Japan
Department of Otolaryngology Head and Neck Surgery, First Affiliated Hospital of Guangxi Medical University, Nanning, China
Center for Oral Biology, University of Rochester Medical Center, Rochester, NY, USA

Ning Ma
Graduate School of Health Science, Suzuka University of Medical Science, Suzuka, Mie, Japan

Liang-Ru Ke, Wei-Xiong Xia, Wen-Ze Qiu, Xin-Jun Huang, Jing Yang, Ya-Hui Yu, Hu Liang, Guo-Ying Liu, Yan-Fang Ye, Yan-Qun Xiang, Xiang Guo and Xing Lv
Department of Nasopharyngeal Carcinoma, Sun Yat-Sen University Cancer Center, 651 Dongfeng Road East, Guangzhou, Guangdong 510060, China
State Key Laboratory of Oncology in Southern China, Collaborative Innovation Center for Cancer Medicine, Guangzhou, Guangdong 510060, China

Lin Yang, Liangping Xia, Yan Wang, Shasha He, Shaodong Hong and Yong Chen
Sun Yat-sen University Cancer Center, 651 East Dong Feng Road, Guangzhou 510060, China
State Key Laboratory of Oncology in Southern China, Guangzhou, China
Collaborative Innovation Center for Cancer Medicine, Guangzhou, China

Haiyang Chen
The Six Affiliated Hospital of Sun Yat-sen University, Guangzhou, China

Shaobo Liang
The First Hospital of Foshan, Foshan, China

Peijian Peng
The Fifth Affiliated Hospital of Sun Yat-sen University, Zhuhai, China

Yorihisa Imanishi
Department of Otorhinolaryngology–Head and Neck Surgery, Keio University School of Medicine, 35 Shinanomachi, Shinjuku, Tokyo 160-8582, Japan
Department of Otorhinolaryngology, Kawasaki Municipal Kawasaki Hospital, Kawasaki, Kanagawa 210-0013, Japan

Hiroyuki Ozawa, Yoshihiro Watanabe, Mariko Sekimizu, Fumihiro Ito, Toshiki Tomita and Kaoru Ogawa
Department of Otorhinolaryngology–Head and Neck Surgery, Keio University School of Medicine, 35 Shinanomachi, Shinjuku, Tokyo 160-8582, Japan

Yoichiro Sato
Department of Otorhinolaryngology, Kawasaki Municipal Kawasaki Hospital, Kawasaki, Kanagawa 210-0013, Japan

Koji Sakamoto
Department of Otorhinolaryngology, Saiseikai Utsunomiya Hospital, Utsunomiya, Tochigi 321-0974, Japan

Ryoichi Fujii
Department of Otorhinolaryngology, Saiseikai Yokohamashi Nanbu Hospital, Yokohama, Kanagawa 234-0054, Japan

Seiji Shigetomi
Department of Otorhinolaryngology, Yokohama Municipal Citizen's Hospital, Yokohama, Kanagawa 240-8555, Japan

Noboru Habu
Department of Otorhinolaryngology, Kyosai Tachikawa Hospital, Tachikawa, Tokyo 190-0022, Japan

Kuninori Otsuka
Department of Otorhinolaryngology, Saiseikai Yokohamashi Tobu Hospital, Yokohama, Kanagawa 230-8765, Japan

Dan-Fang Yan, Wen-Bao Zhang, Feng Zhao and Sen-Xiang Yan
Department of Radiation Oncology, the First Affiliated Hospital, College of Medicine, Zhejiang University, 79 Qingchun RoadHangzhou, Zhejiang 310003, People's Republic of China

Qi-Dong Wang
Department of Radiology, the First Affiliated Hospital, College of Medicine, Zhejiang University, Zhejiang, Hangzhou 310003, China

Li-Song Teng
Department of Oncology, the First Affiliated Hospital, College of Medicine, Zhejiang University, 79 Qingchun Road, Zhejiang, Hangzhou 310003, China

Shan-Bao Ke
Department of Radiation Oncology, Henan Province People's Hospital, Zhengzhou, Henan 450000, China

Hisashi Hasegawa, Takeshi Asakawa, Miyoko Maeda, Tohru Furusaka and Takeshi Oshima
Deparment of Otorhinolaryngology, Head and Neck Surgery, Nihon University School of Medicine, 30-1 Ohyaguchikami-cho, Itabashi-ku, Tokyo 173-8610, Japan

Yoshiaki Kusumi, Toshinori Oinuma and Mariko Esumi
Department of Pathology, Nihon University School of Medicine, 30-1 Ohyaguchikami-cho, Itabashi-ku, Tokyo 173-8610, Japan

Sadayuki Kawai, Tomoya Yokota, Satoshi Hamauchi, Akira Fukutomi, Akiko Todaka, Takahiro Tsushima, Yukio Yoshida, Yosuke Kito and Hirofumi Yasui
Division of Gastrointestinal Oncology, Shizuoka Cancer Center, 1007 Shimonagakubo, Nagaizumi, Sunto-gun, Shizuoka 411-8777, Japan

Yusuke Onozawa
Division of Medical Oncology, Shizuoka Cancer Center, Sunto-gun, Shizuoka, Japan

Hirofumi Ogawa and Tsuyoshi Onoe
Division of Radiation Oncology and Proton Therapy, Shizuoka Cancer Center, Sunto-gun, Shizuoka, Japan

Tetsuro Onitsuka
Division of Head and Neck Surgery, Shizuoka Cancer Center, Sunto-gun, Shizuoka, Japan

Takashi Yurikusa
Division of Dental and Oral Surgery, Shizuoka Cancer Center, Sunto-gun, Shizuoka, Japan

Keita Mori
Clinical Research Center, Shizuoka Cancer Center, Sunto-gun, Shizuoka, Japan

Min-jie Mao, Xue-ping Wang, Pei-dong Chi, Yi-jun Liu, Shu-qin Dai and Wan-li Liu
Department of Laboratory Medicine, State Key Laboratory of Oncology in South China, Collaborative Innovation Center for Cancer Medicine, Sun Yat-sen University Cancer Center, Guangzhou 510060, China

Ning Xue
Department of Laboratory Medicine, Affiliated Tumor Hospital of Zhengzhou University, Henan Tumor Hospital, Zhengzhou 450100, China

Qi Huang
Guangdong Medical University, Guangzhou 523808, China

Camilla K. Lonkvist and Julie Gehl
Department of Oncology, Herlev and Gentofte Hospital, University of Copenhagen, Herlev, Denmark

Simon Lønbro
Department of Experimental Clinical Oncology, Aarhus University Hospital, Aarhus, Denmark
Department of Public Health, Section for Sports Science, Aarhus University, Aarhus, Denmark

Anders Vinther
Department of Rehabilitation, Herlev and Gentofte Hospital, University of Copenhagen, Herlev, Denmark

Bo Zerahn
Department of Clinical Physiology and Nuclear Medicine, Herlev and Gentofte Hospital, University of Copenhagen, Herlev, Denmark

Eva Rosenbom
Nutritional Research Unit, Herlev and Gentofte Hospital, University of Copenhagen, Herlev, Denmark

Hanne Primdahl
Department of Oncology, Aarhus University Hospital, Aarhus, Denmark

Pernille Hojman
Centre of Inflammation and Metabolism (CIM) and Centre for Physical Activity Research (CFAS), Department of Infectious Diseases, Rigshospitalet, University of Copenhagen, Copenhagen, Denmark

Martin McLaughlin, Holly E. Barker, Aadil A. Khan, Malin Pedersen, Magnus Dillon, David C. Mansfield, Radhika Patel and Joan N. Kyula
Targeted Therapy Team, The Institute of Cancer Research, Chester Beatty Laboratories, 237 Fulham Road, London SW3 6JB, UK

Shreerang A. Bhide, Kate L. Newbold and Christopher M. Nutting
The Royal Marsden Hospital, 203 Fulham Road, London SW3 6JJ, UK
Division of Radiotherapy and Imaging, The Institute of Cancer Research, 237 Fulham Road, London, UK

Kevin J. Harrington
Targeted Therapy Team, The Institute of Cancer Research, Chester Beatty Laboratories, 237 Fulham Road, London SW3 6JB, UK
The Royal Marsden Hospital, 203 Fulham Road, London SW3 6JJ, UK
Division of Radiotherapy and Imaging, The Institute of Cancer Research, 237 Fulham Road, London, UK

Sanghyuk Song
Department of Radiation Oncology, Kangwon National University Hospital, Baengnyeong-ro 156, Chuncheon 24289, Republic of Korea

Hong-Gyun Wu
Department of Radiation Oncology, Seoul National University College of Medicine, 101 Daehangno, Jongno-gu, Seoul 110-744, Republic of Korea

Chang Geol Lee, Ki Chang Keum and Mi Sun Kim
Department of Radiation Oncology, Yonsei Cancer Center, 50-1 Yonsei-ro, Seodaemun-gu, Seoul 03722, Republic of Korea

Yong Chan Ahn, Dongryul Oh and Hyo Jung Park
Department of Radiation Oncology, Samsung Medical Center, Sungkyunkwan University School of Medicine, 81 Irwon-Ro Gangnam-gu, Seoul 06351, Republic of Korea

Sang-Wook Lee and Geumju Park
Department of Radiation Oncology, Asan Medical Center, University of Ulsan College of Medicine, Seoul, South Korea

Sung Ho Moon and Kwan Ho Cho
Research Institute and Hospital, National Cancer Center, 323 Ilsan-ro, Ilsandong-gu, Goyang-si, Gyeonggi-do 10408, Republic of Korea

Yeon-Sil Kim and Yongkyun Won
Department of Radiation Oncology, Seoul St. Mary's Hospital, The Catholic University of Korea, 222 Banpo-daero, Seocho-gu, Seoul 06591, Republic of Korea

Young-Taek Oh
Department of Radiation Oncology, Ajou University School of Medicine, Gyeonggi, South Korea

Won-Taek Kim
Department of Radiation Oncology, Pusan National University Hospital and Pusan National University School of Medicine, 179 Gudeok-ro, Seo-gu, Busan 49241, Republic of Korea

Jae-Uk Jeong
Department of Radiation Oncology, Chonnam National University Medical School, 42 Jebong-ro, Dong-gu, Gwangju 61469, Republic of Korea

Chen-Lin Lin
Department of Nursing, National Cheng Kung University Hospital, College of Medicine, National Cheng Kung University, Tainan, Taiwan

Wei-Ting Lee, Chun-Yen Ou, Jenn-Ren Hsiao, Cheng-Chih Huang, Sen-Tien Tsai, Sheen-Yie Fang, Jiunn-Liang Wu, Hsiao-Chen Liao and Yu-Shan Chen
Department of Otolaryngology, National Cheng Kung University Hospital, College of Medicine, National Cheng Kung University, Tainan, Taiwan

Jehn-Shyun Huang, Tung-Yiu Wong, Ken-Chung Chen and Tze-Ta Huang
Department of Stomatology, National Cheng Kung University Hospital, College of Medicine, National Cheng Kung University, Tainan, Taiwan

Yuan-Hua Wu, Wei-Ting Hsueh, Yu-Hsuan Lai, Ming-Wei Yang and Forn-Chia Lin
Department of Radiation Oncology, National Cheng Kung University Hospital, College of Medicine, National Cheng Kung University, Tainan, Taiwan

Chia-Jui Yen and Shang-Yin Wu
Division of Hematology/Oncology, Department of Internal Medicine, National Cheng Kung University Hospital, College of Medicine, National Cheng Kung University, Tainan, Taiwan

Jang-Yang Chang
Division of Hematology/Oncology, Department of Internal Medicine, National Cheng Kung University Hospital, College of Medicine, National Cheng Kung University, Tainan, Taiwan
National Institute of Cancer Research, National Health Research Institutes, 1F No 367, Sheng-Li Road, Tainan 70456, Taiwan

Yi-Hui Wang, Ya-Ling Weng, Han-Chien Yang and Jeffrey S. Chang
National Institute of Cancer Research, National Health Research Institutes, 1F No 367, Sheng-Li Road, Tainan 70456, Taiwan

E. McColl and M. Breckons
Institute of Health and Society, Newcastle University, The Baddiley-Clark Building, Richardson Road, Newcastle upon Tyne NE2 4AX, UK

J. M. Patterson
Institute of Health and Society, Newcastle University, The Baddiley-Clark Building, Richardson Road, Newcastle upon Tyne NE2 4AX, UK
Speech and Language Therapy Department, Sunderland Royal Hospital, Sunderland, UK

M. Fay, C. Exley
Faculty of Health and Life Sciences, Northumbria University, Newcastle upon Tyne, UK

V. Deary
Psychology Department, Northumbria University, Newcastle upon Tyne, UK

Hao Peng, Ling-Long Tang, Xu Liu, Lei Chen, Wen-Fei Li, Yan-Ping Mao, Yuan Zhang, Ying Sun and Jun Ma
Department of Radiation Oncology, Sun Yat-sen University Cancer Center, State Key Laboratory of Oncology in Southern China, Collaborative Innovation Center for Cancer Medicine, 651 Dongfeng Road East, Guangzhou 510060, People's Republic of China

Li-Zhi Liu and Li Tian
Imaging Diagnosis and Interventional Center, Sun Yat-sen University Cancer Center, State Key Laboratory of Oncology in Southern China, Collaborative Innovation Center for Cancer Medicine, Guangzhou, People's Republic of China

Ying Guo
Department of Clinical Trials Center, Sun Yat-sen University Cancer Center, State Key Laboratory of Oncology in Southern China, Collaborative Innovation Center for Cancer Medicine, Guangzhou, People's Republic of China

Akhileshwar Namani and Xiuwen Tang
Department of Biochemistry, University School of Medicine, Hangzhou 310058, People's Republic of China

Md. Matiur Rahaman and Ming Chen
Department of Bioinformatics, College of Life Sciences, Zhejiang University, Hangzhou 310058, People's Republic of China

Yifei Xu, Weilin Zhao, Xue Xiao and Xiaoying Zhou
Department of Otolaryngology-Head and Neck Surgery, First Affiliated Hospital of Guangxi Medical University, 6# Shuangyong Road, Nanning, Guangxi 530021, China

Guangwu Huang and Zhe Zhang
Department of Otolaryngology-Head and Neck Surgery, First Affiliated Hospital of Guangxi Medical University, 6# Shuangyong Road, Nanning, Guangxi 530021, China
Ministry of Education, Key Laboratory of High-Incidence-Tumor Prevention and Treatment (Guangxi Medical University), Nanning, Guangxi, China

Longde Lin and Xiaoyun Zeng
Ministry of Education, Key Laboratory of High-Incidence-Tumor Prevention and Treatment (Guangxi Medical University), Nanning, Guangxi, China
Department of Epidemiology, School of Public Health, Guangxi Medical University, Nanning, Guangxi, China

Jian Liao and Yancheng Li
Cancer Institute of Cangwu County, Wuzhou, Guangxi, China

Yufeng Chen
Department of Otolaryngology-Head and Neck Surgery, First Affiliated Hospital of Guangxi Medical University, 6# Shuangyong Road, Nanning, Guangxi 530021, China
Department of Epidemiology, School of Public Health, Guangxi Medical University, Nanning, Guangxi, China
Department of Medical Epidemiology and Biostatistics, Karolinska Institutet, Stockholm, Sweden

Tingting Huang
Department of Otolaryngology-Head and Neck Surgery, First Affiliated Hospital of Guangxi Medical University, 6# Shuangyong Road, Nanning, Guangxi 530021, China
Ministry of Education, Key Laboratory of High-Incidence-Tumor Prevention and Treatment (Guangxi Medical University), Nanning, Guangxi, China
Department of Medical Epidemiology and Biostatistics, Karolinska Institutet, Stockholm, Sweden

Weimin Ye
Department of Medical Epidemiology and Biostatistics, Karolinska Institutet, Stockholm, Sweden

Carlos Narvaez, Claudia Doemer and Dirk Rades
Department of Radiation Oncology, University of Lübeck, Ratzeburger Allee 160, D-23562 Lübeck, Germany

Christian Idel
Departments of Radiation Oncology and Oto-Rhino-Laryngology and Head and Neck Surgery, University of Lübeck, Lübeck, Germany

Cornelia Setter
Department of Radiation Oncology, Christian-Albrechts University Kiel, Kiel, Germany

Denise Olbrich
Centre for Clinical Trials Lübeck, Lübeck, Germany

Zaza Ujmajuridze and Jesper Hansen Carl
Department of Oncology, Zealand University Hospital, Naestved, Denmark

She-Gan Gao, Jun-Qiang Yang, Zhi-Kun Ma, Xiang Yuan, Chen Zhao, Xiao-Shan Feng and Yi-Jun Qi
Henan Key Laboratory of Cancer Epigenetics; Cancer Hospital, The First Affiliated Hospital, College of Clinical Medicine, Medical College of Henan University of Science and Technology, Luoyang, Henan 471003, People's Republic of China

Guang-Chao Wang
Department of Oral Mucosal Diseases, Shanghai Ninth People's Hospital, Shanghai Jiao Tong University School of Medicine, Shanghai 200011, People's Republic of China

Hua Wei
Huaihe Hospital, Henan University, Kaifeng, Henan 475004, People's Republic of China

Dominic Mcavery
Regional Maxillofacial Unit, University Hospital Aintree, Liverpool, UK

Simon N. Rogers
Regional Maxillofacial Unit, University Hospital Aintree, Liverpool, UK
Edge Hill University, Liverpool and Evidence-Based Practice Research Centre (EPRC), Faculty of Health and Social Care, Road, L39 4QP, Ormskirk, St Helens, UK
Consultant Regional Maxillofacial Unit, University Hospital Aintree, L9 1AE, Liverpool, UK

Derek Lowe
Regional Maxillofacial Unit, University Hospital Aintree, Liverpool, UK
Edge Hill University, Liverpool and Evidence-Based Practice Research Centre (EPRC), Faculty of Health and Social Care, Road, L39 4QP, Ormskirk, St Helens, UK

Cher Lowies
Head and Neck Clinical Trials, University Hospital Aintree, Clinical Sciences Building, Liverpool, UK

Seow Tien Yeo
Centre for Health Economics and Medicines Evaluation (CHEME), School of Healthcare Sciences, College of Health and Behavioural Sciences (CoHaBS), Bangor University, Ardudwy Building, Normal Site, Bangor, UK

Christine Allmark and Anastasios Kanatas
Leeds Teaching Hospitals and St James Institute of Oncology, Leeds Dental Institute and Leeds General Infirmary, Leeds, UK

Gerald M. Humphris
School of Medicine, Medical and Biological Sciences, North Haugh, St Andrews, UK

Robert Flavel
Southway, Guildford, Surrey, UK

Cherith Semple
Macmillan Health and Wellbeing Service, Ulster Hospital, Upper Newtownards Road, Dundonald, Belfast, UK

Steven J. Thomas
Oral and Maxillofacial Surgery Department, University, Bristol, Lower Maudlin Street, Bristol, UK

Index

www.ingramcontent.com/pod-product-compliance
Lightning Source LLC
Chambersburg PA
CBHW080523200326
41458CB00012B/4313